Digital Mammography

IWDM 2002

6th International Workshop on Digital Mammography

Springer

Berlin
Heidelberg
New York
Hong Kong
London
Milan
Paris
Tokyo

Heinz-Otto Peitgen
Editor

Digital Mammography

IWDM 2002

6th International Workshop
on Digital Mammography

Proceedings of the Workshop
June 22–25, 2002, Bremen, Germany

Springer

Heinz-Otto Peitgen, Ph.D.
Professor of Mathematics and Biomedical Sciences
MeVis – Center for Medical Diagnostic Systems and Visualization
at the University of Bremen
Universitätsallee 29
28359 Bremen, Germany

With 282 figures and 78 tables

ISBN 3-540-00523-4 Springer-Verlag Berlin Heidelberg New York

Cataloging-in-Publication Data applied for

Bibliographic information published by Die Deutsche Bibliothek
Die Deutsche Bibliothek lists this publication in the Deutsche Nationalbibliografie; detailed bibliographic data is available in the Internet at <http://dnb.ddb.de>

Springer-Verlag Berlin Heidelberg New York
a member of BertelsmannSpringer Science+Business Media GmbH
http://www.springer.de

Cover-Design: design & production GmbH, Heidelberg
Typsetting: Camera-ready by editor

Printed on acid free paper 21/3150 HS – 5 4 3 2 1 0

Preface

This book comprises the scientific proceedings of the International Workshop on Digital Mammography (IWDM), held in Bremen, Germany, from June 22 to June 25, 2002. Since its inception in 1992, IWDM has grown into the International Forum on Digital Mammography. The uniqueness of IWDM is its attractiveness to researchers, medical practitioners, and industrial developers.

Former workshops were held in San Jose, USA (1992), York, UK (1994), Chicago, USA (1996), Nijmegen, NL (1998), and Toronto, Canada (2000). Each of these scientific events has been combined with very successful and focused industrial and research exhibits, which demonstrated the milestones of digital mammography hard- and software.

Now, that digital mammography is entering routine clinical use, we witness its strong impact on screening and diagnostic mammography, computer aided detection, minimally invasive procedures, and the development of systemic and integrated disease- oriented breast care. In view of this, the 2002 workshop provided a window to give us a glance at the future, and the work which was presented in talks, posters and exhibits has demonstrated that IWDM2002 will take a special place in the very successful sequence of IWDM events.

Finally, as conference chair, I would like to thank all who have helped to prepare and run IWDM2002: the Scientific Advisory Board for its excellent work in guaranteeing scientific significance, the Organizational Board for its hard work to accomplish an appropriate framework for the event, and the industrial exhibitors and sponsors for their generous support.

Bremen, January 2003

Heinz-Otto Peitgen
Conference Chair
Professor of Mathematics and
Biomedical Sciences

Scientific Committee

Susan Astley	University of Manchester, UK
Ulrich Bick	Charit Berlin, Germany/University of Chicago, USA
Michael Brady	Oxford University, UK
Hiroshi Fujita	Gifu University, Japan
Maryellen Giger	University of Chicago, USA
Nico Karssemeijer	University Hospital Nijmegen, The Netherlands
Heinz-Otto Peitgen	University of Bremen, Germany
Etta D. Pisano	University of North Carolina, USA
Martin Yaffe	University of Toronto, Canada

IWDM 2002 was supported by

MeVis BreastCare

SIEMENS medical

General Electric

R2

Display Solutions from SIEMENS

HOLOGIC®

BARCO Filmless Perfection for Digital Mammography

Table of Contents

Imaging Systems and Detectors

Digital mammographic application of a single photon counting pixel detector

Amendolia S. R. [1], Bisogni M.G. [2], Delogu P. [2] Fantacci M. E. [2], Novelli M. [2], Quattrocchi M. [3], Rosso V. [2], Stefanini A. [2], Zucca S. [2]

[1] Istituto di Matematica e Fisica, Universita' di Sassari and Sezione INFN Pisa, Italy
[2] Dipartimento di Fisica, Universita' di Pisa and Sezione INFN Pisa, Italy
[3] Dipartimento di Fisica, Universita' di Napoli and Sezione INFN Pisa, Italy
mariagrazia.quattrocchi@pi.infn.it

Abstract. We present the imaging capabilities of a system based on a single photon counting chip, bump-bounded to a Si pixel detector. The detector is 300 μm thick a matrix of 64 x 64 square pixels with a dimension side of 170 μm. The active area is about 1.2 cm^2. The photon counting chip matches the geometry of the detector so it has 4096 asynchronous read-out cells, each containing a charge preamplifier, a leading edge comparator and a pseudo-random counter. We have tested the image quality and the stability of our acquisition system imaging some phantoms used for mammografic quality checks. Our system allows to see low contrast details with a patient dose comparable with that given in mammographic examinations.

1. Introduction

Our group has reported previously on the imaging capabilities of our single photon counting system [1]. The single photon counting mode implies that a converted incident photon is recorded only when its energy exceeds the selected energy threshold. In our hybrid system the semiconductor pixel detector is bump bonded to the read-out chip called PCC (Photon Counting Chip) developed by the Medipix collaboration [2]. The pitch of the read-out cells is the same as detector's one. Each electronic read-out cell is a 170 x 170 μm^2 pixel and provides a complete electronic chain starting from the charge sensitive preamplifier up to the counter. As semiconductor substrate for this work we use a 300 μm thick silicon crystal. The Si detector pixel are 150 x 150 μm^2 separated by 20 μm for a total 170 μm pitch. The charge induced by the radiation in the 20 μm interpixel zone is collected by adjacent pixel [3]. The chip sensitive area is 1.1837 cm^2.

The main limitation for this acquisition system is the limited detection area that has to be compared with the required one that is 18 x 24 cm^2; so we have acquired different images translating the detector. We present the images obtained using the RMI phantom that has a 8 x 8 cm^2 section.

2. Experimental setup

We have imaged the RMI phantom suggested by American College of Radiology (ACR) for quality checks in mammography. This phantom is 8 x 8 cm^2 and is made up of a wax block in which are positioned 16 various sets of test objects. In the Figure 1a we present a scheme of the location of these test objects in the wax insert. The total thickness of the phantom is composed by a 3.3 cm thick Lucite block in which is inserted the wax block and a 0.3 cm thick cover. All together is approximately the same of a compressed breast (4.2 cm). In the wax there are included five groups of simulated micro-calcifications of different diameter (varying from 0.54 mm to 0.16 mm), five different size tumor-like masses (from 2.00 mm to 0.25 mm) and six different size nylon fibers that simulate fibrous structures (from 1.56 mm to 0.40 mm).

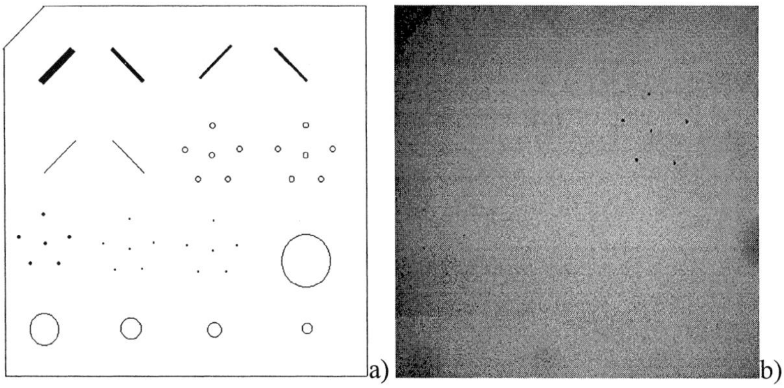

Figure 1 a) Layout of the RMI156 phantom. **b)** Composite image of RMI-156 phantom, constructed from several images of smaller field of view.

In order to obtain an image of this phantom we have exposed the total phantom to X-rays and moved it respect to the detector. The detector was positioned at 1 cm from the end of the Lucite block. We have used a standard mammographic tube with Molibdenum target and Be (1 mm) and Mo (0.025 mm) filters. We used the tube at 30kVp and at 30 mAs anodic current – exposure time. The detector was far away 75 cm from the tube focus.

We have acquired 36 small areas images and each of these is equalized by weighting with a high statistical image acquired in the same beam condition. By composing these images we obtained the total image of the phantom (Figure 1b). We have applied a smoothing filter and contrast enhancement operations. It is possible to distinguish all nylon fibers, the first three groups of micro-calcifications and four of the five tumor-like masses. So the performances of our system are good with respect to the indication of the ACR. We acquired the different images without anti-diffusion grid and irradiating the phantom area completely. In this way the imaging quality is reduced by the photons scattered by Lucite. From previous work [4] we know that reducing the irradiation area we will improve the SNR, so increasing the imaging capabilities of the acquisition system and we plan to apply this method.

In particular we studied the 2 mm mass like tumor (SCR≈1). We analyzed the signal-to noise ratio behaviour as function of the dose. We have acquired five different images of the same detail at 24 kVp and I_{tube} = 24 mAs, then we have calculated the contrast and the signal-to-noise ratio (Figure 2) changing the number of summed images.

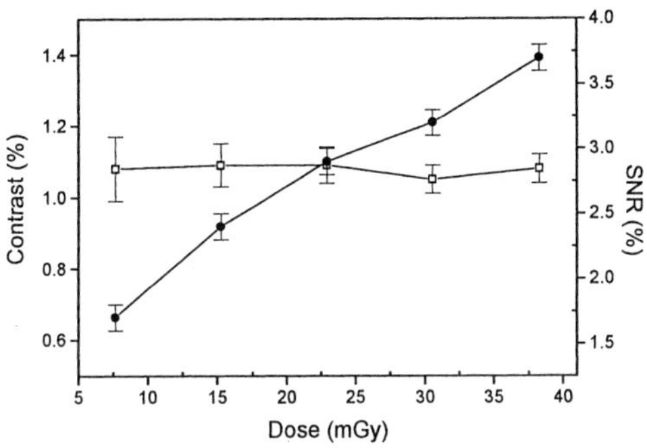

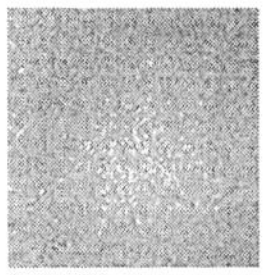
a)

b)

Figure 2. The behaviour of the signal-to-noise ratio as function of the dose, calculated by considering a 5 cm thick Lucite, for 2 mm mass like tumor (a detail of the RMI-156 phantom). On the right we present the image for single exposure (a) and the image obtained summing five single image (b).

As expected the contrast is about independent on the dose, while the SNR increases increasing the dose. On the right of figure 2 we present the single image (a) and the image obtained summed all five acquired images (b). Using a 7.65 mGy dose we can see the detail with signal-to-noise ratio of about 1.7.

3. Conclusions

In this paper we have used a silicon pixel detector with an active area of about 1.2 cm^2 to radiograph a 6 x 6 cm^2 area of our phantom. On the basis of ACR statement the imaging quality of our acquisition system is good. Future developments will be directed toward reducing pixel size (55 μm) and increasing the detection efficiency using 500 μm silicon detector.

References

1. S. R. Amendolia et al., "Evaluation of the imaging properties of a direct detection single photon counting based system", Nucl. Instr. Meth. Phys. Res. A461: 389-392 (2001)
2. Bisogni M. G. et al., "Performance of a 4096 Pixel Photon Counting Chip", Proceedings SPIE **3445**, 298-304 (1998)
3. L. Abate et al., Noise and interpixel dead space studies of GaAs pixellated detectors, Nucl. Instr. Meth. Phys. Res. A458: 164-168 (2001)
4. S. R. Amendolia et al., "Experimental study of Compton scattering reduction in digital mammography", Proceeding IEEE Nucl. Sci. Symp. Med. Im. Conf. **M9B-5** (2001)

Breast Cancer Screening using a Dedicated Breast CT Scanner: A Feasibility Study

John M. Boone, Karen K. Lindfors, James A. Seibert, and Thomas R. Nelson*

Department of Radiology, University of California, Davis, CA 95616 USA
*Department of Radiology, University of California, San Diego, CA 92093 USA

Abstract. Physical measurements of radiation dose, image noise and contrast were performed on a clinical CT scanner, using cylinders of breast dimensions. The contrast to noise ratio and signal to noise ratio were calculated from these measured data. The SNR versus lesion diameter results demonstrate, based on Rose's criterion (SNR $\geq$ 5), that breast CT can produce excellent image quality at mean glandular doses comparable to mammography. The potential to identify smaller lesions may improve early detection performance, which in turn would likely result in a reduction of breast cancer mortality.

1. Introduction

X-ray mammography is used worldwide for screening asymptomatic women for breast cancer. While mammography saves lives, the search for diagnostic techniques which outperform the cancer detection performance of screen-film mammography remains intense.

We have advocated the *study* of dedicated breast CT as an alternative imaging technique for breast cancer screening, and previously demonstrated dose efficacy based on Monte Carlo simulation of breast CT[3]. Here we evaluate breast CT dose using physical measurements performed on phantoms on a clinical CT scanner. We also extend these experimentally-determined results from 10 cm diameter to 10, 13, and 16 cm diameter breasts.

2. Methods

2.1 Dose Measurements

Poly methyl methacrylate (PMMA) cylinders were machined to diameters of 10 cm and 13 cm, and a 16 cm diameter PMMA cylinder was already available. Holes in the cylinders allowed placement of a pencil ion chamber for dose measurement; with one hole at the center and another centered 16 mm from the edge of the cylinder. An MDH 1015 dosimeter (Radcal, Monrovia, California, USA) was used for dose measurements. The phantoms were placed with their centers at the isocenter of a clinical multislice CT scanner (Lightspeed Plus, General Electric Medical Systems,

Milwaukee, Wisconsin, USA), and dose measurements were made at 50 mAs at four kVps (80, 100, 120, and 140 kVp), in both the center and edge positions. The scanner was set to acquire four simultaneous 2.5 mm slices for a total nominal collimation of 10 mm, and the computed tomography dose index (CTDI) values for the 100 mm long pencil chamber, $CTDI_{100mm}$, were computed.

The air dose measurements were converted to glandular dose by multiplication by the ratio of the mass energy absorption coefficients for glandular tissue and air. To estimate the mean glandular dose, the weighted $CTDI_w$ was computed from the glandular center and edge $CTDI_{gl}$ values as:

$$CTDI_{w,gl} = 1/3\ CTDI_{100mm,gl,\ center} + 2/3\ CTDI_{100mm,gl,\ edge}\ .$$

2.2 Contrast Measurements

The half value layer of the CT x-ray beam was measured at acceptance testing, and it was determined by spectral modeling [4] that the HVLs were consistent with ~9 mm of added aluminum. CT spectra were modeled accordingly, and the effective linear attenuation coefficients (μ_{eff}) were determined for 0%, 50%, and 100% glandular breast compositions, and for water. The μ_{eff} value of each breast composition was determined for each spectrum (80, 100, 120, and 140 kVp) and each PMMA cylinder diameter (diameter influences μ_{eff} due to beam hardening). CT numbers (i.e. Hounsfield Units) were computed from the μ_{eff} values.

Johns and Yaffe [5] demonstrated that the μ_{eff} of breast cancer is very similar to that of glandular breast tissue, and to simplify matters and reduce the number of permutations under study, breast cancer lesion contrast was taken as the contrast of 100% glandular tissue on a 50% glandular background.

2.3 CT Noise Measurements

Each of the three PMMA cylinders (10, 13, and 16 cm diameter) was scanned at the isocenter of a commercial CT scanner, at 80, 100, 120, and 140 kVp and at 10, 20, 30, 50, 70, 100, 150, 200 and 300 mAs. Four images, each with 5 mm section thickness, were acquired at each acquisition, using the quad detector array scanner in axial (non-helical) mode. The images were reconstructed using the "standard" convolution filter. For the 10 cm and 13 cm cylinders, the reconstructed field of view (FOV) was 200 mm and the pixel width was 0.39 mm. The 16 cm cylinder had a 250 mm FOV, resulting in 0.49 mm pixel widths.

The images were transferred to a workstation for analysis, and large regions of interest (ROIs) were hand-positioned on each image (to avoid holes), and the mean and RMS standard deviation (σ) of the CT numbers was computed. The mean and standard deviation values were averaged over several ROIs and over all four images acquired at each x-ray technique setting.

2.4 Analysis

The $CTDI_{w,gl}$ was used in this study as an approximation to the mean glandular dose, and the CTDI values could be scaled to any mAs technique for each PMMA cylinder diameter and kVp. The contrast and noise values were also determined at each mAs. The noise values were determined using 5 mm section thickness, however our design goal for breast CT is closer to a 1 mm section thickness. Therefore, the noise measurements were corrected by a factor of $5^{1/2}$ to adjust for the reduction of photons that would occur for a 1 mm section thickness.

Pendant breast diameters of 10, 13 and 16 cm correspond approximately to compressed breast thicknesses of 4.0 cm, 6.8 cm, and 10.4 cm, respectively. Radiation dose levels from two-view mammography for these breast thicknesses were 3.6 mGy, 9.0 mGy, and 17.5 mGy, respectively, based on output measurements performed on clinical mammography systems at our institution. The CNR values corresponding to these doses were used in this study for each breast diameter.

3. Results

The mean glandular dose ($CTDI_{gl,w}$ per 100 mAs) is shown as a function of kVp in Figure 1. As with the DgN values used in mammography for converting from entrance dose to tissue dose, the smaller breast diameters demonstrate higher conversion factors. The CT number is shown as a function of beam energy for CT spectra in Figure 2. Lesion contrast used in this study was taken as the contrast between 50% glandular and 100% glandular tissues (vertical arrow).

The CT image noise was measured for a number of mAs/kVp/diameter permutations, and the results are shown in Figure 3. These results show the measured noise values for the 5 mm section thickness acquisitions. Figure 4 illustrates lesion CNR per pixel as a function of dose. The noise term used in the CNR results of

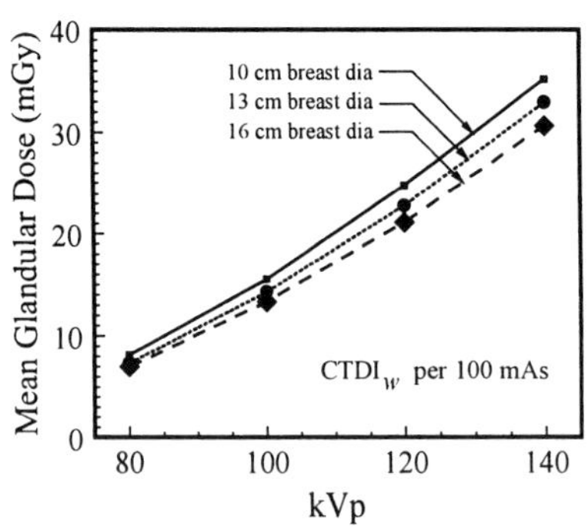

Figure 1: The weighted CTDI (mGy/100 mAs) is shown versus kVp for three breast (PMMA) diameters. The values shown were converted to glandular tissue dose from the air dose measurements.

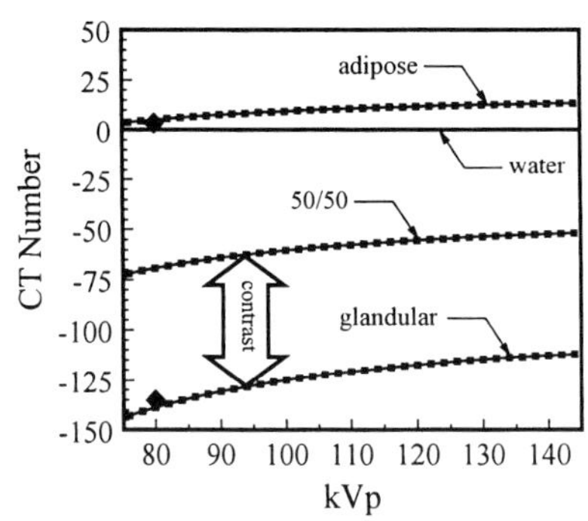

Figure 2: The CT Number was computed using modeled CT x-ray spectra. The two diamonds correspond to measured CT numbers at 80 kVp from a cadaver breast of adipose and glandular regions.

Figure 4 includes the correction from 5 mm to 1 mm slice thickness.

The CNR was used to compute the SNR for a lesion of $area_L$ using the simple assumption that $SNR = CNR_{pixel} \times (N_{pixels})^{1/2}$, where N_{pixels} is the number of pixels on the image which contain the lesion, and thus $N_{pixels} = area_L / area_{pixel}$. CNR values were linearly interpolated from Figure 4, and the lesion diameter corresponding to a lesion SNR of 5 was determined. Since the Rose Criterion states that a lesion should be highly visible when its SNR is ≥ 5, the corresponding lesion diameters represent the dimensions of breast cancers that should be clearly visible on breast CT. Figure 5 illustrates the lesion diameters which should be visible on breast CT based on the Rose Criterion. Depending on breast diameter and beam spectrum, lesions from 3 mm to 6 mm should be detectable.

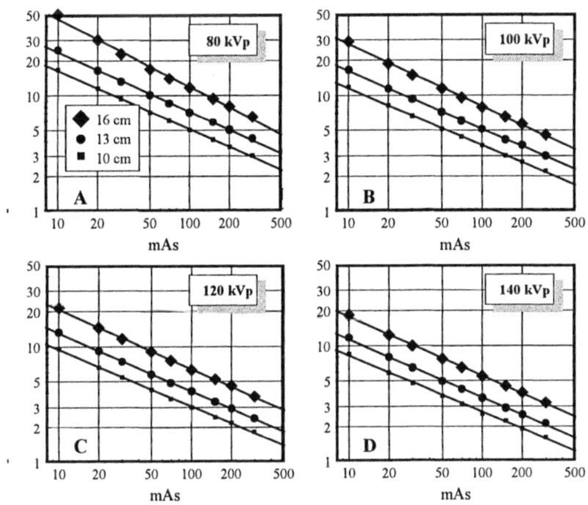

Figure 3: The CT noise (RMS standard deviation on the CT images) is shown as a function of mAs, for four kVps. The $-\frac{1}{2}$ slope of these log-log plots indicates excellent quantum detection performance of the scanner.

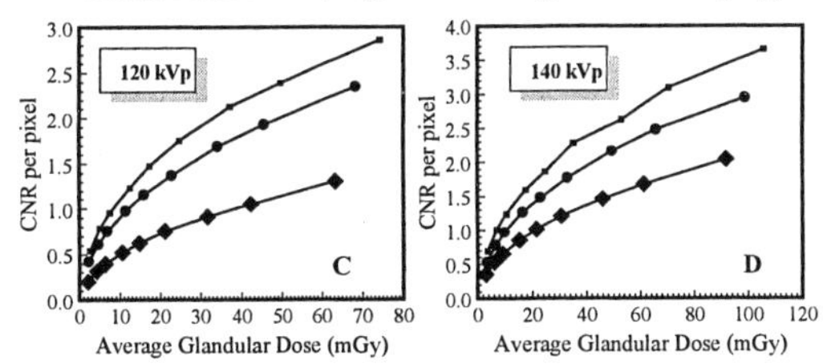

Figure 4: The contrast to noise ratio (CNR) *per pixel* is shown as a function of mean glandular dose. These data confirm the well-known theoretical relationship: $CNR^{1/2} \propto$ dose.

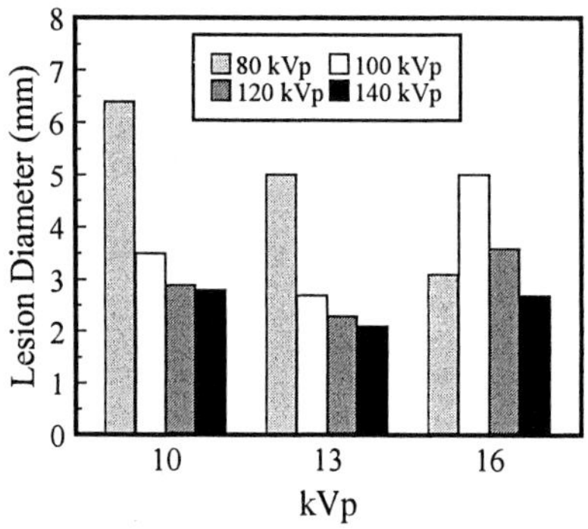

Figure 5: The lesion diameters corresponding to the point where SNR ≥ 5

4. Discussion and Conclusions

Experimentally measured data from a clinical CT scanner demonstrate that highly probable lesion detection (i.e. SNR≥5) would occur at radiation dose levels equivalent to mammography. Compared to the median lesion diameter of 11 mm in mammography, lesion diameters of 3, 4, 5, and 6 mm diameters correspond respectively to 1.54, 1.20, 0.93, and 0.72 years of earlier detection assuming a 100 day tumor volume doubling rate.

The above CNR/SNR calculations are based upon x-ray quantum noise considerations, but it is well recognized that anatomical noise is a more fundamental limitation in mammography, especially in the dense breast. Breast CT vastly reduces anatomical overlap due to its tomographic nature, and this will result in significant (order of magnitude) reductions in anatomical noise.

Based upon the preliminary observations discussed above, we conclude that breast CT has excellent potential for substantially earlier detection of breast cancer than mammography. We remain cautiously optimistic, but recognize that other technical challenges such as cost, the ability to image the axilla, and potentially low specificity remain. The development of a breast CT scanner is underway in our laboratory.

Acknowledgements

This work was funded by grants from the NCI (CA 89260) and the California Breast Cancer Research Program (7EB-0075).

References

[1] Boone JM, Nelson TR, Lindfors KK, Seibert JA. Dedicated breast CT: radiation dose and image quality evaluation. Radiology 221 (2001) 657-667

[2] Boone JM, Seibert JA. An accurate method for computer-generating tungsten anode x-ray spectra from 30 to 140 kV. Med Phys 24 (1997) 1661-1670

[3] Johns PC, Yaffe MJ. X-ray characterisation of normal and neoplastic breast tissues. Phys Med Biol 32 (1987) 675-695

Physical Evaluation of a Prototype for the Sectra Microdose Mammography System

Mats Lundqvist, David Bergström, Björn Cederström, Valery Chmill, Alexander Chuntonov, Mats Danielsson and Magnus Åslund

SCFAB, Kungl Tekniska Högskolan Physics Department, 10691 Stockholm, Sweden
Mats.danielsson@mamea.se

Abstract. The Sectra Microdose mammography system is the first photon counting digital mammography detector system in clinical test. We will discuss fundamental features of the new direct photon counting technique in terms of dose efficiency and present preliminary measurements for a prototype module on physical parameters such as MTF and DQE[1].

1. Introduction

The dose-efficiency of any x-ray imaging system can be defined from the patient dose required to obtain a certain image quality as compared to an ideal system, the lower the required dose the higher the dose-efficiency. The following factors determines the dose-efficiency:

1) Absorption efficiency
2) Noise in readout electronics and detector. Swank noise.
3) How the information from each photon is transferred to the image as a function of x-ray energy
4) Efficiency of scatter rejection.
5) Quality of incident x-ray spectra.

Absorption efficiency and noise is normally accounted for in the Detective Quantum Efficiency (DQE), for film-screen the DQE is typically 20%-40%. Obviously the DQE and the dose-efficiency decreases with noise and increases with absorption efficiency. It is however important to remember that the last three factors are normally not included in the DQE, this is in spite of the fact that they are crucial for the dose-efficiency [1].

A typical mammography x-ray energy spectrum incident on the detector ranges approximately from 15 keV to 30 keV. As is well known contrast increases when energy decreases (Fig 1), the difference in contrast information between the low- and high-energy photons is approximately a factor 10. Thus, the dose-efficiency for an x-ray imaging system that increases the weight of high energy photons at the cost of

[1] This work was supported by Stiftelsen för kunskaps- och kompetensutveckling.

low energy photons will be significantly lower compared to a system that does the inverse[2].

Scattered x-rays is the oldest known and often largest source of noise in x-ray imaging. The two standard ways of minimizing this background is by using a Bucky grid or through scanning x-ray imaging. It is hard to make an efficient grid for low energy x-rays and this translates into a dose efficiency advantage for scanning systems[3]. The difference corresponds to of the order of 50% difference in dose-efficiency. When the DQE is measured on area imaging systems, the Bucky is normally removed to achieve an improved DQE value. When the system is prepared for patients it is put back in position. This corresponds to an overestimation of the DQE relative to the dose-efficiency for area imaging systems [3].

One can calculate that the dose-efficiency in today's film-screen is, depending on breast thickness, between a factor 5 to 100 less than the dose-efficiency for an ideal system [1].

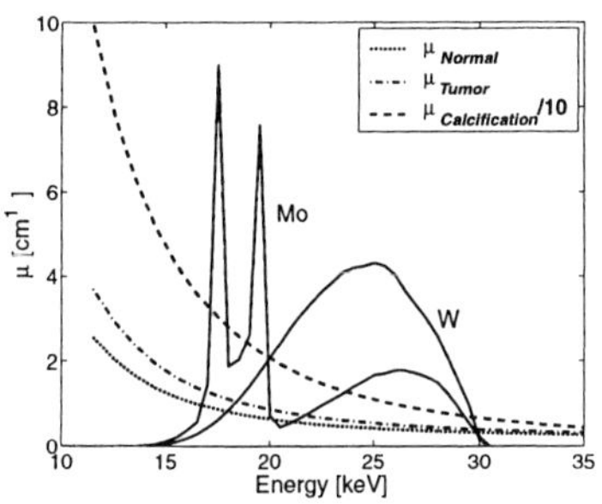

Fig. 1. Typical mammography x-ray spectra and variation in cross-section for absorption of x-rays. Since the variation in cross-section is an order of magnitude the weighting of individual photons will become crucial for the dose efficiency.

2. Sectra Microdose Mammography

The Sectra Microdose Mammography is a full-field digital mammography system with a photon counting scanned-slit detector (Fig 2). The field of view is 26 cm x 24 cm. To acquire the clinical images a prototype detector containing only one quarter of the final detector area was used. The detector consist of crystalline silicon and to obtain a Quantum Efficiency exceeding 90% the silicon detector is oriented edge-on to the incident x-rays. The silicon strips point back to the x-ray source to avoid parallax errors. The detector strips are wired to front-end electronics consisting of custom designed ASIC's. Each channel has its dedicated read-out chain corresponding of a charge sensitive preamplifier, a shaper and discriminators with programmable thresholds. The signal from one individual x-ray photon is, depending on the x-ray energy, typically 5000 electrons and since the noise is around 200 electrons RMS a virtually noiseless operation is possible by adjusting the threshold level to 2000 electrons. The electronics can handle synchronous pulse rates of maximum 5 x10^6 Hz, the rates in mammography is several orders of magnitude lower resulting in negligible dead-time. Several lines are positioned next to each other in a multi-slit geometry resulting in a scan-time of 5 seconds for a full detector. For the prototype detector the scan time was 15 seconds to compensate for the fact that only one quarter of the detector was deployed. Since several lines are used there is a redundancy in image data resulting in increased reliability compared to area imaging systems. A dedicated data processing system is assembling the image and it is transferred to a workstation for display and quality assurance within 20 seconds.

It is important to note that the image acquisition time in any single point in the image is significantly shorter than 5 seconds, even shorter than typical exposure times in area imaging systems. Thus, if one takes into account the possibility to individually process the data from the different detector lines, one may expect a decreased sensitivity to motion artefacts for scanning systems as compared to area imaging systems, inversely to what one may intuitively expect [5].

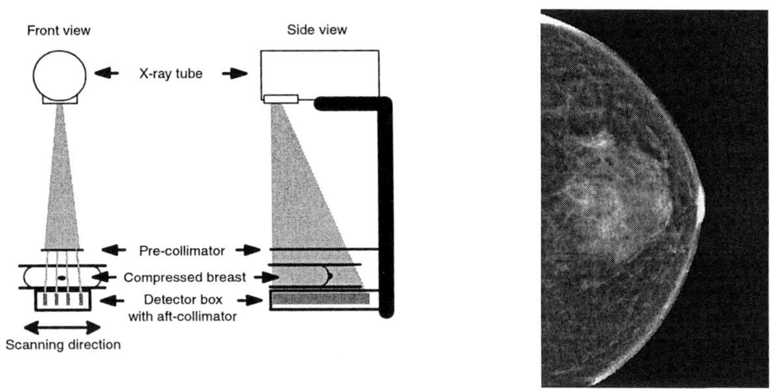

Fig. 2. Sectra MicroDose system outline (not to scale) with clinical image.

A scanning system increases the load on the x-ray tube and a slightly modified mammography tube is used, the modification is mainly that the anode diameter is increased with one inch and that liquid cooling of the tube housing is added. What is important is that the x-ray tube cope with patient flow. The optimum anode material for breast thickness exceeding 2 cm in combination with the Sectra Microdose system is Tungsten in combination with 0.5 mm Aluminium filter.

Photon counting detectors has previously been used in particle physics, bone densitometry and nuclear medicine such as PET imaging [4]. Typically these applications demand that a maximum of information is acquired for each detected photon. With the Sectra Microdose system the photon counting technique is for the first time used clinically in digital mammography. Even if the application is different the bottom line motivation for using it is the same: to extract maximum information from each detected x-ray.

4. Measurement of MTF, NPS and DQE

In all x-ray imaging systems the spatial resolution is dependent on the relative position of the X-ray source, the object and the detector. Normally all measurements resulting in an estimation for the MTF is made in the immediate vicinity of the detector. MTF and DQE refers solely to the detector properties, and parameters such as the x-ray focal spot size are not taken into account. For a scanned slit system the usual definition of the DQE can only be used in one dimension, in the other dimension the MTF is determined by the slit width, in our case 50 um. In the slit dimension we would have to introduce a system MTF [6], in this paper we limit us to measurements on the detector.

We have measured the MTF for a prototype module by performing an edge-scan with 1 um steps, the resulting presampled MTF is indicated in Fig 3. . The effect on the MTF of adding the different detector lines to form the accumulated image is also displayed in Fig 3.

To calculate the Noise Power Spectra (NPS) 256 flat images where acquired under realistic conditions of a 30 kVp Tungsten spectrum filtered with 0.5 mm Al and 45 mm of PMMA, the latter simulating breast tissue. The average pixel value corresponded to 487 counts corresponding to an Average Glandular Dose to the simulated breast of 0.16 mGy. The counts in each pixel was perfectly Poisson distributed. The result is displayed in Fig 3 in the direction parallel to the detector lines and the direction of the scan respectively. In the detector direction the NPS decreases for higher spatial frequencies. This is partly explained by a few percent of charge sharing between adjacent pixels. We have measured the electronic cross-talk between adjacent channels to be zero. In the scan direction the NPS is flat showing no correlations whatsoever. We determined the DQE according to Ref. [7], where the input is the Quantum Efficiency and the EMTF apart from the NPS. Since the number of counts for each pixel was perfectly Poisson distributed the variance of the number of counts equaled the number of counts itself. With the perfect Poisson distribution we would have expected a DQE at zero spatial frequency equaling the Quantum Efficiency, the reason for the lower DQE remains to be investigated. Also indicated in the image is the DQE we expect when energy weighting is introduced, with the current definition of DQE with the ideal SNR defined as the SNR for a perfect photon counting system this means Sectra Microdose may obtain a DQE exceeding 100%.

3. Conclusion

We have measured some basic parameters for a prototype module of the Sectra Microdose full field digital mammography system Because of the non existent electronic noise, high absorption efficiency, counting of individual photons, excellent rejection of scattered x-rays and since the detector enables the use of the optimum x-ray spectra the Sectra MicroDose enables a significant dose reduction while maintaining or improving the image quality. The clinical experience so far has moreover been very promising and the system mainly fulfills our expectations.

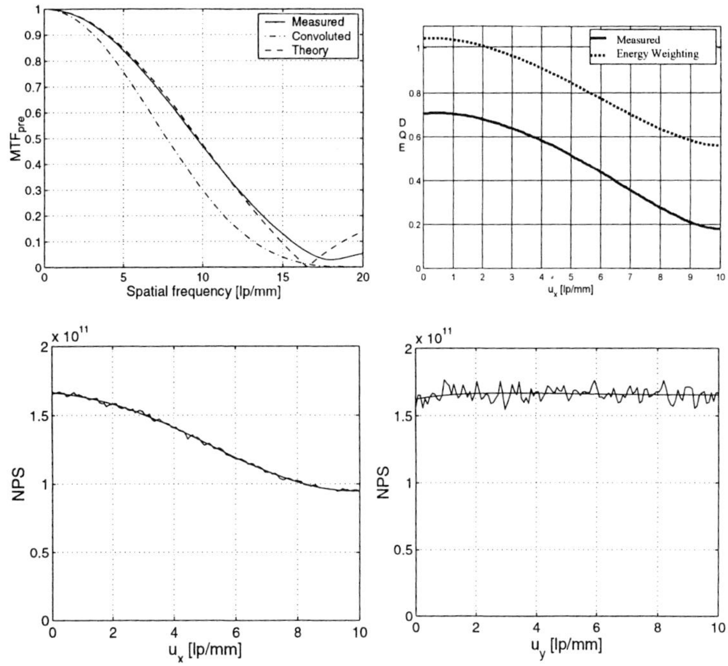

Fig. 3. MTF and DQE for the detector and Noise Power Spectra in the scan and detector direction.

References

1. Danielsson M., Bornefalk H, Cederström Chmill V, Hasegawa B, B., Lundquist M., Nygren D. and Tabar T.: Dose Efficient System for Digital Mammography, "Medical Imaging 2000 Proc. SPIE Vol. 3977 (2000) 239
2. Tapiovaara M.J. and Wagner R.F.: SNR and DQE analysis in broad spectrum x-ray imaging, Phys. Med. Biol. 30 (1985) 519
3. Säbel M and Aichinger H, Phys. Med. Biol. 41 (1996) 315
4. Proc. from the Imaging 2000 conference, Ed. Carlson P., Danielsson M. and Peskov V., Nucl. Instr. Meth. 471 (2001)
5. Boyle E.R., Pak D., Williams W.B.: Motion Artifact Seen on Slot-Scanning Direct Digital Mammography, AJR 172 (1999) 697
6. Nishikawa R.M. and Tahoces P.G.: The Effect of Scatter Radiation and its Removal on the DQE of Digital Mammography Systems , this proceeding
7. Dobbins J.: Med. Phys. 22(2) (1995) 171

Dose Measurements on a Scanning Multi-slit Digital Mammography System

Birgitta Hansson[1], Björn Cederström[2], Mats Danielsson[3], and Magnus Åslund[3]

[1] Department of Nuclear Medicine, Danderyd Hospital, 182 88 Stockholm, Sweden
[2] Physics Department, Royal Institute of Technology, 100 44 Stockholm, Sweden
[3] Mamea Imaging AB, Osquldas väg 6, 114 28 Stockholm, Sweden
mats.danielsson@mamea.se

Abstract. Air kerma and half-value layer were measured and Average Glandular Dose to the patient was calculated for a scanning multi-slit digital mammography system. Dose measurements on this type of system are non-trivial because of the lower dose-rate and the difference in irradiation geometry compared to conventional systems. Methods and results with estimated uncertainties are presented and deviations from standard procedures for conventional systems are discussed.

1 Introduction

To estimate the radiation risk to the patient in mammography Average Glandular Dose (AGD) should be used. AGD can be calculated from measurements of the entrance surface air kerma (ESAK) and half-value layer (HVL) and methods for this can be found in the literature [1]. These methods, however, must be modified on a scanning multi-slit system due to the different irradiation geometry and low dose rate, compared to conventional systems. In this study we use the results from measurements of air kerma and HVL to calculate AGD for 14 patients examined (48 images) with a prototype of the Sectra MicroDose system. The images were evaluated by two experienced radiologists and found acceptable for diagnosis. Image quality will be addressed in a separate study.

2 Description of the system

The Sectra MicroDose mammography system is characterized by an imaging geometry in which several linear arrays of photon-counting silicon detectors are scanned across the breast and combined to a full-field image (Fig. 1). The pre-collimator shapes the radiation field to several narrow beams matching the detector arrays and the post-collimator ensures efficient rejection of scattered radiation. The dose-rate has a pulsed time-structure due to the scanning of narrow beams and the average dose-rate is very low. The dose efficiency does not decrease strongly with energy and the optimal kV for this system is higher than for screen-film systems. Target material is W and the beam is filtered with 0.25 mm Al. To compare tube loading with conventional systems, we introduce an effective tube loading, defined by $I \cdot t_{\text{eff}} = I \cdot w \cdot N/v$, where w is the width of each collimator slit, v is the scan velocity and N is the number of detector lines. For the prototype system used for the measurements we have an effective exposure time of $t_{\text{eff}} = w \cdot N/v$ =(0.065 mm)·7/(8 mm/s)=0.057 s.

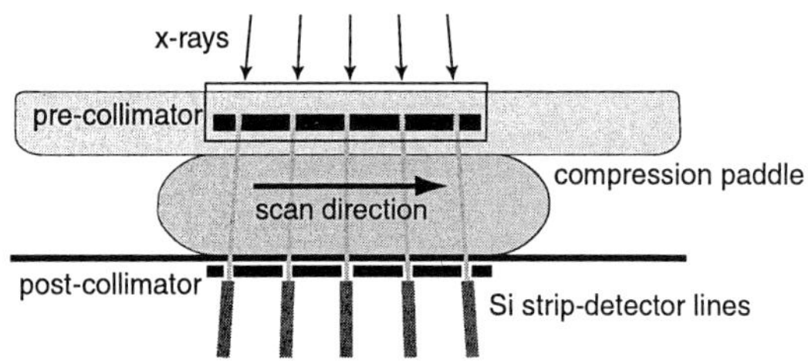

Fig. 1. Schematic of the imaging system. Pre-collimator, post-collimator and detectors are scanned across the image field.

3 Materials and methods

Measurements of air kerma were made using an ionization chamber dedicated for mammography (PTW, type 23344, 0.2 cm^3, connected to dosemeter PTW-Unidos E) and calibrated for the radiation qualities used. The energy dependence was less than one per cent and was neglected. Pressure and temperature were monitored and corrected for. Air kerma was measured by integration of the charge during the entire scan. The low average dose-rate requires very low leakage current. The equipment used had a leakage of less than 0.2 μGy/s. The pulsed time-structure makes the dose-rate vary between almost zero and 0.2 mGy/s. Thus, "smart" dosemeters with trig-levels for start and stop of measurement must be used with caution.

3.1 Measurement of air kerma

Measurements were performed free in air with the chamber 4.5 cm above the patient support, 6 cm from the chest wall edge and centered laterally in the field, in accordance with [1]. Several measurements were made to test reproducibility.

3.2 Measurement of HVL

Half-value layer should be measured in "good geometry" and with high purity aluminum filters [2]. Placing the filter and compression paddle under the pre-collimator resulted in almost 10% over-estimation of HVL due to scatter, and this geometry was therefore ruled out. The pre-collimator rejects scatter efficiently, and good geometry is achieved by placing the Al filters and compression paddle on a separate stationary holder above the pre-collimator. Several measurements of each Al thickness were performed to decrease statistical errors and the series was randomized to exclude systematic drift of the non-monitored tube output. HVL was calculated from interpolation of a semi-logarithmic expression. Thickness of Al filters ($\geq$ 99% purity) was measured with a micrometer. Statistical errors were around 3 μm (1 SD), and an additional uncertainty of 3 μm was added to account for a systematic error of the micrometer.

3.3 Calculation of AGD

AGD for the 48 patient mammograms was calculated from the results of the measurements of air kerma and HVL using standard conversion factors [1] and technique factors used in the clinical study. It was experimentally confirmed that the inverse-square law is valid in this geometry, for scaling of the air kerma to the breast entrance surface.

4 Results and discussion

Results of the measurements of air kerma and HVL together with calculations of AGD for different breast thickness are shown in Table 1. The mean AGD per image in the study was 0.46 mGy. Average breast thickness was 4.2 cm. This is in fact an overestimate of the AGD, since on this prototype the air kerma decreases towards the lateral edges of the field. The effect depends on breast size, e.g. for a 14 cm laterally wide breast the AGD is overestimated by 25%. Reproducibility of air kerma measurements was better than 2.2% (2 SD = 95% confidence). Uncertainty of HVL based on methods in [2] is less than 6%. The uncertainty in AGD is dominated by uncertainties in tabulated conversion factors and breast thickness (about 10% each).

Table 1. Air kerma, HVL and AGD for technique factors used in the clinical study. Values in parentheses were not used for this patient group.

U	$I \cdot t_{eff}$	Air kerma$\pm$2 SD	HVL$\pm$ 2 SD	AGD (mGy)				
(kV)	(mAs)	(mGy)	(mm Al)	2 cm	3 cm	4 cm	5 cm	6 cm
27	7.39	0.634 ± 0.008	0.34 ± 0.02	0.24	(0.18)			
34	6.83	1.117 ± 0.008	0.51 ± 0.02		(0.44)	(0.36)	0.30	0.25
37	6.26	1.28 ± 0.03	0.55 ± 0.03		0.53	0.44	(0.37)	(0.32)
40	5.69	1.40 ± 0.03	0.63 ± 0.02		0.64	0.54	0.46	0.40

References

1. European Commission: European Protocol on Dosimetry in Mammography (1996).
2. Wagner, L.K., Archer, B.R., Cerra, F.: On the Measurement of Half-Value Layer in Film-Screen Mammography. Med. Phys. 17(**6**) (1990) 989-997.

Digital Mammography vs. Screen-Film Mammography: a Phantom Study

Heid P, Pagliuchi C, Séradour B, Motte N, Langlois L, Kurkdjian S, Piana L

ARCADES – Marseille - France

Abstract. The primary aim of this study is to compare the image quality of digital mammography vs. screen-film mammography. The study was performed on the new Fuji imaging plates system (photostimulable phosphors, 50 micron pixel size), implemented on a conventional mammography unit. We conducted a first comparison between laser printed images and 4 different high contrast conventional screen-film combinations. Three specific mammographic phantoms were used to evaluate the quality image. The second step was to evaluate and compare the hard-copy and the soft-copy images on specialized high-resolution displays without magnification or contrast enhancement. The analysis revealed a slightly better performance of the printed digital images compare to the conventional screen-films, with an equal or lower dose. Nevertheless, the results comparison suggests that soft-copy, without the use of computer tools, performs lower results than hard-copy, even on dedicated monitor.

1. Introduction

The technology in Digital Mammography is in constant improvement and various systems are actually proposed to the Radiologist. First, in this study we have compared the FUJI Digital Mammography system by imaging plates with the analogical films in term of quality image. In a second time, we have evaluated the SenoPix diagnostic workstation of FUJI Medical System France.

The first part is specifically based on the comparison between the analogical screen/film combinations and the FUJI laser films by analysing and reading different test objects images on a specific mammography viewbox.

In a second part, the phantoms images are visualised on the Fuji SenoPix workstation monitors to compare the quality image of the hardcopies and softcopies.

2. Materials

All the tests were performed on a General Electric DMR X-ray unit. The analogical films were processed on a KODAK 3000-RA system with a standard processing time and a developer temperature of 35°C. The system was checked by sensitometry during the entire test to verify the stability and accuracy.

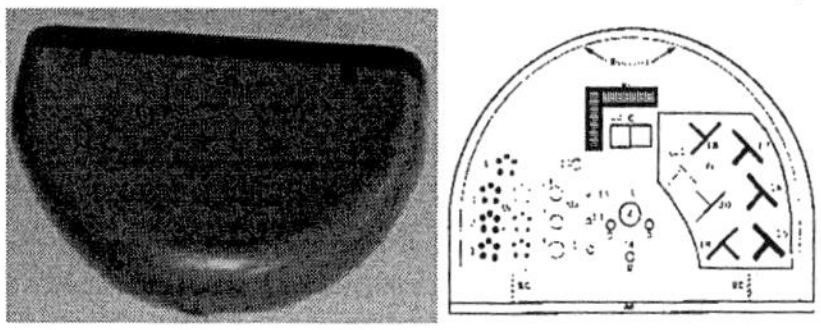

Fig. 1. MTM 100R French accreditation phantom

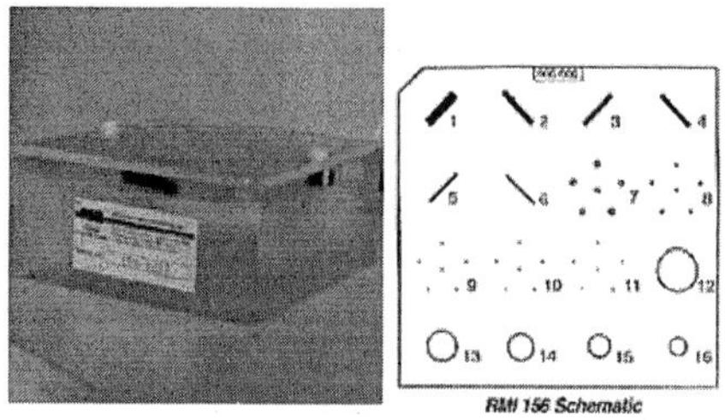

Fig. 2. RMI 156 A.C.R. accreditation phantom

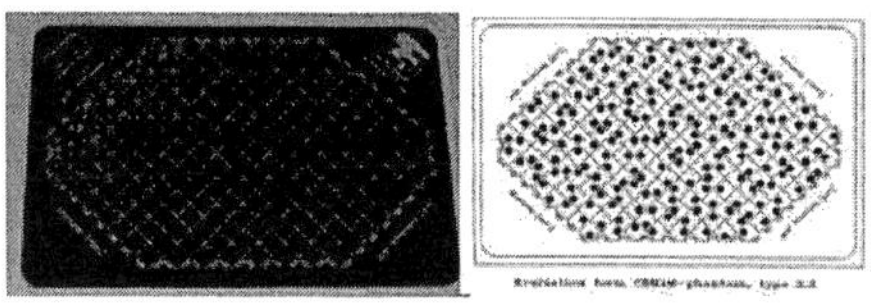

Fig. 3. CDMAM 3.2 European phantom for the contrast/detail evaluation in analogical and digital mammography

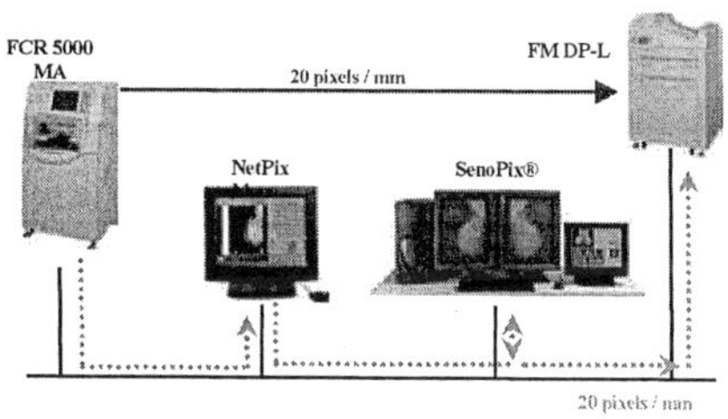

Fig. 4. FUJI digital system

The four high contrast screen/film combinations used are KODAK Min-R 2000/KODAK Min-R 2000, KODAK Min-R 2000/KODAK Min-R L, KODAK Min-R 2000/AGFA Mamoray HDR, FUJI Mammo Fine/FUJI AD M.

A specific mammography viewbox THEZARD DXHM with a maximum luminosity about 7000 Cd/m^2, equipped with masking system and a potentiometer to adjust luminosity according to the film Optical Density, was used to read and analyze films.

All the previous equipment is regularly under technical maintenance and checked by quality control.

The test objects used are accreditation phantoms for the mammography quality control.

The images are printed with the laser FUJI FM-DP L on FUJI DI-AL films and sent to the SenoPix diagnostic workstation where they are visualised on two calibrated monitors.

These monitors are two 5 MegaPixel Portrait Greyscale displays with 5MP1H graphics boards.

Table 1. Technical specifications of the Fuji FCR 5000 MA

FCR 5000 MA	**18*24 Mammo**	**24*30 Mammo**
Reading plates/h	**47**	**39**
Spatial resolution	**20 pixels / mm**	**20 pixels / mm**
	50 µ - 32 Mbytes	**50 µ - 53 Mbytes**
Matrix size	**3540*4740**	**4728*5928**

Table 2. Technical specifications of the BARCO graphic board and display

BarcoMed 5MP1H graphic board	5 MegaPixel Portrait Greyscale display MGD 521
Resolution: 2560*2048 @ 72 Hz Memory: 16 Mbytes Pixel clock rate: 500 MHz 1024 simultaneous grey shades, 12 bit in/10 bit out DAC	Luminosity: 300 Cd/m^2 Resolution 2048 x 2560

3. Methods

The analogical screen/film combinations were exposed using the automatic and full-automatic modes available on the GE DMR X-ray unit, with different tube voltages and target/filter combinations for each test object in order to obtain an Optical Density (included base + fog) in a range of 1.50-1.80.

The FUJI plates were exposed in manual mode with tube voltages, mAs and target/filter combinations determined by the previous results on analogical films in a way to compare the two technologies in term of image quality in a similar or lower range of doses (see table 3).

For all the tests, 3 films were carried out in the same exposure conditions in order to avoid punctual processing problem. For each test object, the scores are performed by 5 readers on a specific mammography viewbox. We have evaluated the score average of all the values. In case of important score discordance, another reading of the films was performed to confirm the first result and eliminated the film whose score is farther of the average.

Table 3. Example of exposures for the CDMAM 3.2

Film type	**Mode on GE DMR**	**Tube Voltage (kV)**	**Dose (mAs)**	**Target**	**Filter**
FUJI DI-AL	MANUAL	26	90	Rh	Rh
FUJI DI-AL	MANUAL	26	100	Rh	Rh
KODAK Min-R 2000	DOSE	26	104	Rh	Rh
AGFA HDR	DOSE	26	106	Rh	Rh
FUJI DI-AL	MANUAL	26	110	Rh	Rh
FUJI DI-AL	MANUAL	26	200	Mo	Mo
KODAK Min-R 2000	CNT	26	221	Mo	Mo
AGFA HDR	CNT	26	224	Mo	Mo
FUJI DI-AL	MANUAL	26	225	Mo	Mo
KODAK Min-R L	CNT	26	248	Mo	Mo
FUJI DI-AL	MANUAL	26	250	Mo	Mo
FUJI ADM	CNT	26	273	Mo	Mo
FUJI DI-AL	MANUAL	26	280	Mo	Mo

4. Results

4.1 Comparison between conventional screen/film combinations and FUJI DI-AL laser films

RMI 156 results

The RMI 156 phantom is used for American College of Radiology accreditation and for others mammography digital systems quality control (GE Senographe 2000D).

According to the tube voltages and target/filter combinations, the score results are at least equal for each type of films and range of doses (Fig. 5 and 6). The RMI 156 phantom scores evaluated on the FUJI DI-AL increase when the dose is higher.

MTM 100R results

The MTM 100R phantom allows measuring the Object Contrast, the optical density, the image quality score and evaluating the Spatial Resolution (lp/mm) [1]. It is the French accreditation test object [2].

We obtain higher scores on the FUJI DI-AL for each screen/film combination, excepted on the FUJI ADM whose score values evaluated on the MTM 100R phantom are at least equal or higher to the FUJI DI-AL film, for each tube voltage and target/filter combination (Fig. 7 and 8).

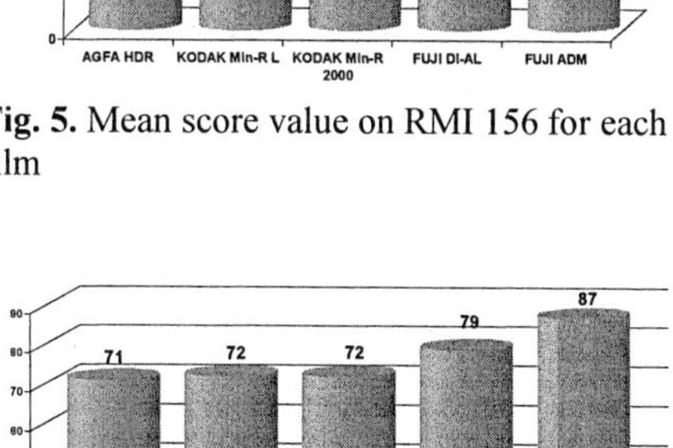

Fig. 5. Mean score value on RMI 156 for each film

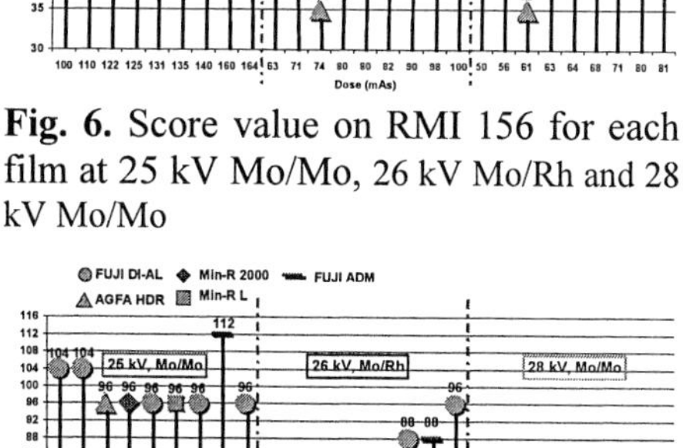

Fig. 6. Score value on RMI 156 for each film at 25 kV Mo/Mo, 26 kV Mo/Rh and 28 kV Mo/Mo

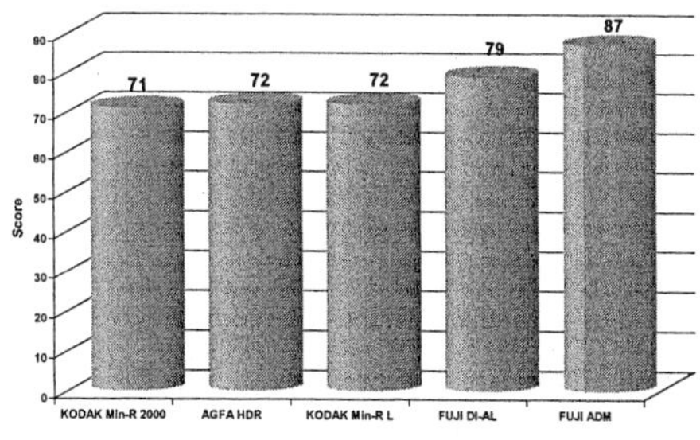

Fig. 7. Mean score value on MTM 100R for each film

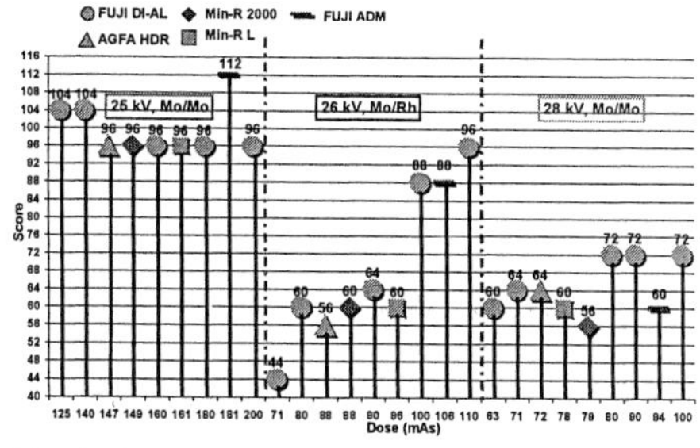

Fig. 8. Score value on MTM 100R for each film at 25 kV Mo/Mo, 26 kV Mo/Rh and 28 kV Mo/Mo

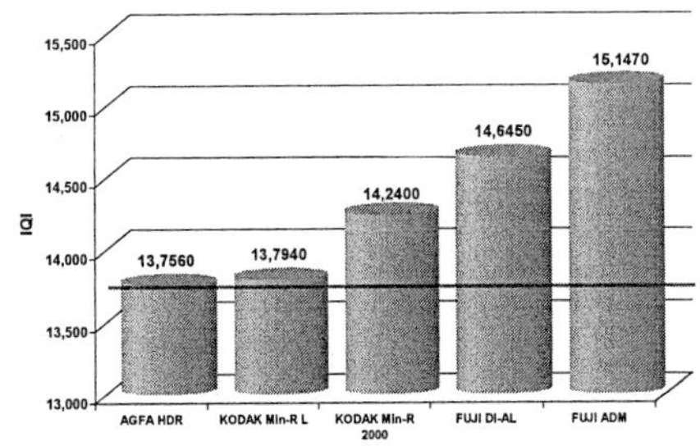

Fig. 9. Mean IQI value on CDMAM 3.2 for each film

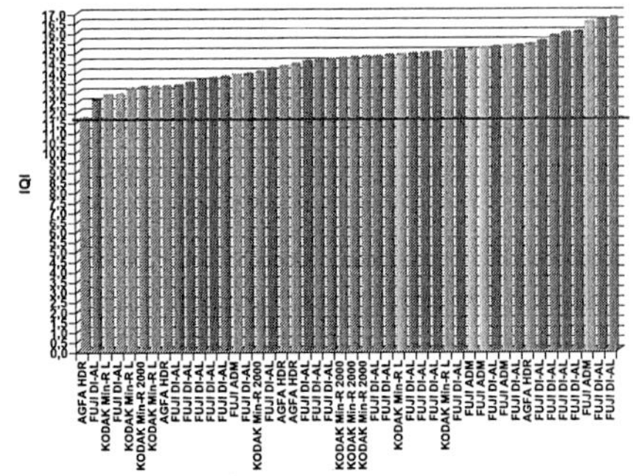

Fig.10. IQI value distribution on CDMAM 3.2 for each film

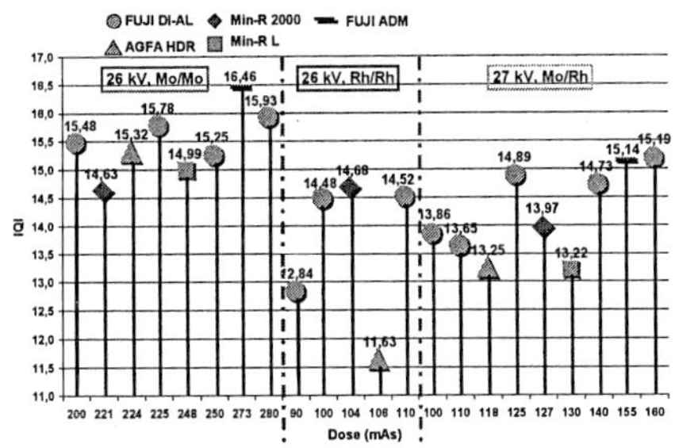

Fig. 11. IQI value on CDMAM 3.2 at 26 kV Mo/Mo and Mo/Rh, and 27 kV Mo/Rh

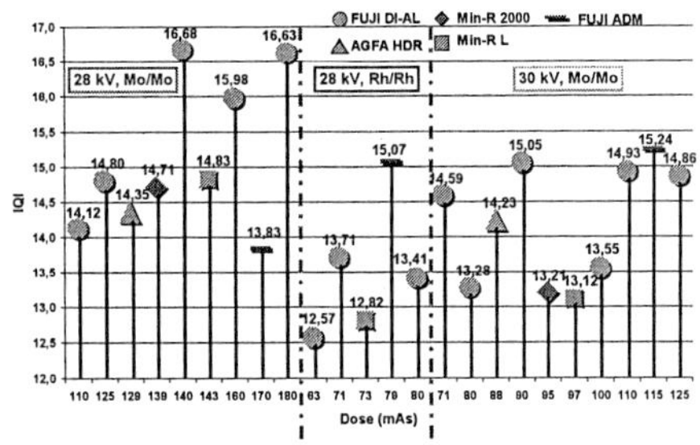

Fig. 12. IQI value on CDMAM 3.2 for each film at 28 kV Mo/Mo and Rh/Rh, and 30 kV Mo/Mo

CDMAM 3.2 results

The CDMAM 3.2 is used in the digital and analogical mammography systems performances evaluation [3]. We have decided to take the inverse of the Image Quality Index (IQI) for presentation reasons [4].

The formula to calculate the IQI value is [equation 1]:

$$\mathrm{IQI} = 16 \,/ \sum_{i=1}^{16} C_i * D_{i,\min} . \quad (1)$$

A higher IQI value represents a better contrast/detail and image quality.

We obtain at least equal or better IQI with the FUJI DI-AL for each tube voltage and target/filter combination with lower or equal dose, except in comparison with the FUJI ADM for 26 kV Mo/Mo, 28 kV Rh/Rh and 30 kV Mo/Mo exposures whose IQI values are higher (Fig. 9, 10, 11 and 12).

4.2 Comparison between FUJI hard- and soft copies

All the following results have been carried out without using the tools available on the SenoPix diagnostic workstation (FUJI Medical System France) like magnifying possibility, contrast and luminosity adjustment.

According to the test object used, hard-copy results are better than soft-copy (Fig. 13, 14 and 15). However, the difference between the image quality scores decreases whereas the dose increases.

More detailed results shows that, with the MTM 100R test object, the difference of detection noted on the SenoPix workstation monitor essentially corresponds to microcalcifications (Fig. 17) and more specifically to masses group, in particular with a lower dose (Fig. 18).

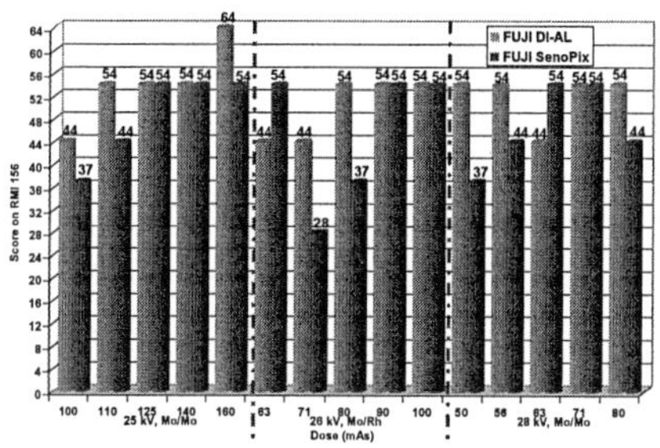

Fig. 13. Results for the RMI 156 test object

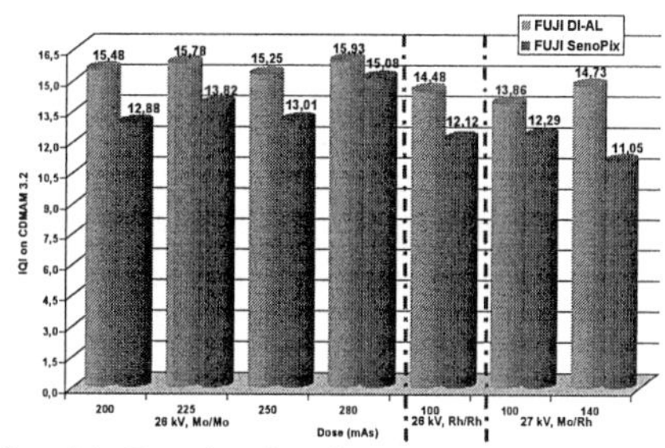

Fig. 14. Results for the CD MAM 3.2 test object

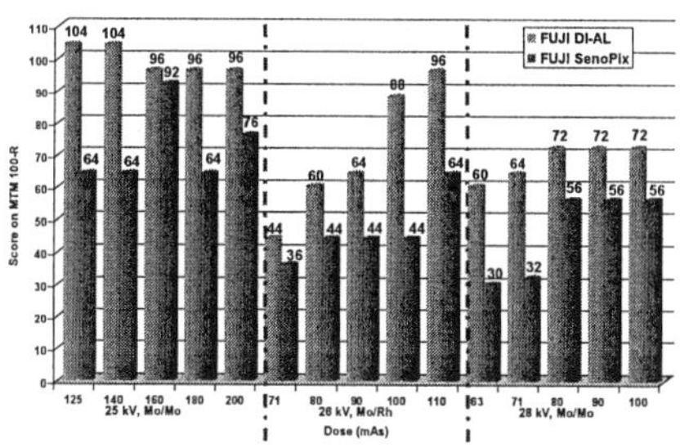

Fig. 15. Results for the MTM 100R test object

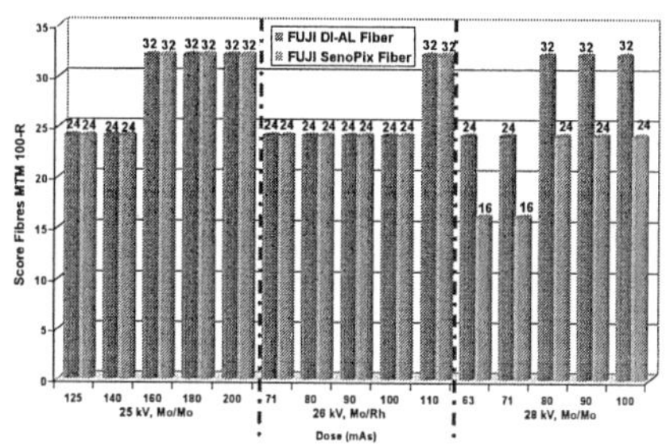

Fig. 16. Results for the fibrous structures (MTM 100R)

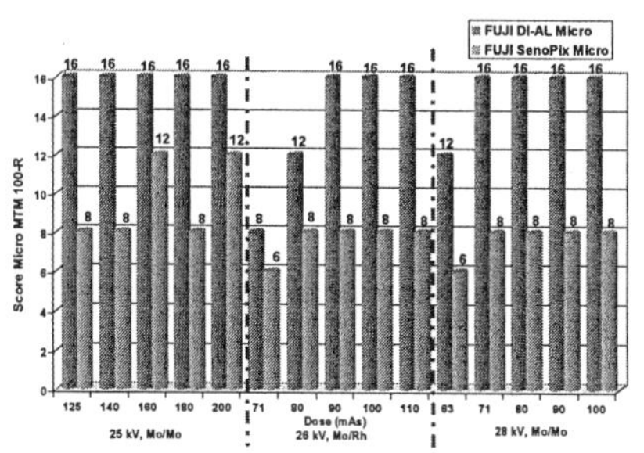

Fig. 17. Results for the microcalcifications (MTM 100R)

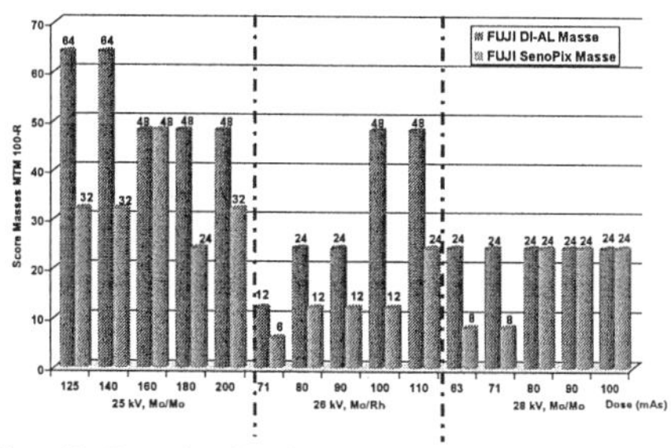

Fig. 18. Results for the masses (MTM 100R)

5. Conclusions

The comparison between results of conventional and laser films show that image quality is at least equal to the different analogical screen/film combinations in the same or lower range of dose.

The detection with the FUJI SenoPix workstation on monitor is clearly lower, in particular in the case of small and low-contrasted structures like powdery microcalcifications or certain type of masses.

In opposition to the others studies on phantoms, we have chosen to not use the workstation magnification and contrast enhancement and read the primary images to directly compare hard- and softcopies in the same conditions, in order to determine the detection threshold of image interpretation on display. But the workstation functionalities (magnifying possibility, colour-reverse, luminosity and contrast adjustments…) improve the interpretation quality on monitor.

In clinical practice the waste of time due to the systematic image review is most important in comparison with an analogical film visualised on a specific mammography viewbox, in particular in a screening programme which is intended to healthy women in the large majority.

The Computer Aided Detection seems to be essential in complement with the reading on workstation for detection. So the ability of direct compatibility between the digital system and the CAD is necessary for a clinical practice, and maybe in a second reading system.

This study is an image quality comparison between phantoms. Further complete tests with other adjustments on the workstation post-treatment, other values of kV have to be carried out. In the same time, clinical studies are in progress in another French centre.

References

1. A. Noel, J. Stines, M. Zerhouni. Développement d'un fantôme en matériau équivalent sein pour la mammographie. RBM (1993) 15,7 421-423
2. A. Noel, I. Desquerre-Aufort, A. Lisbona, P. Heid. Protocole de contrôle qualité des installations de mammographie. Direction Générale de la Santé, édition révisée, juillet 1998
3. Bijkerk, K.R., and M.A.O. Thijssen: The CDMAM-phantom: A contrast-detail phantom specifically for mammography. Radiol. (1993) 185: 395
4. M. Thijssen, W. Veldkamp, R. Van Engen, M. Swinkels, N. Karssemeijer, J. Hendricks. Comparison of the detectability of small details in a film-screen and a digital mammography system by the imaging of a new CDMAM-phantom. Book of the IWDM 2000 proceedings (2000) 666-670

Mammography Taxonomy for the Improvement of Lesion Detection Rates

Daniel Howard[1], Simon C. Roberts[1] and László Tabár[2]

[1] QinetiQ Software Evolution Centre, Building U50, QinetiQ PLC, Malvern WR14 3PS,UK tel: +44 1684 894480 dhoward@qinetiq.com
[2] Falun Central Hospital, Falun, Sweden

Abstract. This work in this paper aims to assist CAD by classifying the context in which lesions can occur. This is achieved by a mammogram taxonomy system which automatically classifies breast parenchyma. The classification engine is an artificial neural network which successfully forms narrow classes to capture the subtleties in parenchyma variation. This paper presents the result of a series of experiments that digitized 628 mammograms at 50 μm from the mammographic archive at Falun Central Hospital.

1 Introduction

The radiographic lesion is a poorly defined object of large variability. Moreover, the variability of the radiological appearance of the parenchyma is even more formidable, and it has been said that a mammogram identifies a woman nearly as uniquely as her fingerprint [3].

Thus, even if it were possible to collect the thousands of breast cancers that have been observed to date, and use machine vision technology to "memorize" every one of them, the resulting tool would fail to detect similar lesions in the future because these may occur in a woman with a different parenchyma. The best that this strategy can do is to produce a large number of false alarms.

The objective of computer-aided detection (CAD) as a primary reader, i.e. the machine acting as a filter prior to human inspection, would be never to miss a lesion. Failing realization of this qualifying requirement, the objective of CAD as a secondary reader is to perform as well as a competent radiologist while producing an acceptable level of false alarms.

While a high number of false alarms is acceptable in screening programmes which practice a high recall rate, e.g. >15%, this level of false alarms is unacceptable to European screening programmes where a <5% recall rate is the norm.

Our solution to the machine as primary and as secondary reader problems is to "memorize" the normal parenchyma and detect the lesion by detecting the "abnormality". To this end our proposal is to use millions of screening examinations to produce a mammogram taxonomy, and once the taxonomy is in place, the abnormal for the class will simply "drop out". Hence, the lesion will be detected in this way.

With respect to the machine as primary and as secondary reader, the taxonomy can be exploited to detect lesions in at least two ways: (1) to allow CAD technology to specialize in a particular taxonomic class (to reduce complexity [4]); and/or (2) to expose the lesion directly as an abnormality of the taxonomic class. With respect to the human as primary or secondary reader the taxonomy can be exploited by presenting specific taxonomic classes to specific human readers. Furthermore, the taxonomy is a form of data-mining of an archive and could thus help to reveal subtle relationships between lesion occurrence and parenchyma appearance. Therefore this may even lead to a revision of the quantitative risks of cancer and of abnormal breast development for patients.

The idea of a classification, taxonomy or organisation of a pattern was established in ancient times and predates scientific explanation. More recently the Victorians developed a taxonomy to organize the field of botany and it was in place to offer examples to support genetic studies. Millions of mammograms exist in archives in breast cancer screening countries, possessing a wealth of information from which to build a taxonomy. Most of this film material is currently redundant other than for longitudinal comparison with the forthcoming examination; older examinations are being destroyed. Our proposal is to save the information contained in these archives, and to use the image features to construct a systematic taxonomy.

2 Computational method for producing the taxonomy

It is difficult to manually classify mammograms based on parenchyma types [3, 5, 7] due to the high variability in appearance of dense, glandular and fatty tissue. Although subjective analysis can identify broad qualitative characteristics in a mammogram, e.g. the approximate position and texture of the parenchyma, the quantification of these characteristics is difficult. Furthermore, the gradual atrophy and involution of the parenchyma causes the subjective classification to be a very ambiguous task. Consequently, the manual classification of mammograms into a precise taxonomy of numerous and narrow classes is infeasible.

The difficulty of subjective classification also means that a computational system cannot be *supervised* to produce desired classifications, because a one-to-one mapping between each mammogram and each potential class cannot be subjectively assigned. Therefore, mammogram taxonomy must be approached by employing an unsupervised method which uses an autonomous system to form classes simply through exposure to a set of mammograms.

An artificial neural network known as Sonnet (self-organizing neural network) is such a system [2]. It is a continually adaptive network of many processing nodes which serve to gradually develop a long-term memory for patterns to which it is exposed. Sonnet does not simply memorise presented inputs but instead it extracts the characteristic features which discriminate each *class* of input. These developing classes compete to classify each new input and in doing so they adapt as Sonnet gains more experience. Consequently, Sonnet is able to generalize any given input as belonging to a class that it has formed. Furthermore, Sonnet outputs the confidence with which the input belongs to each class and so novel inputs will be classified with a low confidence. Eventually, Sonnet will form new classes for uncommon inputs.

Sonnet is applied to mammogram taxonomy simply by exposing it to a set of mammograms. However, as Sonnet is completely data-driven, critical decisions must be made about the type of image information to extract from the mammograms and even the order in which the mammograms should be presented. A number of Sonnet parameters must also be investigated in order to achieve optimum classification coarseness and quality. The most important parameter is learning speed which controls the balance between memorizing input cases and generalizing into classes.

Although Sonnet removes the difficulty of subjective mammogram analysis, a number of performance measures must be manually defined in order to quantify the desirability of Sonnet's classes. These were based both on the input mammograms (e.g. it is expected that a patient's left and right breasts should be classified the same) and on Sonnet's general responses (e.g. Sonnet should maximize its classification confidences). Nevertheless, the ultimate judgment of Sonnet's performance is still explicit subjective analysis, where the mammogram classes should appear to maximize both intra-class homogeneity and inter-class heterogeneity. However, this is far easier to judge subjectively than to manually prescribe training classes to a supervised method.

3 Unsupervised classification

The breast tissue in a mammogram was segmented from the background so that equivalent regions could be extracted from different mammograms. The location of the nipple was estimated to ascertain different regions within the breast and the distance from the chest wall to the nipple was normalized.

Standard image processing techniques were used to extract information from each mammogram to be input to Sonnet. The image features are brightness, contrast and textural features calculated from co-occurrence matrices [1].

The mammogram foreground was separated into three regions: a retroareolar region, an axillar region and a medial region (as shown in figure 1). Brightness and contrast were calculated in a 10mm square which was swept over each region, and the distribution of each computed.

Textural features were calculated by accumulating co-occurrence matrices over each region. A matrix was generated for each of four orientations (0, 45, 90 and 135 degrees) in each region, and nine textural features were calculated from each matrix [1].

The above processing resulted with 132 image features for each mammogram. This dimensionality was reduced to 53 by identifying the strongly correlated features, and then neglecting those that had least variation across the mammogram set. Each image feature type was linearly scaled to range between 0 and 1 across the mammograms, to prevent any particular feature type from dominating in the input vectors presented to Sonnet.

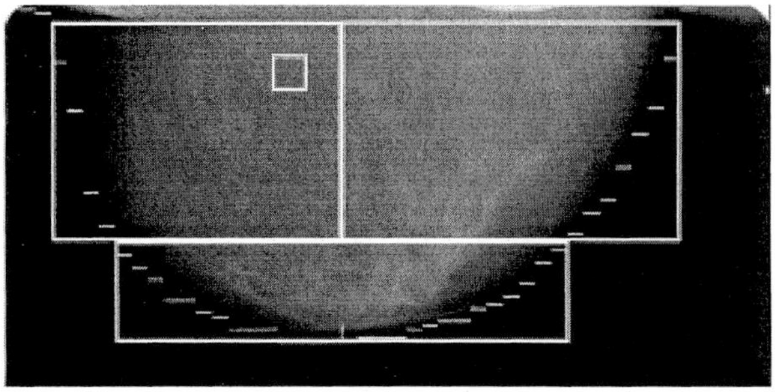

Fig. 1. The mammogram foreground is separated into three regions.

Note that the mammogram for the left breast was flipped horizontally before processing to map the axillar and medial regions onto those for the right breast, and to give the appropriate orientations for the textural features. Sonnet processed the features from CC views only.

4 Sonnet: breast parenchyma classifiers

Sonnet consists of an array of classifiers connected to an input field as shown in figure 2. Sonnet responds to each mammogram in turn and gradually encodes the corresponding input features as follows. The constituent classifiers compete to encode each mammogram such that the classifier with the best match to the current input tends to adapt itself more than the other classifiers. The classifiers consequently diverge so that each responds only to mammograms similar to its encoding.

Each presentation of the mammogram set is known as an epoch. Sonnet typically learns by adapting itself over many epochs until a stable set of classifiers can categorize each mammogram with a significant degree of confidence. Sonnet comprised 80 classifiers which responded to 628 mammograms over 100 epochs. The best epoch was chosen to maximize the number of classifications and the confidence of each classification.

Sonnet possesses many parameters controlling the various aspects of the network's dynamics. The most important of these is the learning rate which specifies how quickly Sonnet will adapt to each input. The fastest learning rate produces one-shot learning where Sonnet simply memorizes each mammogram. Reducing the learning rate allows Sonnet to classify like mammograms, where slower learning produces broader classes.

The 628 mammograms presented the left and right CC views of each patient consecutively. It was expected, but not mandated, that a patient would receive the same classification for the left and right breasts. Consequently, a patient-wise score was deduced to quantify the extent to which this occurred in a Sonnet run. A number of runs were conducted to investigate the interactions between dif-

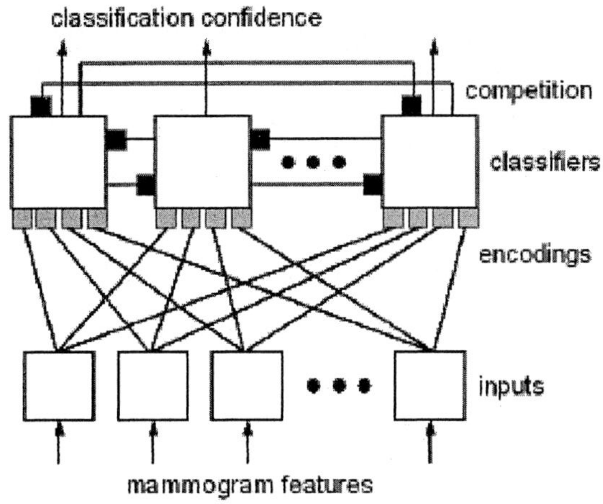

Fig. 2. Sonnet architecture.

ferent Sonnet parameters. The best run was chosen by considering the maximal number of classes encoded and the highest patient-wise score.

The Figure 3 illustrates four classes from the 60 formed by the best epoch on the best Sonnet run. The mammograms in each class are ordered by decreasing classification confidence when viewed from top-left to bottom-right. The classifications were based on subtle variations in mammogram appearance instead of simply quantifying the amount of fatty, dense and glandular tissue. For example, the resulting classes showed that the distribution and orientation of characteristic tissue textures were chief class discriminators.

References

1. C. Gotlieb, H. E. Kreyszig: Texture descriptors based on co-occurrence matrices. Computer Vision, Graphics and Image Processing, vol 51, pp70-86 (1990).
2. A. Nigrin: Neural Networks for Pattern Recognition, ISBN 0-262-14054-3, Bradford Books, MIT Press (1993)
3. Eric. J. Roebuck: Clinical Radiology of the Breast ISBN 0-433-00066-X Heinemann Medical Books (1990)
4. J.-C. Simon: Patterns and Operators. The Foundations of Data Representation. ISBN 0-946536-16-3 North Oxford Academic Publishers Ltd. (1986)
5. L. Tabár: Teaching Course in Diagnostic Breast Imaging: Diagnosis and in-depth differential diagnosis of breast diseases. Mammography Education, Inc., Lucerne, Switzerland, 2001.
6. L. Tabár and P. Dean: Teaching Atlas of Mammography 3rd Edition ISBN 0-86577-962-7 (TNY) Thieme, Stuttgart · New York (2001)
7. J. N. Wolfe, A. F. Saftlas, M. Salane: Mammographic parenchymal patterns and a quantitative evaluation of mammographic densities; a case control study. Am. J. Radiol. 148, 1087-92 (1987)

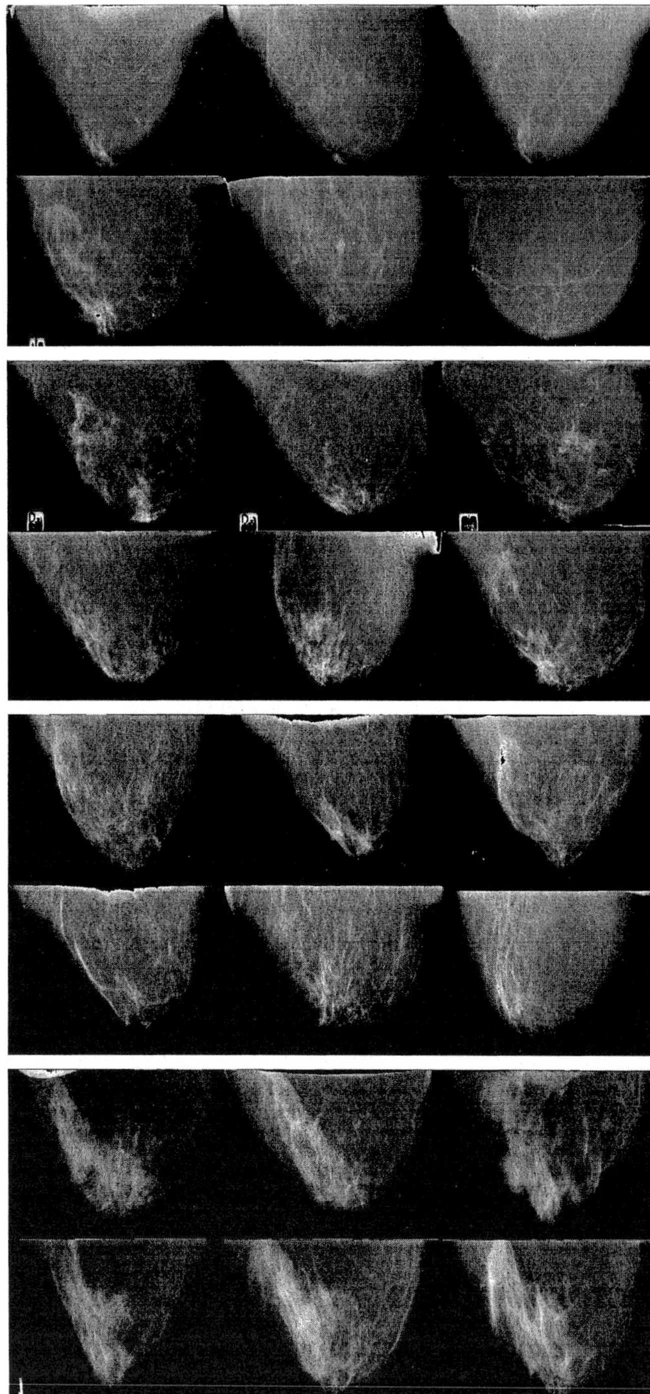

class

class

class

class

Fig. 3. Four classes encoded by Sonnet.

A high resolution (25 μm) hybrid selenium/CCD slot scan detector for digital mammography

DM Hunter[1], G DeCresenzo[1], SO Kasap[2], JG Mainprize[1], GE Mawdsley[1], JA Rowlands[1], C Smith[3], T Tümer[4], S Yin[4], MJ Yaffe[1]

[1]Sunnybrook and Women's College Health Sciences Centre, 2075 Bayview Avenue, Toronto, ON, Canada; [2]University of Saskatchewan; [3]DALSA Semiconductor; [4]Nova R&D
david.hunter@swchsc.on.ca

Abstract. We describe the design and testing of slot scanned digital mammography detectors that utilize 200-μm thick layers of selenium directly deposited on specially-designed CCDs (charge coupled devices) with a 25-μm pixel pitch. The detector element fill factor approaches 100%. We have produced and are testing CCD structures that utilize both surface and buried channel structures. We are developing selenium blocking layers that are optimized for electron signal transfer to a CCD.

1. Introduction

One approach that has been demonstrated to be feasible for digital mammography is based on a slot-beam of x rays which is scanned across the breast in synchrony with a long, narrow, multi-line detector. While this requires a specialized mechanical scanning apparatus and a longer image acquisition time, compared to flat-plate detector systems, and x-ray tube heat loading is much greater, it does have the benefit of dose-efficient scatter rejection and possibly lower detector cost. Typically, the detector used in such a system consists of a CsI(Tl) phosphor, fibreoptically coupled to multiple rectangular CCD arrays operated in time delay integration (TDI) mode. While this detector can produce excellent images, it suffers from some of the limitations common to all phosphor-based or indirect x-ray detectors. The main limitation is the need to compromise between detector thickness (and, therefore, its quantum interaction efficiency) and spatial resolution. This compromise occurs because the spread of light from the phosphor and the accompanying loss of resolution becomes more significant as detector thickness increases.

It is possible to overcome this problem by using a direct conversion detector in which the energy of absorbed x rays is immediately converted to electric charge carriers. In such detectors, an electric field normal to the image plane guides the signal charges directly to a collection electrode. There is little lateral displacement of the charges and the main factor affecting MTF should only be the aperture response function of the detector element (del). A number of direct conversion detector materials are currently under development, including silicon, amorphous selenium (a-Se), cadmium zinc telluride, mercury iodide, lead iodide and gallium arsenide. Here, we discuss our development of a slot-scanned detector based on an a-Se x-ray absorber, directly deposited on a TDI CCD readout device. Our work is proceeding along two parallel, but integrated paths: 1) development and evaluation of a selenium material suited to this application, and 2) design, development and testing of the CCD readout section of the detector.

Current digital mammography systems have detector apertures of nominal dimensions ranging between 40 μm and 100 μm. At present there is no consensus [1] on what del size is required although there is some anecdotal evidence that characterization of microcalcifications is facilitated when the spatial resolution is increased. In any case, in the interpretation of mammograms, it is often desirable to produce images of certain suspicious areas of the breast with very high spatial resolution and we have, therefore, attempted to produce a detector with this capability. For situations when lower resolution is acceptable, this can easily be achieved by averaging the signals from adjacent dels.

2. Design considerations

In order to meet or exceed the resolving capabilities of screen-film mammography we decided that a 25-μm detector element (del) would be sufficient, given that screen-film systems can resolve high contrast objects containing spatial frequencies of 16 cycles/mm. For a variety of reasons, it is very difficult to create a full-field digital mammography system employing flat panel TFT arrays with a 25-μm del. Maintaining a high fill factor is one reason, and another is poor manufacturing yield, due to the large number of dels. On the other hand, such a small del size on a slot-scanned system is technically tractable, in part, because the detector is smaller, so there will be fewer dels.

Typically a digital mammography detector must accommodate a maximum exposure (unattenuated x-ray beam incident on the detector) on the order of 1 Roentgen (~ 3×10^7 quanta/mm^2). The number of electron-hole pairs produced upon absorption of an x-ray quantum is given by: $n_c = h\nu/W$, where W is the mean x-ray energy required to create a free charge pair. For a-Se, W is on the order of 60 eV [2], and for most other direct conversion materials considered for use as x-ray detectors, it is in the range 3-6 eV. Therefore, the maximum amount of charge that must be accommodated by the CCD array can be extremely large (1×10^{10}/mm^2). Unfortunately, the charge storage capability per unit area of CCDs is 10-20x less than the required value, when W = 3-6 eV. The charge storage is limited by the minium practical thickness of the CCD gate oxide layer. We have, therefore, explored different approaches to dealing with the excess charge and have chosen to design a multi-tapped CCD structure that allows readout of fractions of the total charge along several parallel output paths.

Unlike other photoconductors, the W value for a-Se (W_{se}) is field dependent. W_{se} can be decreased or increased by increasing or decreasing the bias respectively. Therefore, it is possible to adjust the effective gain of the system by controlling the bias voltage. Obviously if the signal is reduced in this way, additional attention must be paid to the readout noise to ensure that it never exceeds the intrinsic quantum noise of the x-ray signal. Fortunately, CCD structures can be devised with exceptionally low readout noise, considerably lower than possible with active matrix TFT arrays. Shown in Table 1 are the nominal signal charges that the CCD must accommodate.

Much of our previous work was centred around devices in which the x-ray absorption and readout layers were electrically and mechanically connected by an array of indium bumps [3]. This is expensive and requires extremely precise alignment of the two components. Here we have focused on a system in which the a-Se is deposited directly on an array of del electrodes on the CCD.

In order to refine the new detector technology it is of benefit to be able to make rapid iterations. Most modern CCD manufacturing processes utilize p^+ layers and employ minority carrier electrons as the signal. Since we wish to use standard CCD processes, we must operate a-Se with a negative bias on the "free" surface plane (surface distant to the CCD). Partially because a-Se has a higher mobility for holes than for electrons, to date it generally has been optimized for hole transport and the application of positive bias to the free surface plane. A design goal is the reduction of dark currents with negative biases and the improvement of electron carrier transport (mobility-lifetime product).

Table 1. Calculated parameters for soft and hard Tungsten spectra: Spectrum 1 and Spectrum 2. The exposure was 1 Roentgen. The absorbing a-Se layer was 200 μm thick and W_{se} was 60 eV

Parameter	**Spectrum 1** (30 kV, 15 μm Molybdenum filter)	**Spectrum 2** (45 kV, 1mm Aluminum filter)
Mean energy	17.8 keV	28.8 keV
Quantum interaction efficiency	97%	76.8%
Absorbed energy per del	4.8×10^{-11} J	2.2×10^{-10} J
Charge produced	5×10^{6} electrons	2.2×10^{7} electrons
Noise from 1 x-ray photon interaction	300 electrons	480 electrons
Number of x-ray photons per del	1.7×10^{4}	4.7×10^{4}

The main design features of the new detector design include: the adoption of an adjustable-gain photoconductor (a-Se) such that the signal charge matches the intrinsic CCD storage capacity, direct deposition of the photoconductor on the CCD readout device, adoption of standard, optimized, CCD device fabrication processes which use electron signal carriers, and optimization of a-Se for electron signal generation. These are illustrated in Fig. 1.

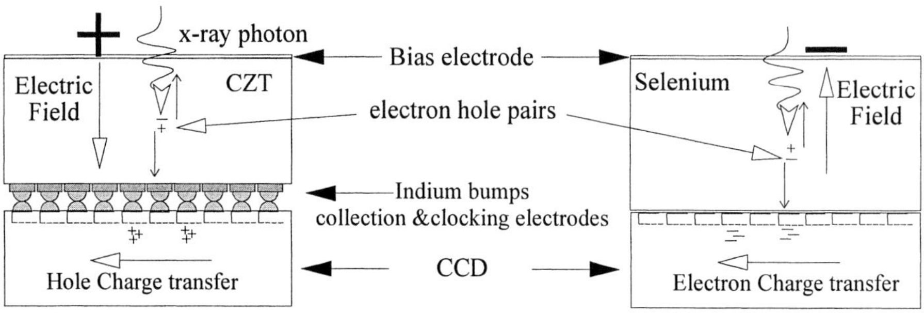

Fig. 1. **Illustration of the primary differences between an existing direct-conversion, slot-scan design (left), and the new design (right).**

3. Design of the linear array test CCDs

Two test CCDs have been designed and are currently under fabrication. The designs differ only in that one operates in surface channel mode, the other in buried channel mode. The surface channel mode has a better signal storage capacity (electrons/mm^2) than the buried channel, but a poorer charge transfer efficiency (CTE) than the buried channel mode. The test CCDs are designed to facilitate tests of the following major parametric factors: signal capacity, CTE, readout noise, and the proper transfer of charge between the a-Se and the CCD. Table 2. summarizes the device characteristics.

Table 2. Parametric factors of the two test CCDs. Readout noise is reduced when correlated double sampling (CDS) is applied

Parameter	**Surface Channel**	**Buried Channel**
Del pitch	25 μm	25 μm
Number of stages	220 active + 11 isolation	Same
Selenium pixel area	25 μm x 1000 μm	Same
Readout register area	25 μm x 100 μm	Same
Signal capacity	1.8 x 10^7 e	6.0 x 10^6 e
Conversion efficiency	0.15 μV/e	0.4 μV/e
Rms dark noise (excluding dark current)	100e (15 μV) with CDS 400e (60 μV) w/o CDS	30e (12 μV) with CDS 220e (88 μV) w/o CDS

4. Design of the slot-scan TDI CCD

The TDI CCD will differ from the linear array test CCDs in that it will have a TDI surface channel image section and a buried channel shift register section. The surface channel TDI dimension will be 1 cm, provided the CTE measured on the test surface channel CCD is sufficiently high. One cm in the scan direction will provide 400 dels, reduce tube loading, while keeping the scatter factor sufficiently low. The mammography scan time of 5 s dictates a TDI transfer frequency of only 1.4 kHz, good for improving the surface channel CTE. The buried channel charge shift register length will be 5.1 cm, providing 2048 dels in the slot direction, and minimize the number (4-5) of CCD devices required in the slot direction. Readout speed is 3 MHz.

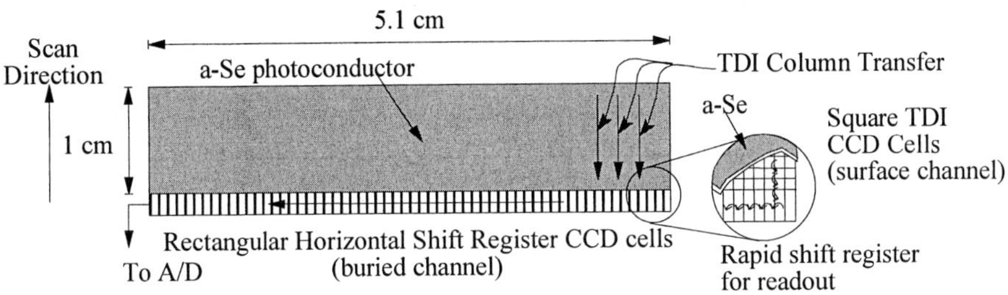

Fig. 2. Simplified schematic of the slot-scan TDI CCD design. The diagram is not to scale.

5. Summary

Amorphous selenium seems well suited for the design of a direct detection slot-scan mammography system based upon CCD readout technology. Materials research is in progress to adapt the properties of a-Se for CCD charge readout. Initial results are promising. Custom CCD test devices with, and without a-Se evaporated on them, will be prepared and tested by the middle of 2002.

References

1. Muller, S., Rick, A., Priday, K., Levy, L.: Analysis of the Influence of Pixel Size on Diagnostic Accuracy in Digital Mammography. IWDM 2000 5th International Workshop on Digital Mammography.
2. Stone, M.F, Zhao, W., Jacak, B.V., O'Connor, P., Yu, B., Rehak, P.: The x-ray sensitivity of amorphous selenium for mammography. Med. Phys. **29**, 319-324 (2002).
3. Mainprize, J.G., Ford, N.L., Yin, S., Tümer, T., Yaffe, M.J.: A slot-scanned photodiode-array/CCD hybrid detector for digital mammography. Med. Phys. **29**, 214-225 (2002).

Co-registered Breast Imaging with 3D X-Rays and 3D Ultrasound

A. Kapur, Ph.D.*, P.L. Carson, Ph.D.**, K. Thomenius, Ph.D.*, J.W. Eberhard, Ph.D.*, M. Goodsitt, Ph.D.**, J.L. Krücker, MS**, M.A. Roubidoux, M.D.**, M. Helvie, M.D.**, O. Astley, Ph.D.*, B. Yamrom, Ph.D.*, B. Claus, Ph.D.*, A. Alyassin, Ph.D.*

*GE Global Research Center, X-ray Systems and Applications Laboratory, 1 Research Circle, Niskayuna, NY, 12309; **University of Michigan, Department of Radiology, 200 Zina Pitcher Place, Ann Arbor, MI 48109
kapur@crd.ge.com

Abstract. A semi-automated prototype compression paddle system has been designed to enable co-registered acquisition of tomosynthesis and 3D breast ultrasound images. The system retrofits to a digital mammography system (Senographe 2000D, GE Medical Systems). A high frequency, linear, multi-row transducer is positioned in mechanical alignment above the paddle. The two-dimensional transducer motion in a plane above the digital mammography detector is controlled and synchronized through dedicated software that resides on a stand-alone computer, that also interfaces with a LOGIQ700 ultrasound system (GE Medical Systems). Following tomosynthesis or standard projection digital mammography exposure, a full-breast ultrasound scan is acquired with multiple linear sweeps of the transducer positioned above the compressed breast. The digital mammograms and sonograms are thus acquired with the same views of the breast, as determined by mechanical design. The images are then transformed into a common coordinate system and reformatted views in orthogonal or oblique planes may be visualized in various ways to compare regions of interest on the two sets of images for combined evaluation. Initial results on 2D ad 3D mammograms combined with 3D ultrasound for anthropomorphic breast phantoms and 2D mammograms combined with 3D ultrasound for patients demonstrate promising potential of this system towards improved breast imaging.

1. Introduction

Currently 2D mammography and clinical breast examination are the only approved procedures for breast screening. Ultrasound is a useful adjunct to mammography.[2,3] The high rate of false positives and false negatives with current breast imaging techniques approved for screening suggests seeking alternative approaches. Some factors that compromise breast imaging are related to the limitations of 2D x-ray imaging with respect to structured noise especially for women with dense breasts. These limitations include sub-optimal radiographic specificity for cystic versus solid masses, operator variability in ultrasound scanning and compromised registration between separate x-ray and follow up ultrasound scans.

With mammograms and sonograms acquired with the patient in a different position, and at a different time, errors in accurate localization and identification of the same regions in the breast may arise, leading possibly to incorrect evaluation. In one study, it was shown that misidentification of regions with non co-registered images occurred in at least 10 % of 50 patients[1]. While a significant percentage of the patients in this study had fatty breasts, misidentification may be anticipated to be greater in patients with dense breasts. There are several reasons why misidentification may occur in such circumstances. There may be multi-centric disease that may render the determination of the location of specific suspicious structures ambiguous in the absence of obvious neighboring anatomic features. There may be mammographically occult cysts that are seen on sonograms. Similarly there may be sonographically occult objects that are seen on the mammograms. Fibrocystic changes may occur over time. Normal parenchyma-mimicking masses may be seen. There may be motion of internal parenchymal structures. The images are acquired in different geometries, and in particular are very dependent on the skill set of the ultrasound operator.

Our approach was to mitigate these factors by designing a prototype compression paddle system that enables the co-registered acquisition of 3-D digital mammograms acquired in tomosynthesis mode and 3D ultrasound images, in a clinical setting. Thus the mammographic limitations of structured noise, cysts versus solid mass differentiation are reduced with this system, by providing tomographic x-ray imaging capabilities and an adjunct co-registered, full breast 3D ultrasound image. The prototype system, with semi-automated ultrasonic probe motion control features was tested on x-ray and ultrasound phantoms. Image quality was compared for x-rays against that obtained with standard compression paddles used in mammography. That for ultrasound was compared on rigid phantoms with and without the compression plate. Co-registered acquisitions were tested on multi-modality anthropomorphic breast phantoms and on an initial set of patients in an IRB-approved research study validated in some cases by biopsy.

.2. Methods

2.1 System design

The prototype compression paddle system has three subsystems[4]. The first is the plastic paddle used for compression; the second is a mechanical probe mover assembly that supports an ultrasound transducer and its motion in a two dimensional plane, and is mechanically mounted above the tray; and the third is acoustic coupling materials that transmit ultrasound energy from the transducer to the breast through the compressing tray. Special software drives the motion of the transducer over the paddle in time with the acoustic frame rate of the ultrasound system that is based on the image acquisition settings such as the center frequency, number of focal zones and depth. The spacing between sequential B-scans is regular and its value is affected by the resolution desired in the scan direction and the elevational resolution of the transducer probes. Typically the resolution is poorest in this direction for the ultrasound scan compared to the other orthogonal planes and is significantly poorer than that of the tomosynthesis images. The lateral and axial ultrasound resolution however is typically significantly better than that of tomosynthesis images acquired with a limited number of angles. The combined images therefore retain the best resolution along all directions.

2.2 Experiments

There were two sets of experiments performed in this work. In the first part, a custom anthropomorphic breast biopsy phantom embedded with masses and cysts 2- 10 mm in size, clusters of microcalcifications 130 – 400 micron large and a set of nylon fibers was imaged to give projection and tomosynthesis mammograms and 3D ultrasound images. In the second part, projection mammograms and 3D ultrasound images of patients with known pathology or features from prior research or clinical studies who consented to this study through an IRB approval process were obtained. Special visualization scripts using the visualization toolkit software and ANALYZE software[5] were used to display the co-registered images.

3. Results and discussion

Figures 1 and 2 show multiplanar tomosynthesis and ultrasound images of the custom breast phantom at specific depths. The projection mammogram is shown for reference. A suspicious region on the projection mammogram may be interrogated either with the tomosynthesis or ultrasound images either individually or in overlay mode with the cursors shown in color in the depth (axial), sagittal or coronal views. Figure 3 shows the corresponding ultrasound orthogonal views for a mass seen on a projection mammogram of a patient.

For the phantoms, the masses and cysts were seen on both the tomosynthesis and ultrasound images but more clearly differentiated on the ultrasound images. The microcalcifications were clearly seen on the mammograms but not as clearly seen on the ultrasound images. Familiar effects of acoustic enhancement and shadowing distal to cysts and masses respectively were observed for these objects, providing additional detail about the acoustic attenuation that occurred. Reverberations of the ultrasound beam both from the coupling gel and the plastic plate were clearly visible in the region within and surrounding the breast that were not in acoustic contact with the transducer probe. The tomosynthesis images were obtained using filtered back projection. Thus tomographic axial slices on these images blur the out-of-focus objects for any specific slice. This was apparent for high contrast fiducial markers that were placed on the phantom.

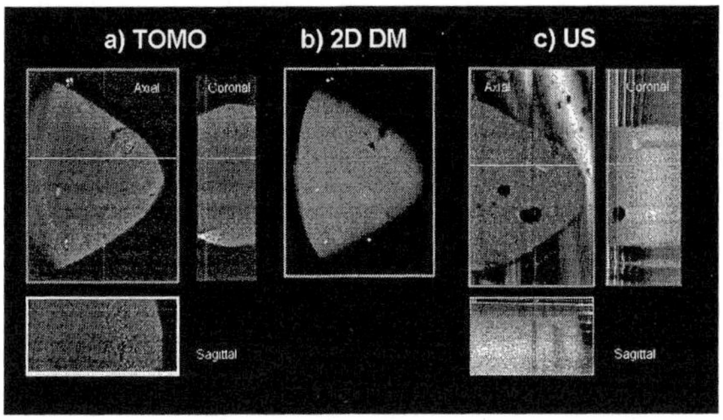

Fig. 1. Co-registered a) Tomosynthesis, b) projection mammogram and c) ultrasound images are shown for a custom CIRS phantom. The red line on the projection mammogram shows the region along which the orthogonal planes are displayed.

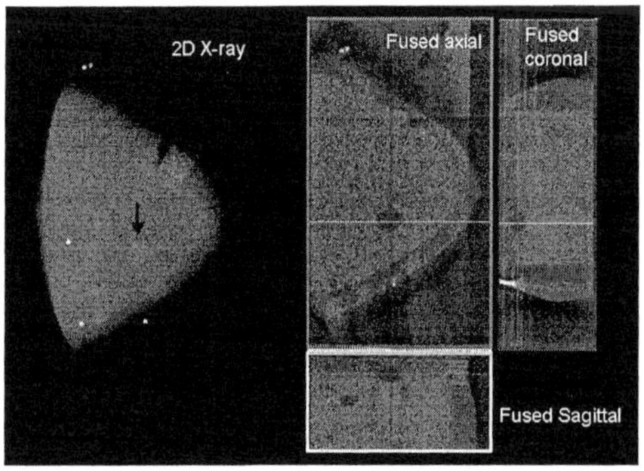

Fig. 2. Fused multiplanar views of the phantom are shown. The tomosynthesis and ultrasound images are blended in the ratio of 4:1 for this display. The red line on the projection mammogram shows the region along which the orthogonal planes are displayed. Note especially the separation of superimposing structures on the sagittal view and the contrast of the regions.

The x-ray and ultrasound image quality obtained with the solid paddle *in vivo* is illustrated from the cranial caudal compression displayed in Fig. 3. The digital x-ray image quality is undiminished from that of the standard Senograph 2000. Ultrasound quality in this case is essentially indistinguishable from that in single, hand held images with no compression plate. The quality is outstanding compared with previous 3D images of the breast, particularly those through compression plates. These contain cysts, probably the most challenging features for reverberation artifacts from a solid-plate scan window. The mammogram shows an 18 mm, well-circumscribed mass. It was confirmed by clinical ultrasound as a circumscribed hypoechoic mass with some internal echoes on a high gain, high dynamic range display. Fine needle aspiration removed 3 cc of yellow fluid and the mass resolved on ultrasound. Colored cross hairs show corresponding locations by electromechanical-registration. The ~2 mm deep C-scan on the right illustrates the exceptional detail visible with this system from within the skin to almost 1 cm depth.

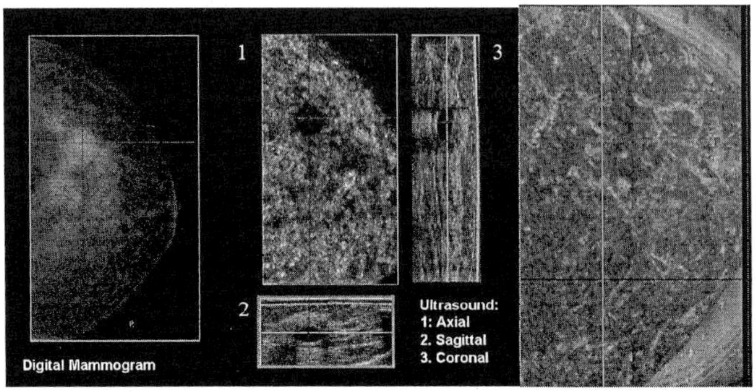

Fig. 3. A projection mammogram shown side by side along with three orthogonal sections of the ultrasound image through the clearly visible mass-like region. Note the acoustic enhancement and striking contrast shown on the ultrasound image.

In summary therefore we have shown that with the prototype compression paddle system, co-registered images may be obtained of the compressed breast that have the potential of significantly adding to the accuracy in localizing structures of interest and therefore of providing better characterization. In addition this provides a powerful platform for the investigation of advanced imaging modes.

Acknowledgements

This work was supported in part by the Office of Naval Research under Grant Number MDA905-00-1-0041.

References

1. "Occult breast masses: Use of a mammographic localizing grid for US evaluation", William F. Conway, Curtis W. Hayes, William H. Brewer, Radiology 1991, 181, 143-146
2. "Occult cancer in women with dense breasts: detection with screening US-diagnostic yield and tumor characteristics", Kolb TM, Lichy J, Newhouse JH, Radiology 1988, 207:191-199
3. "Solid breast nodules: use of sonography to distinguish between benign and malignant lesions", Stavros AT, Thickman D, Rapp CL, Dennis MA, Parker SH, Sisney GA, Radiology 1995, 196:123-134
4. "Fusion of Digital Mammography with Breast Ultrasound – a Phantom Study", A. Kapur, J. Krücker, O. Astley, D.Buckley, J.W. Eberhard, A. Alyassin, B. Claus, K. Thomenius, Heather Myers, Michael Rumsey, Roger Johnson, Steve Karr, *Medical Imaging 2002: Image Processing*, Proc. SPIE **4684**, 2002.
5. Analyze, Comprehensive Visualization for Biomedical Imaging, Mayo Foundation for Medical Education and Research

Imaging Characteristics of a Direct Conversion Full-Field Digital Mammography Detector using Selenium

Denny L. Lee, Ph.D., Jeffery G. Yorker, Ph.D., Zhenxue Jing*, Ph.D.
and Lothar S. Jeromin, Ph.D.

Direct Radiography Corp., a Hologic Company; 600 Technology Drive, Newark, DE 19702
* Hologic Inc., Lorad Division, 36 Appleridge Road, Danbury, CT 06810
leedl@directradiography.com

Abstract. A new flat panel full-field digital mammography, FFDM, system teams a DirectRay® selenium direct conversion detector technology and Lorad M-IV mammography x-ray generator with HTC™ x-ray scatter rejection grid. Modulation transfer function, MTF, approximates theoretical limits for the 70 μm pitch DirectRay® array. Detective quantum efficiency, DQE, approaches the ~70% theoretical maximum at zero-frequency for normal mammography x-ray exposure, and remains excellent at lower doses and higher frequencies. ACR phantom and breast images from production prototypes exhibit unprecedented image sharpness and near quantum noise limited operation. Clinical use of this FFDM system is expected to improve image quality at reduced patient dose compared to screen-film mammography.

1. Detector Structure and Principle of Operation

This flat panel full-field digital mammography detector uses direct-conversion technology[1] with selenium deposited on a thin-film transistor, TFT, array per Fig. 1.

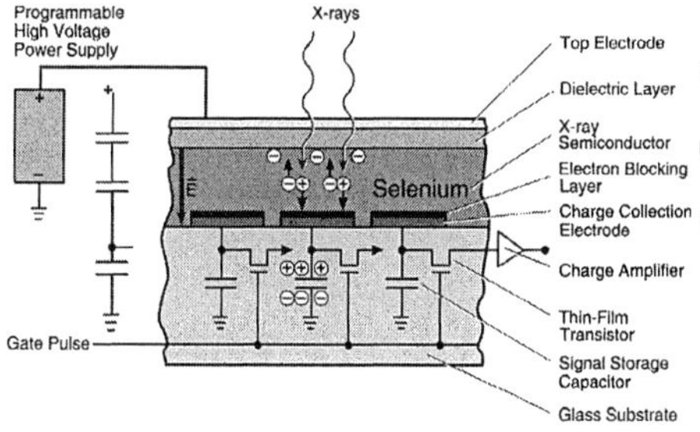

Fig. 1. Layered-structure sensor.

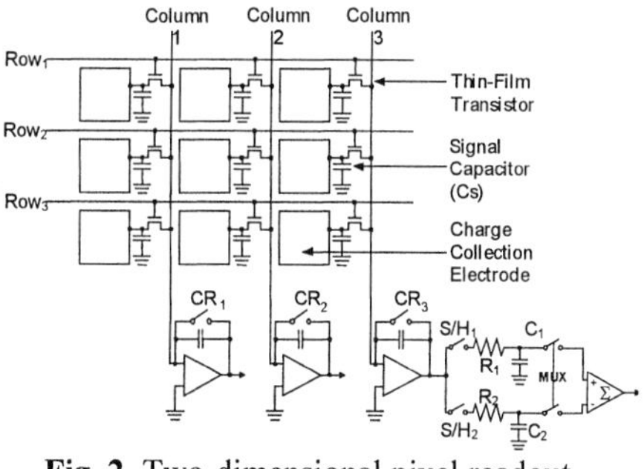

Fig. 2. Two-dimensional pixel readout.

The 251 × 287 mm active imaging area has 3584 × 4096 square pixels on 70 μm centers. They are arranged as a two-dimensional array connected by rows of gate control lines and columns of signal-source output and ground lines per Fig. 2. Each pixel has a storage capacitor to collect and store photoconductor generated charge, and amorphous silicon TFT to direct captured charge to a readout amplifier when gate enabled. Capacitors are connected between ground and a charge-collection electrode adjacent to the selenium layer and connected to the TFT drain electrode. Source lines connect to custom ASIC silicon chips with numerous low-noise integrating charge amplifiers, and include low-pass filtering and correlated double sampling for noise reduction. Source lines extend only halfway across the detector to reduce noise gain due to parasitic capacitance. Amplifiers are arranged and rows of TFT gates are connected together so four sets of 1792 pixels read out simultaneously when a gate line is enabled. Fig. 3 illustrates this detector readout architecture.

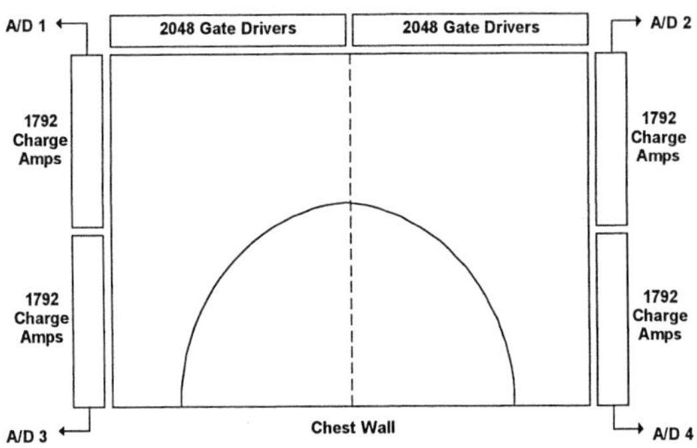

Fig. 3. Detector readout architecture.

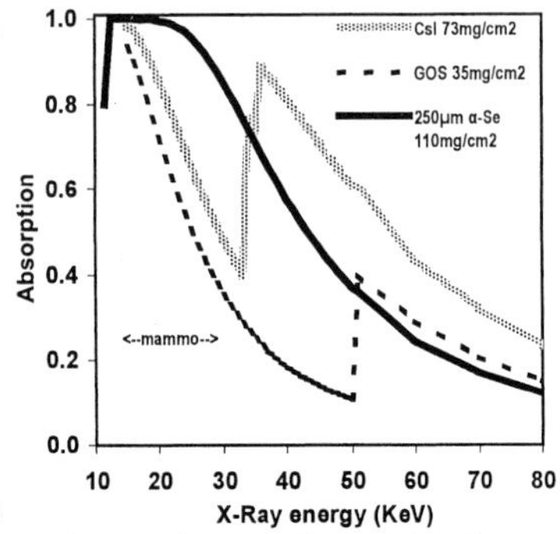

Fig. 4. Photoconductor absorbance.

Selenium's K-absorption edge near 12 KeV makes it a very efficient material for absorbing x-rays in the mammography range of 25 to 32 KVP. This detector's 250 µm thick selenium layer absorbs 90% to 98% of incoming mammography photons. Fig. 4 shows selenium absorbance is superior to two popular x-ray scintillators.

A 1500-2500 high-voltage bias is applied to the top electrode, resulting in an electric field in the selenium of 6 to 10 V/µm. Electron-hole pairs are created in proportion to the number of x-rays incident x-rays absorbed by the selenium.[2] When a positive bias is applied holes are driven along electric field lines to accumulate in the storage capacitors. Later they are read out and converted to pixel image values.

2. Imaging Performance

Fig. 5 and Fig. 6 compare measured MTF and DQE for a prototype selenium direct conversion detector and a CsI-Tapered Optic CCD mammography detector[3].

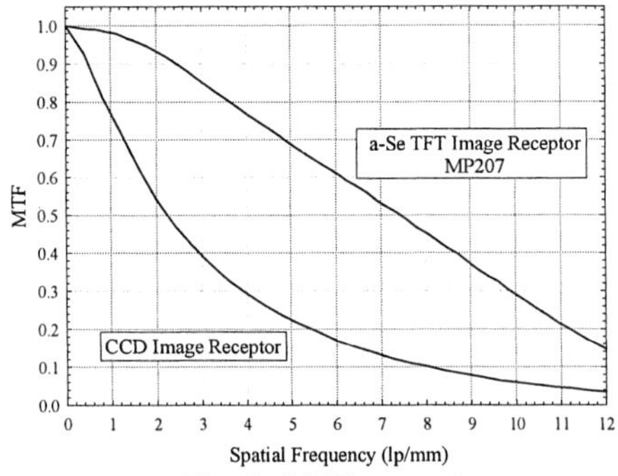

Fig. 5. MTF comparison.

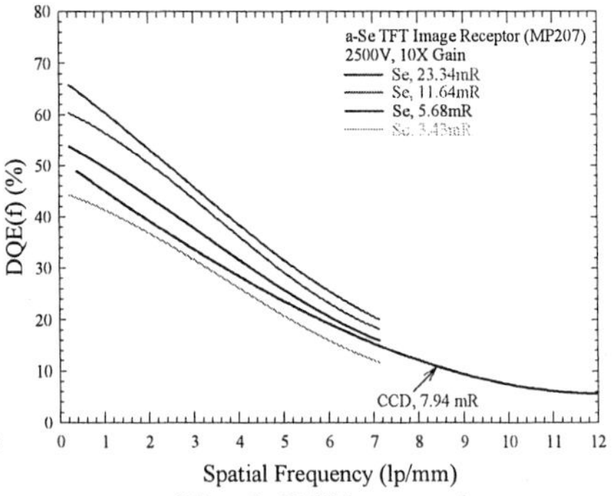

Fig. 6. DQE comparison.

Over the entire range from zero to 7 line pairs per millimeter, the MTF of the selenium detector is substantially higher than that of indirect conversion detector due to the non-spreading nature of selenium detector with captured x-ray information. DQE are also in general higher because of the favorable absorption characteristic of selenium material over the mammography x-ray energy range.

3. ACR phantom image and results

The ACR accreditation phantom was designed as a quality control test tool for screen-film mammography systems. It comprises six fibers, five groups of aluminum oxide specs, and five simulated masses embedded in a body of ~ tissue equivalent acrylic material. An x-ray image of this phantom, such as in Fig. 7, can be used to provide an overall measure of the imaging system performance.

Table 1. ACR phantom scores (25 kVp, Mo filter)

	Fibers	Speck Groups	Masses
DirectRay®	5.5	4	4
CCD	5.5	4	3.5
Screen-film	6	4	3.5

Table 2. ACR phantom scores (28 kVp, Mo filter)

	Fibers	Speck Groups	Masses
DirectRay®	5.5	4	4
CCD	5.5	4	4
Screen-film	4	3.5	3.5

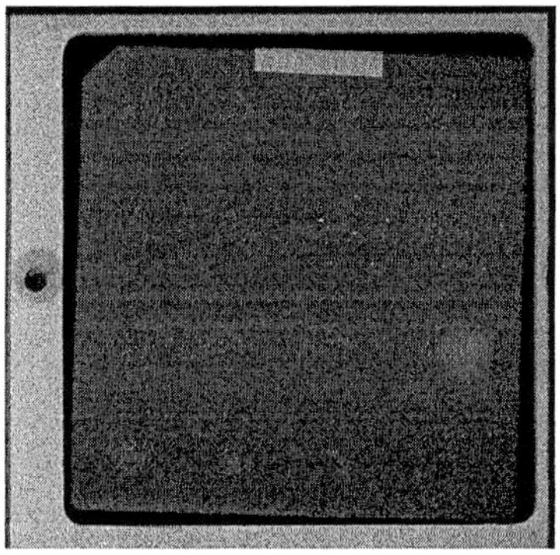

Fig. 7. ACR phantom x-ray image.

ACR phantom images were acquired by a Lorad M-IV system using DirectRay® and CCD digital mammography detectors, and a Kodak Min-R 2000 screen-film image receptor with HTC grid. All images were acquired using the same x-ray exposure techniques, and all were printed to hardcopy film for analysis. Table 1 and Table 2 compare resulting scores at 25 kVp and 28 kVp exposure, where higher indicates better performance. Table 3, Table 4, and Table 5 compare results for 26, 28, 30, and 32 kVp exposure and 1.8X geometric magnification.

Table 3. ACR phantom scores for DirectRay® detector and 1.8X magnification.

kVp	mAs	Fibers	Speck Groups	Masses
26	65	5.5	5	5
28	40	5.5	5	5
30	30	5	5	4.5
32	22	5	5	4

Table 4. ACR phantom scores for CCD detector and 1.8X magnification.

kVp	mAs	Fibers	Speck Groups	Masses
26	64.4	5.5	5	5
28	42.8	5	5	4.5
30	30.3	5	5	4.5
32	22.6	5	5	4

Table 5. ACR phantom scores for Kodak Min-R 2000 screen-film and 1.8X magnification.

kVp	mAs	Film Optical Density	Fibers	Speck Groups	Masses
26	65	1.57	5.5	5	4
28	42	1.69	5	5	4
30	30	1.81	5	5	4
32	22	1.90	5	4	4

4. Clinical Studies

Early clinical trials of a selenium direct-conversion mammography system yielded favorable preliminary results. The magnified region near a biopsy marker in Fig. 9 qualitatively shows DirectRay® MTF is superior to indirect CCD results in Fig. 8.

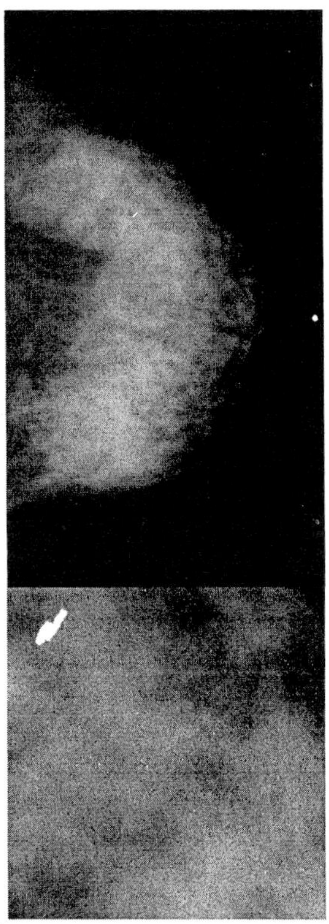

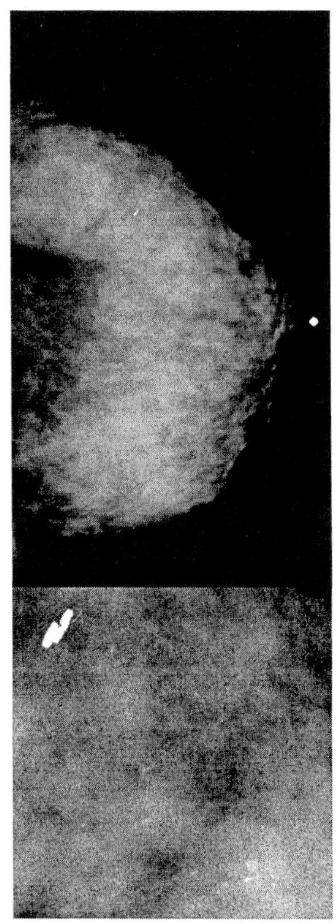

Fig. 8. (left) Mammogram by indirect-conversion CsI+CCD with 40 μm pixels.
Fig. 9. (right) Mammogram by DirectRay® selenium detector with 70 μm pixels.

5. Conclusion

We have developed a selenium-based, direct-conversion x-ray detector suitable for digital mammographic imaging. In this paper, we have presented the results and analysis of quantitative measurements made on key imaging performance characteristics of this detector. These measurements demonstrate high MTF, an intrinsic property of direct conversion technology. DQE measurements show the performance of DirectRay® detectors can approach the theoretical maximum for this technology. Digital mammographic images obtained with this detector in a clinical environment demonstrate the applicability of this technology to mammography.

References

1. D.L.Y. Lee, L.K. Cheung, L.S. Jeromin, "A New Digital Detector for Projection Radiography," *Physics of Medical Imaging 1995*, SPIE Vol. **2432**, pp. 237-249, Feb 1995.

2. S.O. Kasap, V. Aiyah, B. Polischuk, A. Baillie, "X-ray Sensitivity of a-Se for X-ray Imaging with Electrostatic Readout," *Journal of Applied Physics*, vol. **86 (6)**, pp. 2879-2887, 1998.

3. L. Cheung and R. Coe, "Fullfield, Single Exposure Digital Mammography," *Medical Electronics*, 13-21, Oct 1995.

Simultaneous Acquisition of Diffraction, Scattering and Phase-Contrast Images by Means of a Multi-Layer Edge-On Microstrip Detector

Alessandro Olivo[1], Fulvia Arfelli[1], Anna Bergamaschi[1], Diego Dreossi[1], Renata Longo[1], Francesco Montanari[2], Ralf Hendrick Menk[2], Silvia Pani[1], Paolo Poropat[1], Luigi Rigon[1], Erik Vallazza[1] and Edoardo Castelli[1]

[1] Dipartimento di Fisica, Università di Trieste e INFN, Via Valerio 2, 34100 Trieste, Italy
[2] Sincrotrone Trieste SCpA, Strada Statale 14 Km 163.5, 34100 Trieste, Italy
olivo@trieste.infn.it

Abstract. The SYRMEP (SYnchrotron Radiation for MEdical Physics) collaboration has built and is currently operating a synchrotron radiation beamline dedicated to digital mammography at ELETTRA, the Trieste synchrotron radiation facility. A multi-layer, single photon counting edge-on silicon microstrip detector has also been designed by the collaboration. Recently, new imaging modalities have been investigated; namely, phase-contrast, diffraction and scatter imaging. All these techniques result in a relevant increase in image contrast and detail visibility with respect to conventional absorption imaging. Our recent work demonstrates that, with the proper set-up, all these techniques can be implemented making use of the microstrip detector quoted above. Hence, since this device has a very high efficiency, the images can be acquired while delivering a low dose to the sample. Moreover, the single photon counting capability of the device allows the detection of very small contrasts

1. Introduction

Recently, Phase Contrast Imaging has been deeply investigated by several researchers, mainly for the extremely high potential of this technique in the medical field [1-2]. Difficulties arise when digital phase contrast images have to be produced at a dose level compatible with radiographic examinations. The interference pattern resulting from the phase contrast is convolved with the detector pixel Point Spread Function, and this results in a nearly complete smearing of the signal if the pixel dimensions are larger than a few tenths of μm [2]. As it is very well known, spatial resolution and efficiency are counteracting issues: a small pixel size generally results in a low detection efficiency, and consequently in a high dose delivered to the patient. In this paper, an innovative experimental set-up capable of removing the pixel size constraints is described. Furthermore, with a slight change in this set-up, scatter imaging becomes feasible. The advantages of this technique are briefly described.

2. Materials and Methods

All measurements described below were carried out making use of monochromatic synchrotron radiation at the SYRMEP beamline [2-4] at ELETTRA. The SYRMEP detector prototype was used as the imaging device. Basically, this device is a silicon microstrip detector used in edge-on geometry [3]; the resulting active surface (height = 300 μm, length = 5 cm) is matched to the laminar beam cross section. Beam and detector are kept stationary, and the two dimensional images are obtained by scanning the sample through the beam.

3. Results and Discussion

The dimensions of our detector pixel are of the order of a few hundreds of μm: as mentioned above, this is too high for phase contrast imaging. Nevertheless, high quality phase contrast images can be obtained by reducing the thickness of the beam impinging on the pixel. In order to obtain symmetric interference patterns (see ref. [2]), it is necessary to split the beam in two separate thin beams, each one impinging on one of the chip edges. In this way, the centre of the detector active surface (i.e. an off-edge region the dimensions of which are of the order of $0.27x50\ mm^2$) is not illuminated [4]. On the other hand, even higher image contrast can be achieved by utilizing only one thin beam, centred on one of the chip edges (i.e. as in the previous set-up, but removing one of the beams). In this case, high intensity asymmetric patterns, very similar to the ones provided by the so called Diffraction Enhanced Imaging Technique [5], are obtained. Fig. 1 shows an image of a bee obtained with the single beam technique (Fig. 1b), compared to the pure absorption image of the same sample (Fig. 1a). As it can be seen, the improvement in image quality is extremely high.

Finally, by moving the thin beam completely out of the detector active surface, no direct photons are detected and pure scatter images can be collected. Fig 1c shows a scatter image of the bee. As it can be seen, image quality is lower with respect to Fig. 1b, but higher or comparable to the one of Fig. 1a. It is important to notice that with a multilayer detector, such as the one recently developed by our collaboration [6], the scatter image can be collected at absolutely no dose expense by one (non-illuminated) detector layer, while the other (illuminated) layers are simultaneously collecting absorption and/or phase contrast images of the same sample.

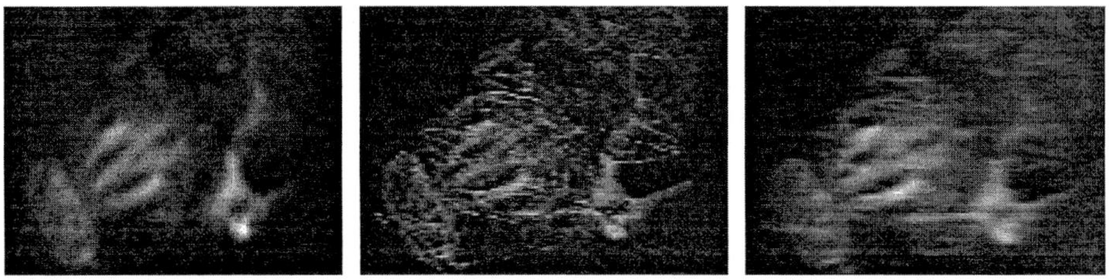

a b c

Fig. 1. Digital images of a bee obtained with different techniques. Beam Energy was equal to 17 keV. 1a is the absorption image, 1b the phase image, 1c the scatter image.

4. Conclusions

An innovative set-up capable of collecting phase contrast images even with a large pixel imaging device has been presented. Some advantages of scatter have been also briefly discussed. By means of the three-layer detector recently developed by our collaboration, the absorption, phase contrast and scatter images of a sample can be achieved all at the same time, with a single scan of the sample through the beam.

References

1 Davis, T.J., Gao, D., Gureyev, T.E., Stevenson, S.W., Wilkins, S.W.: Phase Contrast Imaging of Weakly Absorbing Materials Using Hard X-Rays. Nature 373 (1995) 595-598

2 Arfelli, F., Assante, M., Bonvicini, V. et al.: Low-Dose Phase Contrast X-Ray Medical Imaging. Phys. Med. Biol. 43 (1998) 2845-2852

3 Arfelli, F., Barbiellini, G., Bonvicini, V. et al.: An "Edge-On" Silicon Strip Detector for X-Ray Imaging. IEEE Trans. Nucl. Sci. 44 (1997) 874-880

4 Olivo, A., Arfelli, F., Cantatore, G., et al.: An Innovative Set-up Allowing a Low Dose Approach to Phase Contrast Applications in the Medical Field. Med. Phys. 28 (2001) 1610-1619

5 Chapman, D., Thomlinson, W., Johnston, R.E. et al.: Diffraction Enhanced X-Ray Imaging. Phys. Med. Biol. 42 (1997) 2015-2025

6 Arfelli, F., Bonvicini, V., Bravin, A. et al.: A Multilayer Edge-On Silicon Microstrip Single Photon Counting Detector for Digital Mammography. Nucl. Phys. B 78 (1999) 592-597

Full Field Digital Mammography with a CCD Based Slot-Scanned Detector. Physical Characteristics Measurement

Pablo G. Tahoces[1] and Robert M. Nishikawa[2]

[1] Department of Electronics and Computer Science,
Universidad de Santiago de Compostela
15782 Santiago de Compostela, SPAIN
mrpablo@usc.es
[2] Department of Radiology,
The University of Chicago
5841 S. Maryland, Chicago, IL 60637, USA
r-nishikawa@uchicago.edu

Abstract. We have characterized the performance of a Fischer SenoScan (Fischer Imaging Corporation, Denver CO, USA) fullfield digital mammography system in terms of MTF, NPS and NEQ. Measurements were made using both standard resolution mode (54 microm pixel size) and high resolution mode (27 microm pixel size) at different detector exposures. Result shows that while the MTF for scan and subscan directions are quite similar, differences between colums (scan direction) and rows (subscan direction) appear for NPS and NEQ.

1 Introduction

The SenoScan is a full field digital mammography system, based on the slot-scan concept. The detector and x-ray beam together to scan the breast with a slot of x rays. The collimation dimensions are adjusted to macth the x-ray beam to the sensitive area of the detector. The scanning is accomplished by attaching a rigid arm that swings in an arc to the detector. Scan motion is provided by a stepper motor attached to the scan arm. The total scan time for a 30 cm. image is less than 6 seconds, but the effective exposure time is only 1/30 of the scan time (200 ms.).

2 Material and Methods

2.1 Presampling Modulation Transfer Function.

The presampling modulation transfer function (MTF) was obtained by using the slanted edge method [1]. Images of a squared 10 x 10 mm. size aluminum phantom placed at the center of the detector at a slight angle (less than 4 degrees) to the anode-cathode were obtained. Four line spread functions (LSF) following north, south, west and east directions were obtained from each MTF image.

2.2 Noise Power Spectrum and Noise Equivalent Quanta.

Noise Power Spectrum (NPS) was measureed following the method described by Dobbins et al. [2]. Flat images, at different exposure levels, were obtained by placing a block of Lucite of 4.0 cm. thickness over the compression paddle, situated 23 cm above the detector panel.

To calculate the Noise Equivalent Quanta (NEQ), we computed the expression:

$$NEQ(f) = \frac{MTF(f)^2}{NPS_{norm}(f)} \tag{1}$$

where

$$NPS_{norm}(f) = \frac{NPS_{raw}(f)}{(mean_{s}ignal_{o}f_{t}he_{R}OI)^2} \tag{2}$$

One dimensional NPS curves (NPSraw) were required to compute the NEQ. Those curves were obtained by using the average of the initial 2D NPS for a thick slice of several lines on either side of both axes excluding the lines corresponding to the borders. Each value (u, v) of the slice at the frequency domain of the 2D NPS was compute as for the one dimensional NPS estimated.

3 Results and Discussion

The presampling MTF measured for both low and high resolutions are shown in figure 1. As it can be expected the MTF for higher resolution achieves higher

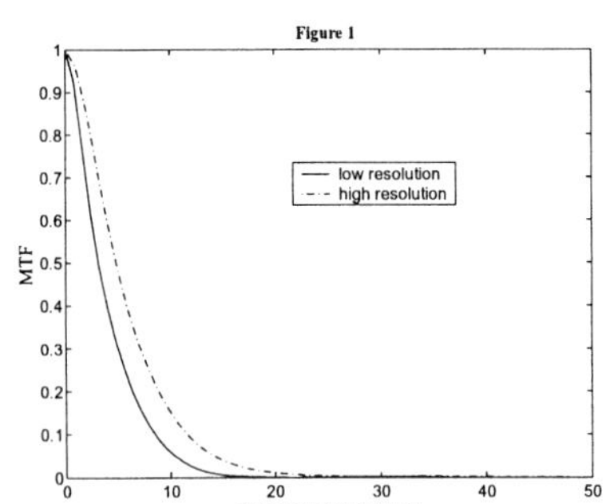

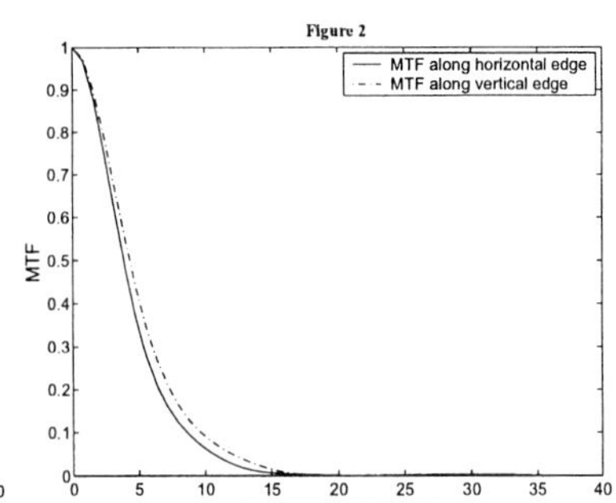

values. Small differences can be appreciated if we compare MTF along vertical and horizontal edges at high frequencies (Figure 2). MTF along vertical edges (scan direction) shows higher values.

NPS for both low and high resolution modes were calculated at different KV (30, 35 and 40) and mA values, resulting different exposure levels ranging from 5.2 mR to 107.5 mR. We verified that the integral of the NPS was equal to the

Figure 3

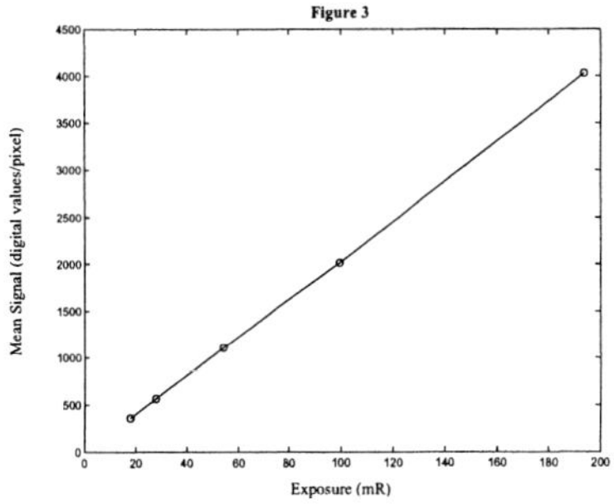

Figure 4

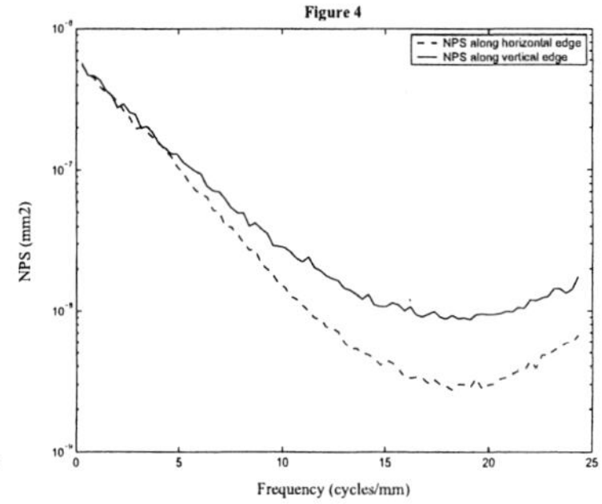

rms variance at each exposure level. The linearity of the system was measured. Results for 35 KV are show in figure 3.

The one dimensional NPS following scan and subscan directions were plotted together for comparisons. The plot demonstrated an increase for noise with the frequency when subscan direction was taken (Figure 4). As exposure increases, values for noise increases as well (figure 5).

Time-delayed integration (TDI) mode was selected by designers for CCD to operate in the SenoScan. The result is a continuously scanning adquisition that provide a reduction in noise for scan directions with a minimal reduction for signal. The result is a better performance of the system along the vertical edge, in terms of signal to noise relation. The plot of the NEQ curve reflect this fact (Figure 6).

Figure 5

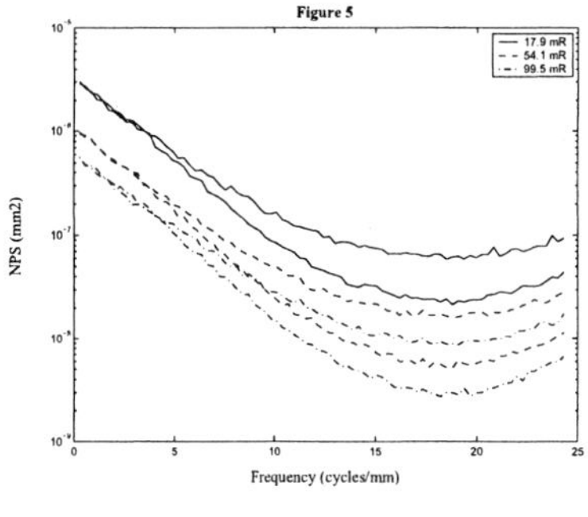

Figure 6

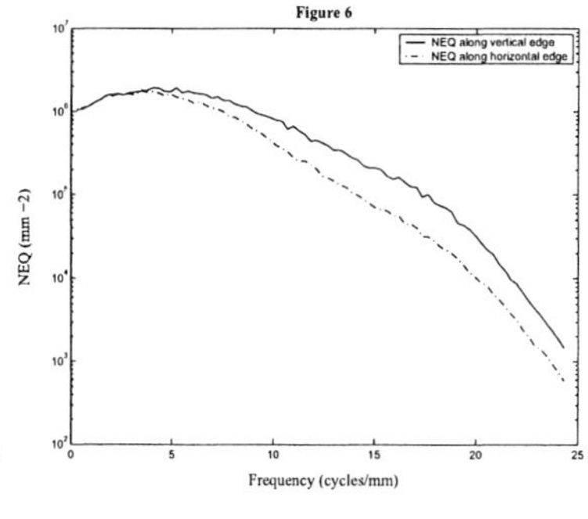

References

1. Reichenbach, S.E., Park, S.K. and Narayanswamy R.: Characterizing digital image acquisition devices. Optical Engineering. **30** (1991) 170–177
2. Dobbins J.T.: Handbook of Medical Imaging. Vol. 1 Physics and Psychophysics. Society of Photo-optical Instrumentation Engineers (2000).

Evaluation of light collection in digital indirect detection x-ray imagers: Monte Carlo simulations with a more realistic phosphor screen model

Nicholas Petrick[*], Tae-Ho Woo[†], Heang-Ping Chan[‡], Berkman Sahiner[‡] and Lubomir M. Hadjiiski[‡]

[*]U.S. Food and Drug Administration, Center for Devices and Radiological Health, Rockville, MD, [†]The University of Michigan, Department of Nuclear Engineering, Ann Arbor, MI, [‡]The University of Michigan, Department of Radiology, Ann Arbor, MI
petrick@cdrh.fda.gov

Abstract. We are performing simulation studies to investigate whether a microlens layer sandwiched between a phosphor screen and a photodetector will improve light collection in indirect-detection x-ray imagers. In this study, we examined the light collection efficiency after incorporating the spatial and angular spread of photons due to the phosphor screen in the model. Monte Carlo simulations of a uniform, planar x-ray source were conducted and the light collection efficiencies of two imager configurations were compared. Imager 1 had the screen in direct contact with the photodetector while Imager 2 had a microlens array sandwiched between the screen and the photodetector. A total of 72% of the scintillation light (31% in the "central" pixel directly below the x-ray interaction point and 41% in the 8 nearest neighbor pixels) was collected by the photodetector for Imager 2 compared with only 56% (28% in the central pixel and 28% by the nearest neighbor pixels) for Imager 1.

1. Introduction

Active matrix, flat-panel imagers (AMFPIs) have recently been introduced into clinical usage as digital radiographic imaging systems. AMFPI development has largely been motivated by the need for a solid state digital imager with real time readout. [1-3] AMFPIs can be subdivided into direct and indirect x-ray detection devices. We will concentrate on indirect detection devices in the study. AMFPIs employing indirect detection couple an array of thin-film switches, one switch per pixel, to photosensitive elements, which detect light generated by an overlying scintillating material. [4] AMFPI arrays with 100 μm pixels and a CsI(Tl) scintillation layer are commercially available for clinical mammography [5] with larger pixel sizes used in other clinical imaging applications. One key limitation of current indirect detection AMFPI devices is a poor optical fill factor (i.e., the fraction of their surface sensitive to light). In a commercial 127-μm device the optical fill factor is only 57%. While the fill factor for these devices is improving and work on the development of a continuous photodiode surface is underway [6], a large percentage of the photons are still lost because of the dead space between the photosensitive regions in the imager. A small fill factor may reduce the total number of x-ray quanta utilized in the output image because x-ray interactions occurring between the light sensitive regions could be lost because of lack of light collection.

Our technique for reducing the effects of a limited fill factor is to direct light from local areas of the phosphor screen, about the size of a photodetector pixel, onto the limited photosensitive area of that detector element using microlenses. [7-9] This has the potential to increase the number of x-ray photons utilized and may improve the detective quantum efficiency (DQE) if the number of detected light photons per x-ray interaction can be maintained or improved in all regions of the imager. In this study, we evaluated light collection and image blur for two different digital imager configurations using Monte Carlo simulations. We have previously reported results under highly idealised conditions [7]. In the current study, we improve the model by incorporating a better approximation of the angular dependent radiance (ADR) and modulation transfer function (MTF) for the phosphor screen into the simulations.

2. Materials and Methods

2.1 Monte Carlo Simulation

A simplified Monte Carlo simulation package was developed previously to track the trajectory of individual light photons produced by an x-ray interacting in a phosphor screen from the interaction location to the photodetector plane. [7; 8] We simulated a uniform parallel x-ray field incident on the phosphor where the x-rays were distributed uniformly in the xy plane and the trajectory of the incident x-rays was in a direction perpendicular to the detector plan (i.e., all x-rays travel in the z-direction). The trajectories of individual light photons produced in the screen were tracked by ray-tracing from their interaction locations through all intervening lenses to the photodetector plane. The goal of the simulation was to compare light collection and added blur for different imager configurations. We made a number of simplifying assumptions about the screen and photodetector in performing the earlier simulations. They included:

(1) x-rays interacted at the same fixed depth in the screen,
(2) a fixed number of light photons, at a fixed energy, were produced by each x-ray interaction,
(3) no spatial spread in light photons produced in the screen,
(4) a Lambertian angular distribution of the light photons at the exit surface of the screen, and
(5) the photosensitive region of each photodetector pixel was central and square.

A total of 1000 x-ray events and 100 light photons per x-ray interaction were used in the initial simulation.

In this study, the screen model has been improved to include both the modulation transfer function (MTF) and a more realistic angular distribution, thus, eliminating assumptions (3) and (4) from above. This substantially improves the accuracy of the simulation results.

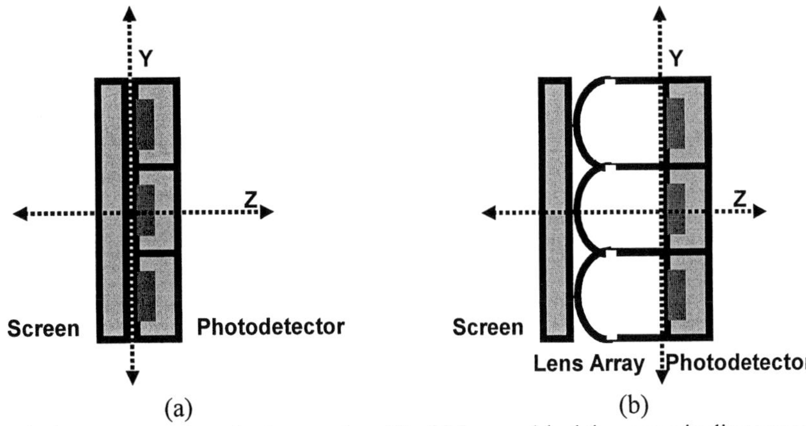

Fig. 1. A yz-cross sections for Imagers 1 and 2. (a) Imager 1 had the screen in direct contact with the photodetector. (b) Imager 2 had a 59.9 μm thick microlens array placed between the screen and the photodetector.

2.2 Imager Configurations

The simulated photodetector consisted of a 7x7 array of pixels (49 elements) with a 127 μm pixel pitch and a 57% optical fill factor. The x-ray conversion screen was based on a Gd_2O_2S:Tb converter with an MTF defined by:

$$MTF(f) = e^{-\frac{|f|}{2.67}}, \tag{1}$$

where f is spatial frequency in lp/mm. This corresponds to a full-width half-maximum of 91 μm for the screen's point spread function. The normalized radiance as a function of angle was taken to be:

$$ADR(a) = \begin{cases} 1: & 0 \leq a \leq 72^\circ \\ 0: & \text{else} \end{cases}, \tag{2}$$

where a is the azimuth angle. The spread was assumed to be uniform in the radial direction. Fig. 1 shows the cross-section of the two imagers simulated in this study. Imager 1 did not employ a microlens array and had the screen placed in direct contact with the photodetector. Imager 2 had a 59.9 μm microlens array placed between the screen and the photodetector. A single f/1.1 microlens was matched to each photodetector pixel. The lenses were spherical and had cross-sectional diameters of 127 μm matching the photodetector pixel size.

3. Results

In this simulation, all 1000 incident x-rays where uniformly distributed within photodetector pixel 25 with 610 of the x-rays falling within the photosensitive region of the pixel. This was done to allow both the light collection and blur to be estimated for the two imager configurations. Fig. 2 shows the pixel numbering used in the simulation. The photodetector pixels were grouped based on their distance from the central pixel. These groupings consisted of the central pixel (pixel 25) located directly below the x-ray interaction region, the 1st neighbor group consisting of the eight nearest neighbors to the central pixel, the 2nd neighbor group consisting of the next 16 nearest neighbors and so on. Table 1 summarizes the percentage of incident and collected light photons in each photodetector pixel. A total of 56% of the scintillation light (28% in the central pixel and 28% in the 1st neighbor group) was collected by the photodetector for Imager 1 compared with 72% (31% in the central pixel and 41% by the 1st neighbor group) for Imager 2. Approximately 5% and 7% of the light was collected by the 2nd and 3rd neighbor groups for Imager 1 and Imager2, respectively. These results indicate that including the microlens array substantially improves light collection in the central and 1st neighbor groups while increasing the amount of blurred light from 4.8% to 6.8% in the 2nd and 3rd neighbour groups.

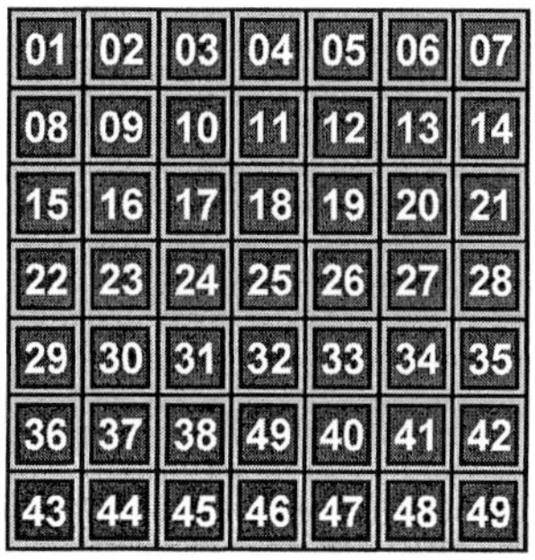

Fig. 2. The photodetector pixel numbering used in the simulation. The light gray area defines the extent of an individual pixel while the dark gray corresponds to the photosensitive area of the pixel based on a 57% fill factor.

4. Conclusions

This study simulated a uniform, planar x-ray field incident on a fluorescent screen and traced the light photons produced by the x-ray interactions from the screen to the photodetector. In, this study, the phosphor screen model was improved by incorporating a model for both the MTF and ADR of the light photons produced by x-rays interacting in the phosphor. With this improved screen model, we found that the light collection in indirect detection AMFPIs can be improved by as much as 29% (72/56=1.29) with only a small increase in blurring when a microlens array is placed between the screen and the photodetector to help direct the scintillation light onto the photosensitive region of each pixel. This predicted improvement was much larger when the ADR and MTF were included in the screen model as compared to our previous simplified simulations. We are continuing to improve the models used in the simulation and are in the process of experimentally measuring the light collection and blur for both of these imager configurations.

Table 1. Summary of the incident and collected light for Imagers 1 and 2. The incident light is defined as the light photons hitting anywhere within a pixel while the collected light includes only the light photons hitting the photosensitive region of a pixel.

Pixel Group	Photodetector Pixels In Group	Incident Light		Collected Light	
		Imager 1	Imager 2	Imager 1	Imager 2
Central Pixel	25	40.4%	36.1%	27.9%	31.1%
1st Neighbors	17-19, 24, 26, 31-33	49.8%	53.4%	28.2%	41.2%
2nd Neighbors	09-13, 16, 20, 23, 27, 30, 34. 37-41	6.3%	6.9%	3.8%	5.4%
3rd Neighbors	01-07, 8, 14, 15, 21, 22, 28, 29, 35, 36, 42, 43-49	1.7%	1.8%	1.0%	1.4%

Acknowledgements

This work is supported by USPHS Grant CA79943. The content of this publication does not necessarily reflect the position of the U.S. government, and no official endorsement of any equipment or product should be inferred.

References

1. Jee, K.-W., Antonuk, L.E., El-Mohri, Y., Maolinbay, M. and Zhao, Q.:Evaluation of direct-detection and indirect-detection active matrix flat-panel imagers (AMFPIs) for digital mammography. Proc. SPIE Med. Img. 4320 (2001) 13-23
2. Antonuk, L.E., El-Mohri, Y., Hall, A., Jee, K.W., Maolinbay, M., Nassif, S.C., Rong, X., Siewerdsen, J.H. and Zhao, Q.:A Large Area, 97 μm Pitch, Indirect-Detection Active Matrix, Flat-Panel Imager (AMFPI). Proc. SPIE Med. Img. 3336 (1998) 2-13
3. Capp, M.P.:Radiological Imaging - 2000 A.D. Radiol. 138 (1981) 541-555
4. Antonuk, L.E., El-Mohri, Y., Huang, W., Jee, K.W., Maolinbay, M. and Street, R.A.:Development of a high resolution, active matrix. flat-panel imager with enhanced fill factor. Proc. SPIE Med. Img. 3032 (1997) 3-13
5. Vedantham, S., Karellas, A., Suryanarayanan, S., Albagli, D., Han, S., Tkacyk, E.J., Landberg, C.E., Opsahl-Ong, B., Granfors, P.R., Levis, I., D'Orsi, C.J. and Hendrick, R.E.:Full bresat digital mammography with an amorphous slicon-based flat-panel detector: Physical characteristics of a clinical prototype. Med. Phys. 27 (2000) 558-567
6. Mulato, M., Lemmi, F., Lau, R., Lu, J.P., Ho, J., Ready, S.E., Rahn, J.T. and Street, R.A.:Charge collection and capacitance in continuous film flat panel detectors. Proc. SPIE Med. Img. 3977 (2000) 26-37
7. Petrick, N., Woo, T.-H., Chan, H.-P. and Sahiner, B.:Microlens focusing for enhanced light collection in digital x-ray detectors. Radiol. 221(P) (2001) 691
8. Petrick, N., Chan, H., Goodsitt, M., Sahiner, B. and Hadjiiski, L.:Digital mammographic imaging using microlens focusing: Estimation of light collection and x-ray utilization. Proc. SPIE Med. Img. 3659 (1999) 276-284
9. Petrick, N., Chan, H.P., Goodsitt, M.M., Sahiner, B. and Hadjiiski, L.M.:A Technique to Improve the Effective Fill Factor of Digital Mammographic Imagers. Proc. SPIE Med. Img. 3336 (1998) 210-218

The Effect of Scatter Radiation and its Removal on the DQE of Digital Mammography Systems

Robert M. Nishikawa

Department of Radiology, The University of Chicago, 5841 South Maryland Avenue MC-2026, Chicago, IL 60637 USA
r-nishikawa@uchicago.edu

Abstract. The detective quantum efficiency (DQE) is often used as a figure-of-merit of imaging systems. The DQE of different digital mammography *detectors* have been measured. However, digital mammography *systems* usually employ some means to reduce the deleterious effects of scattered radiation. There are two different anti-scatter methods being used in full-field digital mammography: anti-scatter grids and slot scanning. These two approaches have different effectiveness in reducing scatter and require different amounts of extra radiation. We calculated the theoretical DQE of an anti-scatter device based on standard performance metrics. The DQE of a grid ranges from 0.4 to 0.6 depending on breast thickness and kVp. The DQE of a slot system ranges from 0.7 to 0.9 depending on breast thickness and slot width. The advantage of the slot-scanning systems in terms of DQE over grid systems disappears if the width of x-ray beam is not closely matched to the width of the detector.

1. Introduction

The detective quantum efficiency (DQE) is often used to characterize an x-ray detector. It is a useful parameter in designing a detector because it indicates how efficiently the detector can use the radiation incident on it to form an image. That is, the DQE of the detector is:

$$DQE = [SNR_{out}/SNR_{in}]^2 , \tag{1}$$

where SNR is the signal-to-noise ratio and the subscripts out refers to the image and in to the x-ray image incident on the detector.

Wagner *et al.* have extended this concept to characterize the efficiency of anti-scatter grids [1]. They have shown that:

$$DQE_g = T_p \, SDF_g , \tag{2}$$

where T_p is the primary transmission factor of the grid and SDF_g is the scatter degradation factor when the grid is used; it is equal to the radiographic contrast when the grid is used to the radiographic contrast if no scatter were present.

In designing a digital mammographic system, it is useful to know how the full system functions, in addition to knowing how the individual components function. We can then define the DQE of the system as:

$$DQE_{system} = DQE\ DQE_g\ . \qquad (3)$$

In this paper, we describe preliminary work on characterizing the DQE of digital mammography systems, which includes the detector and the anti-scatter device.

2. Results

As can be seen in Fig. 1, the DQE_g of a slot system is higher than that of a grid. This is because a slot has 100% transmission of primary, whereas grids have only 70-75% transmission [2]. For grids, primary x-rays can be absorbed in the interspace material (unless it is an air-interspace grid) and some are absorbed by the lead. Also, the amount of scatter reaching the detector is higher for a grid. Figure 2 shows scatter-to-

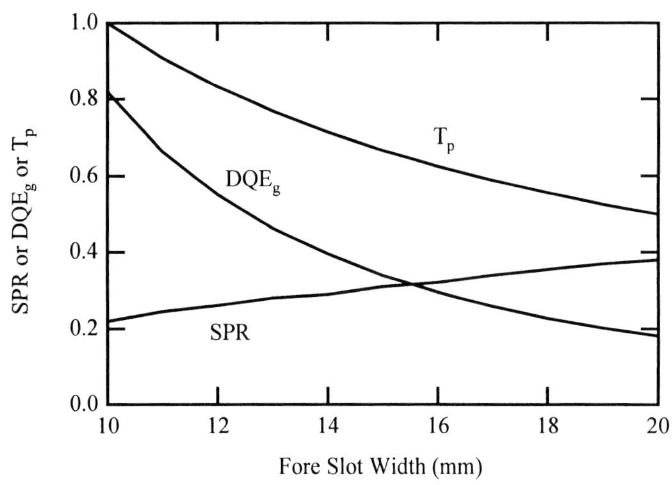

Figure 1. Comparison of DQE_g for a 5:1 grid and a 10-mm wide slot. Based on data taken from Boone *et al.* [3].

primary ratios for the two different approaches. Since the amount of scatter created depends on the volume irradiated, when using a narrow slot a significant decrease in scatter created.

The above results are only true if the aft and fore slots are perfectly matched and aligned. That is, the size of the fore slot projected on the aft slot is the same. If the projected width is wider than the aft slot, then there is radiation that is not recorded by the detector. This has the effect of lowering the primary transmission factor as shown in Fig. 3. In addition, the wider slot results in more scatter being created. As a result, the DQE_g decreases.

3. Discussion

Rose showed over 50 years ago that the SNR correlates with human's ability to see objects [4]. DQE is a measure of how efficiently SNR is passed by the detector or system. Thus DQE is useful in designing a detector or system. However, to compare different imaging systems the appropriate metric to use is the noise equivalent quanta (NEQ) [5]. NEQ can be thought of as the square of the image SNR as a function of spatial frequency. That is, DQE is a measure of the systems efficiency, whereas NEQ is an absolute measure of image quality.

In addition to using NEQ instead of DQE to compare different x-ray systems, one

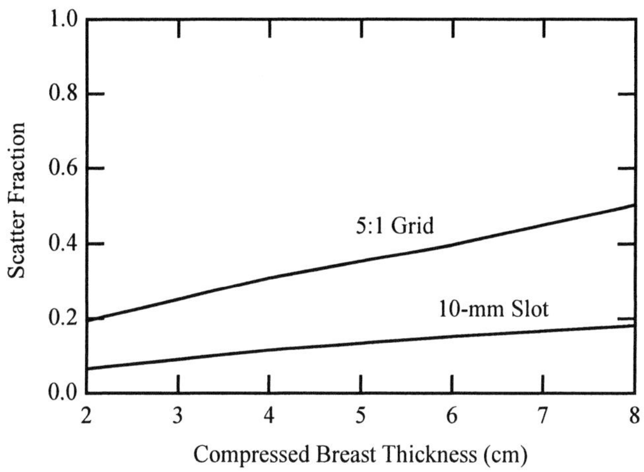

Figure 2. Comparison of scatter fractions for a 5:1 grid and a 10-mm wide slot. Based on data taken from Boone et al. [3].

needs to insure that the measurements or calculations are done using the appropriate x-ray spectrum and exposure. In particular, in this preliminary study, the same spectrum was used independent of the breast thickness. In clinical practice, as the breast thickness increases, a higher kVp is used. The data necessary to calculate DQE or NEQ is not available in the public literature, so such analysis remains to be done in the future.

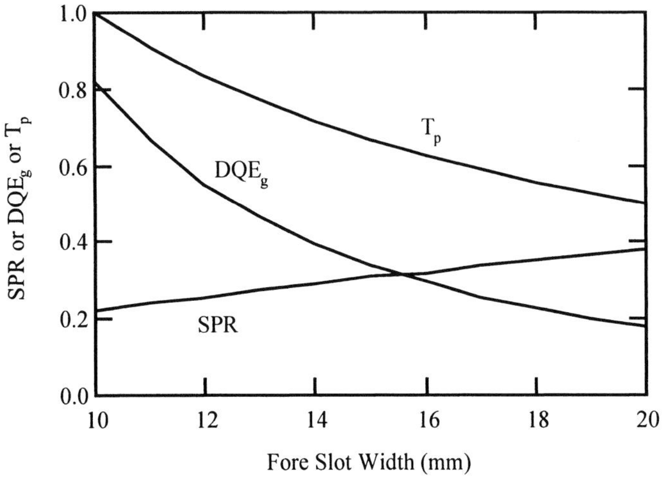

Figure 3. Scatter-to-primary ratio (SPR), DQE_g or T_p for a 10-mm wide aft slot as a function of fore slot width (projected onto the aft slot). This assumes a 40 kVp W spectrum. SPR data was taken from Boone *et al.* [3]

4. Conclusions

Properly designed slot scanning systems have significant advantages over grids. Fewer scattered x rays are created in the breast and fewer are recorded in the image. Grids also attenuate more of the primary beam. As a result, the slot system has higher DQE_g than the grid. If the fore slot is more than 40% bigger when projected onto the aft slot, then the DQE_g advantage is lost. To compare properly the performance of the whole imaging chain (detector, anti-scatter device, x-ray spectrum, etc.), one should use NEQ as a function of spatial frequency (not just the zero frequency value). DQE is not a valid metric for that type of comparison.

References

1. R. F. Wagner, G. T. Barnes and B. S. Askins, "Effect of reduced scatter on radiographic information content and patient exposure: a quantitative demonstration," Med Phys 7, 13-8 (1980).
2. P. S. Rezentes, A. d. Almeida and G. T. Barnes, "Mammography Grid Performance," Radiology **210**, 227-232 (1999).
3. J. M. Boone, J. A. Seibert, C.-M. Tang and S. M. Lane, "Grid and Slot Scan Scatter Reduction in Mammography: Comparison by Using Monte Carlo Techniques," Radiology 222, 519–527 (2002).

4. A. Rose, "A unified approach to the performance of photographic film, television, pickup tubes, and the human eye," Journal of the Society of Motion Picture and Television Engineers 47, 9-30 (1946).
5. ICRU, *Medical Imaging - The Assessment of Image Quality. ICRU Report 54* ed. (International Commission on Radiation Units and Measurements, Bethesda, Maryland, 1996).

Acknowledgments

Thanks to John Boone for providing some of the scatter data used in this project. This work was funded in part by the NIH/NCI (R01 CA60187)

Finding CLS Using Multiresolution Oriented Local Energy Feature Detection

Veit U.B. Schenk and Michael Brady

Medical Vision Laboratory, Dept. of Engineering Science, Oxford University, Ewert House, UK-Oxford OX2 7BZ
{vubs,jmb}@robots.ox.ac.uk

Abstract. In this paper, we present a novel technique for the detection of the curvilinear structures (CLS) in a mammogram based on a multiresolution, oriented local energy analysis. Local energy enables the detection not only of linear structures; but also features of several different kinds in a unified framework. It is possible to distinguish between such feature types using the local phase. In a separate post-processing stage, the behaviour of energy over multiple scales can be used to determine a) whether a response is due to a feature or to noise and b) to estimate at each location the local width of a CLS. Orientation information computed from steerable filters is used in the same post-processing stage to distinguish between curvilinear structures and speck-like responses such as microcalcifications which, on a micro-scale, resemble CLS. By combining scale, phase and orientation information we can distinguish the CLS from non-CLS locally linear features as well as localised structures with high gradients and thus remove only the CLS whilst leaving the remaining important image information intact.

1 Introduction

Curvilinear Structures (CLS) are locally linear structures in mammograms with a well-defined local orientation that changes as the structure curves. CLS correspond physically either to milk ducts, blood vessels, Cooper's ligaments or spicules in the breast. All of these structures, with the exception of spicules, are features of normal, healthy breast tissue. On the other hand, spicules found near the boundary of a mammographic density (or mass), are highly indicative of breast cancer. As regards CAD, the CLS are high frequency structures that complicate, and often defeat, image analysis tasks such as matching (temporal, lateral, CC-MLO) and the detection of masses and microcalcifications (for example: local point operations often respond strongly to the overlap of CLS). The identification, and possibly removal, of the CLS potentially improves CAD algorithms. More importantly, it can make them more robust.

In the ideal case, the CLS appear as thin features that are brighter than the surrounding tissue. Unfortunately, this ideal is frequently not realised, for example near parenchymal regions, so that and the detection of CLS, especially in the vicinity of masses, remains an open problem, though there have been several previous attempts to compute them [1, 2, 6]. From an image processing point of view, the detection of CLS corresponds to the general problem of ridge finding, however standard ridge detection methods do not work well since CLS do not conform very well to their ridge model [1]. A major problem stems from the fact that CLS appear at different depths within the breast, that is, they appear at an unpredictable range of scales and orientations. Cerneaz and Brady's CLS detection method, for example, did not include automatic local estimation of scale.

In this paper, we use local energy to extract the CLS. Exploiting the advantages of local energy over standard gradient-based feature detectors [5], we detect, in a single framework, both the lines (ridges) that correspond to the centre of a CLS and the edges that delimit the CLS on either side. We remove the CLS between the two delimiting edges by interpolating between pixels bordering either edge. The pixels appropriate for interpolation are selected using the orientation information along the central ridge, which has, therefore, to be estimated accurately. Fortunately, this is possible without excessive computation. By using the exact edges of the CLS, we avoid interpolating between inappropriate points and thus potentially introducing artifacts.

In Sect. 2 we describe the multiresolution oriented local energy decomposition used to analyse the mammograms. Sect. 3 shows how the resulting decomposition-coefficients can be analysed and combined in order to detect curvilinear structures in the presence of noise.

2 The Decomposition

The filter banks that we use consist of filters which are polar-separable in the Fourier domain, the radial part corresponding to the local energy component, the angular part corresponding to the orientation computation. Local energy is computed using the following odd and even symmetric quadrature filters: an even-symmetric $R_e(\lambda) = \log(\frac{1}{\lambda}\cos(x)^2)$ and the corresponding odd-symmetric version R_o with a negative going lobe on the negative frequency axis. Local energy amplitude and local phase can be obtained immediately after filtering the image with these filter pairs. For the angular part $A(\phi_n)$ of our filters (at orientations $\phi_n = \pi n/N$ evenly spread at N orientations over the half-circle), we use the raised cosine $A_o(\phi_n) = \cos^3(\phi - \phi_n)$ for the odd-symmetric filter and $A_e(\phi_n) = |\cos^3(\phi - \phi_n)|$ for the even symmetric filter. Both these functions can be implemented easily as a steerable [3] quadrature filter pair. The huge advantage of using steerable filters is that the *exact* filter response can be computed at any arbitrary angle, which is important for example when using phase-angles to distinguish between features.

Decomposition of the Input Image Two filter banks are constructed, an odd symmetric one using the cross-product of R_o and A_o at $N_o = 4$ orientations, evenly spread over $\phi_{n_o} = n\pi/N_o$ and an even symmetric one using the cross-product of R_e and A_e at $N_e = 4$ orientations, evenly spread over $\phi_{n_e} = n\pi/N_e$, each at $S = 3$ scales λ_s resulting in a total of $S * (N_e + N_o) = 27$ orientated and scaled filters. The Fourier transform of the image is multiplied by each of the filters and the results inverse Fourier transformed. At each scale, the local orientation at each pixel is obtained by computing a vector sum weighted by the amplitude of the orientated filter coefficients. The corresponding filter response at the orientation is computed, or *steered* for each pixel at all scales.

3 Postprocessing

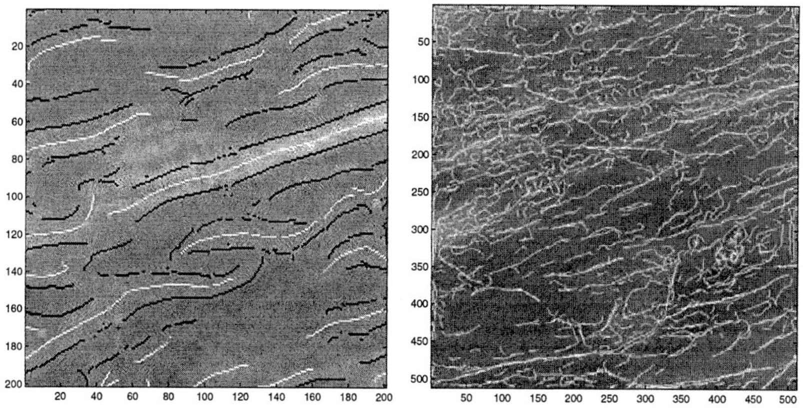

Fig. 1. Left: ridges (white) and step-edges (black) at one scale overlaid onto closeup of mammogram shown in figure 2. Right: all ridge-candidate points at all scales overlaid over mammogram

Our approach to finding CLS is to search for combinations of three parallel lines; a ridge bordered by a positive going step edge on one side and a negative going step edge on the opposite side.

The distribution of energy over scale, in particular energy amplitude and phase is noted. Only those points that correspond to a spatial energy amplitude maximum at at least one scale and have the desired phase-value (i.e. the phase is congruent [4]) over a range of scales are considered for further processing.

When using energy amplitude to detect features of interest it is important to observe that one cannot insist on spatial maxima over *all* scales at a location of a feature. Counter-examples include small features super-imposed onto large features or broad lines which will have maxima at large scales but zero amplitude response at very small scales. Such events are not infrequent in detecting CLS.

The use of phase as a distinguishing characteristic helps eliminate a wide range of unwanted high amplitude responses, often due to noise, but of course also due to other legitimate features such as valleys, roofs or ramps.

At each point x, the approximate width w_x of a (potentially underlying) CLS is determined by selecting that scale which corresponds to the coefficient with the largest magnitude. Due to the coarsely sampled nature of the individual scales, this only yields an approximation to the exact size of the feature. The value w_x is used in further a post-processing stage where the *exact* extent of a CLS is computed.

The left side of Fig. 1 shows the central ridges and the corresponding step-edges of a close-up of the upper right of the original image (figure 2 left) at one particular level. This example illustrates nicely the advantage of obtaining the exact extent of a feature using the step-edges as boundaries as opposed to using an average width for a feature at this scale: has almost the same width throughout and could thus easily be described by an 'average' width. The majority of the features vary significantly in width along their length and selecting one width only for each of these features would always only be a compromise. The right side of Fig. 1 shows all ridge candidate points at all $S = 3$ levels of the decomposition. For each point x on the central ridge, only those points are considered for further processing which have corresponding step-up *and* step-down 'neighbours' in a neighbourhood along the local orientation vector $\overline{o}_x$ at point x. The size of this neighbourhood depends on the width w_a, as described above.

The resulting set of points X_f is used to interpolate between points bordering the step-edges. Our approach is as follows: at each point $x \in X_f$ find both step edges along $\overline{o}_x$ at x. Generate two histograms H_l and H_r of small neighbourhoods just outside the step-edge. Replace the points along $\overline{o}_x$ randomly sampling from H_l and H_r where the sampling is weighted by the distance to either step-edge: the closer to one step-edge, the higher the probability of sampling from 'its' H_x. The result of applying this process to the left image in figure 2 is shown at the right of figure 2.

4 Discussion

We have presented a novel local-energy based method which effectively detects and removes CLS in mammograms. The advantages of local energy methods using steerable filters in the context of CLS detection are a) the behaviour of energy over scale which can be used to distinguish features from noise, b) the use of phase which can be used to distinguish different types of features and which is *congruent* over scale the location of features and c) the use of accurate orientation information to facilitate neighbourhood post-processing and help distinguish between locally linear features (CLS) and other features which at small scales resemble CLS.

The scale-adaptive local energy algorithm for detecting CLS outlined in this paper is described in more detail in [5] and in a forthcoming article, in which we present a ROC analysis demonstrating the superiority of this method to several previously published algorithms for detecting CLS.

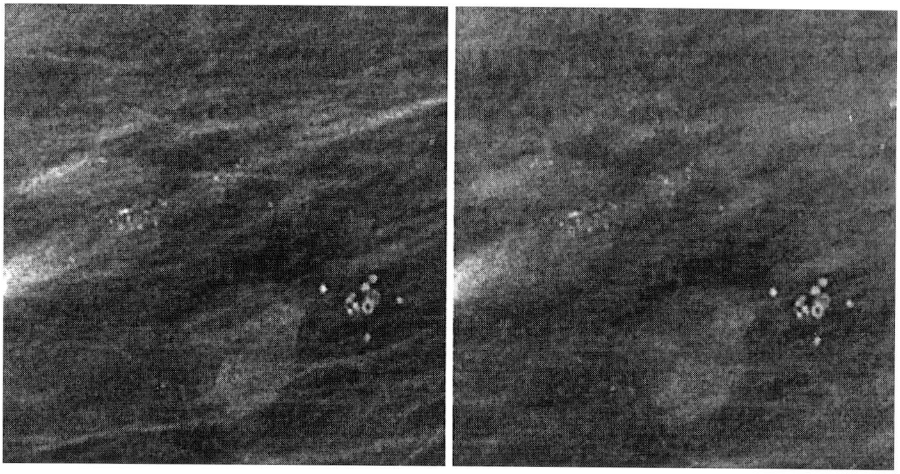

Fig. 2. Left: original mammogram (a 512x512px closeup of a large mammogram). Right: same image after removing CLS. Note that the 3 clusters of calcifications and the large mass near the bottom-centre remain largely unaffected

Acknowledgements

We thank Professor Kimmo Kaski and colleagues of the Helsinki University of Technology for insightful discussions and for providing financial support for this project.

References

1. N. Cerneaz and M. Brady. Finding curvilinear structures in mammograms. In Nicholas Ayache, editor, *Computer Vision, Virtual Reality and Robotics in Medicine*, Lecture Notes in Computer Science. Springer-Verlag, April 1995.
2. C.J. Evans, K. Yates, and Michael Brady. Statistical characterisation of normal curvilinear structures in mammograms. In *Proc. Sixth Digital Image Computing Techniques and Applications DICTA*, Melbourne, Australia, 2002.
3. William T. Freeman and Edward H. Adelson. The design and use of steerable filters. *IEEE Transactions on Pattern Analysis and Machine Intelligence*, 13(9):891–906, September 1991.
4. P. Kovesi. *Invariant measures of image features from phase information.* PhD thesis, University of Western Australia, May 1996.
5. Veit U.B. Schenk. *Visual Identification of Fine Surface Incisions.* PhD thesis, University of Oxford, March 2002.
6. R. Zwiggelaar, T.C. Parr, and C.J. Taylor. Finding orientated line patterns in digital mammographic images. In *Proc. 7th British Machine Vision Conf., Edinburgh*, pages 715–724, Edinburgh, UK, September 1996.

Characterization of an FFDM unit based on a-Se direct conversion detector

Achille Albanese[1], Alessandro Bevilacqua[2], Renato Campanini[3], Emiro Iampieri[3], Nico Lanconelli[3], Massimo Rossi[3], Davide Romani[3], Valerio Salomoni[3] and Paolo Vignoli[1]

1. IMS, Via Sagittario 5, 40044 Bologna, Italy
2. DEIS, University of Bologna, Viale Risorgimento 2, 40136 Bologna, Italy
3. Physics Department, University of Bologna, Viale Berti-Pichat 6/2, 40127 Bologna, Italy
nico.lanconelli@bo.infn.it

Abstract. The aim of this paper is to investigate the properties of a clinical FFDM unit (Giotto - Image MD, IMS Italy). The digital detector consists of a flat panel using the amorphous selenium technology (ANRAD Corporation, Canada). The active area of the imager is 17.4 cm × 23.9 cm (2048×2816 pixels) with a pixel pitch of 85 μm. The direct conversion of X-rays into charge provides excellent imaging performance. In this work we present an objective and complete characterization of such system: detector response, MTF, NPS and DQE calculation will be presented. MTF and DQE at Nyquist frequency (5.88 lp/mm) are equal to 38% and 15%, respectively. The detector linearity is very good under the typical mammographic tested exposure conditions.

Introduction

In the last years advancements have been achieved in digital mammography, by getting a significant improvement in image quality. Several approaches to digital image acquisition have been considered: the most promising are the ones based on amorphous Silicon or amorphous Selenium flat panel detectors [1,2]. Here the photoconductor layer is deposited directly onto a TFT substrate. The electric charges are then collected, amplified, digitized and transferred through a specific electronic chain. In particular, detectors based on a direct-conversion technology seem to give a better performance, especially at high-spatial frequency; the charges are drawn to the surfaces by an applied electric field, without significant image blurring.

In this paper we examine the physical characteristics of a clinical FFDM unit (Giotto - Image MD, IMS Italy). This system is based on a a-Se flat panel digital detector (ANRAD Corporation, Canada): the detector is characterized by a compact size and rapid image readout. The imager is presently undergoing clinical evaluation at the “Maggiore” Hospital in Bologna, Italy. To assess the image quality of the apparatus, its spatial resolution and noise properties are evaluated, by calculating objective functions like as Modulation Transfer Function (MTF), Noise Power Spectra (NPS) and Detective Quantum Efficiency (DQE).

Methods

The X-ray source consists of a Mo-Mo X-ray tube (30 μm Mo filtered) with a Source to Detector Distance equal to 65 cm. No anti-scatter grid and a fixed tube voltage equal to 28 kVp are utilized, for all the measurements. For the achievement of the detector response curve, a 2 cm plexiglas filter is placed in X-ray beam path. The exposure level is then changed, by varying the exposure time; to evaluate the digital signal value, an average of the pixel values included in selected Region Of Interest (ROI) is calculated. The exposure is measured with a calibrated mammographic ionization chamber (PMX-III - RTI).

Pre-sampling MTF is measured by using the slit technique: an oversampled LSF is obtained by a 10 μm tantalum slit [3]. The slit is placed at an angle of about 3°, both in horizontal and vertical directions; 28 kVp, 10 mAs images are then acquired. An exponential fitting of the oversampled Line Spread Function (LSF) is performed, in order to reduce the contribution of the noise on the tails. By Fourier transforming each oversampled LSF, various MTFs are obtained for each image (one MTF for any LSF); the final MTF is then calculated as the average of the single MTFs.

NPS is calculated from flat field images at different exposure levels, with a 4 cm plexiglas filter attached to the generator head. Five images are obtained for each exposure level; and for each image a 256×256 pixels ROI is extracted, Fourier transformed and averaged, for getting the 2D NPS. No low frequency noise reduction algorithm is applied. Four lines above and below the principal axis are selected from the 2D spectrum, for the achievement of the 1D NPS, useful for DQE calculation. The 1D NPS is then normalized for the squared mean signal value of the ROI.

For the determination of the X-ray photon fluence, HVL measurements are made with 4 cm plexiglas filter. From tabulated data [4] we calculate the photon fluence at the considered X-ray average energy, and then the number of photons per unit area at the measured exposure is computed.

The DQE is then calculated as:

$$DQE(f) = \frac{MTF^2(f)}{NPS(f,q)\cdot q} \quad (1)$$

where q is the number of photons per unit area.

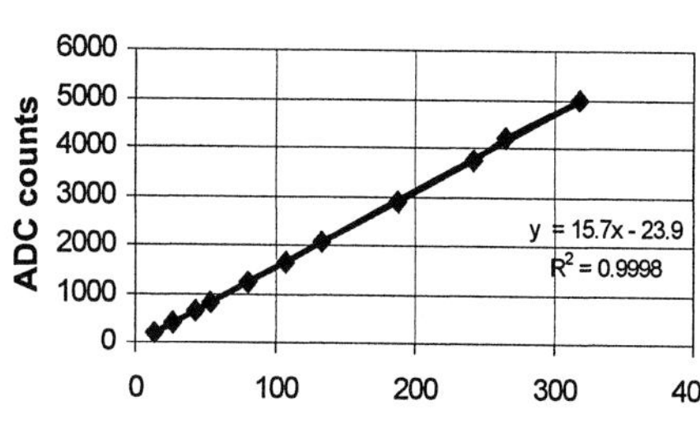

Fig. 1. Detector response.

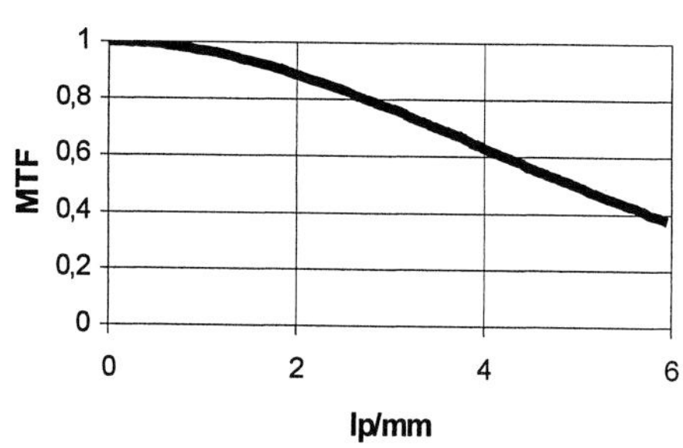

Fig. 2. Pre-sampling MTF.

Results

In figure 1 the detector response is illustrated: it is worth noting that the system maintains its linearity over the entire range of the considered exposures. In figure 2 the pre-sampling MTF is shown: the spatial resolution of the detector is extremely high, even in case of high spatial frequency (at 5.88 lp/mm the MTF is almost equal to 40%). The horizontal and vertical MTFs are nearly identical. In figure 3 there is depicted the 1D NPS: it is possible to note that the noise is almost frequency independent. Finally, in figure 4 the DQE of the system is presented, for three different exposure levels: its value is particularly high, especially for two of the three considered exposures. The DQE(0) is almost equal to 52%, whereas at Nyquist limit its value is about 15%. For the lower exposure level the DQE value is worse; further investigations have to be done, in order to find out if the quantum noise limited condition is not valid here anymore, or if other effects contribute to the reduction of DQE at lower exposures.

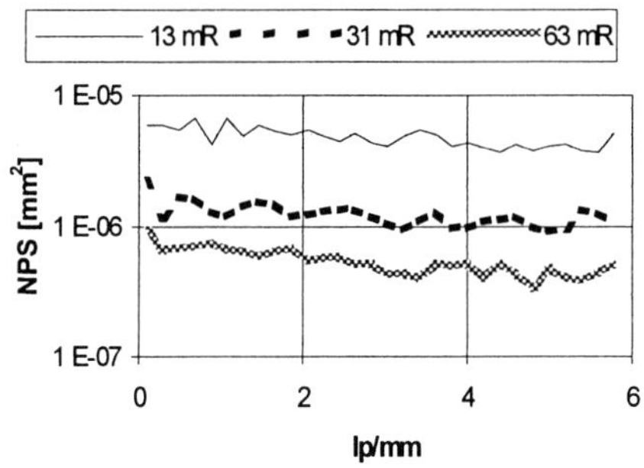

Fig. 3. NPS at different exposures.

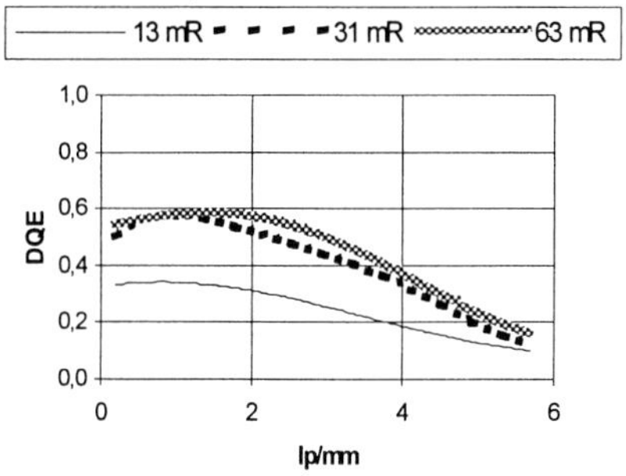

Fig. 4. DQE at different exposures.

References

1. Vedantham, S., Karellas, A., Suryanarayanan, S., Albagli, D., Han, S., Tkaczyk, E. J., Landberg, C. E., Opsahl-Ong, B., Levis, I., D'Orsi, C. J., Hendrick, R. E.: "Full breast digital mammography with an amorphous silicon-based flat panel detector: physical characteristics of a clinical prototype", Med. Phys. 27 (3), 2000, 558-567
2. Debrie, A., Caron, M., Savard, S., Hansroul, M., Wong, K., Loustauneau, V., Shukri, Z., Martin, J.P.: "Quantitative analysis and qualitative performance of flat-panel detector for digital mammography", in Digital Mammography, Proceedings of 5th IWDM, Med. Phys. Pub., 2000, 25-31
3. Fujita, H., Tsai, D., Itoh, T., Doi, K., Morishita, J., Ueda, K., Ohtsusuka, A.: "A simple method for determining the modulation transfer function in digital radiography", IEEE Trans. Med. Imaging, 11 (2), 1992, 34-39
4. Johns, H. E., Cunningham, R. J.: "The Physics of radiology", (Thomas, Springfield, IL), 1983

Comparison of Noise Characteristics between CR System and Full -Field Digital Mammography System

Kobayashi H , Tanikoshi M , Uchiyama N , Suzuki T , Kumazaki T

Department of Radiology ,
Nippon Medical School , 1-1-5 Sendagi, Bunkyo-ku Tokyo, Japan
koba@nms.ac.jp

Abstract. We compared noise characteristics between CR system and full field digital mammography (FFDM) system in raw data to evaluate image quality performances. CR system was performed with a unit (Senographe DMR; GE Medical Systems,Milwaukee, Wis) and a CR (FCR5000MA Plus; FUJI PHOTO FILM,Tokyo). FCR system was able to conduct dual light collection and a pixel density was 20pixels/mm(50μm pixels). FFDM system was performed with a unit (Senographe2000D; GE Medical Systems,Milwaukee, Wis). We also measured NPS values changing the exposure level to evaluate the relationships between the exposure dose and the noise with PMMA phantom. Each system indicated improvement of NPS value in accordance with increase of exposure level.

1. Introduction

The current gold standard for mammography in Japan is an analog system using screen films. However, since the introduction of full-field digital mammography (FFDM) in November 2000, digital mammography has come to be used with increasing frequency. A new CR system with a pixel size of 50 μm (FCR5000MA) has been developed and applied clinically. To ascertain the image quality provided by these two digital mammography systems, we investigated the noise characteristics of images obtained by these two systems at the detector level before subjecting these images to image processing.

2. Materials and Methods

2.1 Measurement item

- o Noise character at the change of dose level of Senographe2000D.
- o Noise character at the change of dose level of FCR5000MA.
- o Noise characteristic comparison of two digital mammography systems.

2.2 Noise measurement codition

Mammography was performed under the following conditions: Mo target/Mo filter, 28 kVp, grid (-), and acrylic filter (40 mm) under the radiation source. The dose level (2.82~74.07mR) was adjusted by varying mAs. In each noise characteristic assessment, a Wiener spectrum was calculated based on digital values, eliminating image processing effects and output printer characteristics. To allow comparison of the two digital systems, the resulting spectrum was converted by the fluctuation level of relative X-ray intensity.

3. Results

Figure 1 shows the raw data obtained using the Senographe2000D by varying the dose level from 3 to 74 mR. At dose levels between 8 and 74 mR, the changes were dictated by quantum noise. Figure 2 shows that the noise characteristics for the FCR5000MA were comparable. In a comparison of the noise characteristics of the two systems at the same incident dose, the Wiener spectrum value of the two systems crossed at frequencies of 1-1.5 cycles/mm. While the noise characteristics of the Senographe2000D were superior at frequencies below 1-1.5 cycles/mm, the noise characteristics of FCR5000MA were superior at higher frequencies. The results were the same at different dose levels.

4. Discussion

Full-field digital mammography systems incorporate a CsI scintillator. They are flat-panel detector systems employing the indirect conversion method. The new CR system is a dual-screen scanning system using an imaging plate having a picture element of 20 pix/mm (50 μm element). We initially anticipated that the noise characteristics of the FCR5000MA, which has smaller pixel size, would be inferior to those of the Senographe 2000D. But the noise characteristics for the Senographe2000D were superior at lower frequencies, while those for the FCR5000MA were superior at higher frequencies. Nonetheless, in clinical settings, the images captured by these systems are processed by their own image processing programs. Thus, these differences do not directly affect the ability of these systems to identify tumors and micro-calcification lesions.

5. Acknowledgements

We would like to express our deepest gratitude to Makoto Iriuchijima at GE Yokogawa Medical Systems and Hiroaki Yasuda, Satoshi Arakawa, and Shigeru Saotome at Fuji Photo Film for their invaluable assistance in the undertaking of this present study.

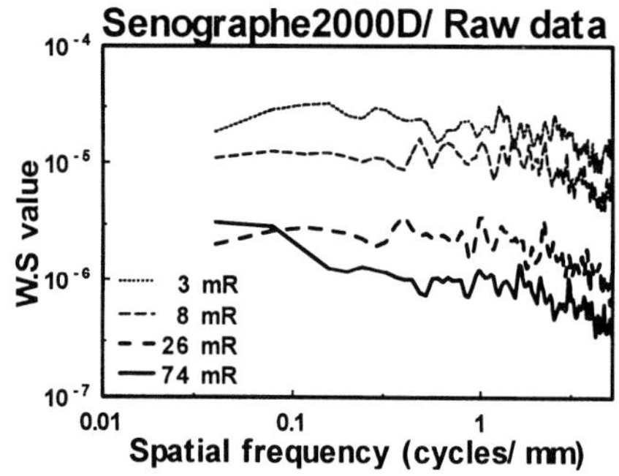

Fig. 1. Digital W.S illustrating the effects of various incident exposure at Senographe2000D

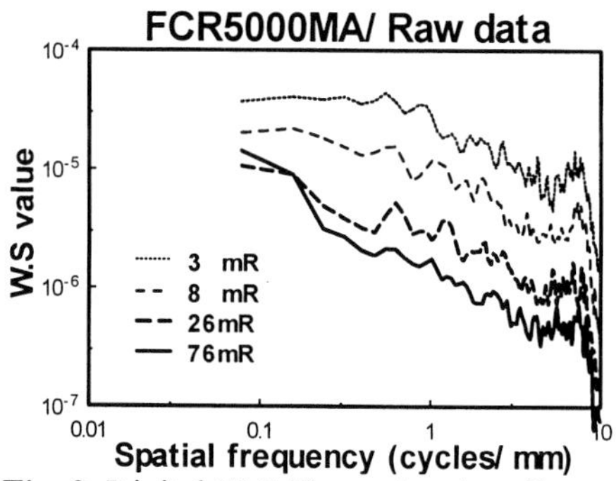

Fig. 2. Digital W.S illustrating the effects of various incident exposure at FCR5000MA.

Physical factors affecting the detection of calcifications in digital mammography

Chris C. Shaw, Chao-Jen Lai, Xinming Liu, S. Cheenu Kappadath, Gary J. Whitman

Department of Imaging Physics, University of Texas M. D. Anderson Cancer Center, Houston, Texas 77030, USA
cshaw@di.mdacc.tmc.edu

Abstract. We are conducting a perception study to investigate the effects of detector design, magnification, and calcification size on the detection of calcifications in uniform as well as structured background. Calcium carbonate grains of various sizes were used to simulate calcifications. Three detectors were studied: a 100 μm aSi:H/CsI(Tl) flat-panel system, a 30 μm CCD based system and an analog screen/film combination. The preliminary results show that the flat-panel system with a 100 μm pixel size outperformed a CCD based system with a 30 μm pixel size and an analog screen-film system. However, in studies with an anthropomorphic phantom as the background, the flat-panel system was outperformed by the other two systems. The presence of tissue structure background substantially reduced the calcification detectability. The use of geometric magnification generally improved the detectability with the exception of smallest and largest calcifications.

1. Introduction

Early detection of breast cancer may improve the mortality rate in cancer treatment. Despite advances in new modalities, x-ray mammography continues to be the main tool for screening and early detection of breast cancer. The two major tasks in screening mammography are the detection and classification of soft tissue masses and microcalcification clusters with the latter often being an important indication of breast cancer in the early stage.

Detection of a microcalcification refers to the recognition of the presence of the microcalcification. In reality, a cancer lesion is often indicated by a cluster of calcifications rather than a single calcification. Both the number and spatial distribution of the calcifications provide important information as to whether they indicate a malignant or benign lesion. Small calcifications can merge together to form a larger calcification grain which may be easy to detect but requires a closer look of the detailed structure for classification.

Visualization of the shape of individual or merged calcifications and their spatial distribution is fundamentally different from detection. However, the task of visualizing and resolving small details in a large calcification structure may be considered as similar to the task of detecting a small calcification.

Detection of microcalcifications is dictated by several factors: contrast, noise, contrast-to-noise ratio, magnification, detector design and tissue structure background. In this paper, we present preliminary results from a perception study to illustrate and discuss the effects of these factors.

2. Contrast-to-noise: detection in uniform background

The contrast of a calcification in the x-ray intensity distribution at the input of the detector is determined by three factors: (1) attenuation of the calcification, (2) blurring of the signal profile through magnification and focal spot blurring, (3) degradation of the overall contrast by the presence of scattered radiation. The contrast of calcifications is further degraded when the x-rays are absorbed and converted into image signals in the detector. Degradation in this process is often characterized by the modulation transfer function (MTF).

Fluctuation of image signals originates first from the detection of x-rays. However, the x-rays detected could be primary, scatter or from focal spot blurring. Despite the origin, the fluctuation follows the Poisson statistics and the noise variance is equal to the mean number of x-rays detected. Additional noises may be introduced as the absorbed x-rays are converted into image signals in the detector. The importance of these secondary noises varies with the x-ray intensity or signal size. If the x-ray noise is the dominating source, the percentage noise or noise ratio is inversely proportional to the square root of the number of x-rays detected. Thus, a more absorbing detector tends to offer lower noise level. Lower system noise (secondary quantum, electronic, etc.) in detector design also helps lower the overall noise level.

The detection of calcifications in a uniform background is mainly determined by whether the contrast of the object is sufficient to overcome the fluctuation of the signals in the object and the background. This phenomenon was first described by the Rose criteria which states that the contrast-to-noise ratio must be above a certain threshold value for an object to be detected over uniform background. The threshold value depends on each individual observer and has been studied in many perception experiments. These experiments have been recently reviewed and indicated that a reasonable estimated threshold values of around 3 [1]. It should be noted that the contrast should be measured and averaged for the entire object and the noise should be measured as that for the average contrast. If the object consists of N pixels, the noise level should be lower than the pixel noise level by a factor of $N^{1/2}$. Thus, a larger object tend to be easier to detect as the fluctuation of the average object signal would be lower due to the larger number of pixels used to represent the object.

3 Breast tissue: detection in structured background

In a mammogram, calcifications generally overlap with tissue structure patterns. These patterns are another source for noise and can affect the detection of the calcifications. However, tissue structures differ from random noise in that they have specific shapes or patterns. These patterns could affect the detection of calcifications in two ways. First of all, if these patterns have similar shape and dimensions as the calcifications, they could obscure the detection of the calcifications. However, the calcifications generally possess such specific shape and dimensions that it would hard to mistake tissue structure patterns for calcifications. Secondly, the tissue structures could generate a background with spatial varying brightness. If the calcifications are located in the region of drastic brightness changes, they can be hard to detect even with adequate contrast-to-noise ratios. This effect is probably a more serious one. In either case, a sharp rendition of the calcification helps distinguish it from the generally less sharp tissue structures.

4. Perception experiment

We are conducting a perception study to investigate the effects of the detector design, calcification size and magnification on detection of microcalcifications in uniform and breast tissue structure backgrounds.

Calcium carbonate grains of various sizes (90-355 µm) were used to simulate microcalcifications. A 5 cm thick slab of 50% adipose/50% glandular simulated breast tissue material was used to provide uniform background. An anthropomorphic breast phantom was used to provide tissue structure background. Ten simulated calcifications from various size groups were imaged with three different mammographic imaging systems: a 100 µm aSi:H/CsI(Tl) flat-panel (FP) (Senographe 2000, GE Medical Systems, Milwaukee, WI)[2], a 30 µm CCD based system (Senovision, GE Medical Systems, Milwaukee, WI)[3] and an analog screen/film (SF) combination (MinR 2000, Eastman Kodak Company, Rochester, NY). (SF). All images were acquired at 28 kVp and 100 mAs Mo-Rh target/filter combination. All digital images were printed onto 8"x10" hardcopies for review. Hardcopy images from each modality were randomized for review by mammographer readers. A 5-scale confidence rating score was given for each calcification in the image.

Preliminary results indicate that with uniform background the FP system performed the best while the SF system did slightly better than the CCD system. With magnification, all detection tasks were improved except for the smallest and largest one or two sizes. In particular, detection in SF and CCD images was significantly improved as compared to the FP system. As the result, the performance difference among the three systems decreased. With tissue structure background, the performance of the FP system was equal or slightly worse than the SF and CCD systems. Improvement with magnification was not as clearly indicated as with the uniform background.

References

1. Barten, P. G. J.: *Contrast Sensitivity of the Human Eye and its Effect on Image Quality*, SPIE Optical Engineering Press, Bellingham, WA (1999).
2 Vedantham, S., Karellas, A., Syryanarayanan, S., et al.: Full breast digital mammography with an amorphous silicon-based flat panel detector : Physicalcharacteristics of a clinical prototype. Med Phys 27(3) (2000) 558-567
3. Vedantham, S., Karellas, A., Syryanarayanan, S., et al.: Mammographic imaging with a small format CCD-based digital cassette : Physical characterization of a clinical system. Med Phys 27(8) (2000) 1832-1840

Image Quality

A first experience of quality control in full field digital mammography

G. Gennaro(1) P. Baldelli(2), C. di Maggio(1), A. Taibi(2), and M. Gambaccini(2)

(1) Department of Oncological Sciences, Padua University, via Gattamelata 64, 35128 Padua - Italy
(2) Department of Physics, Ferrara University, Ferrara - Italy
gisella.gennaro@pd.infn.it

Abstract. A simple phantom for periodic quality control measurement on full field digital mammography systems has been developed. It was employed with three different digital mammography units, by collecting data on detector linearity and uniformity, image contrast and spatial resolution, reproducibility of detector and automatic exposure control device. Results show the phantom is able to give information about some detector characteristics and can detect problems related to the stability of the automatic exposure control system. It is also fast and easy to use, as required in a quality assurance program.

1. Introduction

Digital mammography has revealed that a quality assurance program is still necessary in order to maintain high image quality. Digital imaging systems are more complicated with respect to screen/film systems, mainly due to the great amount of feedback processes which control both the acquisition system and the final output. It becomes difficult to isolate the different parts of the chain whose transfer functions produce the clinical image. In fact, as frequently cited as digital mammography benefit, i.e. acquisition, displaying and archiving are now separated and consequently have to be separately optimized [1, 2, 3].

The digital image availability can permit the automatic calculation of significant parameters such as MTF, NPS and DQE, commonly used for detector characterization [4, 5]. Also the exposure conditions should be revised to take into account the new detector preferences in terms of X-ray spectra, that quite differ from the screen/film behaviour [6].

A simple phantom has been proposed to define the physical quantities that are more relevant in digital mammography images.

2. Materials and Methods

A phantom has been assembled to measure detector linearity, uniformity, image contrast and spatial resolution and to check the stability of both the detector and the automatic exposure control system. The phantom material is PMMA, 45 mm thick; it is divided into three slabs, two of 20 mm and a third of 5 mm, respectively. The thinner slab is marked so that six ROIs are highlighted; particularly, the ROI 5, central and close to the chest wall, is considered the reference ROI. Few details are superimposed: two copper grids for the resolution measurement and three PMMA disks, 3 mm thick, for the contrast ones. A phantom image is shown in figure 1.

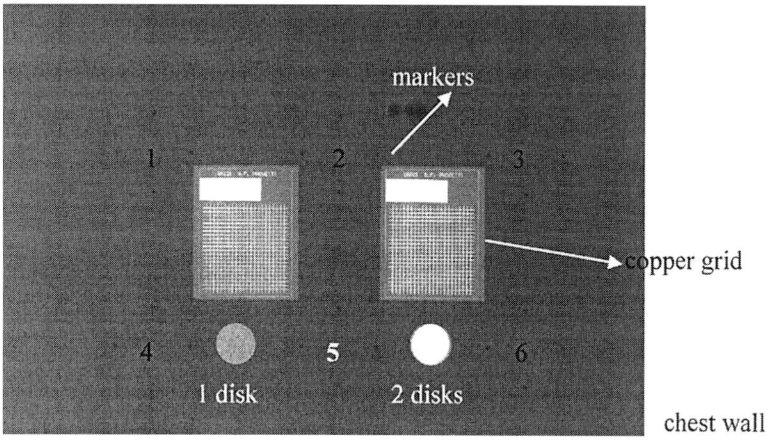

Fig. 1. Phantom image produced by a GE Senographe 2000 D digital unit.

Data provided by three different GE Senographe 2000 D digital mammography units, located in three Italian sites (named FFDM 1, FFDM 2 and FFDM 3, respectively), have been collected and analyzed. The principal results are reported in the following.

The detector linearity was checked by measuring the average gray level of the reference ROI corresponding to five different mAs values (10, 25, 50, 100 and 140 mAs), in two different settings: Mo/Mo – 28 kV and Rh/Rh – 30 kV. The entrance exposure has been measured by a calibrated ionization chamber.

The detector uniformity and contrast have been evaluated from three repeated images obtained by exposing the phantom in automatic/standard mode (AOP/STD) and in manual mode with Mo/Mo – 28 kV – 50 mAs.

The daily measurement in the same conditions permitted us to control the stability of both the detector and automatic exposure control system.

A spatial resolution evaluation is also obtainable from sampling aperture measurements based, for instance, on the grid profile analysis. The detector sampling aperture is related to the MTF according to the formula given in ref. [7]. It can be determined from the contrast reduction factor calculated by measuring the image contrast of an object with known contrast and proper size.

3. Results and conclusions

The evaluated equipment give a linear response over the considered dose range with a high correlation degree, for both the Mo/Mo and Rh/Rh combinations. In figure 2 the linearity measure is shown for the Rh/Rh – 30 kVp setting.

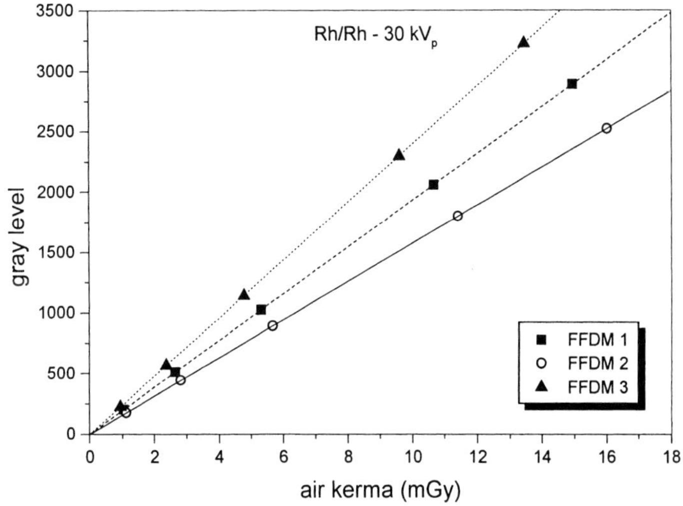

Fig. 2. Gray level response as a function of the air kerma for the evaluated GE Senographe 2000D mammography units (Rh/Rh - 30 kVp).

The detector uniformity is good, mainly due to the flat-field correction commonly applied to flat panel detectors. The signal variations measured in the six ROIs never exceed 5% for both the automatic and the manual exposure modes.

Daily measurements allowed us to check the stability of both detector and automatic exposure control device. The upper plot represented in figure 3 proves that the output stability is slightly fluctuating when the automatic exposure mode is employed, according to the tolerances on the kVp and mAs choice. The lower curve, obtained in manual mode (Mo/Mo – 28 kV – 50 mAs) reveals a good detector stability.

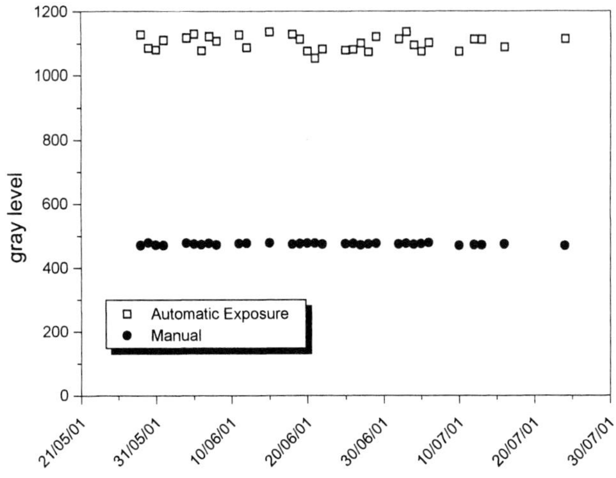

Fig. 3. Lower: detector reproducibility, <0.6%; Upper: reproducibility of the automatic exposure control system, ≈ 2%.

The proposed phantom, in spite of its simplicity, is useful to monitor some quality control parameters in full field digital mammography.

Work is in progress to improve the sampling aperture pattern and to introduce further details able to quantify the digital image quality in a similar way to which normally employed by the QC phantoms applied to screen/film mammography.

References

1. M. J. Yaffe and J. A. Rowlands, "X-ray detectors for digital radiography", *Phys.Med.Biol.* **42**, 1-39, 1997.
2. M. J. Yaffe, "Digital Mammography", *RSNA Categorical Course in Breast Imaging 1999*, 229-238.
3. S. Muller, " Full-Field Digital Mammography designed as a complete system", *Eur.J.Radiol.* **31** (1), 25-34, 1999.
4. S. Vedantham, A. Karellas, S. Suryanarayanan, D. Albagli., S. Han, E. Tkaczyk, C. Landberg, P. Granfors, I. Levis, C. D'Orsi, and E. Hendrick, "Full breast digital mammography with an amorphous silicon-based flat panel detector: Physical characteristics of a clinical prototype". *Med.Phys.* **27** (3), 558-567, 2000.
5. S. Z. Shen, G. Mawdsley, and M. Yaffe, "Automation of quality assurance of digital mammography", *Proceedings of IWDM 2000*, 656-665, Toronto.
6. V. Venkatakrishnan, M. Yavuz, L. Niklason, B. Opsahl-Ong, S. Han, C. Landberg, R. Nevin, L. Hamberg, and D. Kopans, "Experimental and theoretical spectral optimization for digital mammography", *Proceedings of SPIE 1999, Phys.Med.Imag.* **3659**, 142-149.
7. R.F. Wagner, "Toward a unified view of radiological imaging systems. Part II: noisy images", *Med.Phys.* **4**, 279-296, 1977.

Acceptance Testing of Digital Mammography Units for the ACRIN/DMIST Study

Aili K. Bloomquist, Sam Zhongmin Shen, Gordon Mawdsley, Stewart Bright and Martin Yaffe

Sunnybrook and Women's College Health Sciences Centre, 2075 Bayview Avenue, Toronto, ON, Canada
aili.bloomquist@swchsc.on.ca

Abstract. The Digital Mammography Imaging Screening Trial (DMIST) is being conducted by the American College of Radiology Imaging Network (ACRIN) to compare the accuracy of digital versus screen-film mammography in a screening population. 49,500 women are being imaged by both digital and screen-film mammograms at 18 clinical sites. Our group is supervising the quality control program and acceptance testing for 19 digital systems being used in the DMIST trial. Tests were designed to evaluate the detectors from 4 manufacturers. A summary of acceptance tests results will be presented and discussed, including exposure technique factors, estimates of mean glandular dose, modulation transfer function (MTF) and 2-D noise power spectra (NPS).

1. Introduction

Digital mammography has progressed significantly over the past few years, to the point where it is feasible to carry out a large screening study to evaluate the efficacy of the technology. To this end, the American College of Radiology Imaging Network (ACRIN) is conducting the Digital Mammography Imaging Screening Trial (DMIST), which aims to compare digital and screen-film technology for screening on 49,500 women. These women are being imaged on 19 digital mammography units across North America [1]. The quality control program for this study is being supervised by the X-Ray Imaging Research group at Sunnybrook and Women's College Health Sciences Centre. Initial training in the QC protocol and initial acceptance testing of the digital mammography units was performed at each site. Some of the results of the acceptance testing are discussed here.

The DMIST study uses five different system designs from four manufacturers. The key characteristics of the different systems are summarized in Table 1. It should be noted that only a small number of units from each system (5 or less) were tested. As such the results do not necessarily reflect the typical performance of each system type, particularly as manufacturers periodically make design modifications and software changes to their systems.

Table 1. Digital Mammography Units evaluated for DMIST

System	Del Size (μm)	Matrix Size	Technology	Anode/ Filter	Grid	# of Units
A	50	4096x 5625	phosphor coupled by fiber-optics to CCD, slot-scan geometry	W /Al	No	5
B	50	4728x 5928	dual side read computed radiography used with conventional unit	Mo,W/ Mo, Rh	Yes	5
C	100	1914x 2294	cesium iodide on amorphous silicon	Mo, Rh/ Mo, Rh	Yes	5
D	40	4800x 6400	phosphor coupled by fiber-optics to tiled CCDs	Mo/ Mo,Rh	Yes	3
E	70	3328x 4096	amorphous selenium	Mo/ Mo, Rh	Yes	1

2. Methods

2.1 Entrance Exposure and Mean Glandular Dose

The entrance exposures were evaluated for properly exposed images of 2,4, 6 and 8 centimeters of BR12 or acrylic material (PMMA).

Entrance exposures were estimated from the exposure and the tube output measurements (mR/mAs) made during the physics survey. Where it was available, the automatic exposure control was allowed to select the exposure parameters, otherwise the posted technique chart was followed. Based on the measured half-value layer of the system at the selected kV, the entrance exposure (mR) for 4 cm of lucite (equivalent to 4.2 cm 50-50) was converted to mean glandular dose (mGy) using published conversion factors or those supplied by the manufacturer [2][3][4].

2.2 Modulation Transfer Function (MTF)

For each unit, images of slanted edges were obtained in all four directions with a test tool positioned 4.5 cm above the table top. Each image was taken at a clinically relevant kV, with the mAs chosen to ensure that no pixels within the image of the tool were saturated or without signal. A custom software program was run on each image to calculate the MTF following the method outlined by Fujita et al [5][6]. Where possible, the MTF was calculated on the raw (unprocessed, pixel values linear with x-rays detected) images. The MTFs for each direction were then averaged together.

Since a logarithmic transform and rescaling is applied to the CR images, an antilog transform had to be applied to the images from system B before the MTF could be calculated. The manufacturer supplied the transform used, which takes into account the sensitivity number of the original image.

2.3 Noise Power Spectrum

The noise power spectrum for each system was calculated using four images of a 4 cm uniform block of PMMA imaged at a clinically relevant technique following the algorithm described by Dainty and Shaw[7] and then normalized by the square of the average pixel value within the calculation region and an estimated fluence based on entrance exposure, kV and mA settings. The calculations were performed on "raw" image data. For system B, the image data were transformed by an antilog function to return the data to a state where ADU values scale linearly with x-rays detected.

3 Results and Discussion

3.1 Entrance Exposure and Mean Glandular Dose

The average of the mean glandular dose estimates for each system type and all systems as a whole are given in the table below:

Table 2. Mean Glandular Dose for the 4.2 cm average breast

System	Entrance Exposure in R	Range in R	MGD in mGy	Range in mGy
A	0.51	0.41-0.64	1.2	1-1.5
B	1.3	0.98-1.6	2.2	1.8-2.6
C	0.84	0.64-0.88	1.4	1.1-1.7
D	1.3	0.9-1.6	2.0	1.7-2.6
E	1.4		2.1	
All	*0.95*	*0.41-1.6*	*1.7*	*1-2.6*

Table 3. Entrance Exposures for 2, 4, 6 and 8 cm in R

	2 cm		4 cm		6 cm		8 cm	
System	Avg	Range	Avg	Range	Avg	Range	Avg	Range
A	0.24	0.20-0.30	0.48	0.40-0.59	0.76	0.64-0.86	1.1	0.89-1.3
B	0.27	0.18-0.49	0.99	0.69-1.3	2.1	1.6-2.5	3.5	1.9-4.4
C	0.22	0.16-0.28	0.76	0.57-1.3	0.91	0.69-1.3	2.5	1.7-3.7
D	0.34	0.33-0.40	1.3	0.86-1.8	3.40	1.5-5.3	5.4	3.6-7.5
E	0.35		1.5		1.8		3.1	
All	*0.26*	*0.16-0.49*	*0.66*	*0.40-1.8*	*1.1*	*0.64-5.3*	*2.1*	*0.89-7.5*

The mean glandular dose for system A is the lowest because it does not use a grid and operates with a harder spectrum (higher kV, tungsten target and aluminum filter). There is a broad range in exposures and doses among the other systems because techniques are not standardized. The higher entrance exposures and doses measured on systems B, D and E may be the result of sub-optimal technique factors.

3.2 Modulation Transfer Function

The average MTFs for each system are plotted in Figure 1.

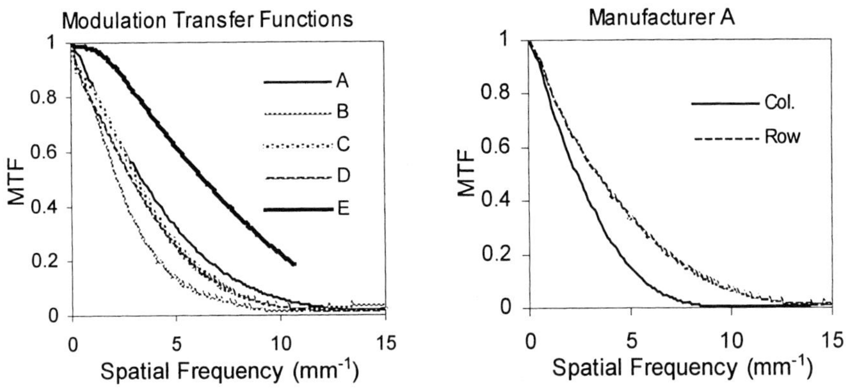

Fig. 1. Modulation Transfer Functions for the different systems, Sample MTF for a system from Manufacturer A

System A occasionally demonstrated a difference between the North-South (row) and East-West (column) directions, as shown in Figure 2, due to poor synchronization between the motion of the detector (scan speed) and the data acquisition (time domain integration). This results in a drop in the MTF for the east and west edges (lower resolution in the column direction).

The MTFs of Systems A and B, both 50 μm systems, drop quite rapidly, comparable to System C, a 100 μm system. This shows that the MTF is limited by factors other than the del size. Clinically, System B employs edge enhancement and other image processing algorithms that can improve the conspicuity of small details. These algorithms were not applied to the images of the MTF tool.

The MTF of System D also drops quite rapidly, considering it is a 40 μm system. The de-warping algorithm applied to correct for distortions introduced by the fiber-optic tapers probably reduces the effective resolution of the system. Note that the test tool edges cross the interfaces between the tiled detectors. A superior MTF could be calculated by ensuring the slanted edge went through the middle of a single detector, minimizing distortion. However, this does not reflect how the system is used clinically –the breast covers multiple detectors.

The highest MTF was seen for System E, which is a direct conversion detector. Without light scattering in the phosphor, and limited blurring due to charge diffusion, direct conversion systems are able to achieve very high resolution, limited primarily by the del aperture.

3.3 Noise Power Spectrum

Typical noise power spectra in the transverse (orthogonal to grid lines) direction for each manufacturer are plotted below.

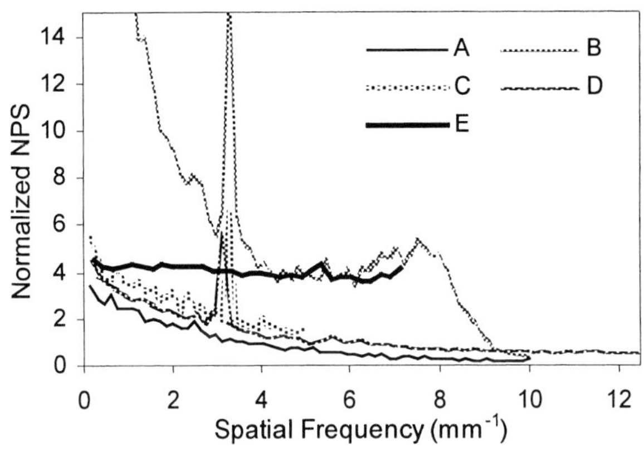

Fig. 2. System Noise Power Spectra

The spike at approximately 3 mm^{-1} visible on systems B, C and D is due to the grid. Elevated low frequency noise may be due to low frequency non-uniformities such as heel effect, beam hardening and path-length differences not fully corrected by flat fielding. Because the fluence values used to normalize the spectra are estimates, the relative magnitudes of the spectra are inaccurate.

References

1. Pisano, E., Hendrick, R. E., Masood, S., Gatsonis, C.: American College of Radiology Imaging Network - ACRIN 6652 - Digital vs. Screen-Film Mammography, ACRIN (2001)
2. Dance, D. R., Skinner, C. L., Young, K. C., Beckett, J. R., Kotre, C. J.: Additional factors for the estimation of mean glandular breast dose using the UK mammography dosimetry protocol. Phys. Med. Biol. 45 (2000) 3225-3240
3. SenoScan Full Field Digital Mammography System Operator Manual. Issue 1. Revision 2. Fischer Imaging Corporation, Denver (2001)
4. Hendrick, R. E., Berns, E. A.: Full-Field Digital Mammography Quality Control Manual. PhantomImage, Chicago (2001)
5. Fujita, H. et. al: A simple method for determining the modulation transfer function in digital radiography. IEEE Trans. Med. Imaging 11 (1992) 34-39
6. Shen, S. Z., Mawdsley, G., Yaffe, M.: Automation of Quality Assurance of Digital Mammograpy. IWDM 2000 5th International Workshop on Digital Mammography. Medical Physics Publishing, Madison (2000) 656-665
7. Dainty, J. C., Shaw, R.: Image Science. Academic Press, Toronto (1974)

Evaluation and Modelling of Detection, Location and Discrimination of Lesions in Mammograms

Arthur Burgess, Francine Jacobson and Philip Judy

Brigham and Women's Hospital, 75 Francis St., Boston MA, USA
burgess@bwh.harvard.edu

Abstract. Previously we described mass detection results for human and model observers using mammogram and filtered noise backgrounds with the same power spectrum. The results were unusual in that threshold amplitudes (contrasts) increased as mass size increased. We were able to predict these results using mathematical observer models. When observers had to search for the mass, human thresholds were identical for both backgrounds. This suggests that breast structure in the image is equivalent to random noise. In mass discrimination experiments, thresholds for masses larger than 4 mm were about 1.5 to 2 times higher than for detection. We conclude that detection, localization and discrimination of masses in mammograms are limited by statistical variation in normal breast structure in the image, rather than imaging system noise.

1. Introduction

X-ray mammography is the primary method of detecting breast cancer. However, tumors are often extremely difficult to detect because of the complex and highly variable normal tissue background in the images. Our work was designed to develop a quantitative understanding of the effect of breast structure on tumor detection, localization and discrimination. It is based on signal detection theory (SDT) models [1], [2], [3] that include statistical properties of image noise and normal patient structure in the images.

As the projected area of signals gets larger, observers usually require less contrast to achieve a particular detection accuracy. In image noise, this leads to an idealized relationship between contrast threshold, C_T, and area, A, of the form $C_T = B/\text{sqrt}(A)$, where B is a constant. This model and our intuition about detectability are based on random processes that are uncorrelated or have a fixed correlation length. As signal size increases, its contributions sum coherently while the interfering noise sums incoherently. The signal contributions grow more rapidly than the noise effects, so the signal becomes more detectable as size increases. The situation is quite different for detection in mammograms because of the unusual image spatial statistics.

2. Lesion Detection Experiments

We did 2AFC experiments using a hybrid image method [3] with masses extracted from specimen radiographs, Figure 1, added to digitized normal mammograms. The masses (a fibroadenoma and 3 ductal carcinomas) were re-scaled to sizes from 0.5 to 16 mm. An example display is shown in Figure 2. We also did experiments using white noise backgrounds. Three observers participated, 2 physicists and a radiologist.

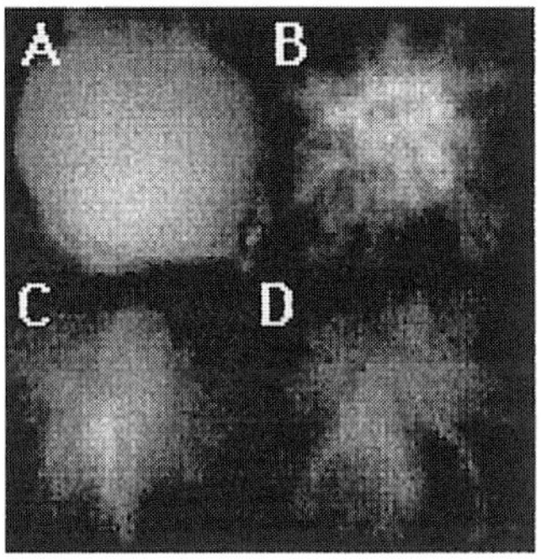

Fig. 1. The masses used.

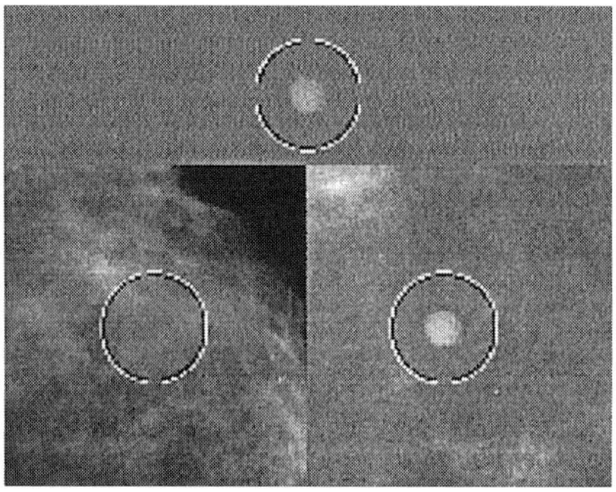

Fig. 2. Example experiment display.

Figure 3 (a contrast-detail or CD diagram) shows thresholds in mammographic backgrounds increasing with size for masses larger than 1 mm. These unusual results are due to the particular power spectrum of breast tissue in mammograms: average radial frequency dependence, $P(f) \approx K/f^3$, (Figure 4). The threshold increase below 1 mm is due to image noise dominance at high frequencies. The CD diagram slope for signal detection in white noise agrees with the expected value of –1 over most of the size range.

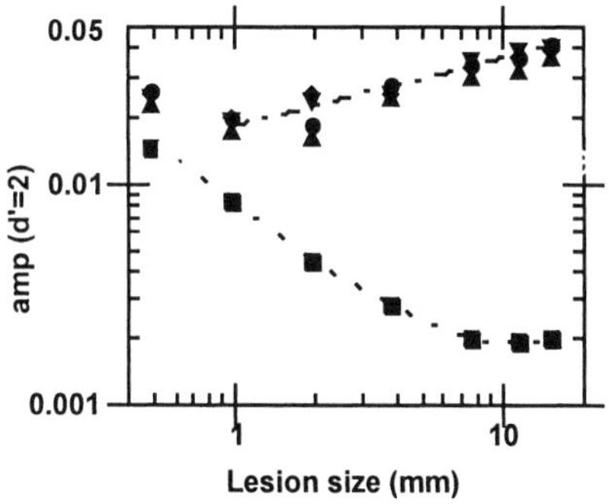

Fig. 3. CD diagrams for mammograms (upper) and white noise (squares).

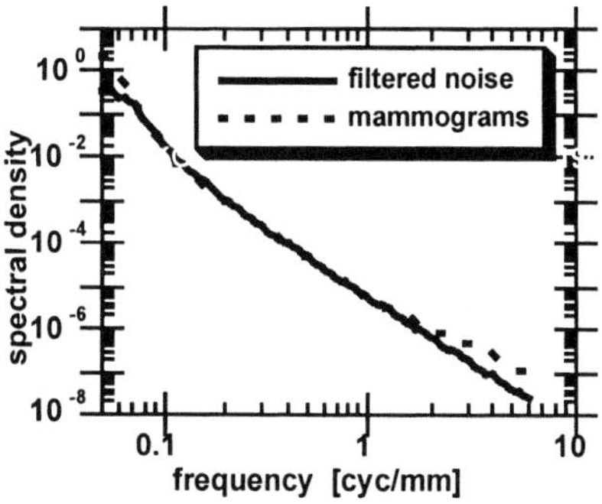

Fig. 4. Power spectra.

We also did 2AFC experiments using a simulated mass in both mammograms and filtered noise with a $1/f^3$ spectrum. Calculated observer model performance was almost the same for the two backgrounds. Human thresholds were about 50% higher with filtered noise. This suggests that, for humans doing the 2AFC detection task, normal structure in mammograms does not act purely as noise. Rather, we can make some use of anatomical knowledge in the decision task [3], [4]. We next did experiments where observers had to search for a known mass within a defined image area. The human thresholds were higher than for 2AFC detection, but were identical for both background types – suggesting that mammogram backgrounds are equivalent to filtered noise for the search task. We were able to account for threshold changes using a simple probability theory-based model that accounted for the effect of location uncertainty. The results of these experiments are reported elsewhere [3].

3. Theory of Lesion Detection for Model Observers

The equation describing the CD diagram for the Bayesian ideal (prewhitening matched filter) observer [3] will be presented for a special case to show the general form of the result. The signal is isotropic with spatial polar equation, $s_R(r) = As(r/R)$, where r is radial distance from the center, R is a positive real-valued size scaling factor, s(0) = 1, and A is signal amplitude. The 2D Fourier transform of this scalable signal is $S_R(f) = AR^2S(Rf)$, where $R^2S(Rf)$ is the 2D Fourier transform of s(r/R). The detectability index {d' or signal-to-noise ratio (SNR)} equation for the 2AFC signal known exactly condition with scaling and noise spectrum $P(f) = K/f^b$ is:

$$(d')^2 = 2\pi \int_0^{\infty} \frac{|S_R(f)|^2 f df}{Kf^{-b}} = \frac{2\pi A^2 R^4}{K} \int_0^{\infty} |S(Rf)|^2 f^{(1+b)} df . \qquad (1)$$

It can be shown [3] that if the integrand converges and form of the signal profile does not change during scaling, then the amplitude threshold, A_T, is given by

$$\log(A_T) = \text{Constant} + m\log(R), \text{ and } m = (b-2)/2 . \qquad (2)$$

The above model requires the assumption that image statistics are stationary (do not depend on spatial position). Since this is violated for mammographic backgrounds, we also investigated performance for the Fisher-Hotelling observer model [1], [2], [3] with spatial frequency channels (FH_C). The detectability index for this observer is calculated in the spatial domain using a vector description of the signal and a covariance matrix description of noise and background spatial statistics. We found that FH_C model observer performance predictions with mammogram backgrounds and filtered noise for the simulated nodule signal were very similar. This indicates that non-stationarity of mammogram statistics in the compressed breast region is not a serious problem. We also evaluated performance of a number of other models: a non-prewhitening matched filter and a FH model with different channels. The CD diagram slopes for all these models were similar. However, there were differences in the offset constant value. These models and results are discussed elsewhere [3].

4. Mass Discrimination Experiments

We also did 2AFC mass discrimination experiments. In this task, the observer was given two mammographic backgrounds (as in Figure 2) but with two different masses present rather than one. The masses were randomly assigned to the left and right fields. Given the mass pairs, (A, B) for example, the observer was asked to select the field that contained mass A. Amplitudes of the masses in a pair were adjusted so that they were equally detectable. With reference to Figure 1, the pairs were, (A, B), a fibroadenoma versus a ductal carcinoma and, (C, D), two ductal carcinomas. The discrimination threshold results for the pair (C, D) are plotted in Figure 5 together with the average detection thresholds for the two masses. For sizes of 4 mm and larger, the discrimination CD diagram slope is similar to that for detection but thresholds are about twice as high. For sizes smaller than 4 mm, the discrimination thresholds increase as size decreases. Similar results were obtained for discrimination between masses A and B, except that threshold elevation for large sizes was only about 1.5 times detection.

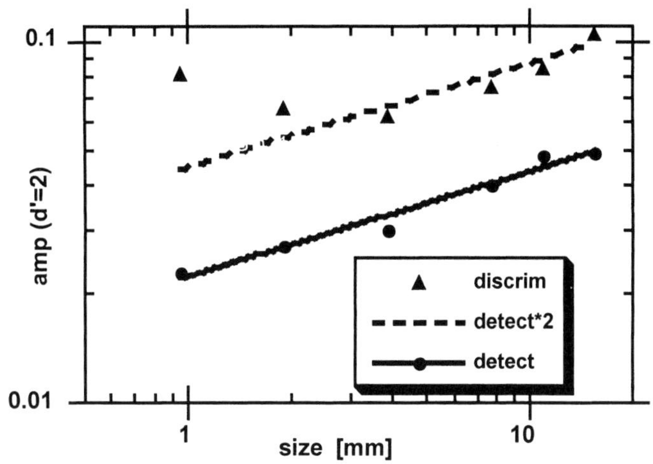

Fig. 5. Amplitude thresholds for 2AFC discrimination (triangles) and detection (circles) for mass pairs C and D, both ductal carcinomas (see Fig. 1). The dashed line is for twice the 2AFC detection threshold amplitudes.

5. Discussion

We found novel CD diagrams for detection of masses larger than 1 mm in mammographic backgrounds. The positive slope means that contrast needed for detection increases as lesion size increases - determined solely by variation in normal background structure in the images. The results also suggested that microcalcification detection is limited by a combination of image noise and breast structure variation. These results are consistent with previous findings by Bochud et al. [4]. We could predict the results using several observer models. The main difference between model predictions was the absolute threshold levels rather than CD diagram slope. The FH_C model with spatial frequency channels gave best agreement with human results. In the 2AFC detection experiments, human amplitude (contrast) thresholds were lower with mammographic backgrounds than with filtered noise. This suggests that we can make some use of anatomical knowledge for that task. There was no difference in thresholds for search experiments with the two background types. This suggests that for more complex decision tasks, mammographic backgrounds can be modeled as random power-law noise. Details of the models, human results and comparisons are presented elsewhere [3]. Experimental results for 2AFC discrimination between masses show positive CD diagram slopes for lesion larger than 4 mm with thresholds about 1.5 to 2 times higher than for detection. The difference in CD diagram slopes for smaller sizes indicates that additional refinement of observer models is needed.

Acknowledgements

We thank Maria Kallergi for providing the digitized mammograms and Jack Beutel for digitizing the specimen radiographs. This research was funded by NIH grant CA58302.

References

1. Eckstein, M., Abbey, C., and Bouchud, F.: A practical guide to model observers for visual detection in synthetic and natural noisy images. In: Handbook of Medical Imaging. Physics and Psychophysics, Beutel, J., Kundel, H., van Metter, R.: (eds.) Vol. 1. SPIE Press, Bellingham WA, (2000) 593-628.
2. Abbey, C., Bouchud, F.: Modeling visual signal detection tasks in correlated image noise with linear observer models. In: Handbook of Medical Imaging. Physics and Psychophysics, Beutel, J., Kundel, H., van Metter, R.: (eds.) Vol. 1. SPIE Press, Bellingham WA, (2000) 629-654.
3. Burgess, A., Jacobson, F., and Judy P.: Human observer detection experiments with mammograms and power-law noise. Med. Phys. 28 (2001) 419-437
4. Bochud, F., Valley, J., Verdun, F. et al.: Estimate of the noisy component of anatomical backgrounds," Med. Phys. 26 (1999) 1365-1370

Effect of Detector Noise on Phantom Image Quality in a Number of FFDM Systems

K. Chakrabarti[*+], R.V. Kaczmarek[*], J.A. Thomas[+] , M. Mahesh[++], and R. C. Fleischman[**]

* Center For Devices and Radiological Health,
US Food and Drug Administration, Rockville, MD 20850
+ Uniformed Services University of The Health Sciences, Bethesda, MD 20814
++Johns Hopkins University School of Medicine, Baltimore, MD 21287-0856
** Memorial Sloan- Kettering Cancer Center, New York, NY 10954
KXC@CDRH.FDA.GOV

Abstract. We have assessed phantom image quality from a number of commercially available Full Field Digital Mammography (FFDM) systems. Image quality, contrast to noise ratio (CNR) and signal to noise ratio (SNR) were evaluated at various technique factors to assess the effect of detector noise on image quality, detector dynamic range and quantum limited operating region.

I. Introduction:

At present the US Food and Drug Administration has approved marketing clearance of three manufacturers' FFDM systems for use in non interventional mammography. These systems are the General Electric (GE) Senographe 2000 D, Fischer Imaging's SenoScan and LORAD's LDBI system. All three systems are "indirect" digital system in which wide band gap phosphor materials are used for x-ray induced light emissions. The emitted visible light is then detected by the narrow band gap solid state digital detectors. All three manufacturers developed quality control test criteria which must be followed by the facilities using any of these systems under the Mammography Quality Standards Act (MQSA). While we believe that QC test procedures when carried out properly provides adequate assurance of quality of image produced by these systems, we also consider that proper care must be taken by the facilities to use these systems in optimum techniques for patient examinations. Unlike in the case of the screen film systems, because of the wide dynamic range and non-existence of film blackening, these systems can be operated in extreme technique ranges. As a part of our on going studies on the effects of signal to noise ratio (SNR) and contrast to noise ration (CNR) on image quality from FFDM systems at high and low exposure ranges, we have studied the detector noise and detector dynamic ranges of all three systems from the knowledge of exposures, SNR, CNR and phantom image quality. From these results it was possible to generate imaging technique charts, at which the system can be operated within the x-ray quantum limited region.

II. Experimental:

We imaged RMI-156 Mammography Accreditation Phantom at various clinical techniques and measured phantom score, CNR and SNR using all three systems. The selected techniques were both higher and lower than the technique given in the manufacturer's MQSA quality standards procedure manuals[1-3]. We focused our study on the effects of detector noise on phantom image quality. Data were acquired using several different mammographic quality control phantoms. The phantom images were scored by a number of ACR trained reviewers. For GE Senographe 2000D, and LORAD LDBI we began with the technique factors recommended by the manufacturers. We then varied technique factors widely so that a large variance of SNR and CNR could be generated. The images were captured at those technique factors and scored along with CNR and SNR measurements. For GE Senographe 2000 D, the CNR was calculated using the largest mass as GE prohibits use of added contrast disc with a phantom in AOP mode. The SNR values were calculated from the surrounding background regions of the largest mass. For Fischer SenoScan and LORAD LDBI the contrast disk was used for CNR calculations. The SNR values were calculated from the surrounding region of the contrast disk. In all cases automated method was used for CNR and SNR calculations to avoid error due to the positioning of the region of interest (ROI) on the contrast objects and on the background. Phantom images were scored by the four ACR trained reviewers under similar conditions (window level, window width, and other viewing conditions).

III. Results and Discussions:

In order to observe the effect of a wide range of SNR and CNR on phantom scores we calculated SNR, CNR at different techniques and scored phantom on those images. Figure 1 shows the plots of SNR and CNR as a function of mAs for the GE Senographe 2000D. Depending on the technique factors chosen, both SNR and CNR values fall non-linearly beyond a certain mAs value. This value shifts to lower mAs as kVp is increased. A similar behavior is noticed for the LORAD LDBI system also, as shown in figure 2. Depending on the system and the technique factors used, the linear part of the SNR or CNR vs mAs plot indicate the region where the system is quantum limited. The non-linear region of the plot indicates the region where the detector noise plays a significant role and the system should not be operated at those techniques. A convenient way to establish a characterstic mAs value for the non-linear behavior to be apparent is the mAs at which the extrapolated straight line part of SNR (or CNR) versus mAs curve deviates by more than 2% from the actual curve. For each of these systems then, a cross cut can be drawn through these points which can show the technique factors for which the system can be operated in the quantum limited region.

The Fischer SenoScan can be operated at limited techniques. Because of lack of adequate data, we could not determine the non-linear region at low mAs values that were available for the system. However, at high mAs value the detector appear to show some saturation. These results are shown in the plot of SNR and CNR as a function of mAs in figure 3. Fischer requires that for a standard size breast, the system be run at 30 kVp. The system seems to operate well at the manufacturer recommended techniques.

Figure 4 shows the mean total phantom scores of four reviewers with different SNR values for the GE Senographe 2000 D. Figure 5 shows the mean total phantom score as a function of CNR. From figures 4 and 5 it can be observed that below 50 SNR and CNR below 2, the phantom scores fall non linearly. These results indicate that image quality may be compromised if the images are acquired at SNR values below 50 or CNR value below 2. The same pattern can be determined from the LORAD LDBI system as shown in figures 6 and 7 which represent respectively SNR and CNR as a function of the mean total phantom scores of four observers. For the LORAD LDBI system, below an SNR value of 45 and CNR value of 2, the phantom scores fall non linearly. Although manufacturers do not specify a minimum requirement for CNR the CNR must not remain within a certain specified percentage of the established base line value. GE does require that the SNR value must not be below 50 and LORAD requires that the SNR value must not be below 45. Our results clearly indicate that below those values phantom scores fall non-linearly, indicating that the system is operating in the non-quantum limited region where the detector noise has a significant impact on image quality. With the data available for the Fischer SenoScan no significant change in phantom score could be observed.

IV. Summary:

We have observed that from the CNR, SNR and phantom image studies, FFDM machine specific technique charts can be determined through which the system can be operated to produce high quality images. Operating above the manufactured required SNR value is extremely important. Image quality may be seriously compromised if adequate importance is not given to this parameter and the system is operated below the action limit.

References:

1. Senographe 2000D Quality Assurance Procedures, GE Medical Systems
2. SenoScan Full Field Digital Mommography System Operator Manual, Fischer Imaging Corporation
3. Loral LDBI Full Field Digital Mammography System Quality, LORAD /Hologic Corp.

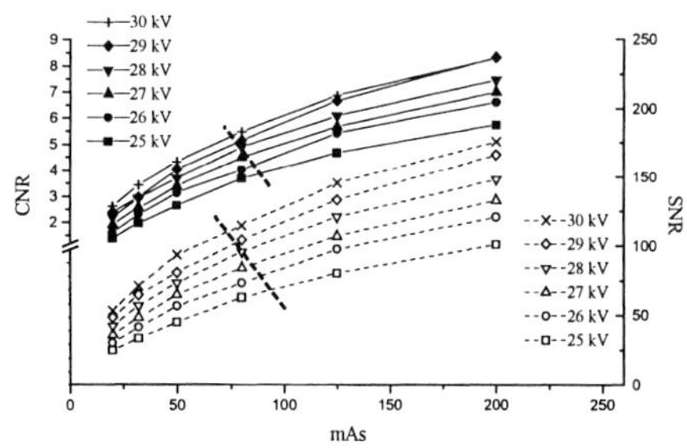

Fig. 1. GE. SNR and CNR vs mAs

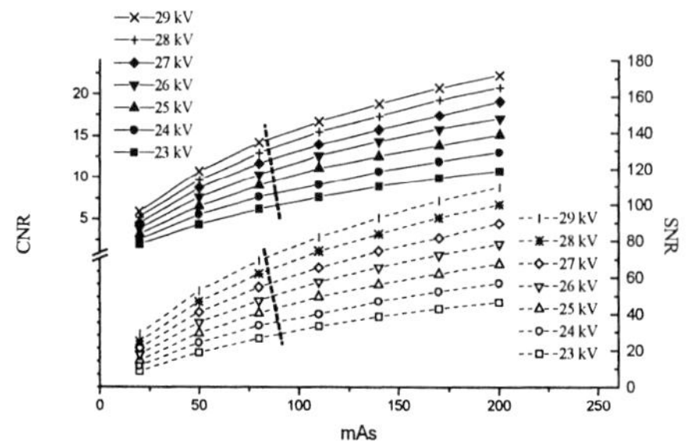

Fig. 2. LORAD. SNR and CNR vs mAs

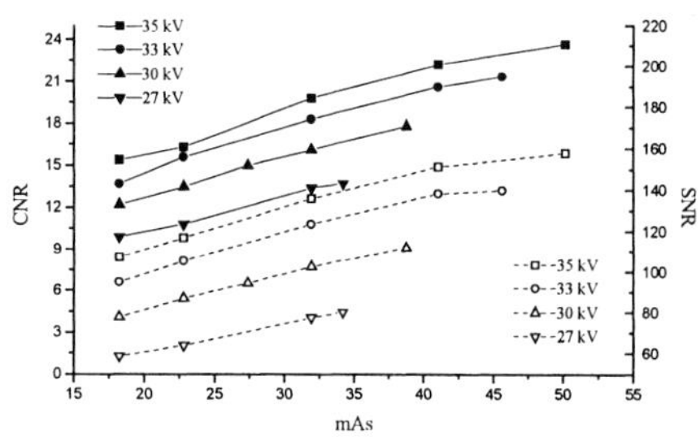

Fig. 3. Fischer. SNR and CNR vs mAs

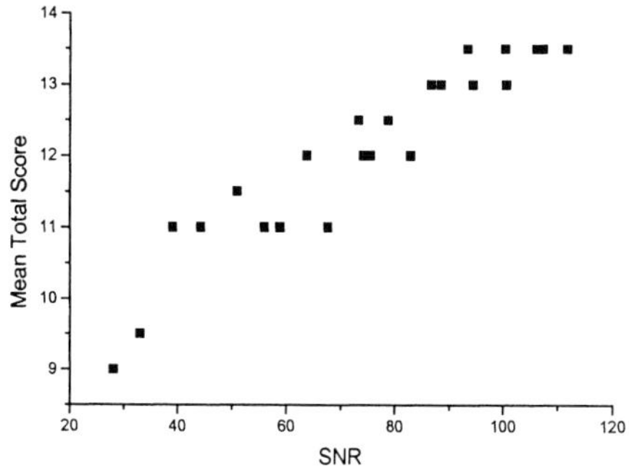

Fig. 4. GE. Mean Total Score vs SNR

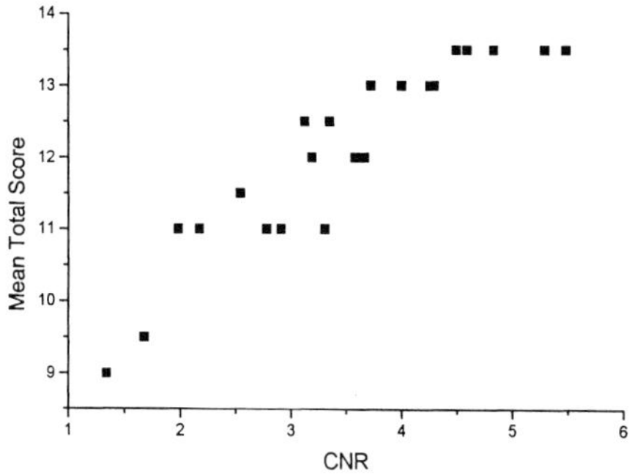

Fig. 5. GE. Mean Total Score vs CNR

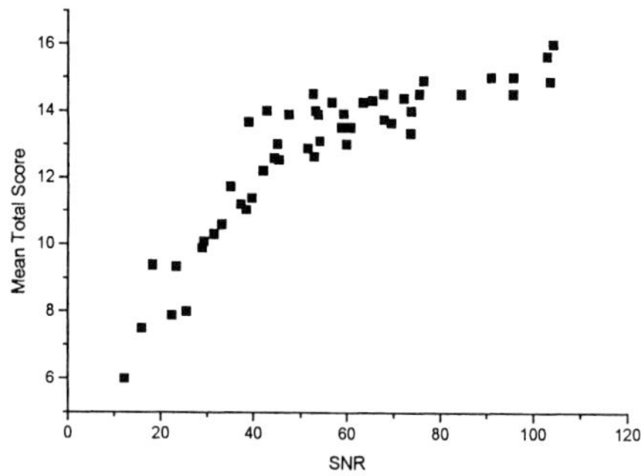

Fig. 6. LORAD. Mean Total Score vs SNR

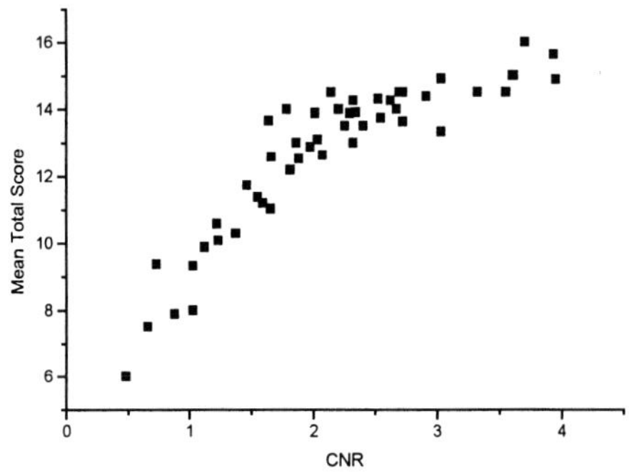

Fig. 7. Lorad. Mean Total Score vs CNR

Features analysis comparison of charge-coupled device (CCD) and amorphous selenium* (aSe) full-field digital mammography (FFDM) systems

Joel E. Gray[1], Zhenxue Jing[1], Laurie L. Fajardo[2], Daniel B. Kopans[3], Barbara Levit[2], and Richard H. Moore[3]

Lorad Corporation, 36 Apple Ridge Road, Danbury, Connecticut 06810, USA,
Johns Hopkins University Hospital, Baltimore, Maryland, USA
Massachusetts General Hospital, Boston, Massachusetts, USA
MammoMan@LoradMedical.com

Abstract. The purpose of this clinical study was to establish the non-inferiority of amorphous selenium (aSe) digital mammographic images to charge-coupled device (CCD) images. A features analysis was carried out to compare the quality of the images produced with a scintillator-CCD-fiber optic system to an aSe system. Six radiologists compared six features from the mammographic images, all of which contained suspected pathology, for 60 patients. The results indicate that the aSe images are similar to or better than the CCD images 94.0% of the time.

1.0 Introduction

There are two types of detectors used in full-field digital mammography systems: 1) Indirect detectors; and 2) Direct detectors.

Indirect detectors use a scintillator or other material to convert the x-ray photons into visible light photons which are then used to generate electrons and produce a digital image. The light produced by the scintillator with indirect detectors scatters within the scintillator or optics. This results in degradation of image quality as the point spread function typically covers multiple pixels.

Direct detectors convert x-ray photons directly to electrons eliminating the x-ray-to-light conversion step. These systems do not suffer the degradation in image sharpness associated with the light in indirect detection systems. The x-ray photons are absorbed and electron-hole pairs are produced directly in the amorphous selenium (aSe) layer. A field of approximately 2 kV is applied across the aSe layer (approximately 250 μm thick) which attracts the electron-hole pairs to the appropriate electrodes before there is any opportunity for them to migrate laterally in the aSe layer. Consequently, the point spread function is limited to a single pixel.

The thick aSe layer provides for a high efficiency in x-ray photon absorption (~ 95%) and a high detective quantum efficiency (~ 0.67 at 0 c/mm). The inherent

---

* The amorphous selenium imaging system described in this paper is an investigational device and not approved for sale in the United States.

sharpness due to the lack of light scatter or electron-hole pair migration in the aSe layer results in a high modulation transfer function (~ 0.80 at 4 c/mm compared to ~ 0.40 for indirect detection systems).

In this study the Lorad Selenia system with an aSe detector was evaluated clinically to determine the non-inferiority of it to the Lorad charge-coupled device (CCD) system. A features analysis was carried out with clinical images.

2.0 Materials and Methods

2.1 Digital Imaging Systems

The two systems compared in this clinical study consisted of a Lorad Digital Breast Imaging (LDBI) system using a cesium iodide scintillator coupled to CCDs through fiber optic tapers. The imaging area was 18 x 24 cm and used an array of 3 x 4 fiber optic taper-CCDs to produce the digital image with ~ 40 μm pixels. (1) Image data were digitized to a depth of 14 bits.

The aSe Lorad Selenia FFDM system utilized a large, 24 x 29 cm detector with an aSe layer thickness of 250 μm and a pixel size of 70 μm. (2) Image data were digitized to a depth of 14 bits.

2.2 Mammographic X-Ray System

The mammographic x-ray system used as part of the FFDM systems was a Lorad M-IV consisting of a conventional molybdenum x-ray anode and molybdenum filter (30 μm thick). The screen-film bucky was removed and the M-IV system was fitted with the CCD or aSe image receptor.

2.3 Subjects

Subjects were recruited into this clinical study based on their screen-film examination (screening or diagnostic). The patient screen-film studies were read by the investigators (LLF or DBK) in the normal clinical approach used at these two institutions. Patients which were determined to have a Breast Imaging Reporting and Data System (BIRADS) classification of 3, 4, or 5 were recruited as subjects for this study. BIRADS 3 indicates a probably benign finding; 4 is a suspicious abnormality; and 5 represents a finding which is highly suggestive of malignancy.

Inclusion criteria were—

- Female, 40 years of age or older, of any ethnic or racial origin
- Screen-film mammogram categorized as a BIRADS classification of 3, 4, or 5
- Subject or legal guardian is willing and able to understand, sign, and date the study specific Patient Informed Consent, approved by the Institution Review Board (IRB).

Exclusion criteria were—

- Subject was unable or unwilling to give informed consent for any reason (i.e., psychiatric or neurological disability)
- Subject had breast implants
- Subject was pregnant or has reason to believe that she may have been pregnant
- One or more of the screen-film images were acquired using a rhodium filter.

2.4 Subject Demographics

Seventy-five subjects were recruited into the study between November 16, 2001, and February 18, 2002. Thirteen patients were not eligible for the features analysis for three reasons: 1) 3 did not meet the eligibility criteria; 2) 4 had their images lost due to technologist errors; and 3) 6 had different image technique factors for their CCD and aSe images. Sixty patients were randomly selected from the remaining 62.

The average age of the patients was 57.4 (± 11.4 SD) years of age. The most suspicious findings included mass (45%), architectural distortion (7%), calcifications (40%), and focal asymmetry (8%). BIRADS scores were 3 (33%), 4 (57%), and 5 (10%).

2.5 Image Acquisition

Clinical images were obtained at two institutions—Johns Hopkins University Hospital and Clinics and Massachusetts General Hospital. Both the CCD and aSe FFDM systems were placed in the same room at both institutions. This allowed for sequential imaging of subjects on these two systems by the same technologist and within a few minutes on each system.

Craniocaudal (CC) and mediolateral oblique (MLO) views were obtained on the affected breast using each system. Technique factors (kVp, mAs, compression force, mean glandular dose, etc.) were similar for the aSe and CCD images of each patient and were selected manually based on those used for the screen-film examination.

All film images were printed and processed at Lorad Corporation's facility to minimize variability due to these variables.

2.6 Participating Radiologists

Six radiologists participated in the features analysis portion of the study. All were board certified and qualified under the Mammography Quality Standards Act (MQSA) regulations. All had previous experience reading full-field digital mammographic images produced by Lorad's CCD system or other manufacturer's equipment. Reimbursement was provided for travel, hotel, and living expenses. In addition, each radiologist received an honorarium for participation in the features analysis study.

2.7 Features Analysis Sessions

Six radiologists were shown side-by-side CC and MLO film images from the 60 subjects. The evaluations were carried out at the Lorad facilities in Danbury, Connecticut under controlled conditions. No room lighting was used. A multiviewer was used to display the images. The luminance of the multiviewer was 3200 nit. All patient identification information was removed from the film images. Viewboxes were masked so that no light would reach the radiologist unless it came through a mammographic film. Lesion type and position were provided to each radiologist to assure that all radiologists evaluated the same suspected pathology. Use of a 2X magnifying glass was permitted.

The radiologists viewed the images starting in early morning without any interruptions. They continued until they requested a break. Most radiologists completed the comparisons in 3 to 5 hours. A research assistant assisted the radiologists in completing forms and monitoring the viewing sessions.

The radiologists were asked to evaluate six features of the images including lesion conspicuity, lesion detail, tissue visibility at chest wall (volume of tissue), tissue visibility at skin line, overall density, and axillary details (MLO views only). The radiologists were asked to assign a score of –3 to +3 to the sets of images indicating the difference in image quality (Table 1).

Table 1. Image quality difference scores and criteria

Score	Image Quality Difference
+3	aSe is much better than CCD
+2	aSe is better than CCD
+1	aSe is slightly better than CCD
0	aSe is similar to CCD
-1	CCD is slightly better than aSe
-2	CCD is better than aSe
-3	CCD is much better than aSe

3. Results*

The results are summarized in Table 2. The radiologists rated the amorphous selenium images similar to or better than the CCD images 91.4% of the time for lesion conspicuity, 93.1% of the time for lesion detail, 93.5% of the time for tissue visibility at the chest wall, 98.2% of the time for tissue visibility at the skin line, 97.4% of the time for overall density, and 87.5% of the time for axillary details. The estimated proportion of scores greater than 0, adjusting for correlations among these scores, is 94.0%, with a 95% lower confidence bound of 92.7%. Thus we formally conclude that the amorphous selenium images are not inferior to the CCD images.

* Statistical analysis provided by Alicia Y. Toledano, Ph.D., Brown University, Providence Rhode Island, USA.

Individual 95% lower confidence bounds exceeding 85% were obtained for each feature except axillary details (95% LCB: 83.3%) and for each radiologist, indicating that non-inferiority is consistent across features and readers.

Table 2. Features analysis score distributions: –3 to –1 favors CCD images; +1 to +3 favors amorphous selenium images.

Feature	-3	-2	-1	0	1	2	3
Lesion Conspicuity	1%	2%	5%	51%	24%	11%	6%
Lesion Detail	1%	1%	5%	35%	32%	19%	8%
Tissue Visibility at Chest Wall	0%	1%	6%	71%	16%	5%	1%
Tissue Visibility at Skin Line	0%	0%	2%	48%	39%	10%	2%
Overall Density	0%	0%	2%	32%	45%	16%	4%
Axillary Details (MLO Only)	0%	2%	11%	59%	19%	7%	2%
Overall	0.5%	0.9%	4.6%	48.2%	30.2%	11.8%	3.8%

References

1. http://www.fda.gov/cdrh/pdf/p010025b.pdf
2. Yorker, J., Jeromin, L., Lee, D., Palecki, E., Golden, K., Jing, Z.: Characterization of a full field digital mammography detector based on direct x-ray conversion in selenium. Proceedings of the SPIE, 2002 (in press).

Comparison of screen-film, imaging plate and direct digital mammography with CD phantoms

Hemdal B[1], Bay TH[2], Bengtsson G[3], Gangeskar L[2], Martinsen AC[2], Pedersen K[4], Thilander Klang A[5], Mattsson S[1]

[1]Malmö University Hospital, Sweden, [2] Ullevål University Hospital, Oslo, Norway, [3] Lund University Hospital, Sweden, [4] Norwegian Radiation Protection Authority, [5] Sahlgrenska University Hospital, Göteborg, Sweden

Abstract. Low contrast-detail phantoms of glandularity 30, 50 and 70%, and thickness 3, 5, and 7cm were imaged. Screen-film (SF), imaging plate (CR), and full-field digital mammography (FFDM) systems were studied. Images were acquired for a range of anode/filter/tube potential/dose (AGD) combinations. The number of perceivable objects (score) was recorded and AGD determined. For FFDM, image scores similar to those with SF can be achieved at 20-60% of the SF dose. The largest dose reduction potential was found for the thickest phantoms and highest glandularity. With CR, a dose reduction of 10-20% was found, the largest reduction appearing for the thinnest phantom thickness.

Introduction, Material and Methods

With the gradual introduction of digital mammography, it becomes of interest to compare the performance of the new technologies to that of the current screen-film technique. A contrast-detail (CD) phantom (CIRS Model 83, thickness 1cm, 50% glandularity) was placed in stacks of breast tissue equivalent material of glandularity 30, 50 and 70% respectively. Phantoms of thickness 3, 5, and 7 cm were arranged for each tissue composition. The CD insert was a 7x7 array of low-contrast circular objects (diameter 1.5-4.5 mm, object contrast 0.10%-1.8% at 20 keV). The systems investigated were: *SF* = Siemens Mammomat 3000 Kodak Min-R 2190/Min-R 2000 (36°C, 90s), *CR* = Siemens Mammomat 1000 with high resolution, Fuji imaging plate HR-BD, pixel size 50 x 50μm^2, image reader FCR 5000MA, dry laser imager FM-DP L and *FFDM* = General Electric Senographe 2000D.

For the SF and CR systems the optical density was 1.40±0.05. Anod/filter/tube voltages used were Mo/Mo/25kV/27kV/29kV/31kV and Mo/Rh/25kV/27kV/29kV. For SF also W/Rh/25kV/27kV/29kV and for CR Mo/Rh/31kV. For the CR system, only the 50% glandular composition was investigated and images were acquired at the AEC dose level and 30 and 60% of that level; for Mo/Mo/27kV and Mo/Mo/29kV also at 20, 45, 80, 125, 150 and 200% of the AEC dose. The FFDM system has an automatic selection of exposure parameters (AOP), based on a short pre-exposure at 4mAs. Three modes are available, Standard (STD), Contrast (CNT) and Dose (DOSE). The STD mode was used clinically. All phantom combinations were imaged with all three automatic modes. Anod/filter/tube voltages used were Mo/Mo/25kV/26kV/27kV/28kV, Mo/Rh/28kV/31kV and Rh/Rh/28kV/29kV/31kV/

32kV. Additional images were acquired at 30 and 60% of the AOP dose. For the three 5cm phantoms, doses at 20, 45, 80, 125, 150 and 200% of the AOP STD dose level where included. Six images at Rh/Rh/29kV were collected at average glandular dose (AGD) 0.8-4.3mGy for the 7cm 30/70 phantom. All images were read by six readers in a randomized order; SF and CR images on light boxes, FFDM images on the GE Senographe 2000 Review Workstation. The mean scores for all the images were plotted as functions of AGD [1, 2]. The function

$$\text{Score} = a_0 \cdot (1 - \exp(-a_1 \cdot AGD)), \tag{1}$$

where a_0 and a_1 are constants representing the maximum possible score and the relative dose, respectively, was fitted to the experimental points (STATISTICA 5.1). Statistical significance in the difference between the scores of two images at the same AGD level was determined by a paired two tailed t-test ($p<0.05$).

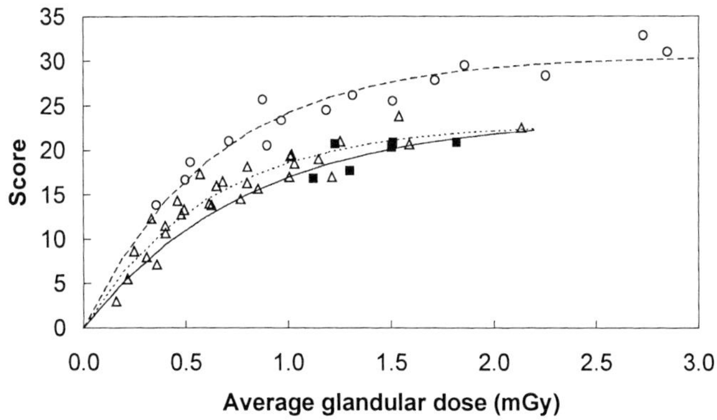

Fig. 1. The mean score from six readers as a function of AGD for the phantom with 50% glandularity and a total thickness of 5cm for images from *SF* (*squares, unbroken line*), *CR* (*triangles, dotted line*) and *FFDM* (*circles, dashed line*).

Results, Discussion and Conclusion

An example of curves fitted to the experimental data points (5cm, 50% glandular phantom) is shown in Fig. 1. SF scores calculated from these functions are presented in Table 1. From the derived functions, the doses required with CR and FFDM to achieve the same image scores as for SF were calculated (Table 1).

With FFDM, scores similar to those with SF can be achieved at 20-60% of the dose. The largest differences are found for the thickest phantoms with the highest glandularity. It is clear that it would be possible to reduce doses, particularly for thin and medium thick phantoms, and still get increased detection of low contrast details for all phantoms as compared to SF. For CR, images with the same score as SF can be obtained with 80-90% of the AGD. The largest dose reduction was seen for the thinnest phantom. The better performance of the FFDM system can alternatively be utilized to achieve increased detection of low contrast details. Table 2 summarizes results of the paired two-tailed t-tests. The low contrast detail detection for FFDM was better than for SF at about the same dose level for seven out of the nine phantoms ($p<0.05$). Such details are difficult to perceive with screen-film systems, especially in thick and dense breasts.

Table 1. Typical AGD levels and corresponding scores for SF, CR and FFDM. All scores are calculated from the estimated functions.

Contrast-detail phantom		SF		Same score as SF		FFDM STD	
Thickness (cm)	Glandularity (%)	AGD (mGy)	Score	AGD_{CR}/AGD_{SF}	AGD_{FFDM}/AGD_{SF}	AGD_{FFDM}/AGD_{SF}	Score
3	30	0.60	22.5		0.48	1.81	33.1
	50	0.65	23.8	0.80	0.58	1.78	32.4
	70	0.70	21.8		0.50	1.80	30.6
5	30	1.2	20.7		0.58	1.43	27.7
	50	1.4	19.6	0.83	0.47	1.08	27.7
	70	1.7	17.2		0.30	1.02	27.5
7	30	3.0	18.7		0.35	0.65	23.2
	50	3.5	17.5	0.90	0.33	0.65	24.0
	70	4.0	14.6		0.23	0.66	23.7

Table 2. Average scores and standard deviation, and results from t-test at comparable dose levels for the 5 cm phantoms.

Contrast-detail phantom						
Thickness (cm)	Glandular/ adipose (%)	AGD (mGy)	System	Score ± SD	p-value	Results of t-test
5	30/70	~1.5	SF	23.2±4.0		
			FFDM	29.8±3.3	<0.05	Better
	50/50	~1.5	SF	20.3±1.9		
			CR	23.8±3.1	<0.05	Better
			FFDM	25.5±3.6	<0.05	Better
	70/30	~1.8	SF	19.2±2.7		
			FFDM	27.5±2.6	<0.05	Better

Acknowledgement

This study was partly supported by grants from the Swedish Radiation Protection Authority (P 1062.98).

References

1. Dance, D.R., Skinner, C.L., Young, K.C., Beckett, J.R., Kotre, C.J. Additional factors for the estimation of mean glandular breast dose using the UK mammography dosimetry protocol. Phys. Med. Biol. 45, 3225-3240 (2000).
2. Zoetelief, J., Fitzgerald, M., Leitz, W. Säbel, M. European protocol on dosimetry in mammography. EUR 16263 (1996).

Optimizing full-field digital mammography techniques: The influence of target-filter and peak voltage settings on lesion detection and average glandular dose

Klaus-Peter Hermann, Silvia Obenauer, Matthias Funke and Eckhardt Grabbe

Department of Diagnostic Radiology, Göttingen University Hospital, Robert-Koch-Str. 40, 37075 Göttingen, Germany
kherman@gwdg.de

Abstract. The goal of this study was to assess the influence of the target-filter combination and the tube voltage on lesion detection and average glandular dose (AGD) in digital mammography using a flat-panel X-ray detector based on amorphous silicon technology. For the assessment of image quality images of the ACR mammographic accreditation phantom were obtained. Increasing peak voltage by 2 kVp decreases breast dose by 7% for the same target-filter combination. Changing the target-filter combination from Mo-Mo to Mo-Rh decreases AGD by approximately 10% and changing from Mo-Mo to Rh-Rh decreases the AGD by approximately 30% at the same peak voltage values. In the peak voltage range between 25 and 35 kVp there was no difference in lesion detectability for different tube voltages at the same detector dose between Mo-Mo and Mo-Rh .

1. Introduction

In screen-film mammography typical X-ray tube voltages range from 25 to 30 kVp and occasionally higher when thick, dense breasts are encountered. Increasing the peak voltage increases the penetrating quality of beam incident on the breast. With a more penetrating beam there is less attenuation by the breast and less dose. But it also decreases attenuation differences i.e. the object contrast. In screen-film radiography the contrast is determined by the object and the film characteristic. In digital radiography with image processing technology you can amplify the contrast and the detectability of subtle details is limited only by noise. Therefore we expected a potential of full-field digital mammography to achieve better image quality at lower dose compared to screen-film mammography.

2. Methods and Materials

The study was performed using the full-field digital mammography unit Senographe 2000D (GE Medical Systems, Waukesha, USA). The image receptor of this system was a cesium iodid coupled flat-panel amorphous silicon detector with a pixel pitch of 100 μm. The system has a dual track X-ray tube with a molybdenum (Mo) and a rhodium (Rh) track on the anode and either a 0.03 mm Mo or a 0.025 mm Rh filtration.

Decreasing the dose for reasons of radiation protection is only justified when the information content of the image remains sufficient. To quantify the detection capabilities of the system the ACR mammographgic accreditation phantom was used. The phantom is an acrylic block containing 16 objects. Each object simulates an anatomical structure which may be found in breast tissue (fibrous structures, microcalcifications, tumors or masses). The phantom images were evaluated directly from a high resolution workstation monitor by counting the correctly detected objects.

3. Results

The resulting correctly detected lesions for different radiation qualities are shown in fig. 1. To eliminate the effects of noise the detector dose was fixed at 80 μGy. Increasing kVp causes a significant decrease in lesion detection. When scores were averaged over all target/filter combinations the correctly detected lesions decreased by 1 object per 3 kVp.

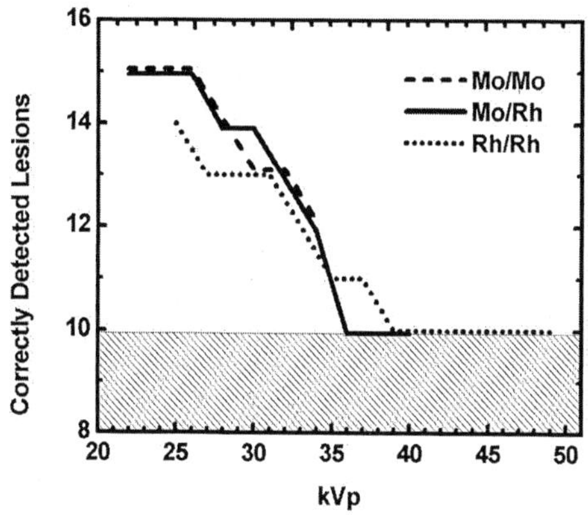

Fig. 1. Correctly detected lesions as function of the kVp for 3 target-filter combinations

The present criteria for the number of objects to pass the ACR mammography accreditation program is a minimum of ten objects.This demand was fullfilled in every case. Given, that peak voltage has a significant effect on lesion detection, use of the lowest possible peak voltage seems preferable. But peak voltage also has a significant effect on X-ray output. With higher kVp decreases exposure time (or tube loading) for fixed detector dose. For example, obtaining the same detector dose with the Mo-Mo combination required a significant higher mAs at 25 kVp than at 28 kVp. This indicates that the preference for using lowest possible peak voltage must be modified by the requirement that exposure times be kept reasonably short, that is less than 2 seconds.

The selection of target-filter materials and peak voltage affects breast dose too. Fig. 2 shows the average glandular dose (AGD) to maintain the same detector dose for the 4.5 cm thick phantom. Increasing peak voltage by 2 kVp decreases breast dose by 7% for the same target-filter combination. Changing the target/filter combination from Mo-Mo to Mo-Rh decreases mean glandular dose by approximately 10%, while changing from Mo-Mo to Rh-Rh decreases the mean glandular dose by approximately 30% at the same peak voltage values.

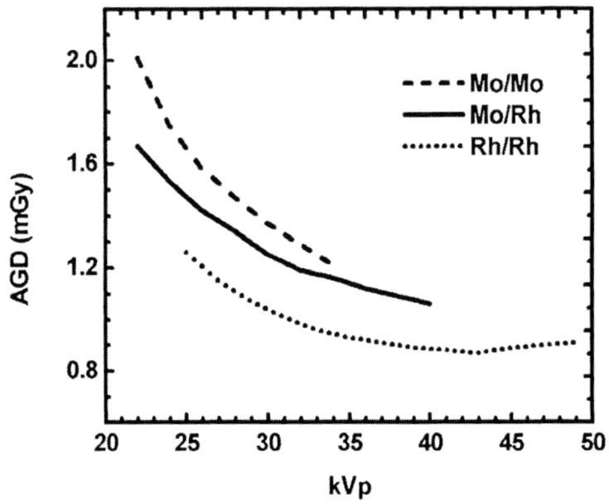

Fig. 2. Average glandular dose AGD as function of the kVp for 3 target-filter combinations

4. Conclusion

With conventional screen film mammography we reached 12 correctly detected lesions at an average glandular dose of 1.25 mGy. The full-field digital mammography system provides an increased number of correctly detected lesions. The lower detection level of screen-film mammography is achieved by the digital system at a 30% lower dose.

The slope of the characteristic curve of the mammographic film determines the contrast properties and the attenuation difference between lesions and the surrounding tissue which can be seen in the image. By contrast with the film-screen technique, in digital mammography with the help of the windowing technique the detectability of subtle details is limited only by noise. Digital mammography thus has the potential for improving the display of poorly contrasted details and/or reducing the dose.

A new CR based system for high resolution mammography: Experimental analysis of low contrast detectability

Klaus-Peter Hermann, Silvia Obenauer, Anne Zach-Enk and Eckhardt Grabbe

Department of Diagnostic Radiology, Göttingen University Hospital, Robert-Koch-Str. 40, 37075 Göttingen, Germany
kherman@gwdg.de

Abstract. The goal of this study was to compare lesion detection of low-contrast objects on images taken with a new photostimulable storage phosphor versus images taken with conventional screen-film mammography. The measured system spatial resolution was 8.5 lp/mm for the CR system compared with 13 lp/mm for the screen-film system. However, the lower spatial resolution did not limited the more important contrast resolution. The fraction of correctly identified objects was higher with CR mammography than with screen-film mammography at every exposure setting.

1. Introduction

The use of photostimulable storage phosphors in mammography has hitherto hampered by the limited spatial resolution achievable with image plates which represented the available technology. The systems employ a 100 μm laserscanning spot that permits a theoretical maximum spatial resolution of 5 lp/mm. Conventional mammographic screen-film systems reach a peak resolution of approximately 20 lp/mm. For this reason, few workers in the field actually use computed radiography (CR) for routine mammographic work. Some groups have either completely rejected its use in mammography or have tried to overcome the limiting spatial resolution by using direct magnification technique [1,2].

In 2001 Fujifilm (Tokyo, Japan) introduced a new image reader with dual-side reading and 50 μm capability for digital mammography. The purpose of our survey was to study the contrast-detail resolution of this new CR based mammographic system in comparison to conventional screen-film mammography.

2. Methods and Materials

All experiments were performed with a contrast-detail phantom consisting of 205 squares, each containing two gold platelets with the same size and thickness. The size of the platelets ranges from 0.1 to 3.2 mm, the thickness from 0.05 to 1.6 μm.

Images of the phantom were obtained using both the new transparent imaging plate and a conventional screen-film system as image receptors. The computed radiography system consisted of a single plate image reader (FCR 5000MA, Fujifilm), which includes dual-side reading and 50 μm capability in 18cm x 24cm and 24cm x 30cm cassettes, and a dry laser imager (FM-DP L, Fujifilm) with 50 μm pixel size. The dual-side reading capability allows captured X-ray information to be read from both sides of the imaging plate simultaneously [3].

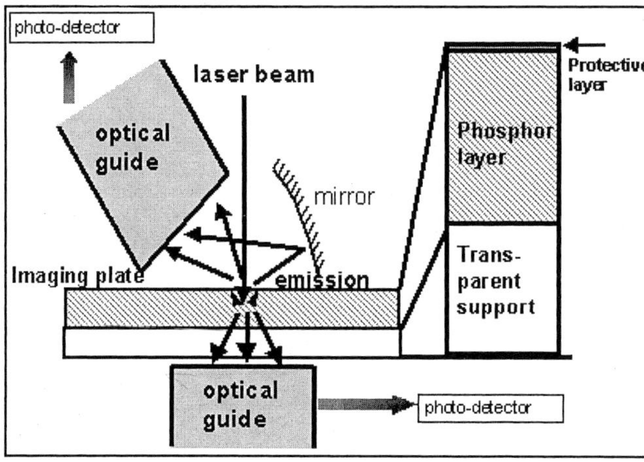

Fig. 1. Dual-side reading method and a thick imaging plate with transparent support

A state-of-the-art mammography unit was used (Mammomat 3000, Siemens, Erlangen, Germany). The system has a dual track X-ray tube with a molybdenum (Mo) and a tungsten (W) track on the anode and either a 0.03 mm Mo or a 0.025 mm rhodium (Rh) filter. Conventional mammograms were produced with Fuji UM-MA film in combination with Fuji Mammo fine screen.

3. Results

The measured system spatial resolution was 8.5 lp/mm for the CR system compared with 13 lp/mm for the screen-film system. However, the lower spatial resolution did not limited the more important contrast resolution. The fraction of correctly identified gold platelets was higher with CR mammography than with screen-film mammography at every exposure setting. The measured contrast-detail curves showed a shift to smaller details and contrasts (fig. 2).

The CR system reached the optimal performance level of the screen-film system already at 30% to 50% lower dose. The advantage of the digital system was more pronounced for larger, low contrast objects. Performance for small objects with a diameter of less than 0.2 mm was similar with both techniques.

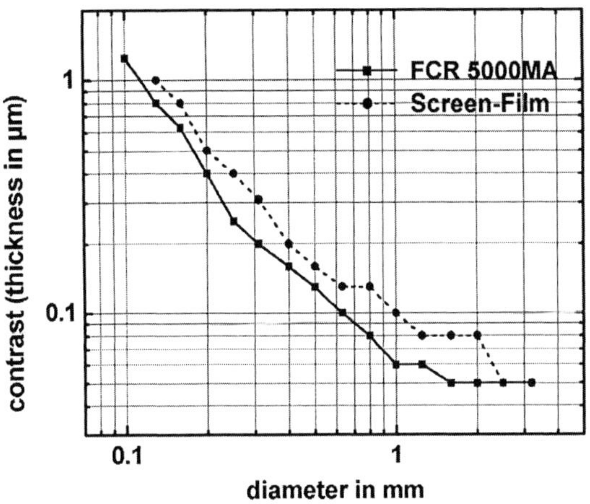

Fig. 2. Contrast-detail curves (phantom + 30 mm PMMA ≈ 40 mm PMMA) at 27 kVp with Mo anode, Mo filter and a tube loading of 90 mAs, showing a better performance for the CR system

4. Discussion

The new reading method that permits detection of emission from both sides of an imaging plate and the transparent support with a thicker phosphor layer work together to achieve 30% to 40% improvement of the detective quantum efficiency, a measure which strongly influences the dose required for adequate image quality. Along with the addition of the 50 µm image reader, the new CR system further enhances spatial resolution, resulting in digital mammograms with high image quality.

In summary we can say that digital mammography uitilizing computed radiography with dual-side reading should be a further powerful tool for detecting low-contrast lesions in the breast.

References

1. Funke M, Breiter N, Hermann K-P, Oestmann JW, Grabbe E. Storage phosphor direct magnification mammography in comparison with conventional screen-film mammography – a phontom study. Br J Radiol 1998, 71: 528-534
2. Fiedler E, Aichinger U, Böhner C, Säbel M, Schulz-Wendtland R, Bautz W. Image quality and radiation exposure in digital storage plate mammography with magnification technique. Fortschr Röntgenstr 1999, 171: 60-64
3. Arakawa S, Itoh W, Kohda K, Suzuki T. Novel computed radiography system with improved image quality by detection of emissions from both sides of an imaging plate. Physics of Medical Imaging 1999, SPIE Vol. 3659:572-581

Digital luminescence mammography (CR) without magnification in clinical routine (n = 1.363)

R. Schulz-Wendtland, U. Aichinger, I. Kuchar, M. Tartsch, W. Bautz

Institute of Diagnostic Radiology, University of Erlangen-Nürnberg
91054 Erlangen, Germany
Ruediger.Schulz-Wendtland@idr.imed.uni-erlangen.de

1. Introduction:

The digital mammography with high resolution phosphor storage plate / luminescence mammography (CR) has the lower spatial resolution (9 lp/mm) in contrast to screen film mammography (SFM) (12 lp/mm) but the advantages of a higher DQE (Detective Quantum Efficiency) (0.33 versus 0.20), a large dynamic range (4.000 : 1 versus 100 : 1), reduction of dose (entrance surface air kerma: 7,60 mGy versus 9,64 mGy), post-processing and CAD [1, 2].

Since 11/2000 such a digital mammography unit is available and after an experimental phantom study, which demonstrated that according to a low contrast phantom (Wisconsin RMI phantom) [3] screen film mammography (SFM) and digital technique are equal in the detection of details (grains, strings, round lesions) [4], we wanted to investigate if the digital luminescence technique can be used in clinical routine.

2. Material and Method:

The preconditions for the digital luminescence mammography (CR) are the European Guidelines for Quality Assurance in Mammography Screening [5] and especially in Germany the German Quality Assurance [2]. They are fulfilled by the combination of Mammomat 3000 N (Siemens) with a molybdenum anode, grid, no magnification and the image reader FFDM-CR (Fuji / Siemens). The imaging processing and the printing of the hardcopies were carried out at a Dry View TM 8600 Laser Imaging System (Kodak).

3. Results:

Between 03/2001 and 08/2001 we examined at our department of Gynaecological Radiology (Institute of Diagnostic Radiology, University of Erlangen-Nürnberg) 1.363 patients. The reasons of examination: preventive examination, screening, afterare. The evaluation of our digital images demonstrates: dose, contrast and noise were in accordance with the Guidelines [2, 5] at every time. The image quality was

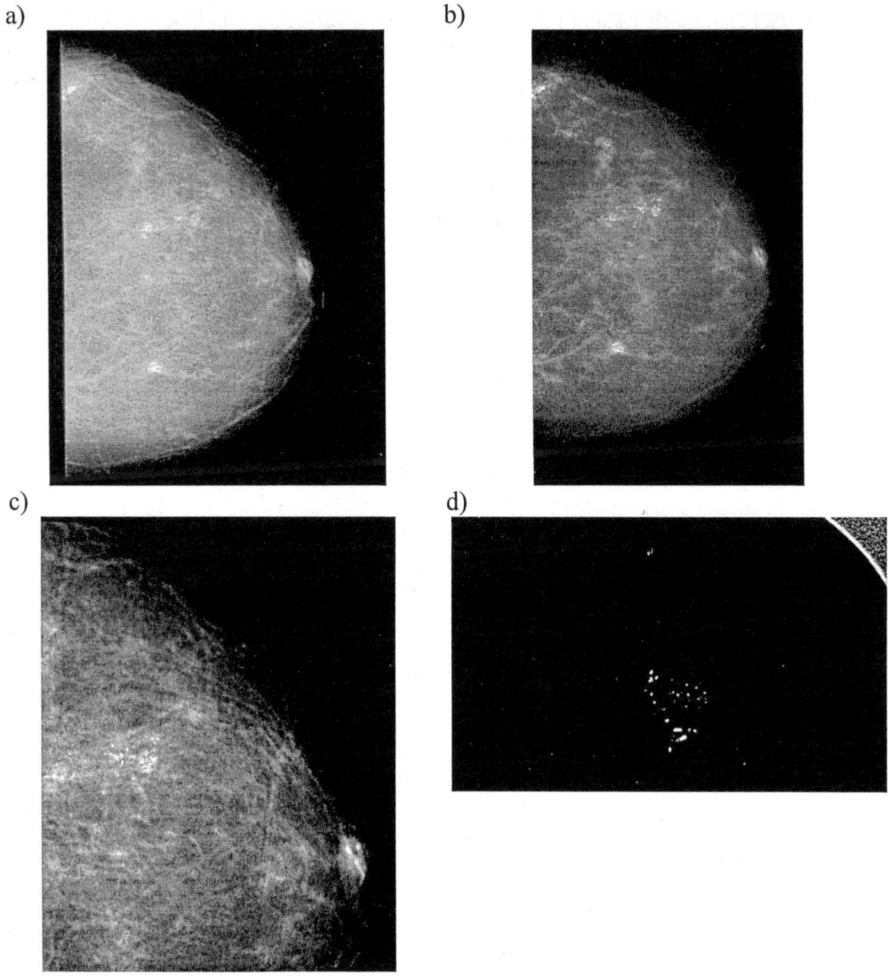

Picture 1a – d: Digital luminescence mammography (CR) without magnification (high resolution), post-processing with edge enhancement, zooming and changing of the grey scale.

classified by all radiologists as good. By the post-processing (work-station) it was not necessary to make new images (picture 1a-d). The higher necessarity of time for the development of digital in contrast to conventional analogue mammography hardcopies could be compensated by 8 cassettes.

4. Discussion:

On the basis of the technical preconditions, the phantom (RMI)-examinations the high resolution phosphor storage plate / digital luminescence mammography (CR)

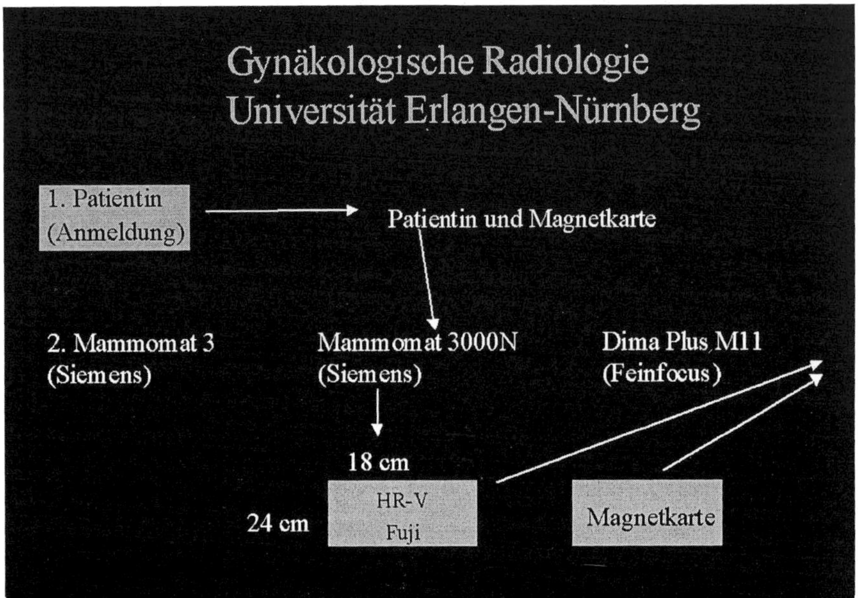

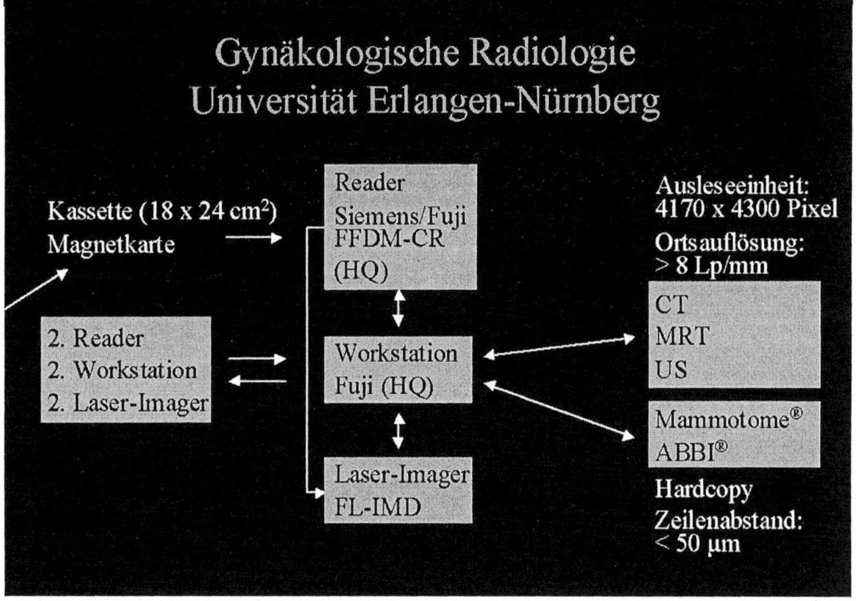

Picture 2a, b: The Gynaecological Radiology of the Institute of Diagnostic Radiology, University of Erlangen-Nürnberg.

(without magnification technique) can replace the conventional analogue screen film mammography (SFM) and be used in clinical routine. By this way we have reconstructed our department (picture 2a, b) to step into the digital world also now in mammography.

5. Literature

1. Pisano, E., Yaffe, M., Hemminger, B., Hendrick, R., Niklason, L.: Current Status of Full-Field Digital Mammography. Acad Radiol 7, 266 – 280 (2000).
2. Säbel, M., Aichinger, U., Schulz-Wendtland, R., Bautz, W.: Digitale Vollfeld-Mammographie: Physikalische Grundlagen und klinische Aspekte. Röntgenpraxis 52, 171 – 177 (1999).
3. Kimme-Smith, C., Bassett, L., Gold, R.: A review of mammography test aobjects for the calibration of resolution, contrast and exposure. Med Phys 16, 758 – 765 (1989).
4. Schulz-Wendtland, R., Aichinger, U., Säbel, M., Böhner, C., Dobritz, M., Wenkel, E., Bautz, W.: Experimental investigations of image quality in X-ray mammography with conventional screen film systems (SFS), digital phosphor storage plate in / without magnification technique (CR) and digital CCD-technique (CCD). Röntgenpraxis 54, 123 – 126 (2001)
5. Perry, N., Broeders, M., de Wolf, C., Törnberg, S. (Eds.): European guidelines for quality assurance in mammography screening. EUREF, 2001, Third Edition.

Digital luminescence mammography: A phantom study before clinical use

R.Schulz-Wendtland, U.Aichinger, C.Böhner, M.Dobritz, M.Tartsch, W.Bautz

University of Erlangen-Nürnberg, Institute of Diagnostic Radiology
91054 Erlangen, Germany
ruediger.schulz-wendtland@idr.imed.uni-erlangen.de

Introduction

Since 02/1998 we use at the Institute of Diagnostic Radiology, Gynaecological Radiology, University of Erlangen-Nürnberg, digital phosphor storage plate mammography in magnification technique (Fuji) in clinical routine (n=12.668) [4, 12, 13, 14].

Experimental investigations for detection and diagnosis of microcalcifications and round lesions demonstrate the same results in view of the diagnosis with conventional film screen system and digital phosphor storage plate in magnification technique[1].

Since 11/2000 a digital phosphor storage plate without magnification (8 – 9 lp/mm) exists (Fuji/Siemens). To receive a first impression of the image quality, we used for our investigation a quality control method which is performed in the USA since many years [6].

Material and Method

The object for radiography was the Wisconsin Mammographic Random Phantom (RMI-phantom), Model 152 A (Radiation Measurements Inc. Wisconsin, USA) [6]. The phantom is constructed of 16 wax blocks which can be variably arranged in 4 columns and rows. 5 blocks contain aluminiumoxide grains with a diameter between 200 μm and 740 μm, 6 wax blocks contain nylon strings with a diameter between 0.4 and 1.6 mm, 4 wax blocks contain round lesions with blurred margin and a thickness between 5 and 14 mm, 1 wax block was empty. The thickness of the phantom was 45 mm in agreement with the standard phantom in the European Protocol on Dosimetry in Mammography [16].

The dosimetry with this standard phantom was performed with the procedure described in literature [7, 16]. The radiation exposures were measured as entrance surface air kerma (table1). After primary dosimetry we compared 2 modalities of investigation (table2):

1. Film Screen System (FSS): The grid images were taken at the Mammomat 3000 (Siemens) with the molybdenum anode under using a 30 μm molybdenum filter at a voltage of 28 kV (resolution 12 lp/mm). For exposure

we chose the film screen combination UM mammo Fine (screen) and UM-MA (film) (Fuji), for development of the films the day light system MF FPM 2100 (Fuji).

2. Digital phosphor storage plate: The X-ray images were exposed at a Mammomat 3000 (Siemens) with a molybdenum anode using a 30 µm molybdenum filter with a grid but without a magnification at a voltage of 28 kV (resolution 8 – 9 lp/mm). Digital phosphor storage plate was the type IP HRV (Fuji). The exposed plates were read at the image reader FFDM – CR (Fuji/Siemens). The image processing and the printing of the hardcopies were carried out at a Dry View TM 8600 Laser Imaging System for digital mammography (Kodak) with a resolution of 12,9 lp/mm.

To avoid learning effects of the investigators we radiographed for every experimental condition always three different phantom configurations. All X-ray images showed an optical density of about 1.3.

The X-ray images were coded by numbers and demonstrated in accidentally sequence to five investigators. The investigator group consisted of 4 radiologists with long time experience in mammography and one physicist well-trained in the evaluation of phantom X-ray images. The analysis of the X-ray images took place under standardised conditions for all investigators at the same viewing box. It was possible to use a magnifying glass. The time of viewing every X-ray image was limited to 5 minutes. The observations of the investigators were noted for every finding of the 16 wax blocks: „g“ for grains, „l“ for round lesions, „s“ for strings and „e“ for empty. The results of the investigators were compared with the true arrangement whereby the test for recognition was planned only for true positive results, i.e. the sensitivity of all 2 systems was proved. For that reason there was recognizable for every modality the maximum of 18 strings, 15 grains and 12 round lesions, the maximum of 45 true positive results possible.

Results

In table 3 the results of the evaluation are demonstrated, analysed to modalities, findings and investigators with the corresponding summaries. The summaries (s) and the averages (a) of all details and investigators (FSS: s 191/a 38.2 ; CR : s 193/a 38.6) show that the 2 modalities, the conventional film screen and the digital phosphor storage plate system without magnification technique, receive nearly the same results.

Discussion

In conventional film screen mammography the quality of the image system will be specified by the limiting resolution, described by line pairs / mm. Until this time all systems of full field digital mammography are limited by lower resolution [3, 9,15]: digital phosphor storage plate mammography a resolution of 5 lp/mm, in magnification technique 8 lp/mm [14], other systems (for example Senograph 2000 D,

GE) 5 lp/mm. In discussion is the use of full field digital systems with a lower resolution (5 lp/mm corresponding to 100 μm pixel) than the demand of the German Quality Assurance [10]. Some investigators [4, 5, 8] could demonstrate that the recognition of details in phantom examinations was the same in spite of lower resolution and also in published clinical studies - this was no problem for the diagnosis [1, 2, 11].

Our results demonstrate that the digital mammography with phosphor storage plates without magnification technique and a resolution of 8-9 lp/mm receive the same detectability of details as the conventional film screen system (table 2 and 3). It is important that the dose of the digital mammography with phosphor storage plates without magnification technique is lower than with the conventional film screen system [14].

Our phantom study proves that it is possible to replace equivalent the conventional film screen system by digital mammography with storage phosphor plate without magnification technique and with this system we have the possibilities of post-processing, teleradiology and archiving.

If these results could be transmitted to clinical mammographies than it exists the chance to change the conventional equipment and to step into the digital world also now in mammography.

Table 1. Entrance surface air kerma of the phantom [16] for the 2 different modalities of investigation

Modalities of investigation	Entrance surface air kerma in mGy
Film screen system (FSS)	9,64
Digital phosphor storage plate (CR)	7,60

Table 2. Technical specifications of 2 different modalities of investigation

Technology	Equipment	Manu-facturer	Anode	Filter	kV	Grid	Magnifi-cation
Conventional film screen system	Mammomat 3000	Siemens AG	Mo	30μmMo	28	yes	no
Digital phosphor storage plate	Mammomat 3000	Siemens AG	Mo	30μmMo	28	yes	no

Table 3. Description of the true positive results of the 5 investigators (A-E) to the 7 modalities of investigation (FSS=film screen system, CR = digital phosphor storage plate without magnification technique) analysed to details, opposed to the maximum of the possible numbers (max). The last column demonstrates the summary of details of the 5 investigators

Modality		**max**	**A**	**B**	**C**	**D**	**E**	**Summary** (225 numbers possible)
FFS	strings	18	13	12	13	12	14	
	grains	15	15	12	15	15	14	
	round lesions	12	12	9	12	11	12	
	summary	45	40	33	40	38	40	191
CR	strings	18	13	14	14	12	13	
	grains	15	14	14	14	15	13	
	round lesions	12	12	11	12	12	12	
	summary	45	39	39	40	39	38	195

Literature

1. Aichinger U, Schulz-Wendtland R, Dobritz M, Mitze M, Bautz W(1999) Mikrokalkanalyse welche Vorteile zeigt die Speicherfolientechnik gegenüber konventionellen Film-Folien-Systemen? RöFo 170: 129
2. Cowen AR, Launders JH, Jadav M, Brettle DS (1997) Visibility of microcalcifications in computed and screen-mammography. Med Phys Biol 42: 1533-1548
3. Feig SA, Yaffe MJ (1998) Digital Mammography. Radio Graphics 18: 893-901
4. Fiedler E, Aichinger U, Böhner C, Säbel M, Schulz-Wendtland R, Bautz W(1999) Bildgüte und Strahlenexposition bei der digitalen Mammographie mit Speicherfolien in Vergrößerungs-technik. RöFo 171: 60-64
5. Funke M, Hermann KP, Breiter N, Hundertmark C, Sachs J, Gruhl T, Sperner W, Grabbe E (1997) Digitale Speicherfolienmammographie in Vergrößerungstechnik: Experimentelle Untersuchungen zur Ortsauflösung und zur Erkennbarkeit von Mikrokalk. Fortschr Röntgenstr 167: 174-179
6. Kimme-Smith C, Bassett LW, Gold RH(1989) A review of mammography test objects for the calibration of resolution, contrast and exposure. Med Phys 16: 758-765
7. Klein R, Aichinger H, Dierker J, Jansen MTJ, Joite-Barfuß S, Säbel M, Schulz-Wendtland R, Zoetelief J (1997) Determination of average glandular dose with modern mammography units for two large groups of patients. Phys Med Biol 42: 651-671
8. Obenauer S, Hermann KP, Schorn C, Funke M, Fischer U, Grabbe E (2000) Digitale Vollfeldmammographie: Phantomstudie zur Detektion von Mikrokalk. Fortschr Röntgenstr 172: 646-650
9. Pisano ED, Yaffe MJ, Hemminger BM, Hendrick RE, Niklason LT (2000) Current Status of Full-Field Digital Mammography. Acad Radiol 7: 266-280

10. Säbel M, Aichinger U, Schulz-Wendtland R, Bautz W(1999) Digitale Vollfeld-Mammographie: Physikalische Grundlagen und klinische Aspekte. Röntgenpraxis 52: 171-177
11. Schönhofen H, Arnold W, Hess T, Allgayer B(1998) Digitale Mammographie: Erfahrungen bei klinischer Anwendung. Fortschr Röntgenstr 169: 45-52
12. Schulz-Wendtland R, Aichinger U, Fiedler E, Böhner C, Säbel M, Bautz W (1999) Digitale Mammographie mit Speicherfolientechnik im täglichen klinischen Einsatz (n = 5.150). RöFo 170: 128-129
13. Schulz-Wendtland R, Aichinger U, Fiedler E, Säbel M, Bautz W (1999) Digital luminescence mammography in clinical use (n = 4.500). BJR 72: 94
14. Schulz-Wendtland R, Aichinger U, Säbel M, Böhner C, Dobritz M, Bautz W (2001) Experimentelle Untersuchungen zur Bildgüte konventioneller Film-Folien-Mammographie, digitaler Mammographie mit Speicherfolien in Vergrößerungstechnik und voll digitaler Mammographie in CCD-Technik. Fortschr Röntgenstr 173: 1-4
15. Thunberg S, Sklebitz H, Ekdahl B, Bätz L, Lundin A, Möller H, Fleischmann F, Kreider G, Weidner T (1999) OPDIMA: Large – area CCD – based X-ray image sensor for spot imaging and biopsy control in mammography. SPIE 3659: 150-158
16. Zoetelief J, Fitzgerald M, Leitz W, Säbel M (1996) European protocol on dosimetry in mammography. EUR 16263 Brüssel. European Commission.

Interpreting System MTF and NPS Measured on Clinical Digital Mammography Systems

Shen SZ, Mawdsley GE, Bloomquist AK, Mainprize JG, Yaffe MJ

Sunnybrook & Women's College Health Sciences Centre, Room S632, 2075 Bayview Ave., Toronto, Ontario, Canada M4N 3M5
Sam.Shen@SWCHSC.on.ca

Abstract. A set of phantoms and a software program have been developed to calculate MTF and NPS conveniently for digital mammographic systems. Phantom images have been collected from 19 digital mammography units from four major commercial manufacturers. MTF and NPS are analysed to relate their shape to design and operational factors of each system.

Introduction:

Modulation transfer function (MTF) and noise power spectrum (NPS) are useful measures of performance of radiological imaging systems. We have developed a method to evaluate the MTF and NPS of a variety of state-of-the-art commercial digital mammography systems used in the ACRIN DMIST trial funded by NIH/NCI [1]. MTF and NPS are measured on these systems under conditions that are as close as possible to those used in daily clinical practice.

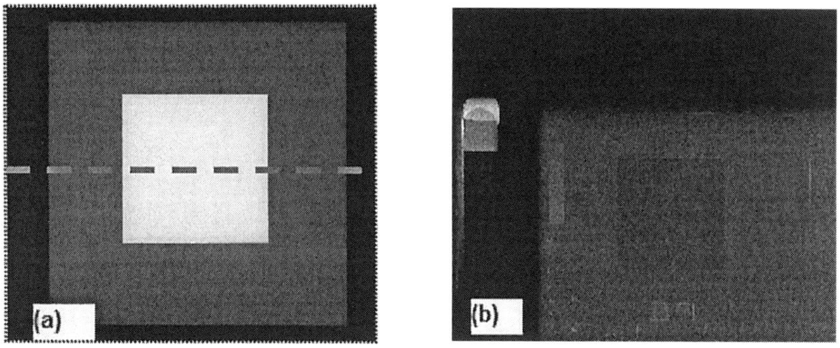

Figure 1: Radiographs of (a) MTF test tool and (b) IDMDG phantom.

The current commercial digital mammography systems are based on several different technological approaches and include: (A) GE: amorphous silicon-based flat panel; (B) Lorad: Phosphor/Fibre Optic Taper/CCD; (C) Lorad: Selenium flat panel; (D) Fuji: Photostimulable Phosphor; (E) Fischer: Slot-Scan with CsI-Fibre Optic Coupled/CCD [2].

The machines were tested during the initial medical physics visits to each of the 19 DMIST study sites. The images of an MTF test tool (Fig 1a) and the IDMDG phantom (Fig 1b) were analyzed with our software. Additional experiments to verify accuracy were done on a GE 2000D machine at our site.

Methods:

The details of methods used for measuring MTF and NPS have been published previously [1,3,4]. For System D, linearization of the logarithmic image data is performed with parameters provided by the manufacturer. The MTF tool is a square brass foil mounted on a larger, 1mm thick aluminum square. Our "standard" method (Method I) to measure MTF is to place this tool at the centre of the table top close to the chest wall. Two other methods were used to analyze the effect of scattered x-rays. In Method II, the brass foil is placed directly on the surface of the detector, with the compression plate and tabletop-grid assembly removed. In Method III, the brass foil was placed between the tabletop and a 2.5cm thick slab of PMMA that covered the entire x-ray field. NPS calculations were performed both on data from the IDMDG phantom and from images of a larger, uniform slab of PMMA.

Results and Discussion:

A. MTF

The system MTF measured with our method appears to have a greater degree of low frequency drop (LFD) than noted previously on similar systems [1,5,6].

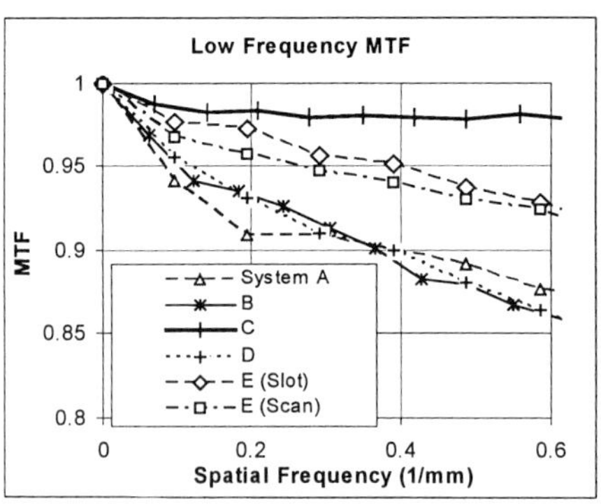

Figure 2: MTF on five systems illustrating LFD with Method I.

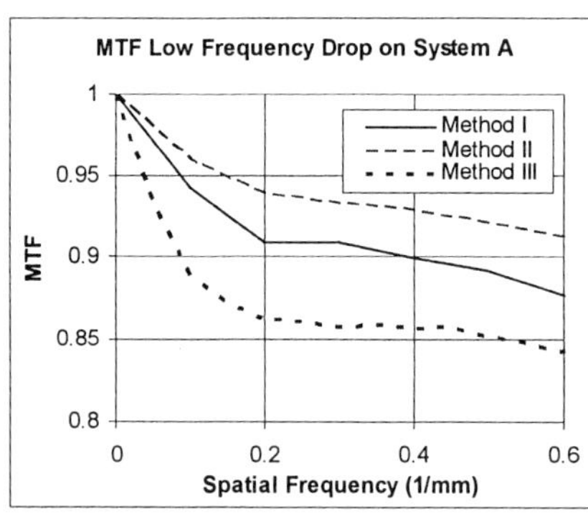

Figure 3: Effect of measurement setup on LFD.

All of the tested systems demonstrated an LFD. This varied from less than 2% to up to 9% using Method I (Fig 2). The lowest value was found in System E. Possible causes of LFD include incomplete flat fielding, x-ray scatter, beam hardening, displaced K-fluorescence re-absorption in the detector, and scattering of light photons. In our experiments, when scatter sources are added to the x-ray field (Fig 3 Method III), the LFD is much more significant. However, even when all extraneous scattering materials are removed from the x-ray field (Method II), LFD persists, although reduced in magnitude. This suggests that LFD is caused both by scattered x-rays entering the detector and scattered light inside phosphor-based detectors. The effect of the scattered signal is appreciable on both the bright and dark sides of the edge in the digital image of the MTF tool (Fig 4). Phosphor-based detectors have greater LFD than the direct conversion detector (Fig 2). This suggests that a significant part of the LFD arises from long distance light spreading in the phosphor. In a slot-scan system, both optical and x-ray scattering play a less important role because collimation reduces the source of scattered x-rays and the narrow geometry of the detector results in less collection of scattered light in the scanning direction. For such systems, signal lag in the scanning direction as well as imperfect TDI synchronization may be the dominant causes of the LFD seen in Fig 2 (System E – "scan").

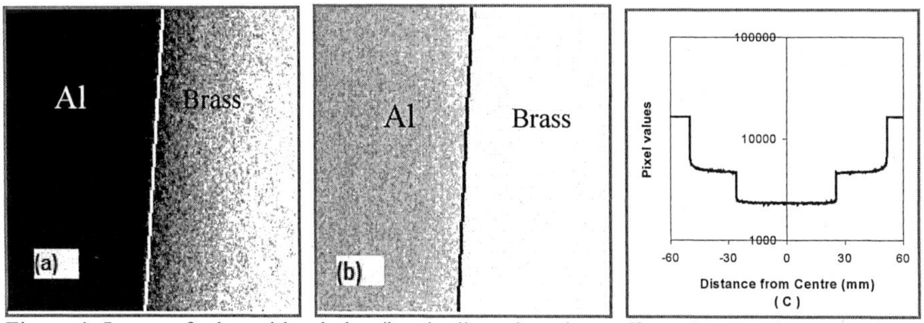

Figure 4: Image of edge with window/level adjusted to show effect of scatter (a) on the brass side, (b) on the aluminum base side. The white line in (a) and the dark line in (b) show the position of the edge. (c) shows the intensity profile of the image of the MTF tool in Fig1a along the dashed line.

To study the components of the LFD, we plotted a smoothed version of the line spread function (LSF) convolved with a 1 mm *rect* function (Fig 5a). There are roughly-symmetric broad tails. The LFD can be corrected by subtracting a wide Gaussian function from the original normalized LSF. We ignore the slight positive trend along the x-axis due to heel effect because preliminary results show that it is of minor importance. Using trial-and-error methods, we found that a Gaussian function (amplitude 0.17% of the LSF peak, FWHM - 7.1mm) can roughly correct the LFD contributing no appreciable change for frequencies greater than 0.2 cycles/mm (Fig 5b).

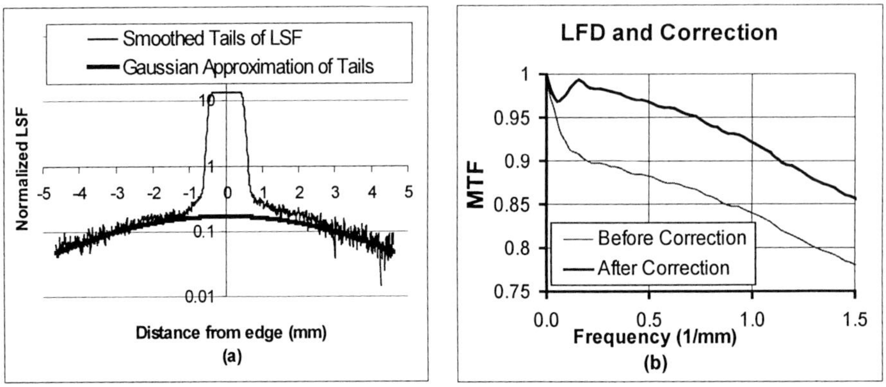

Figure 5: Correction of LSF. (a): Smoothed presampled LSF derived from an edge of system A and a Gaussian approximation for the spreading tails. (b): subtracting the Gaussian approximation from the raw presampled LSF removes the LFD.

B. NPS

It is difficult to compare the magnitudes of NPS on different systems, because the x-ray spectra have not yet been well characterized. However, the shape of the curves can provide insight regarding each system.

1. Enhanced low frequency power, as shown in Fig 6, is found in images from most of the systems. We find this with imperfect flat fielding, when the trend is not completely filtered away, *e.g.* when the heel effect is not completely removed. This may occur because the flat field image used for calibration is taken with a different thickness phantom than used for our NPS measurement. Another effect occurs when differential scatter levels from regions outside the ROI introduce a trend in the ROI. This may occur in the IDMDG phantom due to adjacent test objects. Although attempts to remove such trends by low-pass filtering are partially successful [7] residual power may affect the NPS at low spatial frequency.
2. Superimposed on the NPS curve, there are spikes seen at the frequencies of about 3 mm^{-1} and 6 mm^{-1} (Fig 6). Removing the grid makes these spikes disappear. On System C which uses a 2-dimensional grid, the spikes are much less significant, but seen in both directions. Grid oscillation requires the grid to start and stop when changing directions. For grids with 31 - 32 lines/cm (approx 3.2 lp/mm), even a small amount of signal will provide a very high power in the NPS, because contributions come from the entire area of the image. Higher harmonics of the grid frequency exist and may be aliased. In Fig. 6 we see two spikes, that may represent the fundamental and 1st harmonic of the grid frequency below the Nyquist frequency on a 0.04mm system (System B).

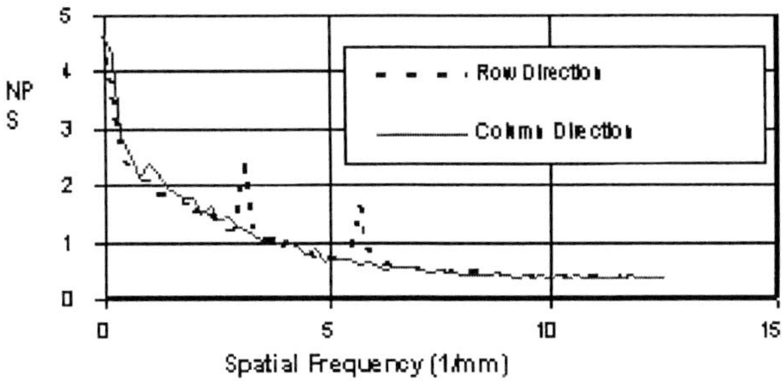

Figure 6: NPS of System B with both grid line noise and residual trend noise at low spatial frequency.

Conclusions:

MTF and NPS measurements provide useful information regarding the performance of digital mammography systems. High quality testing tools and methods are crucial to reveal authentic system image quality. Low frequency drop appears to be caused both by x-ray scattering and light spreading within phosphor detectors. Grid artifacts and imperfect flat fielding are detectible in NPS measurements. The impact of these effects on clinical utility of the images is not yet clear.

References:

1. Shen, S.Z., Mawdsley, G., Yaffe, M.: Automation of Quality Assurance of Digital Mammography. IWDM 2000 Proceedings (2000):656-665 Medical Physics Publishing, Madison WI
2. Yaffe, M.J., Rowlands, J.A.: X-ray Detectors for Digital Radiography. Phys. Med. Biol. 42 (1997) 1-39
3. Dainty, J.C. and Shaw, R.: Image Science. Academic Press, London (1976) 276–298
4. Samei, E., Flynn, M., Reimann, D.: A Method for Measuring the Presampled MTF of Digital Radiographic Systems Using an Edge Test Device. Med. Phys. 25 (1998) 102-113
5. Williams, M.B., Simoni, P.U., Smilowitz, L. *et al.*: Analysis of the Detective Quantum Efficiency of a Developmental Detector for Digital Mammography. Med.Phys 26 (1999) 2273-2285
6. Vedantham, S., Karellas, A., Suryanarayanan, S. *et al.*: Full Breast Digital Mammography with an Amorphous Silicon-based Flat Panel Detector: Physical Characteristics of Clinical Prototype. Med.Phys. 27 (2000) 558-576
7. Williams, M.B., Mangiafico, P.A., Simoni, P.U.: Noise Power Spectra of Images from Digital Mammography Detectors. Med.Phys. 26(1999)1279-1293

Automated Method for Measuring Contrast-to-Noise-Ratio (CNR) and Signal-to-Noise-Ratio (SNR) on a Full Field Digital Mammography System (FFDMS)

Thomas JA, Chakrabarti K, Kaczmarek RV and Romanyukna A

Uniformed Services University of the Health Sciences
Department of Radiology and Radiological Sciences
4301 Jones Bridge Road
Bethesda, MD 20879-4799
United States of America

Abstract. A newly developed automated procedure for contrast-to-noise-ratio (CNR) and signal-to-noise-ratio (SNR) calculations is proposed. Essential precision improvements are achieved with the new procedure. The impact of the variations in the CNR and SNR test procedures is discussed. Possible application of the procedure to different mammography systems is demonstrated.

I. INTRODUCTION

An important element of Quality Assurance Procedures of the United States Mammography Quality Standards Act (MQSA) is a periodic check of CNR and SNR. For example, General Electric (GE) requires weekly checks of CNR and monthly checks of SNR for the Senographe 2000D. According to the Senographe 2000D Manual the change in CNR must not exceed 0.2 and the value of SNR must exceed 50. Other manufacturers have similar requirements for periodic CNR and SNR monitoring.

New product releases are often accompanied by claims of considerable improvement in CNR and SNR in comparison with previous or competing mammography systems. This assumes the use of well-defined and highly reproducible procedure for CNR and SNR determination, which could provide meaningful comparisons of these parameters for different systems of the same model or even different mammography systems produced by different companies. However, currently there is no standardized methodology for measuring CNR and SNR on full field digital mammography systems (FFDMS).

There exist two potential sources of problems with the creation of this type of methodology. The first is associated with the absence of standardized recommendations for the selection of the region of interest (ROI) for CNR and SNR tests, and some variation in the object used for CNR determination (i.e., GE recommends calculating CNR based on image measurements of the largest mass of the FDA approved phantom whereas some companies (Lorad, Hologics Inc.) suggest using an image of an acrylic contrast disc, which can be placed on the phantom surface). The second potential source is connected with limited ability of humans to consistently reproduce the recommended procedure (i.e., to select the ROI exactly in the same location on different images obtained with different mammography systems or to center it precisely with the center of the object's image used for CNR or SNR calculations.

The aim of this paper is twofold - first to investigate the possible impact of these variations in the CNR and SNR test procedures; and, second to describe the newly developed automated procedure, which improves reproducibility of CNR and SNR calculations and can be applied to different mammography systems.

II. EXPERIMENTAL

Two types of experiments were conducted. The first, which was made with a GE Senographe 2000D sought to:

- Compare results of the manual and automated evaluation of CNR and SNR.
- Investigate the impact of the variation of the ROI size on these parameters.

The second was made with 49 FDA approved phantom images taken with a Lorad mammography system and aimed to check the applicability of the developed software to CNR and SNR evaluation on images obtained with this system.

In order to calculate CNR and SNR, 39 raw images of the FDA approved RMI 156 phantom were acquired with a Senographe 2000D FFDM system at the National Naval Medical Center, Bethesda, MD. SNR and CNR were calculated for every image in two ways. One based on the GE recommended manual procedure and the other with the newly developed automated procedure.

The GE recommended procedure for CNR and SNR determination consisted of the selection of the ROI with an ellipse tool on the image of largest phantom mass. GE requires that this ROI must be completely within and centered on the image of the largest mass. The second ROI should be of the same size as the first one, but it must be located on the background with its center at half the distance between the center of the largest mass and the center of the group of the largest specks. Then mean and standard deviation values are determined automatically for each ROI. CNR can be calculated as the difference between mean background and mean mass divided by the background standard deviation. SNR is the quotient of the mean background and its deviation.

The automated procedure is based on the highly reproducible selection of the ROIs' positions and sizes. It was done through the use of the subsequent iterations of the ROIs with different radii to accurately:

- Determine the position of the largest mass center.
- Measure the distance between largest mass of the phantom and one (but always the same) of the largest specks.

III. DEPENDENCY OF THE CNR AND SNR ON THE ROI AREA SELECTION

Figure 1 plots results of the dependency of CNR on ROI area selection for one of the 39 studied raw images. The other images yielded similar results. As seen from Figure 1, CNR depends essentially on the ROI area. Results obtained from the manual and automated methods are very close to each other and can be fitted well with a linear fit. With the exception of the CNR for the smallest areas, the automated procedure yielded considerably less deviation from linear dependence than the manual one. It is interesting to note that for the zero ROI area both methods gave about the same CNR.

Similar results were obtained for SNR determination. Again results of automated calculations had less scatter than manual ones, but both methods gave very close SNR values for the zero ROI area. Stronger ROI dependence of SNR obtained with automated calculations can be explained by its higher accuracy when compared with the manual method. Comparison of the data on mean background and its standard deviation obtained with GE manual and automated procedures shows that in the case of manual evaluation SNR size dependence is flattened by higher scattering of the above mentioned values.

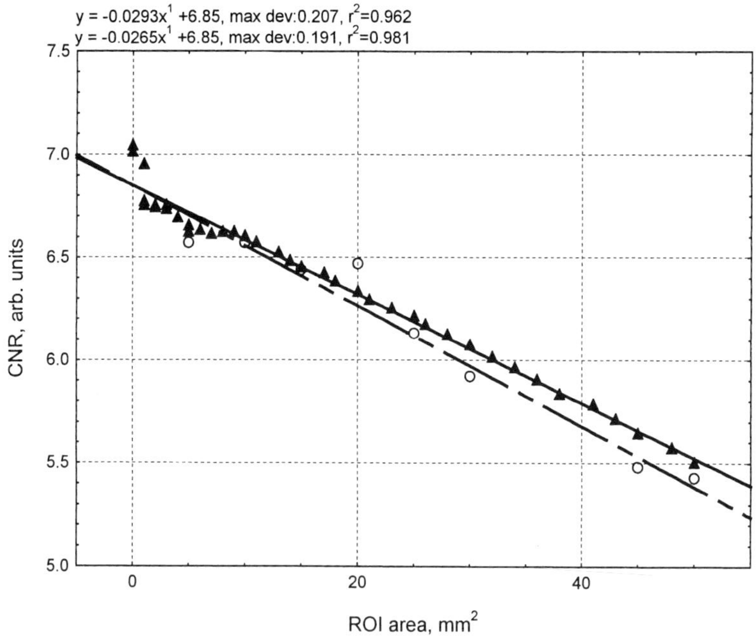

Figure 1. Correlation of CNR results obtained with manual (o) and automated ( ) procedures. Lines show least square fits of experimental data by linear functions (on top).

IV. COMPARISON OF THE MANUAL AND AUTOMATED CNR AND SNR EVALUATION

Comparison of the manual and automated calculation of CNR is shown in Figure 2. These data were obtained from the evaluation of 39 phantom images. Generally, results of the manual CNR calculation are higher than ones obtained with automated procedure. This was caused by the ROI for manual evaluation always being (for all studied images) the same area, 35 mm^2. Whereas, for the automated procedure ROI area was determined by subsequent iterations focused on the whole image of the largest mass and typically it was between 50 and 55 mm^2. Taking into account the observed dependence of CNR on ROI area (Figure 1) one should expect this reduction. Even better correlation for SNR evaluated by both methods was achieved.

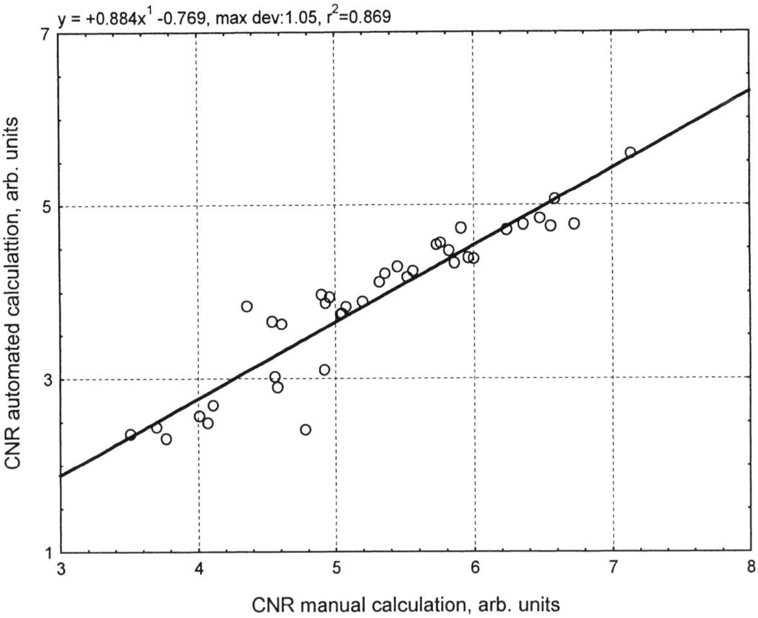

Figure 2. Correlation of CNR calculations by manual and automated methods. Solid line shows least square fit of experimental data by linear function (on the top).

V. APPLICATION OF THE AUTOMATED PROCEDURE TO A LORAD MAMMOGRAPHY SYSTEM

The Lorad mammography system is very different from GE Senographe 2000D and that is why it was selected to check the utility of the developed software for CNR and SNR automated calculation. Lorad mammography systems use a full-field detector that is fabricated as a mosaic of 3 x 4 of the detectors modules; each of which consists of a phosphor X-ray absorber on the surface of a square de-magnifying fiber optic taper. The taper couples the phosphor to an area CCD array. Demagnification leads to signal loss, which reduces the SNR of the images when compared with a GE system where there is no demagnification. The dimension of Lorad individual detector element is approximately 40 μm whereas the GE Senographe 2000D is 100 μm. Perhaps because of lower SNR for Lorad, it was suggested to use an acrylic contrast disc, which is brighter than phantom wax inserts, for SNR and CNR measurements. The newly developed automated procedure was able to calculate SNR and CNR based on both contrast disc and phantom largest mass (as GE recommends). Figure 3 shows high correlation between CNR values calculated by the two methods from 49 phantom images taken with Lorad mammography system. Similar correlation was observed between SNR values calculated by these two methods for the same Lorad images.

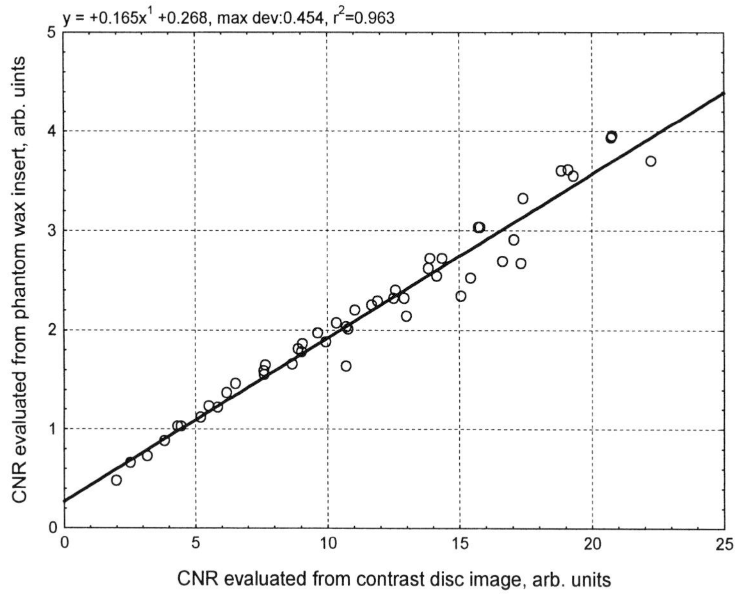

Figure 3. Correlation of CNR calculations with automated procedure based on the measurements of the largest phantom mass (GE methodology) and contract disc (Lorad methodology) image intensities. Solid line shows the least square fit with linear function (on the top).

VI. CONCLUSIONS

These experiments have demonstrated a strong dependence of CNR on the selected ROI area. In order to avoid the impact of this effect when comparing CNR data obtained from different sources one could consider to use its limit to the zero ROI area instead of current practice of the use of some fixed ROI area.

The newly developed automated procedure of CNR and SNR evaluations has shown good correlation with results of their determination by manual method. However, it has superior precision, which gives potential to study finer effects of image quality. Another result of the procedure is that it can be applied to CNR and SNR tests on more than GE mammography systems.

Interpretation of Contrast Detail Images in Digital Mammography: Human Observer versus Computer Detection

K.R. Bijkerk, L.J. Oostveen, R.E. van Engen, M.M.J. Swinkels and W.J.H. Veldkamp

National Expert and Training Centre for Breast Cancer Screening, University Medical Centre Nijmegen, LRCB 451, P.O. Box 9101, 6500 HB Nijmegen, the Netherlands
r.bijkerk@lrcb.azn.nl

1. Introduction

To evaluate the image quality of digital mammography systems, a contrast-detail phantom (CDMAM 3.4) was developed at our institution [1]. The phantom has been designed to enable image quality assessment by a human observer, by determining threshold contrast of an imaging system as a function of object diameter.

Because human assessment of phantom images is rather time consuming, and observers tend to differ in detection capabilities (making readings by a team of observers necessary), a computer program was developed for this task [2]. However, until now investigation of the correspondance of this method with human observer assessment has been limited to digitized film-screen images at one X-ray setting, assessed by a single observer.

In this article, possible differences between the two methods have been evaluated for direct digital mammography, at settings leading to various image quality. Both hard- and softcopy human readings have been compared to computer detection.

2. Method and Materials

Phantom images were made on a GE Senographe 2000D digital mammography unit (a-Si detector with 100 μm pixel size). The 14 bit, unprocessed images were used for the evaluation. Eight images were made at each of the settings mentioned in table 1. The phantom was centered between the additional plexiglass plates. It was repositioned after each exposure, to obtain images with various phantom-object positions with respect to the pixels of the detector. Softcopy images were evaluated on a GE Senographe 2000D Review Workstation (2K CRT's). Hardcopy images were printed with a Kodak DryView 8600 Laser Imager (40 μm pixel size) and evaluated on a viewing box. Two images per setting were evaluated by 4 experienced observers, at an optimized contrast representation (optimum window width and level), giving a total of eight hardcopy and softcopy readings per setting. Eight images per setting were assessed by the computer program. The program, described in detail by Karssemeijer [2], uses the ideal observer model for detection of the phantom objects.

3. Results and Discussion

Contrast-detail curves of computer and human readings (both hard- and softcopy) at different settings are shown in figure 1A - D. The computer curves are plotted at a contrast detection threshold of 62.5 %, halfway the psychometric curve described by Karssemeijer [2]. The human readings (mean values of eight observations) are plotted through the lowest correctly indicated disk thickness at each diameter, as described in the phantom manual [3]. Contrast detection thresholds are not plotted when either the whole column of disks or no disks at a certain diameter were correctly detected.

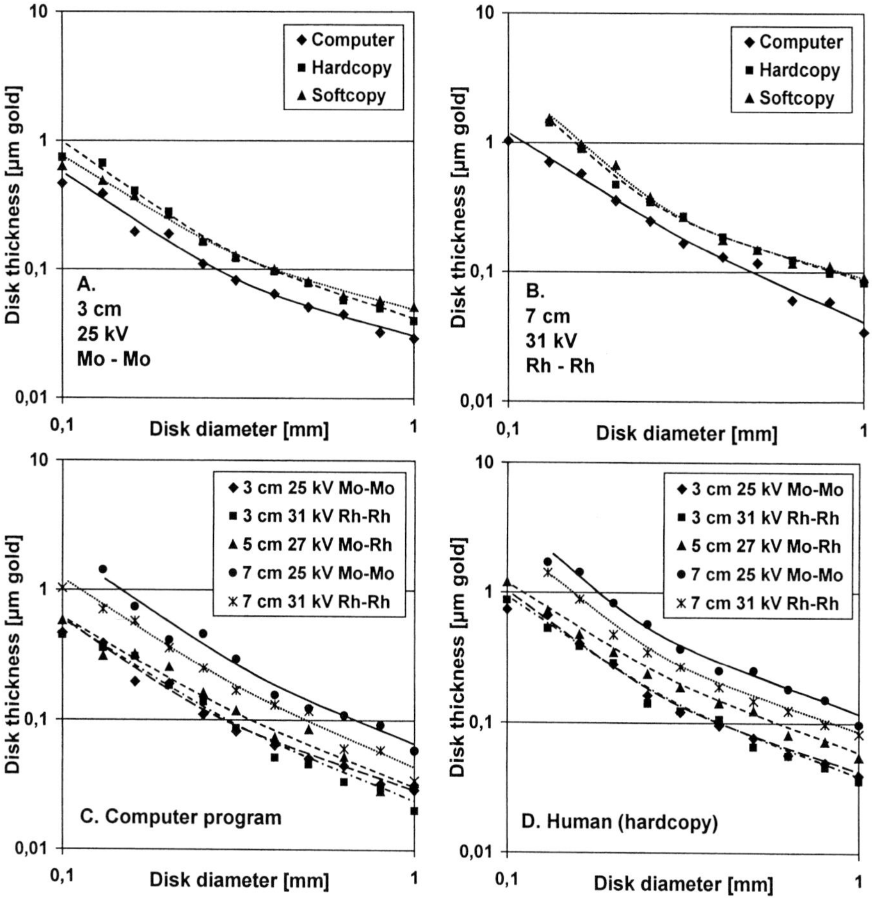

Fig. 1. CD-curves of the GE 2000D for different X-ray spectra and plexiglass thicknesses.

From figure 1A and B, where CD-curves of 3 and 7 cm plexiglass are shown for the softest and hardest X-ray spectra respectively, it appears that the performance of the computer program is significantly better than that of the human observers, as was also found by Karssemeijer [2] for digitized FS-images. Hard- and softcopy readings appear to be reasonably comparable, although there might be a difference in curve shape (see for example figure 1A). From figure 1C and D, where computer program and human (hardcopy) CD-curves are compared for all settings, it appears that both methods give the same ranking of image quality. This is also shown in table 1, where the contrast detail curves are quantified by calculating the Image Quality Figure (IQF, described in the phantom manual [3]) for all reading methods. Additionally, table 1 shows that the computer detects no significant difference in image quality at 3 cm plexiglass for the different X-ray techniques used (see also figure 1C), and the hardcopy and softcopy readings give a different ranking in image quality.

Table 1. Image Quality Figures of the three reading methods at the different X-ray settings

X-ray settings and Entrance Exposure				Computer	Hardcopy	Softcopy
3 cm	Rh-Rh	31 kV	3.0 mGy	0.303	0.446	0.501
3 cm	Mo-Mo	25 kV	4.1 mGy	0.308	0.479	0.474
5 cm	Mo-Rh	27 kV	8.7 mGy	0.381	0.640	0.719
7 cm	Rh-Rh	31 kV	12.9 mGy	0.602	0.981	1.064
7 cm	Mo-Mo	25 kV	18.2 mGy	0.917	1.434	1.627

4. Conclusions

It is reasonable to assume that the differences between the human and computer CD-curves are not entirely caused by a superiority in detection capabilities of the computer program. The computer only has to deal with the image produced by the digital detector, whereas human perception is influenced to some uncertain extent by the medium used for presentation of the information (in this case CRT-display and viewing box), as well as the viewing conditions. Consequently, adaptation of the program to the perception of a human observer, for instance by changing the computer contrast detection threshold level, is not desirable nor correctly possible.

The presented results show that computer detection can be used efficiently to evaluate image quality differences as far as the digital detector is concerned (see figure 1C and D and table 1). However, to evaluate the quality of the whole imaging chain, including representation of the images and viewing conditions, human assessment of CDMAM-phantom images appears to be necessary.

References

1. Bijkerk, K.R., Thijssen, M.A.O., Arnoldussen, Th.J.M.: Modification of the CDMAM Contrast-Detail Phantom for Image Quality Evaluation of Full-Field Digital Mammography Systems. In: Yaffe, M.J. (ed.): IWDM 2000 5th International Workshop on Digital Mammography. Medical Physiscs Publishing, Madison, Wisconsin (2001) 633-640
2. Karssemeijer, N., Thijssen, M.A.O.: Determination of contrast-detail curves of mammography systems by automated image analysis. In: Doi, K., Giger, M.L., Nishikawa, R.M., Schmidt, R.A. (eds.): Digital Mammography. Elsevier, Amsterdam (1996) 155-160
3. Bijkerk, K.R., Thijssen, M.A.O., Arnoldussen, Th.J.M.: Manual CDMAM-phantom type 3.4 University Medical Centre Nijmegen, 6500 HB Nijmegen, the Netherlands (2002)

Automated scoring for CD-MAM phantom on digital mammography

Serge Muller[1], Cybèle Ciofolo[1], Guillaume Peter[1], Alain Noël[2], Joseph Stinès[2]

[1] GE Medical Systems, 283 rue de la minière, 78533 Buc, France
serge.muller@med.ge.com
[2] Centre Alexis Vautrin, avenue de Bourgogne, 54511 Vandoeuvre-les-Nancy cedex, France
j.stines@nancy.fnclcc.fr

Abstract. We developed an automated scoring algorithm for the CDMAM phantom on digital mammography. The Non-Pre-Whitening observer has been implemented. For each phantom cell, the entropy of the corresponding log-likelihood function calculated around each potential insert location is minimised to determine the location of the insert. Using several images, the detection of an insert is accepted if the lower bound of the 95% confidence interval for the correct detection proportion is superior to 0.25, making the scoring more robust. The standard Image Quality Factor is estimated to compare the image quality of a Senographe 2000D™ under different acquisition conditions. Correlation with human observer scores is established.

1. Introduction

Quality control is of paramount importance in mammography. Protocols have been established to monitor the quality of each step in the image chain generation and display. Phantom scoring is widely used to assess the detection performance of human readers from images acquired with a given imaging system and reviewed on a given image display equipment. However, phantom scoring presents some drawbacks. A limited discrimination capability between system configurations may happen with phantoms composed of a low number of inserts (e.g., RMI, MTM100[1]). On the other hand, phantoms with large number of inserts are leading to time consuming and tedious experimental protocols (e.g., CDMAM). Replacing human observers with mathematical observers makes automated scoring of phantom a potential alternative to the assessment and the comparison of system imaging performance.

2. Automated scoring of CDMAM phantom

To assess the performance of the detection task, we used the CDMAM 3.4 contrast-detail phantom developed in Nijmegen for quality control of mammography systems [2]. The CDMAM phantom consists of a matrix of squares. Each square contains two identical gold disks of given thickness and diameter. One disk is placed in the center and the second in a randomly chosen corner. The observer has to indicate the corner where the eccentric disk is located. The phantom covers a range of object sizes and thicknesses representing microcalcifications and small masses. The object diameters range between 60 microns and 2 mm. The object thickness range between 0.03 and 2 microns of gold.

The cells are first localized using morphological openings with linear structuring elements. We implemented a mathematical Non-Pre-Whitening (NPW) observer for the detection task. Better results were obtained using this observer compared to either the Hotelling or the ideal Bayesian observers. The NPW observer is represented with the following log-likelihood function, which is estimated for the four corners of each phantom cell:

$$\lambda_{NPW} = \left(\bar{g}_a - \bar{g}_b\right)^t \cdot g \tag{1}$$

where $\bar{g}_a$ is the mean signal estimated on a ROI including the central disk of a given phantom cell, $\bar{g}_b$ is the mean background estimated on a ROI including no insert, and g is the tested signal corresponding to a ROI including successively one of the four corners of the current phantom cell.

The λ_{NPW} value is sensitive to the exact insert position, especially for small diameter disks. To overcome this issue, we estimate λ_{NPW} for each cell corner at 49 positions (7x7 pixel matrix) around the nominal position of the expected disk insert. We select the corner with the lowest entropy calculated from the λ_{NPW} surface as the one containing the insert. This approach makes robust the scoring to positioning uncertainties in the range of $\pm$ 300 μm.

Using several images acquired under the same conditions, it becomes possible to make the detection more robust to statistical fluctuations. We accept the detection of an insert if the lower bound of the 95% confidence interval (CI) for the correct detection proportion is strictly superior to 0.25, which corresponds to a blind decision. The CI is calculated with the Wilson method that is well suited for small number of images [3].

Finally, the standard CDMAM correcting rules are applied to eliminate detection made by chance in some cells. The results can be presented through curves representing the smallest detected insert diameter versus insert thickness. The Image Quality Factor (IQF) is used as a global indicator of performance with the highest values related to highest scores:

$$IQF = 16 / \sum_{i=1}^{16} C_i . D_{i,\min} \tag{2}$$

where $D_{i,\min}$ is the smallest diameter perceived in column i corresponding to a gold thickness C_i.

Series of images have been recorded on a GE Senographe 2000D™ [4] for 4.5 cm equivalent breast thickness, different entrance doses (32 and 100 mAs) and for calibrated and non-calibrated detector of the mammography unit. Under each imaging condition up to 12 images have been recorded and our automated scoring algorithm has been applied. Five human observers, including 2 radiologists, read 3 times one image of each series in random order.

We find $IQF = 10.96$ for images of the CDMAM phantom acquired at 100 mAs and $IQF = 8.16$ at 32 mAs, demonstrating the ability of our automated scoring algorithm to differentiate image quality variations related to dose modifications.

We find $IQF = 10.96$ for images of the CDMAM phantom acquired on a calibrated system at 100 mAs and $IQF = 8.99$ on a non calibrated system, demonstrating the ability of our automated scoring algorithm to differentiate calibrated from non calibrated digital mammography systems. An analysis of variance demonstrated that the only significant source of variability is the inter-observer variability (p=0.02). The intra-observer variability is the second leading source of variance (p=0.1) before the calibration variability.

We observe correlated results between the mean human observer and the mathematical observer. Higher IQF values for the mathematical observer lead to higher detection sensitivity.

3. Conclusion

We developed an automated scoring algorithm for the CDMAM phantom on digital mammography that correlates with human observer scores. Using this algorithm, it is possible to differentiate images acquired at different dose levels or with different detector calibration status. Further experimentation are needed to determine the sensitivity of our algorithm to various acquisition parameters in order to validate its use for quality control in screening mammography.

Acknowledgements

This work has been supported by the French Ministry of Research under Grant N° 00B018001.

References

1. Noël, A., Stinès, J., Zerhouni, M.: Développement d'un fantôme en matériau équivalent-sein pour la mammographie. RBM, Vol. 15-7 (1993) 412-423
2. Thijssen, M., Veldkamp, W., Van Engen, R., Swinkels, M., Karssemeijer, N., Hendricks, J.: Comparison of the detectability of small details in a film-screen and a digital mammography system by the imaging of a new CDMAM-phantom. IWDM 2000, Toronto, Yaffe, M. ed, Medical Physics Publishing, Madison, Wisconsin, 666-672.
3. Brown, L.D., Cai, T., DasGupta, A.: Interval estimation for a binomial proportion. Technical report, Department of Statistics, Purdue University, 1999.
4. Muller, S.: Full-field digital mammography designed as a complete system. Eur. J. Radiol. Vol. 31-1 (1999) 25-34

Comparison of experimental and theoretical assessments of detail visibility in digital mammography

David R Dance[1], Roger A Hunt[1], Anthony M Sajewicz[2], Walter Huda[2], Kent M Ogden[2], Michael Sandborg[3] and Gudrun Alm Carlsson[3]

[1]Joint Department of Physics, The Royal Marsden NHS Trust, Fulham Road, London SW3 6JJ, United Kingdom
[2]Department of Radiology, SUNY Upstate Medical University, 750 E Adams Street, Syracuse, NY 13210, USA
[3]Department of Radiation Physics, IMV, Faculty of Health Science, Linköping University, SE-581 85 LINKÖPING, Sweden
d.dance@icr.ac.uk

Abstract. An experimental and modelling study is being made of the influence of tube voltage, target material and exposure on the performance of digital mammography systems. Digital images of the ACR accreditation phantom at 80 mAs, 25-32 kV and at 28 kV, 5-500 mAs were read by eight observers, and the numbers of fibres, specks and masses visible determined. The computer model simulates photon transport through phantom, anti-scatter grid and image receptor. It calculates image pixels and the signal-to-noise ratio per pixel (SNR) for the phantom details. For exposures below 100 mAs, the numbers of fibres and masses visualised were found to be consistent with a constant SNR threshold for detection. For the visualisation of specks, the product of SNR and speck area was approximately constant. At higher mAs, the number of objects visualised was little influenced by exposure, due to the limited dynamic range of the phantom. The results validate the use of computational models to predict performance for simple detection tasks against a uniform background.

1. Introduction

In digital mammography it is possible to modify the image prior to display so that contrast requirements associated with screen-film mammography may be relaxed. In addition, because of the improved dynamic range and DQE, it may be possible to reduce the dose for imaging with a given radiation quality or to use a different radiation quality, with further dose saving.

We are making an experimental and computer modeling study of the influence of user-controllable parameters such as exposure, tube voltage and target material on the performance of digital mammography systems. In this paper[1] we present the results of measurements and calculations of detail visibility for the ACR accreditation phantom (Gammex-RMI, Middleton, WI) imaged with a LoRad (Danbury, CT) digital mammography system at a series of tube voltage and exposure values.

[1] This work is supported in part by US Army grant No DAMD 17-00-1003375.

2. Materials and Methods

An ACR accreditation phantom was exposed using the LoRad digital mammography system and an x-ray spectrum from a Mo target/Mo filter. Images were acquired at 28 kV for 12 values of the exposure between 5-500 mAs and at 80 mAs for 8 values of the tube voltage between 25-32kV. The phantom contains sets of details which simulate fibrils (six nylon filaments with diameters between 0.40 - 1.56 mm), calcifications (six groups of alumina specks with sizes between 0.16 - 0.54 mm) and masses (water density objects of thicknesses between 0.25 - 2.00 mm). The soft-copy images were viewed under controlled conditions by eight readers and the number of objects of each type which were visible were scored [1].

The model used was based on a Monte Carlo computer program developed for modeling mammographic systems [2], and extended to treat the 'patient' as an array of voxels. For this case each voxel was composed of polymethyl methacrylate apart from a 5 mm layer of wax which contained the test details. The phantom was 45 mm thick and rested on a 2 mm thick carbon fibre support. The anti-scatter grid had ratio 5 and 31 lines.cm^{-1}. The x-ray spectra were adapted so that they matched measured HVL values. The image receptor was 73 mg.cm^{-2} CsI. The program could calculate mean glandular breast dose, entrance air kerma, the energy imparted per image pixel, image contrast and signal-to-noise ratio per pixel (SNR). In this way the SNR per pixel was calculated for each detail size and type, exposure and tube voltage.

In its present form, the model makes no allowance for image unsharpness. This will affect the estimation of contrast for the smallest details and of the fractional noise per pixel, both of which will decrease.

3. Results and Discussion

Figure 1 shows the calculated (normalised) SNR per pixel for the smallest detail detected by the observers at 28 kV for exposures between 5 and 160 mAs. The results are for the detection of nylon filaments (left) and masses (right). The central value of the SNR at each mAs corresponds to the size of the smallest detectable detail averaged over observers. The error bars represent one standard deviation. The different data points thus correspond to the detection of objects of different sizes. The size of the smallest detectable object and the associated image contrast become smaller as the exposure increases because there is an associated decrease in the image noise.

In both cases, for exposures of 80 mAs and below, the SNR for the smallest detail visualised is consistent with a constant value. In other words, objects are detected when the SNR exceeds a threshold value. Above 80 mAs, some observers see all 6 filaments and the calculated SNR increases and no longer represents the threshold value. A similar comment applies to the masses. In this case, only 4 out of 5 of the masses were generally seen at the higher exposures, which may relate to the fixed display window used for the experiments and the low contrast of the smallest mass (1% at 28 kV). The absolute values of the threshold SNR per pixel are different for the masses and filaments. This is because the imaging tasks are different. The first involves the detection of long thin cylinders of low contrast (where the detection task may involve integration along the length of the cylinder) whereas the second involves the detection of circular, medium to large diameter low contrast objects.

The results for the specks differed from those for the filaments and masses. In this case, the objects are small and circular and it was found that for low mAs values, the product of the SNR per pixel and the area for the smallest detectable speck was approximately constant. In other words for small round objects, the total signal (integrated over the image of the detail) is strongly correlated with dectability.

The calculations of SNR for the smallest details detected in the experiments where the kV was varied show similar behaviour to those where the mAs was varied.

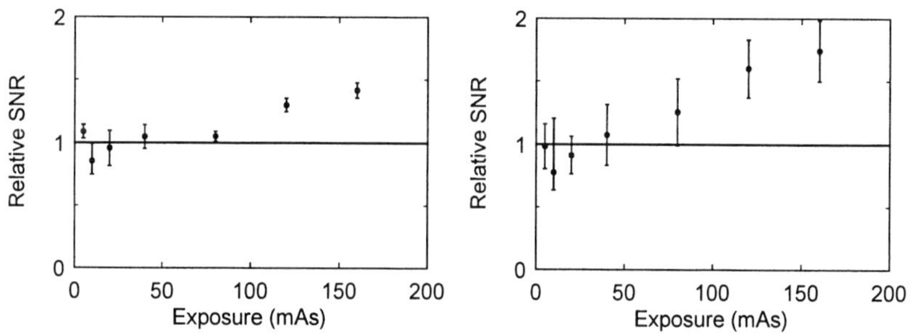

Fig. 1. Relative values of the calculated SNR corresponding to the smallest detectable filament and mass (*left and right figures*) as a function of exposure at 28 kV. Values are normalised to the mean of the first five data points (*horizontal line*).

4. Conclusion

The SNR calculated by the computer model can be used to predict the detectability of simulated fibrils, calcifications and masses against a uniform background. Since the model can also estimate mean glandular dose, it forms a useful tool for the optimisation of the exposure conditions (mAs, kV, target material and filter) so that dose can be minimised for these simple detection tasks. How these tasks relate to the detection of abnormality against a structured background needs to be established.

References

1. Huda, W., Sajewicz, A.M., Ogden K.M., Scalzetti, E.M., Dance, D.R.: How good is the ACR accreditation phantom for assessing image quality in digital mammography? Acad. Radiol. (2002) In press
2. Dance, D. R., Thilander-Klang, A., Sandborg, M., Skinner, C. L., Castellano Smith, I., and Alm Carlsson, G.: Influence of anode/filter material and tube potential on contrast, signal-to-noise ratio and average absorbed dose in mammography: a Monte Carlo study, Br. J. Radiology 73 (2000) 1056-1067

Comparison of objective and subjective methods to assess imaging performance in digital mammography

Walter Huda[1], Kent Ogden[1], Anthony Sajewicz[1], David Dance[2], Ernest Scalzetti[1]

[1]Radiology, SUNY Upstate Medical University, Syracuse NY 13210
[2]Joint Department of Physics, The Royal Marsden NHS Trust, London SW3 6JJ
hudaw@mail.upstate.edu

Abstract. Digital images were acquired of an anthropomorphic breast phantom (Rachel) at mAs values that ranged from 40 to 120 mAs. Digital mammograms were obtained with/without added lesions, which permitted the generation of a digital version of the lesion alone. The lesion was added back to the digital image of the Rachel phantom at varying levels of contrast. A subjective method of lesion visibility was compared to an objective method used Four Alternate Forced Choice (4AFC) methodology. Both methods showned observer performance for detecting a mass lesion to be *independent* of x-ray tube output between 40 and 120 mAs. The objective approach results in a higher precision, but alo requires many more images.

1. Introduction

The assessment of imaging performance in digital mammography is important for selecting the optimum technique factors (kVp/mAs) and for evaluating the utility of new image processing algorithms. For example, it is of considerable interest to determine the effect of x-ray tube output (mAs) on observer performance [1]. In this study, we compared a subjective imaging performance approach with an objective method for assessing how lesion detection changes with increasing mAs in digital mammography.

2. Method

2.1 Digital image acquisition

Digital images were obtained of an anthropomorphic breast phantom (Rachel) using a Lorad Full Field Digital Mammography imaging system at four mAs values (i.e., 40, 60, 90 and 120 mAs). Digital mammograms were made with/without added lesions, which permitted the generation of a digital version of the lesion alone. The 1 cm diameter lesion was added back to the digital image of the Rachel phantom alone at varying levels of contrast. The threshold contrast level for detection was investigated as a function of the mAs using three observers.

2.2 Observer assessment

For a given mAs, the lesion intensity (Scaling Factor/SF) was modified to produce six images where lesion visibility (i.e., contrast) ranged from the "extremely difficult" to "easily seen". Five copies of these 24 different images (4 mAs values & 6 SF factors) were generated to produce a series of 120 images which were presented to each observer in a single reading. Observers specified a probability of a lesion being present on a scale ranging from 0 to 100% which permitted the subjective scaling factor value for a 50% probability to be obtained at each mAs value [2].

The objective method used Four Alternate Forced Choice (4AFC) methodology with an observer identifying which one of four images actually contained the lesion. The results permitted the objective scaling factor to be determined as the value at which the observer accuracy was 92% at each mAs value. An accuracy of 92% corresponds to a theoretical signal to noise ratio of 2.5 (d') [3].

3. Results

3.1 Objective results

Figure 1 (left) shows the results obtained in the objective 4 AFC experiment, where SF for 92% accuracy is plotted as a function of mAs, with each datum the average (± standard deviation) for three observers. The coefficient of determination for the least squares linear fit to the four data points (r^2) was 0.59.

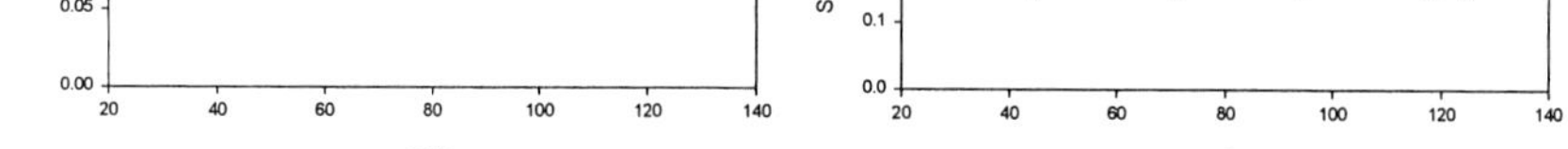

Figure 1. Comparison of objective (4 AFC) and subjective assessments of observer performance.

These data also show no significant correlation between SF(92%) and mAs. The average SF for a 92% correct score was 0.20, and the average coefficient of variation at the four mAs values was 8%.

3.2 Subjective results

Figure 1 (right) shows the results obtained in the subjective experiment, where SF at 50% observer confidence level is plotted as a function of mAs. The coefficient of determination for the least squares linear fit to the four data points (r^2) was 0.18, and these data clearly show that changing the mAs had no effect on observer performance. The average SF for a confidence score of 50% was 0.46 for this mass lesion, and the average coefficient of variation at the four mAs values was 24%.

4. Discussion

The results of both subjective and objective methods of assessing observer performance gave similar trends of performance as a function of the mAs used to acquire these digital images. There was no evidence of any significant change in observer performance as the x-ray tube output increased by a factor of three from 40 to 120 mAs.

The precision (coefficient of variation) in the subjective method was a factor of three larger than the corresponding precision with the 4 AFC approach. In part, this is due to the fact that the subjective method required an observer to read 30 images, whereas the 4 AFC approach required 128. The absolute level of scaling factor differed markedly between the two approaches; the subjective method requiring an SF value of 0.46 to achieve a confidence score of 50%, whereas a SF of 0.21 resulted in a observers achieving a 92% correct score.

Both subjective and objective modes of evaluating observer performance have advantages. The 4AFC method is clearly superior, but is also much more labor intensive. The subjective approach can be performed quickly, with *all* the images read in a random manner in a single sitting that will minimize systematic errors. The most appropriate method thus depends on the specific scientific task at hand, with the subjective approach useful for performing pilot studies and the objective method ideal for obtaining definitive scientific results.

Acknowledgement. This work was supported in part by a US Army Grant No. DAMD 17-00-1003375. AE Burgess provided invaluable assistance in the development of the four AFC method.

References

1. Huda W, Sajewicz A, Ogden KM, and Scalzetti EM. "How good is the ACR accreditation phantom for measuring image quality in digital mammography?". *Academic Radiology* (2002) *(In press)*

2. Sajewicz A, Huda W, Hseuh D, Ogden KM, Scalzetti EM. "Observer performance and radiographic technique factors in digital mammography." SPIE Medical Imaging (2002) *(In press)*

3. Burgess AE. Comparison of receiver operating characteristic and forced choice observer performance measurement methods. *Medical Physics* 22 (1995) 643-655.

Dose Reduction in Full-Field Digital Mammography – An Anthropomorphic Breast Phantom Study.

Silvia Obenauer, Klaus-Peter Hermann and Eckhardt Grabbe

Department of Diagnostic Radiology, Georg-August-University Göttingen, Robert-Koch-Str. 40, 37 075 Göttingen, Germany
soben@med.uni-goettingen.de

Abstract. The goal of this study was to evaluate the potential of radiation dose reduction in full-field digital mammography (FFDM) compared to screen-film mammography (SFM). An anthropomorphic breast phantom with superimposed microcalcifications (50-200μm) was used to evaluate the detectability of microcalcifications. Images were exposed automatically (AEC mode) using a Mo/Mo anode-filter-combination (protocol A). Dose reduction in digital mammography was achieved by using protocol B with Mo/Rh and protocol C with Rh/Rh. The detectability of microcalcifications was assessed by 3 well-experienced readers with a confidence level ranging from 1 to 5. A receiver operating characteristic (ROC) analysis was performed. Compared to screen-film mammography the digital mammography system allows an equivalent detection rate for microcalcifications at a lower radiation exposure.

1. Introduction

Screen-film mammography systems reach a spatial resolution of approximately 12-15 lp/mm whereas spatial resolution of digital systems is about 5 lp/mm (Feig et al 1995; Hermann et al. 2000; Muller 1999, Pisano 2000, Shtern 1992, Yaffee et al. 1997). As shown previously a dose reduction by lowering mAs results in an immediate loss of microcalcification detectability due to increasing noise (Muller 1999; Obenauer et al 2000). The presented study compares the potential for patient dose reduction by use of other anode-filter-combinations and higher tube voltages in full-field digital mammography (FFDM) compared to a state-of-the-art conventional screen-film system and analyses the effect on the detectability of microcalcifications in an anthropomorphic breast phantom.

2. Material and Methods

The study was performed using an FFDM (Senographe 2000D) and a conventional system (Senographe DMR, both GE Medical Systems, Buc, France). The digital detector is composed of a cesium iodide scintillator with an amorphous silicon detector. The pixel size is 100 μm. After exposure, the images are displayed on the high resolution monitors (2k x 2.5k) of the review workstation. For the conventional screen-film system, a dedicated mammographic screen-film combination (UM-MA film with UM-MA fine screen, Fuji Photo Film, Tokyo, Japan) was used. An anthropomorphic breast phantom with superimposed microcalcifications was used to evaluate the detectability of microcalcifications with a confidence level ranging from 1 to 5. A breast specimen proven to be free of microcalcifications was embedded in a 4 cm paraffin block and superimposed with an acrylic test plate. 13 of the 25 pits were chosen randomly and filled with a variable number of eggshell fragments of a defined size between 50 and 200 μm to simulate clusters of microcalcifications. By rotating the plate, a set of four images with different patterns of microcalcifications was obtained providing a total number of 100 test fields. Contact mammograms and magnification views (m=1.8) obtained with both the digital and the screen-film system were compared. The digital images were obtained at a radiation dose equivalent to that selected by the AEC mode of the screen-film system (protocol A). Digital images acquired at a lowered radiation dose were performed using protocol B with Mo/Rh and protocol C with Rh/Rh anode-filter-combination (table1). A receiver operating characteristic (ROC) analysis was performed by 3 readers.

Table 1: Different dose values for the protocol A-C.

System	Technique	Anode/filter kVp/mAs	ESAK (mGy) = %
SFM	m=1.1	Mo/Mo 27/63	5.30 = 100
	m=1.8	Mo/Mo 28/63	15.56 = 100
FFDM-A	m=1.1	Mo/Mo 27/63	5.19 = 98
	m=1.8	Mo/Mo 28/63	13.89 = 89
FFDM-B	m=1.1	Mo/Rh 31/28	3.04 = 57
	m=1.8	Mo/Rh 31/36	9.13 = 59
FFDM-C	m=1.1	Rh/Rh 32/20	2.48 = 47
	m=1.8	Rh/Rh 32/18	5.89 = 38

3. Results

The ROC analysis demonstrated a higher performance of the digital images compared to the screen-film mammograms. The ROC curves indicate that the digital imaging technique represented the better diagnostic method than the screen-film mammography with the curves running more closely to the left upper corner. The ROC curves of the digital system for the protocols A - C are plotted for contact and magnification views in comparison to the conventional system (figure 1a+b).

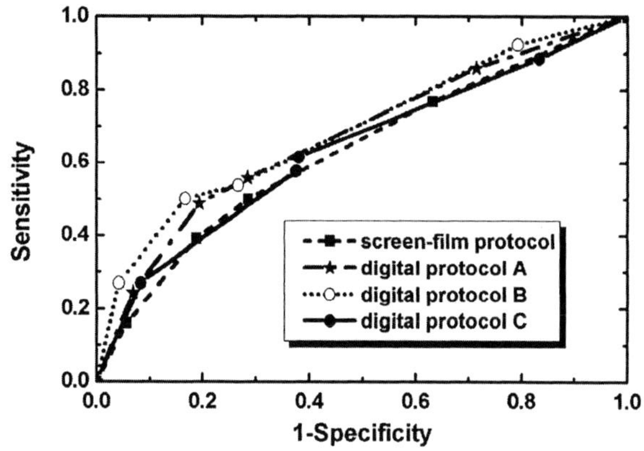

a)

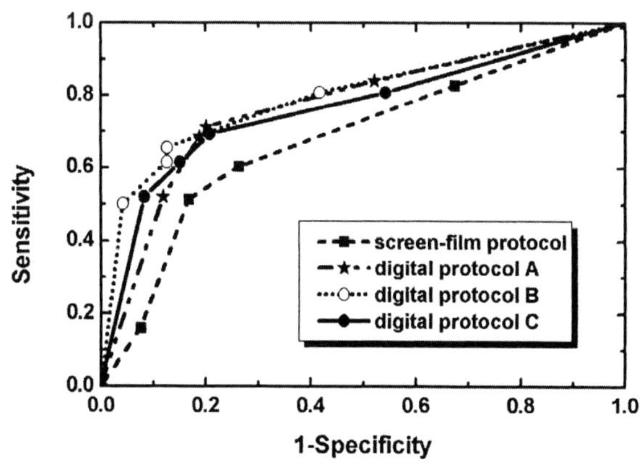

b)

Figure 1a+b ROC curves of the dose reduction protocols B (Mo/Rh/31kVp) and C (Rh/Rh/32kVp) in comparison to the ROC-curves in screen-film and digital mammography at 100% dose (protocol A). Contact (a) and magnification views (m=1.8) (b).

4. Discussion

Lowering dose by just reducing the mAs has been shown to result in a diminished detectability of microcalcifications (Obenauer et al. 2000). In the presented study, therefore, patient dose was reduced by varying the radiation quality and the effect on the detectability of microcalcifications was analysed. With this method the dose to the patient is reduced without changing the dose to the detector. Our preliminary results suggest that this modification has an advantage over just lowering the tube current. Microcalcification detectability was equivalent to that in conventional images at about 50% of the radiation exposure.

References

1. Feig S.A., Yaffe M.J. Digital mammography, computer-aided diagnosis, and telemammography. Breast Imaging (1995) 33: 1205-1230
2. Hermann K.-P., Obenauer S., Grabbe E. Comparison of radiation exposure between a digital amorphous silicon and a screen-film based mammography system. Fortschr Röntgenstr (2000) 172: 940-945
3. Muller S. Full-field digital mammography designed as a complete system. Eur. Radiol. (1999) 31: 25-34
4. Obenauer S., Hermann K.-P., Schorn C., Fischer U., Grabbe E.. Full-field digital mammography: dose–dependant detectability of simulated breast lesions. Fortschr. Röntgenstr. (2000) 172: 1052 - 1056
5. Pisano E.D. Current status of full-field digital mammography. Radiology (2000) 214: 26-28
6. Shtern F. Digital mammography and related technologies: a perspective from the national cancer institute. Radiology (1992) 183: 629-630
7. Yaffe M.J., Rowlands J.A. X-ray detectors for digital radiography. Phys. Med. Biol. (1997) 42: 1-39

Evaluation of the exposure dose reduction in Full-Field Digital Mammography System

Tanigoshi M, Kobayashi H,Uchiyama N,Suzuki T, Kumazaki T

Department of Radiology , Nippon Medical School , 1-1-5 Sendagi, Bunkyo-ku Tokyo, Japan m-tani@nms.ac.jp

Abstract. We evaluated image quality characteristic of full-fielddigital mammography (Senographe 2000D ; GEMS , CR-AL film ;FUJIFILM) system in comparison with screen film mammography(Senographe DMR+ ;GEMS , Min-R 2000/Min-R 2000 ; Kodak) systemand investigated the possibility of exposure dose reduction in FFDMsystem. To evaluate each systems image quality characteristics, wemeasured characteristic curve, modulation transfer function (MTF)value , and wiener spectrum (W.S) value. image qualities and observer performance by RMI-156 phantom and CDMAM phantom were alsoevaluated in accordance with the change of exposure dose. W.S value of FFDM become equal to that of SFM system in the amount of 60% exposure dose . The phantom studies reveled that the observer performance of FFDM system was also superior to that of SFM system. Those results indicated the possibility of exposure dose reduction in FFDM.

Introduction

The use of high DQE(u) for full-field digital mammography (FFDM) is generally preferable to the use of screen-film mammography (SFM). This suggests the possibility of reducing the exposure dose for FFDM; however, its image qualities are dependent on the radiation dose. In the present study, we physically and visually investigated exposure-dose reduction in FFDM. As diagnostic imaging is generally performed using hard copies rather than CRT monitors in Japan, the overall performance of these two systems was assessed through a comparison of hard copies.

Material and method

Table 1 shows both screen-film and FFDM systems. For physical assessments, the overall digital-characteristic curves, overall W.S values, and overall MTF values were measured. With FFDM, in order to determine the relationship between radiation dose and noise characteristics, the overall W.S values were measured by varying the radiation dose from 4 mAs to 125 mAs. For visual assessments, the relationship between radiation dose and visual characteristics was investigated using RMI-156 and CD-MAM phantoms.

Table 1. Comparison of System

FFDM	Screen Film
Fuji FM-DRL	Fuji CEPROS M2 32.5° 90sec
Fuji CR-AL	Kodak Min-R2000/Min-R2000
Senographe 2000 D	DMR

Results

At a comparable radiation dose, the noise characteristics for FFDM were clearly superior to those for SFM. In addition, the results of W.S analyses showed that a similar level of noise was seen with FFDM when only approximately 60% of the SFM dose was used (Figure 1). When a grid and the RMI-156 phantom were used to simulate mammography in clinical settings, the detection of calcified lesions and tumors for FFDM was comparable when only approximately 60% of the incident SFM dose was used. Furthermore, with the CD-MAM phantom, the results for FFDM were comparable when 90% of the SFM dose was used.

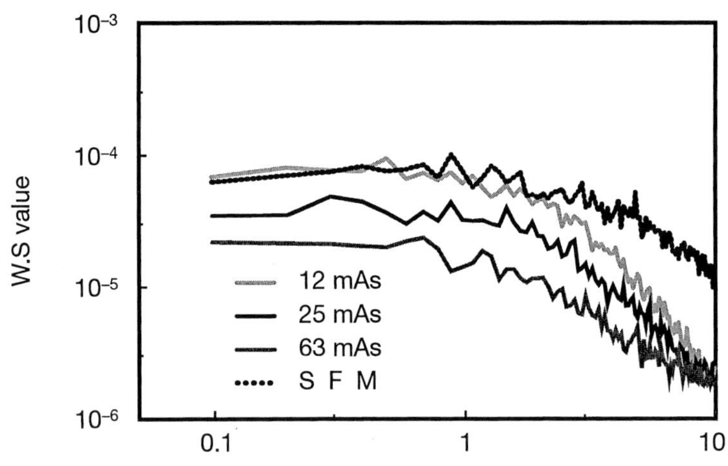

Figure 1. Comparison of overall W.S values in relation to different radiation doses and SFM

Discussion

The results of the physical assessments showed that the noise characteristics of FFDM were more favorable than those of SFM, and that a comparable noise level was obtained by FFDM using approximately 60% of the SFM dose. Nonetheless, from the viewpoint of S/N, as the MTF value for FFDM was lower than that for SFM, the radiation dose of FFDM cannot simply be lowered. The results of the CD-MAM analysis supported this view. In addition, there were differences in the degree of radiation dose reduction between the two phantoms, and one study found that the detection of small calcified lesions was determined by the limits on X-ray quantum statistics [1]. As a result, the range of clinically effective dose reduction requires investigation.

Acknowledgements

We would like to express our deepest gratitude to Makoto Iriuchijima at GE Yoga Medical Systems for his valuable assistance in conducting the present study

References

Roehrig H, KrupinskiEA, DallasWJ.Necessary spatial resolution indigital mammography. In: Lemke HU et al., editors. Computer Assisted Radiology.Elsevier Science,1996;53-59

Optimization of Digital Subtraction Mammography using Monte Carlo simulation of the imaging chain

Gustaf Ullman[1], Michael Sandborg [1], David R Dance[2], Martin Yaffe[3], Mia Skarpathiotakis [3], Gudrun Alm Carlsson[1]

1. Department of Radiation Physics, IMV, Faculty of Health Sciences, Linköping University, SE-581 85 LINKÖPING Sweden
2. Joint Department of Physics, The Royal Marsden NHS Trust, Fulham Road, London SW3 6JJ, UK
3. Department of Medical Imaging and Medical Biophysics, Sunnybrook and Women's College Health Science Centre, University of Toronto, Ontario, M4N 3M5, Canada

gusul@imv.liu.se

Abstract. The aim of this work was to search for the optimal x-ray tube voltage (20-55 kV) and anode-filter combination (Mo/Rh, Rh/Cu, W/Cu) for digital iodine subtraction mammography. The optimum was defined as the combination minimizing the average glandular dose, AGD, for a fixed signal-to-noise ratio, SNR, for detecting an iodine contrast detail. For a 4 cm thick breast (50% glandularity) and conventional Mo/25μmRh spectrum, two shallow dose-minima were found at 28 kV and 47 kV. Using W/0.3mmCu, two local minima were also found at 23 kV and 46 kV; the AGD at the higher tube voltage was significantly lower and results in 3.8 times lower AGD (for SNR=5) than the Mo/Rh combination. The results for Rh/0.3mmCu are similar to W/Cu. The dose advantage using copper filtration is larger for thicker breasts. We conclude that an increase in tube voltage and added Cu-filtration will result in significant dose-advantage in digital iodine subtraction mammography.

1. Introduction

Digital radiological imaging make quantitative analysis of the images possible. Digital iodine subtraction mammography (or contrast digital mammography) is one such example, and its utility is being studied experimentally [1]. It is of interest to find the optimal x-ray spectrum for this examination. Several theoretical and experimental studies have been made for mammography in search for the optimal tube voltage and filter combination [2, 3], when the task was to detect micro-calcifications or tumors. In this work, we focus on the detection of iodine contrast media, injected in the patient during the mammography examination. Because of the energy of the K-edge in iodine (33.2 keV), the tube voltages in this study were increased beyond those usually employed in mammography imaging. To minimize the patient dose, additional filters of 0.3 mm Cu were used. For the simulations, we use a modified Monte Carlo computer program based on a model originally developed for conventional mammography [2].

2. Materials and Methods

The simulated imaging geometry is as follows. A 60 cm focus-detector distance was used. X-ray photon cross sections and soft tissue compositions were taken from [4] and [5], respectively. The model of the compressed breast consists of a homogeneous mixture of glandular (1.04 g/cm^3) and adipose (0.93 g/cm^3) tissue in the central region surrounded by 5 mm thick adipose shield, all in a semi-circular shape. The breast glandularity was kept constant at 50%, but the compressed breast thickness was varied between 2-8 cm. A small (2 mm) iodine detail was added in the model as the object for which the image quality was calculated. It had a projected density of 6 mg/cm^2 and a volume density of 1.027 g/cm^3. The anti-scatter grid had 18 μm lead strip width separated by 300 μm fiber material and a grid ratio of 5. The image detector consisted of 36 mg/cm^2 CsI with a pixel area of 0.01 mm^2. A computer program [6] generated the x-ray spectra using either Mo, Rh or W as anode material. Additional filters of 25 μm Rh or of 0.3 mm Cu were used.

In digital mammography, where the contrast can be adjusted, the most relevant measure of physical image quality is the signal-to-noise ratio, SNR here computed as

$$SNR = \frac{\left|\langle N_{p1}\rangle \cdot \langle \varepsilon_{p1}\rangle - \langle N_{p2}\rangle \cdot \langle \varepsilon_{p2}\rangle\right|}{\sqrt{\langle N_{p1}\rangle \cdot \langle \varepsilon^2_{p1}\rangle + \langle N_s\rangle \cdot \langle \varepsilon^2_s\rangle}} \tag{1}$$

where $\langle N_i\rangle$ is the expectation value of the number of photons incident at (i=1): a pixel adjacent to the contrast detail, and (i=2) a pixel within the shadow of the detail. The quantity $\langle N_s\rangle$ is the mean value of the number of scattered photons, here assumed equal for the two cases (i=1,2) above. The quantities $\langle \varepsilon\rangle$ and $\langle \varepsilon^2\rangle$ are the mean and mean squared value of the energy imparted to the image detector per incident photon. Only the quantum noise is considered here; other additional noise sources were assumed negligible. The effect of system unsharpness was also ignored.

The average glandular dose, AGD, was calculated in the following manner. The energy imparted for each interaction was shared between the glandular and adipose tissue in accordance to the tissue cross-sections and the breast composition. Finally, the AGD was normalized to a SNR of 5.

3.Results and discussion

Figure 1 shows the AGD in a 4 cm thick breast with 50% glandularity for a fixed SNR using the W/Cu, Rh/Cu and Mo/Rh anode/filter combinations. For the Rh/Cu and W/Cu spectra, there is a wide minimum in AGD for tube voltages around 46 kV. This is because of the increased contrast (hence signal) for photons above 33.2 keV (iodine's K-edge). Using the conventional Mo/Rh combination results in 3.8 larger minimum AGD than with W/Cu or Rh/Cu. The AGD using Mo/Rh anode/filter compared to using W/Cu or Rh/Cu is 5 times larger for breasts of 6 and 8 cm thickness but only 2 times larger for thin breasts (2 cm).

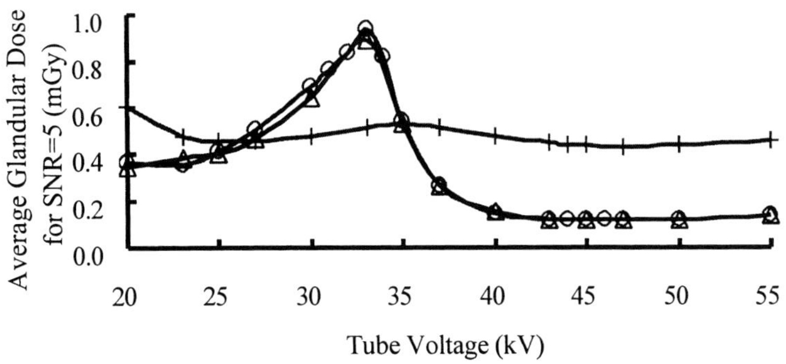

Figure 1. Average glandular dose AGD for SNR equal to 5 for detecting the iodine contrast detail as function of tube voltage for a breast of 4 cm thickness. Three different anode/filter combinations were used: +: Mo / 25 μm Rh, Δ: Rh / 0.3 mm Cu, o: W / 0.3 mm Cu.

4. Conclusions

The use of tube voltages 40-50 kV combined with Cu filtration results in a significant lower AGD for fixed SNR in iodine subtraction mammography compared to conventional Mo/Rh combination. The dose-advantage of using for example W/0.3mmCu or Rh/0.3mmCu instead of Mo/25μmRh is larger for thicker breasts.

References[1]

1. Skarpathiotakis, M., Bright, S., Yaffe, M., Jeunnehomme, F., Muller, S., Mainprize, J.: Selection of Technique Factors for Contrast Digital Mammography, SPIE Proc. (2002)
2. Dance, D. R., Thilander-Klang, A., Sandborg, M., Skinner, C. L., Castellano Smith, I., and Alm Carlsson, G.: Influence of anode/filter material and tube potential on contrast, signal-to-noise ratio and average absorbed dose in mammography: a Monte Carlo study, Br. J. Radiology 73 (2000) 1056-1067
3. Venkatakrishnan, V., Yavuz, M., Niklason, L. T., et al.: Experimental and theoretical spectral optimization for digital mammography, SPIE Proc. 3659 (1999) 142-149
4. Berger, J., Hubbell, J. H., and Seltzer, S. M.: XCOM: Photon Cross Section Database, URL: www.physics.nist.gov
5. Hammerstein, G. R., Miller, D. W., White, D. R., et al.: Absorbed Radiation Dose in Mammography, Radiology 130 (1987) 485-491
6. Birch, R., and Marshall, M.: Computation of Bremsstrahlung x-ray spectra and comparison with spectra measured with Ge(Li) detector, Phys. Med. Biol. 24 (1979) 505-517

[1] The European co-authors were supported by a grant from the CEC (FIGM-CT2000-00036).

Image quality of a dual side reading Fuji computed mammography system compared to the GE FFDM system and a film/screen mammography system

R.E. van Engen, W.J.H. Veldkamp, L.J. Oostveen, M.A.O. Thijssen, N. Karssemeijer

University Medical Centre Nijmegen, LRCB 451, P.O.Box 9101, 6500 HB Nijmegen, the Netherlands
R.vanEngen@LRCB.azn.nl

Abstract. Contrast detail analysis has been performed to compare the image quality of the Fuji FCR 5000MA CM system to the image quality of the GE Senographe 2000D and the Kodak Min-R 2000/Min-R 2190 film/screen combination. The dose of the images was kept identical between the X-ray units. For the comparison of both digital systems 8 phantom images (CDMAM version 3.4) have been made at each exposure setting and have been read-out by a computer programme. For the comparison of the Fuji and Kodak system two CDMAM images have been made at a number of exposure settings and have been read-out by experienced readers. Results show that image quality of both digital systems is fairly comparable. For small details there is no better performance with the Fuji system, despite its smaller pixel size. The image quality of the Fuji system is slightly superior to the image quality of the Kodak system.

1. Introduction

Recently Fuji introduced the FCR 5000 MA Computed Mammography reader. Due to the double-sided reading of the imaging plates the efficiency of this new CM system has increased considerably compared to previous types[1]. In this presentation the image quality of this Fuji CM system is compared to the image quality of an existing digital mammography X-ray unit (GE Senographe 2000D) and to the image quality of a widely used film/screen combination (Kodak Min-R 2000/Min-R 2190).

2. Materials and methods

Contrast-detail analysis using the CDMAM phantom (version 3.4) [2] has been performed to evaluate image quality. In this analysis image quality is expressed by the contrast detail curve relating the treshold contrast of an imaging system as a function of object diameter.

For the comparison of the image quality of the Fuji system (in combination with a GE Senographe DMR X-ray unit) and the GE Senographe 2000D eight CDMAM images have been made at each chosen exposure on each system. A standard setting has been chosen (5 cm PMMA, molybdenum target, molybdenum filter, 27 kV). From this setting PMMA thickness has been varied from 3 to 7 cm, target/filter combination has been varied (Mo/Mo, Mo/Rh and Rh/Rh) and tube voltage has been varied from 25 to 31 kV. Glandular dose was kept identical for both systems and for each simulated breast thickness [3]. The CDMAM images have been read-out by a computer programme, which detects the gold dots on the phantom images using an ideal observer model and calculates contrast-detail curves. The 100 μm pixels of the GE images have been scaled to 50 μm pixels using bilinear interpolation to allow identical processing by the detection algorithm.

For the image quality comparison of the Fuji CM system and the Kodak film/screen combination (both systems have been used in combination with a GE Senographe DMR) two CDMAM images have been made at a number of exposure settings on each system. A standard setting has been chosen (5 cm PMMA, molybdenum target, molybdenum filter, 27 kV). In this setting the dose of the images has been varied. CDMAM images have been also made in the Mo/Rh target/filter combination (5 cm PMMA, 27 kV). Glandular dose of the images was kept identical for both systems [3]. Four experienced readers have read the images. All individual readings of an exposure setting have been combined and contrast-detail curves have been calculated. Soft-copy reading was used for the digital images and window levelling was allowed to optimise the visibility of the gold dots.

3. Results

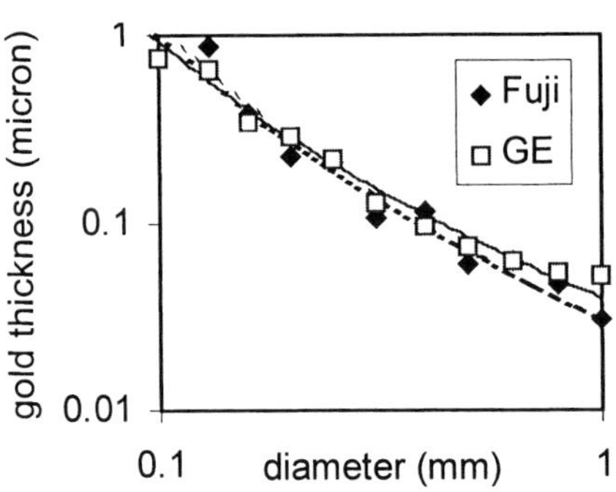

Fig. 1. Contrast detail curves of the Fuji and GE system using 5 cm PMMA, Mo/Mo target/filter and 27 kV

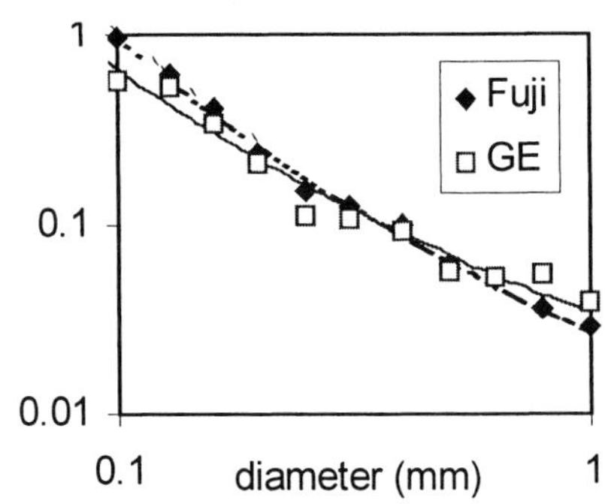

Fig. 2. Contrast detail curves of the Fuji and GE system using 5 cm PMMA, Rh/Rh target/filter and 27 kV

In all settings, except for one, the contrast detail resolution of the Fuji and GE system was found to be comparable (see figure 1 and 2). In one setting (5 cm PMMA, Mo/Rh, 27 kV) the contrast detail resolution of the GE system was slightly superior.

The contrast-detail resolution of the Fuji system is superior to the Kodak system at lower glandular dose (1.31 and 1.80 mGy) due to the low gamma at low optical density on films, see figure 3. At higher glandular dose (2.62 and 4.09 mGy) and at the molybdenum-rhodium target-filter combination (using 5 cm PMMA, 27 kV and glandular dose of 1.80 mGy) contrast-detail resolution was comparable, see figure 4.

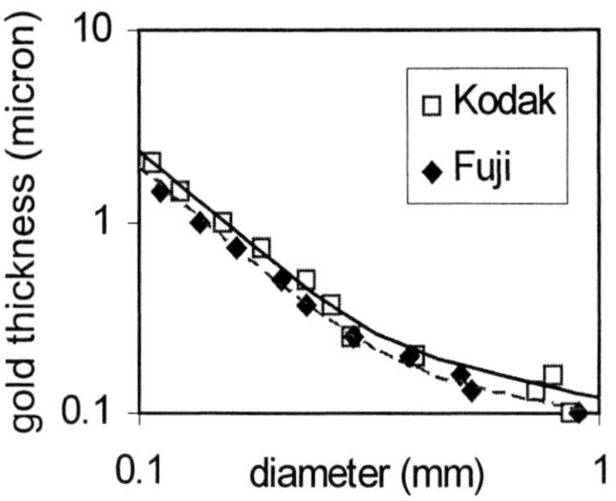

Fig. 3. Contrast-detail curves of the Fuji and Kodak system, 5 cm PMMA, Mo/Mo target/filter, 27 kV, glandular dose 1.80 mGy

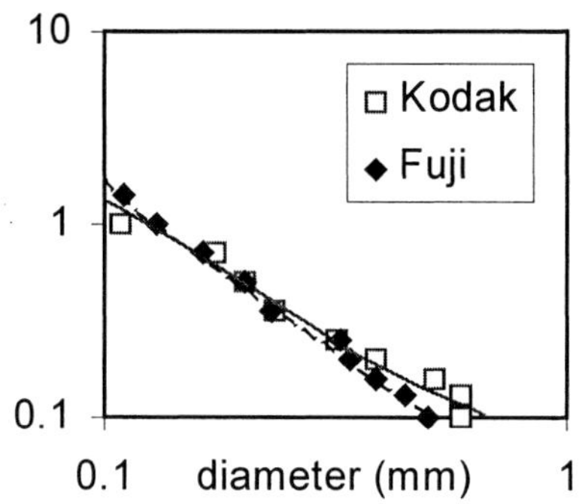

Fig. 4. Contrast-detail curves of the Fuji and Kodak system, 5 cm PMMA Mo/Mo target/filter, 27 kV, glandular dose 2.62 mGy

4. Conclusions

This study of the image quality of the Fuji FCR 5000 MA system has been limited but it can be concluded that the image quality of the Fuji system is fairly comparable to the image quality of the GE Senographe 2000D. Despite its smaller pixel size, the Fuji system is not better for small details. The image quality of the Fuji FCR 5000 MA system is slightly superior to the image quality of the Kodak Min-R 2000/Min-R 2190 film/screen combination. Previous studies on the GE system at our institution showed improved image quality using harder X-ray beams at high PMMA thickness (7 cm) [4]. This PMMA thickness and X-ray settings have not been included in this study. Therefore further study at other PMMA thicknesses and spectra is recommended to compare mentioned systems more in detail.

References

1. S. Arakawa et al.: Novel computed radiography system with improved image quality by detection of emissions from both sides of an imaging plate. In: SPIE Proceedings vol. 3659, Medical Imaging 1999: Physics of Medical Imaging
2. K.R. Bijkerk et al.: Modification of the CDMAM contrast-detail phantom for image quality evaluation of full-field digital mammography systems. In: M. Yaffe (ed.): Digital mammography. Medical physics publishing, Madison, 2001 633-640
3. D.R. Dance et al.: Additional factors for the estimation of mean glandular breast dose using the UK mammography dosimetry protocol. In: Physics of Medicine and Biology, 2000, 3225-3240
4. W.H.J. Veldkamp, N. Karssemeijer, R. van Engen, Optimized spectrum in direct digital mammography, abstract in: Supplement 1 op vol 12. European Radiology (2002), 232

Image Processing and Display

An Automatic Scheme to Breast Region Segmentation

Mouloud Adel, Monique Rasigni, Georges Rasigni,
*Brigitte Seradour, *Patrice Heid

INTERFACE PHYSIQUE - BIOLOGIE - MEDECINE
Faculté des Sciences et Techniques de Saint Jérôme, case EC1, 13397 Marseille cedex 20
France
*ARCADES, Hôpital de la Timone, rue Saint Pierre, 13005 Marseille cedex 5, France
mouloud.adel@univ.u-3mrs.fr

Abstract. An automatic scheme for breast region segmentation is presented. It is based on global automatic thresholding, region growing and merging. Thirty digitized mammograms including different kinds of breast parenchymal patterns were used for this study: 14 as training set and the remaining 16 others as testing set. The segmentation results are compared to those obtained manually by radiologists. The method achieved good results in the case of mammograms where the pectoral muscle was separated from the fibroglandular region. In the other cases, a fitting model was applied in order to get rid of the pectoral muscle. The segmentation results were still valid.

1. Introduction

The segmentation of a digital mammogram into regions of interest is needed for studying the relation between the improvement of cancer detection and the film optical density range. Many studies have been devoted to tackling this problem [1-4]. The aim of such studies is first to exclude the background area from the further processing and then to evaluate within the breast region the areas and the density range of the adipose and fibroglandular tissues. The main idea of this work is to segment a digitized mammogram into four regions : The background, fibroglandular and fatty regions and the pectoral muscle.

2. Methods

The automatic scheme we developed consists of three major steps :

- separating the background from the breast region.
- finding seeds for the region growing process.
- segmenting the fibroglandular tissue and the pectoral muscle.

2.1 Background separation

First the image was first filtered by a 5x5 median filter. Let design by I this filtered Image and h(i) its histogram; i belongs to the interval [g_{min} , g_{max}] the minimum and the maximum gray level of image I respectively. To separate the background from the breast region, an automatic thresholding method based on the histogram was used. It consists in finding the gray level T_0 where the maximum of histogram h(i) occurs. The threshold value is taken as the gray level $T_b > T_0$ which correspond to the first local minimum after maximum $h(T_0)$. Breast region correspond to pixels belonging to the interval [Tb , g_{max}]

2.2 Finding the initial seeds

To begin the region growing process, initial seeds have to be determined. These seeds are the representatives of each region we want to segment. As the pectoral muscle and the fibroglandular tissue appear much brighter than the fatty tissue, another threshold T_{reg} is determined using the statistical parameters of the breast region. Its value depends on the mean gray level μ_{reg} and the standard deviation σ_{reg} of the breast region as follows:

$$T_{reg} = \mu_{reg} + k\,\sigma_{reg} \tag{1}$$

where k is a weighting parameter the value of which will be determined in the next section. The binary image obtained after thresholding shows two major regions belonging to the pectoral muscle and the fibroglandular tissue respectively. A connected component labeling is used to assign each of the detected region a different label. The barycenter of each detected region is then used as an initial seed.

2.3 Segmenting the fibroglandular tissue and the pectoral muscle

The initial seeds found in the previous step are used to start a region growing segmentation for both pectoral muscle and fibroglandular region. This well known segmentation method is an iterative process in which, in step i, a pixel with gray level p is added to a region R if :

$$|p-\mu(R)|<T_{gro} \tag{2}$$

where $\mu(R)$ the mean gray level of region R and T_{gro} is a fixed threshold.
Finally a region merging is applied to the image in order to reduce the number of regions to be considered.

2.4 Threshold determination

The scheme described above needs the use of two thresholds. T_{reg} depend on parameter k (see Eq.1) which has been determined manually over a 30 image data base. Parameter k was found to equal approximately μ_{reg} / σ_{reg} which leaded to a threshold parameter :

$$T_{reg} \approx 2\,\mu_{reg} \qquad (3)$$

Threshold T_{gro} also depended on μ_{reg} and σ_{reg}. Using a supervised learning method, T_{gro} was found to depend on μ_{reg} and σ_{reg} according to equation :

$$T_{gro} = a\,(\mu_{reg} + \sigma_{reg})^2 + b \qquad (4)$$

where a and b are determined using the image data base.

3. Results

A set of thirty images were used to evaluate the automatic scheme developed in this paper. Fourteen digitized mammograms served as a training subset for determining T_{reg} and T_{gro}. The sixteen other images were used as a test subset. Segmentation results were compared to those obtained by a radiologist, who was asked to manually surround the pectoral muscle and the fibroglandular disc on a screen, using a graphical user interface. In the case of mammograms where the pectoral muscle was separated from the fibroglandular region, automatic scheme achieved good results in 10 over 12 tested images. Further processing was needed on mammograms where the pectoral muscle and the fibroglandular region are not well separated. It consisted on detecting one part of the muscle border. The remaining part of the border was then evaluated as being the line (using a least square estimation) passing through the first points detected in the previous step. Results obtained on 3 over 4 tested images were still valid.

4. Conclusion

In this paper an automatic scheme to segment the fibroglandular disc, the pectoral muscle and the breast region is presented. A larger image data base is now needed in order to test the robustness of this algorithm which achieved good segmentation results on a small number of images.

References

1. Miller, P., Astley, S.: Automated detection of mammographic asymetry using anatomical features. Int. Jour. Patt. Recog. Artif. Intel. 7 (6) (1993) 1461-1476
2. Chandrasekhar, R., Attikiouzel, Y.: A simple method for automatically locating the nipple on mammograms. IEEE Trans. Med. Imag. 16 (5) (1997) 483-494
3. Karssemeijer, N.: Automated classification of parenchymal patterns in mammograms. Phys. Med. Biol. 43 (1998) 365-378
4. Ferrari, R.J., Rangayyan, R.M., Desautel, J.E.L., Frère, A.F.: Segmentation of Mammograms : Identification of the Skin-Air Boundary, Pectoral Muscle, and Fibroglandular Disc. Proceeding of Int. Work. Digit. Mammography June 2000 Toronto Canada. Medical Physics Publishing Madison Wisconsin (2000)

A Universal Segmentation Platform for Computer-Aided Detection

Brent H. Allen, Mark E. Oxley, and Michael J. Collins

Qualia Computing, Inc., 2689 Commons Blvd., Beavercreek, OH, 45431 (USA)
Brent_Allen@qualia-computing.com

Abstract. One of the fundamental image processing challenges that a mammographic computed-aided detection system faces is to reliably segment a wide variety of objects from complicated backgrounds regardless of the input source. Rather than develop a completely new approach for each segmentation task and each source of data, we have found that it is possible to use a single active-contour segmentation engine for each problem. The segmentation engine does most of the work for a given application and can easily be interfaced with problem-specific algorithms that define the engine's input and adapt its operation to the problem at hand. In this paper, we describe the segmentation engine and discuss how we apply it to the segmentation of densities, pectoral muscles, and computed tomography images of lungs.

Introduction

Mammographic computer-aided detection (CAD) systems such as Second Look® (CADx Medical Systems, Quebec, Canada) are now being used clinically to aid radiologists in the reading of mammographic films, and will soon be applied to full-field digital mammography. One of the primary challenges that a CAD system confronts is to reliably segment a variety of objects from noisy backgrounds. For example, it is typically necessary to segment the breast from the mammogram, as well as masses, microcalcifications, and the pectoral muscle from the breast itself. A brute-force approach would be to develop a unique algorithm for each task, but this is inefficient and would likely lead to a complicated system. A better approach is to develop a single segmentation engine that can be applied to most (if not all) of a CAD system's segmentation problems.

We have developed a segmentation engine based on the active contour model in Ref. [1]. This engine can be used in many areas, including mammography and computed tomography (CT). The segmentation engine does most of the work for a given application. It can easily be interfaced with problem-specific algorithms that define the engine's input and adapt its operation to the problem at hand. In this paper, we describe the engine and discuss its application to the segmentation of densities and pectoral muscles in mammography images, and to the segmentation of lungs in CT images.

Active Contour Engine

To segment an object from an image with an active contour model, one defines an initial guess for the object's boundary and evolves the boundary under the influence of a set of image-specific forces until the boundary converges. There are many distinct active contour models (see Ref. [1] for an extensive list). They differ in their mathematical representation of the boundary, the forces that are used, and the method for evolving the boundary.

Our segmentation engine uses a level-set implementation of active contours. This means that the boundary is represented as the set of points (x, y) that satisfy the equation $\phi(x, y) = 0$, where ϕ is some function (called the "level set function"). The set of points that solves this equation is ϕ's zero level set. In a three-dimensional sense, ϕ can be thought of as a surface, and the contour is where the surface crosses the $x - y$ plane. By convention, $\phi > 0$ inside the object and $\phi < 0$ outside.

For the model we use, the boundary of the object in an image $I(x, y)$ is given by the zero level set of ϕ_{min}, where ϕ_{min} is the level set function that minimizes the following energy:

$$\begin{aligned} E &= \mu \int dx\, dy\, \delta(\phi(x,y))\,|\nabla\phi(x,y)| + \nu \int dx\, dy\, H(\phi(x,y)) \\ &+ \lambda_{\text{in}} \int dx\, dy\, |I(x,y) - m_{\text{in}}|\, H(\phi(x,y)) \\ &+ \lambda_{\text{out}} \int dx\, dy\, |I(x,y) - m_{\text{out}}|\,[1 - H(\phi(x,y))]. \end{aligned} \tag{1}$$

H is the Heaviside (step) function, and m_{in} is the mean of the image inside the object:

$$m_{\text{in}} = \frac{\int dx dy I(x,y) H(\phi(x,y))}{\int dx dy H(\phi(x,y))}. \tag{2}$$

m_{out} is m_{in} with $H \to 1 - H$, i.e. the mean of the image outside the object.

Each of the four terms in Eq.(1) acts as a force on the contour during its evolution. The first term is the contribution from the perimeter length of the object. It forces the perimeter to stay smooth. The second term is the contribution from the area of the object. It forces the object to grow or contract as a whole. The third and fourth terms are the contributions from the variances of the intensity inside and outside the object. They force the intensities inside and outside the object to be homogeneous. Each of the four terms competes with the others, and their relative strengths are determined by the parameters $\mu, \nu, \lambda_{\text{in}}$, and λ_{out}.

Using the calculus of variations, one can show that minimizing Eq.(1) is equivalent to solving a differential equation. If we consider ϕ to be a function of time, then $\phi_{\min}(x,y) = \phi(t=\infty, x, y)$, where $\phi(t,x,y)$ is the solution to the differential equation

$$\frac{\partial \phi}{\partial t} = \delta(\phi)\left[\mu \,\mathrm{div}\left(\frac{\nabla \phi}{|\nabla \phi|}\right) - \nu - \lambda_{\mathrm{in}}(I - m_{\mathrm{in}})^2 + \lambda_{\mathrm{out}}(I - m_{\mathrm{out}})^2\right] = 0. \quad (3)$$

In principle, the initial condition $\phi(t=0,x,y)$ can be chosen arbitrarily, although if the image is very noisy or contains multiple objects, it is necessary in practice to choose the initial contour wisely. Our segmentation engine solves Eq.(3) by smoothing the Heaviside and delta functions, quantizing the equation on a discrete grid, and using an iterative procedure [2].

Density Segmentation

The first application that we discuss is the segmentation of densities in mammograms. The purpose of segmenting densities is to allow the system to compute discriminating region-based features that can aid in the classification of detections as cancer or non-cancer. Our density detection system was developed on a database of 905 screen-detected biopsy-proven cancers.

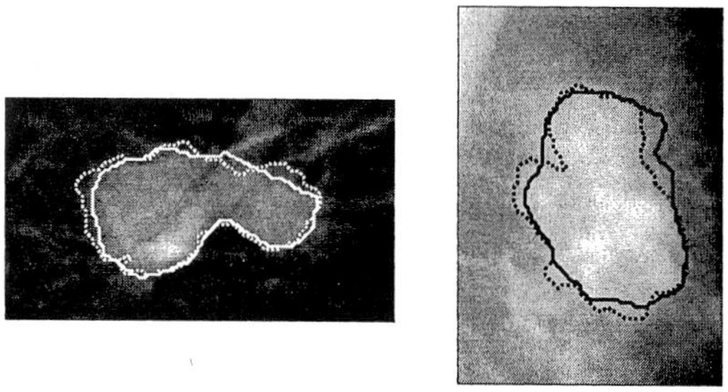

Fig. 1. Example density segmentation results. The solid lines represent the algorithm's output, and the dotted lines represent the true extents of the densities.

For a given image, the input to the density segmentation routine is a set of detections from a detector that is based on matched-filter response. Each detection is a crude estimation of the extent of a region of interest (ROI). The density segmentation routine's first step is to use the detection to define the bounds of a rectangular portion of the image (a chip) on which to perform the segmentation. Then it normalizes the chip by adaptively subsampling it to achieve a standard chip area (in pixels), removing the local background, and re-mapping the chip's dynamic range. The normalization process is important because it allows the same set of active contour parameters to be used for each ROI.

Once normalization is complete, the algorithm defines an initial level set function $\phi(t=0,x,y)$ whose zero level set is a small circle within the ROI. It then computes the steady-state solution to Eq.(3) using an iterative procedure. Figure 1 shows the results of the algorithm on two densities.

Given the region R as defined by the segmentation routine, and the true region T as defined by a qualified technician, we quantify the quality of the region R using the XOR score:

$$\text{XOR score} = \text{Area}\left(R \cup T - R \cap T\right) / \text{Area}\left(T\right). \tag{4}$$

This score measures the amount that the region R overshoots and undershoots the true region, relative to the area of the true region. A perfect score is zero, and for a bad result, the score can be arbitrarily large. We have found that a good score is 0.7 or less, and rate a segmentation system on the percent of its segmentations that are good, as well as the mean XOR score of its good segmentations.

To score the segmentation algorithm, we limited the set of 905 densities to the 624 that had a detection that overlapped the true region and whose true region had a medium or high confidence from the truthing technician. Table 1 shows the XOR scores for our baseline and active contour segmentation algorithms. The baseline system is based on a iterative adaptive-threshold floodfill algorithm.

Table 1. Performance comparison of density segmentation systems

System	**% Good Segmentations**	**Mean of Good XOR Scores**
Baseline	85.7	0.35
Active Contour	91.1	0.31

Other Applications

Other segmentation tasks to which we have applied our active contour engine include the segmentation of the pectoral muscle from the breast in mammogram images, and the segmentation of the lungs in CT images. We have used the same segmentation engine for each task (including density segmentation); only the pre- and post-processing steps and active contour parameter values differ.

Figure 2 shows an example active contour pectoral muscle segmentation on a digital mammogram that was captured with a Fischer sensor. We generated these results with no pre- or post-processing. However, when we apply the algorithm to more challenging images in which the muscle is overlaid with parenchyma, extra processing may be necessary.

Figure 3 shows an example lung segmentation in a CT image that was captured with a Marconi MxTwin. In the case of lung segmentation, some pre- and post-processing is necessary. This processing prevents the engine from segmenting the whole body and fills holes in the segmentation results from bright objects inside the lungs. In this example, we used two independent level set functions to allow the engine to segment the lungs simultaneously.

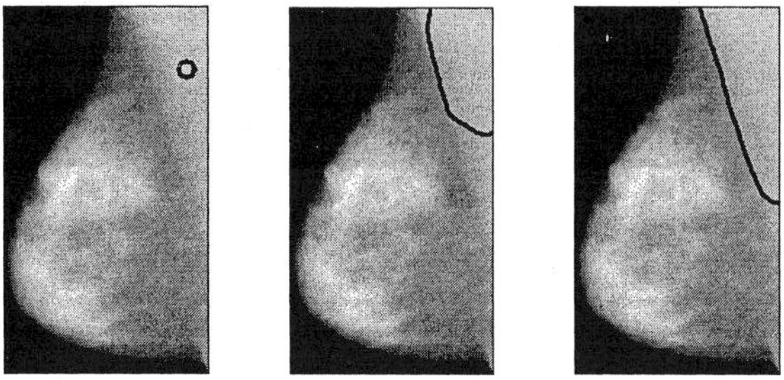

Fig. 2. Example of pectoral muscle segmentation results. The initial contour, an intermediate result, and the final result are shown.

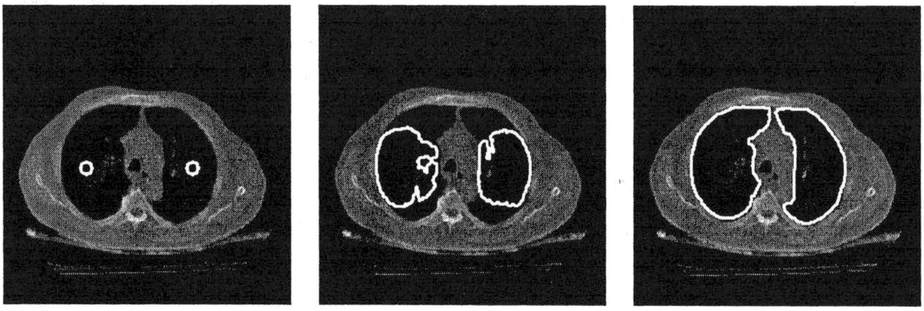

Fig. 3. Example of segmentation of lungs on a CT image. The initial contour, an intermediate result, and the final result are shown.

Conclusion

Segmentation is one of the most difficult and common challenges facing CAD systems. We have found that by applying a single active contour engine to many of these tasks, we can simplify the development process and produce high-quality results.

References

1. T.F. Chan and L.A. Vese, "Active Contours without Edges," *IEEE Trans. Image Processing*, vol. 10, no. 2, pp. 266-277, Feb. 2001.
2. G. Aubert and L.A. Vese, "A Variational Method in Image Recovery," *SIAM J. Numer. Anal.*, vol 34, no. 5, pp. 1948-1979, 1997.

Improved Aids For Image Comparison

Ancelin B, Highnam RP and Brady JM

Mirada Solutions Limited
Oxford Centre For Innovation
Mill Street, Oxford, OX2 OJX.
Corresponding author: bruno.ancelin@mirada-solutions.com

Abstract. In previous publications (mainly [HB99]), we have developed a standardized mammogram representation - the h_{int} representation - for images that were taken with any conventional film-screen equipment. This representation can greatly help radiologists by providing them with images that have a standardized appearance based on the anatomical information contained in h_{int}.
In this paper, we show how the standardization process can be generalized to the new directly-digital equipments such as the Senographe GE2000D from General Electric. We also show how we can simulate images from one modality to another. Thus, ensuring comparison of images no matter on what imaging system they were performed.

1 Introduction

The proliferation of different types of mammographic digital systems is presenting radiologists, radiographers and other imaging professionals with unique and difficult challenges:

- How do you reliably compare an image taken on a digital machine with a film-screen image taken 3 years previously ?
- How do you create a teaching database of images when you have a large mix of images from different machines ?
- How do you create a CAD algorithm which can work equally as well on film-screen and all the digital modalities ?
- How do you learn to read digital mammograms after being trained on film-screen ?

The problem is so serious, that some radiologists have been quoted as saying that they feel each new digital system is effectively a new modality and therefore requires extensive re-training for all radiologists.

We have been working to develop a set of transformations that allow an image from a film-screen system or any of the digital systems to be transformed into a standard form. This standard form, which we have termed Standard Mammogram Form (SMF), allows the user to view all mammograms in an identical way. Thus, for example, we could take a database containing GE digital mammograms, Fischer digital mammograms, digitized film-screen mammograms and we can convert them all to a standard representation. These transformations are based on the physics of mammography and the relevant imaging systems and have been well documented in the past for film-screen mammograms [HB99]. In this paper, we extend our system of transformations to cover digital mammograms.

2 The Problem

Even with film-screen mammography, pictures of the same breast can look very different depending upon the exact imaging parameters used:

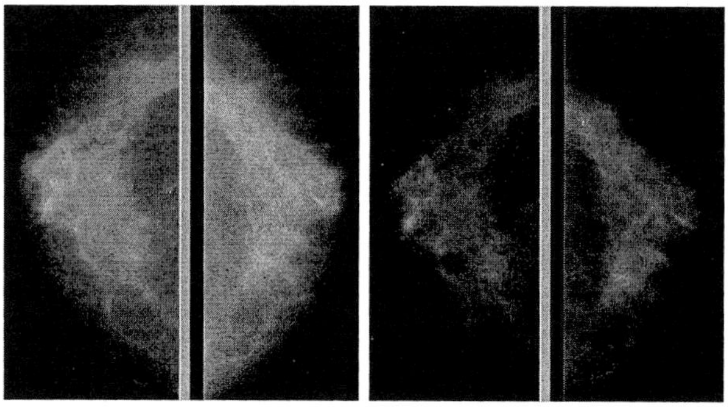

Fig. 1. Same breast on two pairs of mammograms taken with different parameters (exposure, film-screen curve, etc.). Images simulated using VirtualMammo(R)

Figure 1 shows the same pair of breasts on both the left and right hand side - but the exposure parameters have been manipulated by use of an x-ray simulation package to illustrate the potential differences in appearance (the x-ray simulation package used is Mirada Solution's VirtualMammo(R).

Imagine now some of the comparisons which will need to be done between old film-screen systems presented on light boxes and digital mammograms displayed on soft-copy reading workstations. We've been working towards easing this comparison by firstly converting all mammograms to the standard form and then simulating the relevant images for comparison. In particular, and as we demonstrate in this paper, we have been working on converting film-screen mammograms into GE look-alike digital mammograms.

3 Standard Mammogram Form

The aim of SMF is to estimate the height of non-fat tissue over each pixel by modelling each of the degrading factors in the acquisition chain. This involves the following steps:

1. Convert digital image to film density using digitizer characteristics.
2. Convert film density to energy using film characteristic and exposure parameters.
3. Compensate for anode-heel effect and slant.
4. Compensate for phosphor screen blur and noise by optimal deconvolution.
5. Estimate total thickness if not available.
6. Compute and remove scatter component.
7. Convert the obtained primary energy image into height of non-fat tissue using tabulated attenuation coefficient values.

Step 4 is particularly important as it conditions the noise present in the final image. Noise on mammographic images is very specific as it highly depends on signal in an inverse-multiplicative manner. Details of the optimal deconvolution method will be published in the future. As explained in section 5.1, directly-digital images are energy images. Thus, they can be inserted at step 4. The deblurring step then involves the inverse filter of what is described in section 5.1. The h_{int} image should be regarded as a surface that conveys relevant information on the breast structure. An example surface is shown on figure 2.

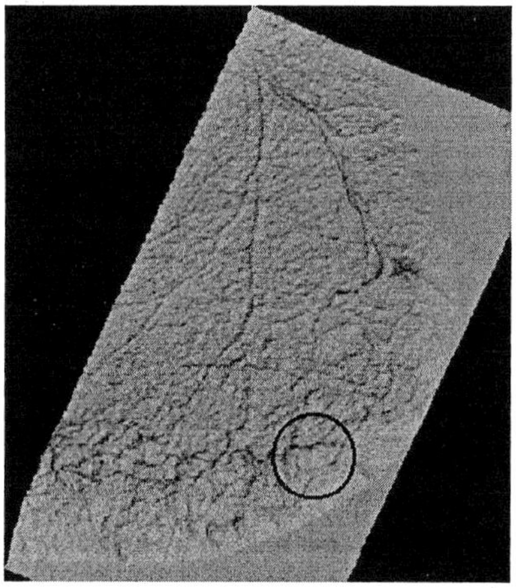

Fig. 2. Example h_{int} surface. The circled area indicates a mass.

4 GE Senographe 2000D

The GE Senographe 2000D uses a flat panel digital detector (14 bits raw, 12 bits processed). The size of the cells is 100 microns but the actual sensitive area is 87 microns wide. Different tube and filter combinations can be selected by the operator. The detector has a linear response. An anti-scatter grid is used. Images are systematically processed before display using a thickness-equalization technique (see section 5.2). Modulation transfer functions have been measured.

5 Conversion of SMF to GE Senographe 2000D

5.1 Simulation

Starting from a standardized mammogram, the simulation involves the following steps:

1. Convert the h_{int} values to energy using a fixed set of exposure parameters (reversible).
2. Compute and add the scatter component according to the model (reversible).
3. Halve resolution to 100 microns by adding pixel energies by groups of four.
4. Add X-ray sensor blur.
5. Optionally, simulate electronic noise.
6. Convert energy to sensor pixel values.
7. Apply post-processing (see section 5.2).

The steps marked as *reversible* do not involve any loss of information. In practice, the simulation can be performed directly from film-screen image, to energy image with scatter, to final simulated image.

The sensor blur is modelled by a spatial linear filter. We use the square-product filter of the measured modulation transfer function as the sensor cells are square and arranged in a matrix. For the time being, we do not take into account the limited size of the sensitive area (87 microns edge) compared to the full size of the cell (100 microns edge). Constant energy spectrum is assumed at the sensor level over the whole image which leads to a linear relationship between energy and pixel value. Under this assumption, directly-digital images are basically energy imparted images and thus fit very well the proposed model for acquisition systems outlined in section 3.

5.2 Post-processing

The simulation described in section 5.1 produces an image that is equivalent to the direct output of the X-ray sensor. In a directly-digital full workstation, the images are processed before being displayed. Typically, the energy scaled is reversed so that the mammogram appears on the screen with bright areas corresponding to low energies. Also, a breast-thickness equalization is performed on the GE2000D images. Here, we describe an equivalent method that, in fact, gives less artifacts than the method actually used on the GE2000D. Full details can be found in [BCY97]. Final results are shown in figure 3.

The idea is to rescale energies in the breast edge area. More precisely, this is the area contained between the inner edge (where the thickness of tissue starts to decrease) and the outer edge (where the thickness of tissue is zero). At each pixel in this area, assuming the breast edge is mainly fat, one can estimate the relative thickness of tissue over that pixel (actual thickness divided by total thickness) by applying a low pass filter on the energy image and comparing with the inner's edge spatially closest pixel. The pixel's energy is then rescaled so that it appears as if there had been a full thickness of tissue. This ensures the visualization of the whole breast structure by the human eye on a single display.

6 Examples and results

Figure 3 shows simulation results. The post-processing step is particularly interesting as it makes the structure of the breast edge visible even on a basic display system. These results are of a preliminary kind as they would require validation through comparison of phantom images or registered images of the same breast.

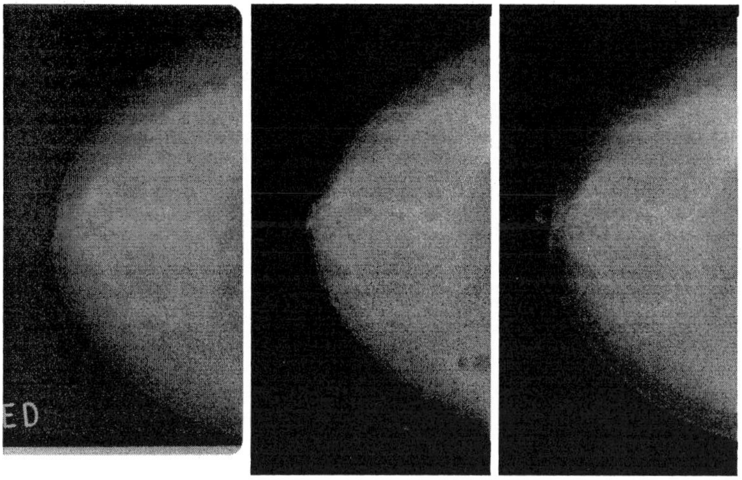

Fig. 3. From left to right: original film-screen mammogram, GE2000D sensor image (scale reversed), GE2000D-like post-processed image.

7 Conclusion

In this paper, we have presented an extension of our existing model for mammographic image acquisition systems to directly-digital systems. This enables simulation of images from one system to another which should help radiologists in comparing images and let them choose to visualize images with much more flexibility. This preliminary study also shows the potential of mammogram simulation. With the introduction of digital mammography, comparison, registration and analysis of mammograms from different equipments will play a key role in computer aided diagnosis.

References

[BCY97] J. W. Byng, J. P. Critten, and M. J. Yaffe. Thickness-equalization processing for mammographic images. *Radiology*, 203:564–568, 1997.

[HB99] R. Highnam and M. Brady. *Mammographic Image Analysis*. Dordrecht: Kluwer Academic Publishers, 1999.

Film-Screen Artefact Detection in Mammograms

Ancelin B, Yam M, Highnam RP, Brady JM

Mirada Solutions Ltd, Oxford Centre for Innovation
Mill St, OXFORD OX2 0JX, United Kingdom

Abstract. Shot noise is the result of "foreign bodies" such as dust or hairs being present on the intensifying screen or on the film during the acquisition. Shot noise is an important potential source of false positives in the detection of micro-calcifications. As such, there has been interest in its detection and labelling which is the aim of the work in this paper. In this paper, we give a clearer and better mathematical justification for our previous work in this area which uses the inherent blur in the imaging system to identify what is noise and what is real calcification. In doing so, we develop a new algorithm with a more mathematically correct approach which is iterative. This ensures that not only are individual pixels correctly marked as shot noise, but the whole area of noise is marked as such.

The new algorithm due to its iterative nature is slower than the old method, but reduces the number of false positives even further in subsequent CAD algorithms by being based on firmer theory and detecting the whole noise region.

1 Introduction

Shot noise in the context of this paper appears when there is an artefact transparent to X-rays (but not to light) that happens to be between the intensifying screen and the film (there is a gap between these two of around 10 to 50 microns). This shot noise blocks out light generated from the screen and causes a bright white mark to appear on the film which can replicate the appearance of a microcalcification.

Other shot noise might appear when there is dust and dirt on the film at digitization time. In this case, the shot noise is black and not white. Our technique does not mark these points as noise as they will not be picked up as potential microcalcifications in subsequent processing steps.

In a conventional mammographic acquisition system, X-ray photons pass through the breast and through the film onto the intensifying screen which converts that beam to a visible light spread beam. Throughout this process there is blurring on the information, not least due to the intensifying screen.

Shot noise, as defined in this paper, only enters the imaging chain at the end whereas real signs such as microcalcifications are present right the way through. Hence, shot noise apppears as relatively non-blurred objects whereas microcalcifications appear as blurred objects. The algorithm described in this paper aims at differentiating the *post-blur* component by using the information in the energies imparted to the intensifying screen (we call this the energy image).

2 Our previous shot noise detection algorithm

2.1 Description

The algorithm works on the image obtained by converting the original digitized image (which we call a film density image) into an energy image using a film response curve as described in [HB99] and other calibration data. This image will be referred as $b(x,y)$ as it has been blurred by the intensifying screen. Our previous work involved noting that when $b(x,y)$ is deconvolved (ie. *deblurred*) using the point spread function for the film-screen system described in [HB99], pixels with negative energies represent shot-noise.

A negative energy in the deconvolved image obviously means something was wrong in the assumption under which the deconvolution was done. As shot noise is added *after* the screen blur, it does not deconvolve properly. That's basically why the deconvolution does not really make sense and wrongly reveals pixels that were attenuated after the screen blur.

2.2 How does it work?

As the light energy response of the intensifying screen is a linear function of the X-ray energy imparted to the screen, we will only refer to *energy* images. Let $i(x,y)$ be the X-ray image (ie. before blur), $b(x,y)$ be the light image and p the point spread function. We therefore have: $i(x,y) * p = b(x,y)$. The *observed* image is then:

$$b(x,y) + s(x,y) \tag{1}$$

where $s(x,y)$ designates the shot noise component. The direct blur deconvolution of (1) is:

$$\mathcal{F}^{-1}(\frac{B+S}{\hat{P}}) = \hat{i} + \mathcal{F}^{-1}(\frac{S}{\hat{P}}) \tag{2}$$

where capital letters designate the Fourier transforms of the images or point spread function and $\mathcal{F}$ designates the Fourier transform operator. The first term is the estimated deconvolved image $\hat{i}$ (without shot noise) and the second term represents how the shot noise has been processed by the deconvolution (assuming our point spread function is accurate).

If s is a single pixel with a unit value, the shot noise term shows as a single peak (with a slight Gibbs ringing around it) with a 8-12 central value (depending on the parameters used for $\hat{P}$). This means that an isolated pixel that received a 4keV decrease after screen blur because of shot noise appears with a 32-48keV decrease after deconvolution, which most of the time can create negative energies.

3 Algorithm extension

3.1 Using energy ratios

It is now clear that the zero-thresholding in [HB99] is a rather arbitrary criterion. From the description we have made of the shot noise phenomenon, a better criterion would be to measure the decrease amplification ratio (deconvolved decrease divided by original shot noise decrease). Ideally this ratio should be around 8-12 (values mentionned above) for shot noise, zero for non shot noise. However, this involves the *a priori* knowledge of the image without shot noise and is therefore not suitable as this image is not known.

Rather than that, we use a direct energy ratio (ie. deblurred energy divided by original energy, for each individual pixel). We can then get similar results to those obtained with the original algorithm using a point spread function with more realistic parameters (screen gap and thickness) which was one of the concerns of our previous work. The energy ratio image may be interpreted in the following way (the values presented here are empirical):

- below 0: definitely shot noise.
- 0 to 0.25: most likely to be shot noise.
- 0.25 to 0.5: usually shot noise but we may come across calcifications.
- 0.5 and above: non shot noise pixel.

From the pictures we have processed and fully manually checked, it appears that using a 0.25 threshold is very safe (no micro-calcification was marked as shot noise on 20 images with known micro-calcifications).

3.2 Iterative detection and correction

The algorithm gives good results for detecting single-pixel-wide shot noise areas. On wider areas (up to 5 pixels wide and a few dozens of pixels long), not all pixels are marked as shot noise. This is because the presence of shot noise minimizes the probability of detecting surrounding shot noise pixels. Hence, if we correct the marked pixels so that their energy looks blurred and re-run the algorithm, it is very likely that surrounding shot noise pixels will give lower energies after deconvolution and be detected by the algorithm. This is the basis for our iterative algorithm which stops when no new pixels are marked as noise.

Energy correction is done on the blurred image: pixels marked as shot noise are replaced by the local mean energy of valid surrounding pixels. Practically, on 50 microns images, the algorithm stabilizes within less than ten steps. An illustration of the iterative process in given in figure 1. Here is a summary of the process:

1. Do the deconvolution and compute the energy ratio image.
2. Mark pixels that are below the selected threshold on the shot noise map image.
3. Correct the energies of all marked pixels using a local-mean estimator.

4. Repeat these steps until no more pixels are detected.

Now, whole shot noise areas are properly marked as shot noise. For large areas, the very border is usually not detected (and thus not corrected). One can circumvent this by performing an energy correction on pixels that are next to marked pixels for large areas.

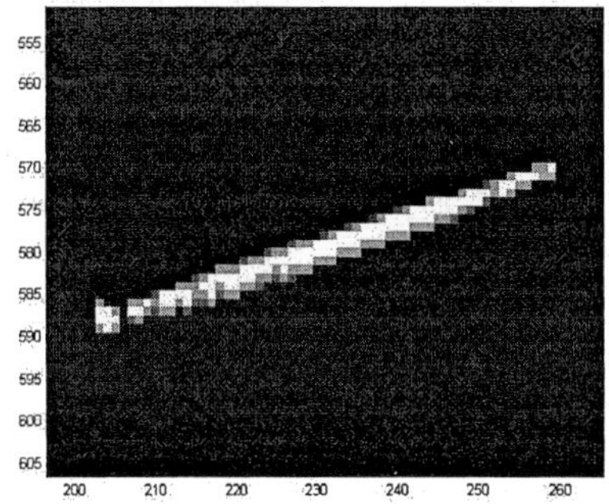

Fig. 1. Illustration of the iterative detection. The gray level indicates the step at which the pixel was marked as shot-noise (bright pixels were detected first).

4 Results and discussion

Previous publications on this subject ([SE98] and [HB99]) mentionned a single *detection rate*, forgetting accuracy in the detection of the border of a shot noise area. In fact, if the iterative detection scheme is not used, the algorithm correctly labels only a subpart of non single-pixel shot noise areas (that is usually below 50 percent of the actual area for artifacts larger than ten pixels). On these originally detected areas, our new iterative detection scheme gives borders as good as what an experienced human eye can see.

The energy ratio criterion described in section 3.1 enables us to detect accurately more than single-pixel-wide artifacts. The algorithm does have susceptibility to film and digitizer saturation around the edges of the breast which make the energy values less reliable and more noisy.

We are using the screen point spread function described in [HB99]. This model uses several physical parameters leaving a choice for the PSF we use. The shot noise amplification coefficient given in section 2.2 is valid if we assume the point spread function is ideal. Computing the energy ratio with a different PSF gives different values but also different deblurred image estimates. Therefore, the algorithm highly depends on the PSF accuracy.

Our algorithm performed well on twenty real images with calcifications. No calcifications were marked as shot noise. Detected shot noise areas have accurate borders. On the four images that we fully manually checked, more than 80 percent of all of the artifcats are detected.

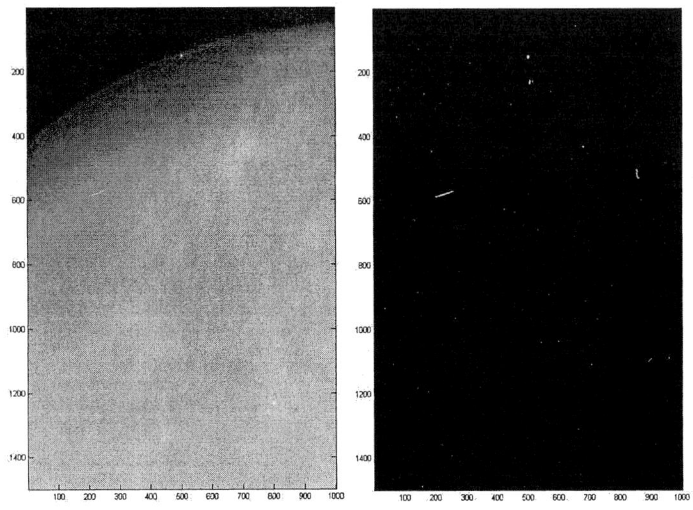

Fig. 2. Sample energy image and map of detected shot noise pixels

5 Conclusion and further work

In this paper, we have developped a math-based justification of the shot noise detection scheme described in [SE98]. As an enhancement to this algorithm, an iterative detection method has also been described that enables detection of whole, well-defined shot noise areas. Further work will include stronger noise modelling for the phosphor screen and for the digitizer as well as measured point spread functions for different equipments.

Acknowledgements

This work has been carried out as part of an internship at Mirada Solutions Ltd, Oxford, UK. Margaret Yam did the visual inspection of the images. I also wish to thank Jerôme Declerck for reviewing the article and for his constant support during the internship.

References

[HB99] R. Highnam and M. Brady. *Mammographic Image Analysis*. Dordrecht: Kluwer Academic Publishers, 1999.

[Kar93] N. Karssemeijer. Adaptive noise equalization and recognition of microcalcification clusters in mammograms. *Journal of pattern recognition and artificial intelligence*, 7:1357–1376, 1993.

[SE98] M. Poissonnier R. Highnam M. Brady B. Shepstone and R. English. Integration of low-level processing to facilitate microcalcification detection. *International Workshop on Digital Mammography*, 1998.

Learning the Optimal Contrast Enhancement of Mammographic Breast Masses

Keir Bovis and Sameer Singh

PANN Research, Dept. of Computer Science, University of Exeter, United Kingdom

Abstract. We propose a methodology to predict the optimal contrast enhancement for a mammogram by learning the non-linear mapping of lesion grey-scale statistics with enhancement and segmentation performance. For the unseen mammogram on test, we identify a suspicious region and using a series of Artificial Neural Networks (ANN), determine the enhancement that will maximise segmentation performance. For accurately defined suspicious regions on test we obtain a rank-ordered correlation coefficient of 0.701 compared with the target enhancement.

1 Introduction

Image enhancement is a necessary component of any Computer Aided Detection (CAD) mammography system [3]. Enhancement improves the poor signal-to-noise ratio found in many images and is a pre-processing step to improve the performance of lesion segmentation. We present a methodology supporting the learning of the optimal contrast enhancement method for a given of mammogram, such that on test for the unseen mammogram, a contrast enhancement method is selected that will maximise segmentation performance. To achieve this, we aim to learn a mapping based on grey-scale features from a given mammogram, with segmentation performance following image transformation, using a given enhancement method m, where $1 \leq m \leq M$ from a set of M enhancement methods. In this study we simplify the training process and improve testing performance by using *two* different ANN's learning the following sub-mappings:

net^m_{enh} For an original image I, enhanced using enhancement method m, learn the mapping between grey features ($f_1, f_2, \ldots, f_n$) taken from a single suspicious area and a set of p quantitative measures (E_1, E_2, ... ,E_p) of enhancement performance [1].

net^m_{seg} For an original image I, enhanced using enhancement method m, learn the mapping between quantitative measure of enhancement performance (E_1, E_2, ... ,E_p) and a set of r measures quantifying the performance of lesion segmentation (S_1, S_2, ... ,S_r) [2].

We evaluate our methodology using the following commonly used enhancement methods; Adaptive Contrast Enhancement (*ace*), Density Weighted Contrast Enhancement (*dwce*), fuzzy enhancement (*fuzzy*), global histogram equalisation (*global*), and two novel variations; adaptive contrast enhancement using local entropy (*lentropy*) and adaptive contrast enhancement using local fractal dimension (*lfractal*). The methodology comprises a separate training and testing phase for each of the set of neural networks $\{net^m_{enh}, net^m_{seg}\}$ that exist for each enhancement method.

2 Experimental Method and Results

Our methodology is evaluated on 200 mammograms from the Digital Database of Screening Mammograms (DDSM) comprising 50 image each containing circumscribed or spiculated masses from one of four mammographic breast types (from fatty through to dense). Each ANN is tested and trained using 5-fold cross validation and optimised by varying the number of hidden nodes to select the optimal model order.

2.1 Training *and Testing Neural Network* net^m_{enh}

For an individual mammogram within our training set we define two disjoint regions; pixels comprising an abnormal *target* region (T) and pixels encircling within a normal *background* (B) region. From each mammogram we compute five features; the target to background ratio of the mean, standard deviation, skewness, kurtosis and entropy of grey-scales comprising each region. Target regions are ground-truths accompanying each abnormal image redefined using a ballooning snake to improve performance. The background region is constructed to comprise only normal tissue and is of the same area as the redefined abnormal. We subject each training mammogram to each of the contrast enhancement methods and extract quantitative measures of enhancement performance [1]; *DSM*, TBC_V and TBC_ε for each image / enhancement combination. For a given enhancement method m, we train network net^m_{enh} using back-propagation with momentum and 22 hidden nodes. To test an unseen mammogram on test, we first segment the image using a Gaussian Mixture Model (GMM) regularised with a Markov Random Field (MRF) and assign each pixel to one of n disjoint regions. Using a separate neural network trained to learn the mapping between region shape and area, we determine the single most likely suspicious target region (T). Around this we construct a background region (B) and from both extract each of the five grey-scale features. We apply these features as inputs to each network net^m_{enh}, associated with each enhancement method m. The Mean Squared Error (MSE) on test for each neural network is shown in Table 1(a). The increased error for net^{fuzzy}_{enh} is related to the increased variability in enhancement measures obtained for this method. This can be attributed to the a property of the *fuzzy* method in enhancing the contrast of local densities containing normal tissue equally as compared with target lesions especially in non-fatty breast types.

2.2 Training *and Testing Neural Network* net^m_{seg}

This ANN aims to learn the mapping of enhancement performance given by *DSM*, TBC_V and TBC_ε with segmentation performance by computing two quantitative measures [2] indicating the percentage of the actual region overlapping the target. For a given enhancement method using the enhancement performance measures, we extract the segmentation measures from the segmented enhanced image. For each enhancement method m, we train network net^m_{seg} using back-propagation with momentum and 10 hidden nodes. To test the unseen mammogram we take the output of net^m_{enh} as the input to network net^m_{seg} for each enhancement method m. The Mean Squared Error (MSE) on test for each ANN is shown in 1(b). We again find that the variability of the fuzzy method is harder to learn indicated by the increased MSE on test.

3 Conclusion

In order to validate the experimental results obtained in this study, we include a performance analysis of the segmentation of each original image following the application of each enhancement method. If our proposed methodology selects the optimal enhancement for a given test image with respect to segmentation performance, we should obtain a high positive rank-ordered correlation coefficient with the error from each network net^m_{seg} with the target segmentation performance. If we test the network net^m_{seg} using test images containing accurately identified suspicious regions (i.e. where there is an overlap with the target) we obtain a rank-ordered correlation coefficient of 0.701. This result shows that we are able to accurately predict the optimal contrast enhancement method if our suspicious region overlaps the target lesion. For our complete test set we obtain a rank-ordered correlation coefficient of 0.430.

Table 1. MSE on test for each of the networks in net^m_{enh} (a) and net^m_{seg} (b)

	Method	ace	dwce	fuzzy	global	lentropy	lfractal	Mean
(a)	$test_{mse}$	0.0009	0.0121	0.0364	0.0088	0.0009	0.0027	0.0101
	Method	ace	dwce	fuzzy	global	lentropy	lfractal	Mean
(b)	$test_{mse}$	0.0544	0.0545	0.0753	0.0602	0.0552	0.0532	0.0587

References

1. K. J. Bovis and S. Singh. Enhancement technique evaluation using quantitative measures. *Proceedings of the 5th International Workshop on Digital Mammography, Toronto, Canada*, pages 547–553, 2000.
2. M. Kallergi, G. M. Carney, and J. Gaviria. Evaluating the performance of detection algorithms in digital mammography. *Medical Physics*, 26(2):267–275, 1999.
3. S. Singh and K. J. Bovis. *Advanced Algorithmic Approach to Medical Image Segmentation: State-of-the-Art Application in Cardiology, Mammography and Pathology.*, chapter Digital Mammography Segmentation, pages 440 – 540. Springer-Verlag Ltd., 2001.

Automatic Evaluation of Mammographic Adequacy and Quality on the Mediolateral Oblique View

Ramachandran Chandrasekhar[1], Sze Man Kwok[1], and Yianni Attikiouzel[2]

[1] Australian Research Centre for Medical Engineering (ARCME)
The University of Western Australia
35 Stirling Highway, Crawley, WA 6009, Australia
{chandra, kwok-sm}@ee.uwa.edu.au
http://www.arcme.uwa.edu.au
[2] Murdoch University
South Street, Murdoch, WA 6150, Australia
yianni@murdoch.edu.au

Abstract. A digitized mammogram is considered to be adequate and of sufficient quality when its extent and appearance, respectively, satisfy certain criteria that enable radiologists to make diagnoses of high specificity and sensitivity. Criteria related to breast positioning, suggested by radiologists, include: inferior extent of the pectoral muscle relative to the level of the nipple; curvature of the anterior pectoral margin; whether the nipple is in profile; and inclusion of all the breast tissue on the mammogram. We present here a systematic approach to automatically determine by computer the adequacy and quality of mammograms. First, landmarks such as the breast border, nipple, and pectoral margin were extracted by automatic algorithms. Compliance with the positioning criteria was then determined from these landmarks. Finally, adequacy of film exposure was assessed from the optical density histogram of the breast region. This approach has been applied to mammograms in the MIAS database. Automatic, computerized evaluation of mammographic adequacy and quality by computer is useful to highlight poor positioning and inadequate exposure, and to alert mammographic radiographers (technicians) to the need for additional exposures or views. It is also an important quality assurance step in any automated analysis of mammograms for computer-assisted diagnosis.

1 Introduction

It has been observed that "an excellent mammogram is a prerequisite for a correct radiological diagnosis" [1, p 8]. Stated another way, the mammogram must be of sufficient *quality* to enable the radiologist to identify abnormalities with high sensitivity and specificity [2]. Unfortunately, it has been noted that "there is no ideal, accurate, or reproducible method for assessing image quality" [2].

Nevertheless, there is a consensus in the literature [2–4] on how ideal mammograms in the mediolateral oblique (MLO) and craniocaudal (CC) views should look like.

Chief among the factors influencing the final image is correct *positioning,* which enables to the best possible *compression* [5]. Indeed, it has been observed that mammography is "the science of imaging and the art of positioning" [3]. Moreover, in a very recent study on clinical image quality and the risk of interval cancer, Taplin et al. conclude that "invasive breast cancer detection by mammography may be improved through attention to correct positioning" [6].

This paper introduces methods for determining automatically by computer some aspects of mammogram adequacy and quality on the mediolateral oblique view. It focuses on those attributes of a good mammogram that may be objectively and unambiguously assessed by machine. Most of these are related to the correctness of positioning during the procedure, as assessed from the completed mammogram. The reasons for doing this include the following. Firstly, in routine mammographic screening, if a mammogram is assessed by machine to be inadequate before the subject leaves the screening centre, a repeat examination may be undertaken immediately, without the need for another visit. Secondly, in computer-aided diagnosis, all mammograms assessed to be inadequate may be identified and flagged for attention by the attending radiologist, rather than be subjected to further automatic analysis that may be of dubious benefit. Thirdly, automatic adequacy assessment may be useful in training mammographic radiographers (technicians) and may also be one facet of an ongoing quality assurance program at a facility.

2 The mediolateral oblique view mammogram

The mediolateral oblique view is considered the more important of the two standard mammogram views because it is the view that best images the upper outer quadrant of the breast in which the majority of cancers occur [5, 7]. In a well-positioned MLO view, it is possible to visualize almost all of the breast [2, 3]. The Mammographic Image Analysis Society (MIAS) digital mammogram database [8], used in this study, also contains only the MLO view. For these reasons, this study is restricted to MLO view mammograms.

2.1 Attributes of a high quality MLO view

A high quality mammogram will incorporate correct positioning, optimal compression, good contrast, adequate exposure, low noise, sharpness, absence of artifacts, and exhibit overall quality [6]. A consistent superset of the quantifiable attributes of a high quality MLO mammogram may be distilled from the current literature [2–6] so: (1) the pectoral muscle should be visible in the image to at least the level of the nipple; (2) the anterior pectoral margin should be convex to indicate relaxation of the muscle; (3) the inframammary fold should be included at the bottom; (4) the nipple should appear in profile; (5) the retroglandular should be visible between the posterior glandular margin and the back of the image; and (6) upper glandular tissue projecting over the pectoral muscle should be included in the image; and (7) the mean optical density of the non-pectoral breast region should lie within the range [1.4, 1.8]. In addition, the MLO view is used to assure the quality of the CC view by requiring that the perpendicular distance from the nipple to the posterior image edge in the CC view should be within 10 mm of the perpendicular distance from the nipple to the pectoral margin on the MLO view. The algorithms presented below assess only attributes (1), (2), (4) and (7) above.

3 Adequacy assessment algorithms

We have previously described automatic methods to determine the breast border [9], locate the nipple [10], and delineate the pectoral margin [11] using a *straight line estimate* in the first instance (referred to as the straight line estimate, hereafter), and a more accurate final *fitted curve* in the second (referred to as the fitted curve hereafter). These algorithms were used to determine the respective landmarks on the mammogram before the adequacy assessment algorithms described below were invoked.

A horizontal straight line was drawn from the nipple to the posterior border of the mammogram. If the inferior margin of the pectoral muscle, determined by the straight line estimate, extended to or below this level, the criterion was met; and not otherwise. The depth of tissue seen on this view may be estimated by the perpendicular distance from the nipple to the straight line estimate of the pectoral edge. This may be used later to determine adequacy of the companion CC view.

The concavity or convexity of the pectoral margin is determined by drawing a straight line from the inferior and superior extents of the fitted curve and comparing the area of this triangle with the area enclosed by the image edges and the fitted curve. If the latter area is larger, the margin is convex; if smaller, concave.

The nipple location algorithm itself yielded information about the nipple being in profile or not.

The inclusion of all breast tissue in the mammogram could not be tested in its entirety, but obvious exclusions of the anterior and inferior breast, resulting in incomplete breast images were identified. This was done by tracking 10 mm segments of the breast border, determining whether the normal direction for all segment pixels was horizontal or vertical, and whether the border segment was closer than 5 mm to the image edges.

Adequacy of exposure was determined by converting all MIAS image pixel values in the non-pectoral breast region to optical densities. If the mean optical density lay within [1.4, 1.8], the image was adequate; otherwise it was not.

4 Experiments and results

Mammograms from the MIAS digital mammogram database at the original 8-bit depth and a resolution of 400 μm per pixel in both orthogonal directions were used. The MLO view is to be implicitly understood in this and the next section. Typical results are shown in Figure 1.

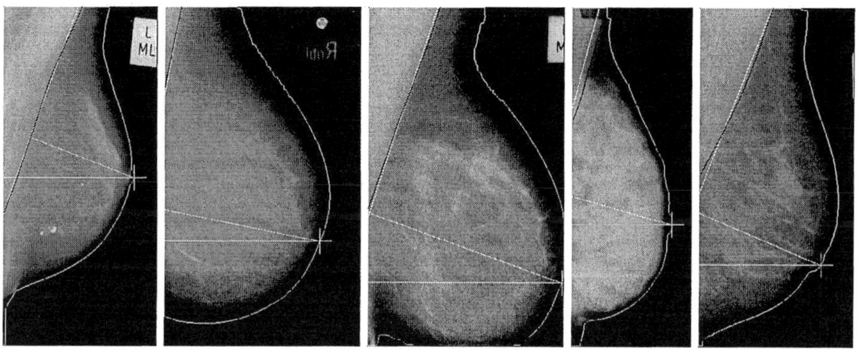

(a) (b) (c) (d) (e)

Fig. 1. All images show the breast border [9], nipple position [10] indicated by a cross, and two estimates of the pectoral margin [11]: the white line is the straight line estimate and the black one is the fitted curve. (a) image is adequate and nipple is in profile. (b) image is not adequate and nipple is not in profile. (c) anterior and inferior portions of breast lie outside image; the relevant border segments are outlined in grey. (d) image is either very dense or underexposed, with mean optical density of 1.15. (e) image is either very fatty or overexposed with mean optical density of 1.86.

5 Discussion

There were relatively few images in the MIAS database which complied with the criterion that the pectoral margin should extend to the level of the nipple. At present, this assessment is a go/no go binary determination, that perhaps should be refined in future to an analog scale of acceptability as suggested in some studies [4]. The algorithms were reliable for detecting exclusion of the anterior and inferior breast but new methods must be developed for detecting the retroglandular fat and axillary tail. Curvature of the anterior pectoral margin could not be reliably estimated by the proposed algorithm because it depends critically on the accuracy of the fitted curve. The importance and usefulness of this measure should be re-assessed and a better method devised if need be.

6 Conclusions

Several simple criteria for assessing the adequacy of positioning on the MLO view, suggested by radiologists, and measurable on the mammogram, have been developed into quantitative algorithms for automatically determining aspects of mammogram adequacy and quality. These measures are related principally to the adequacy of positioning and are by no means exhaustive. They must be extended in future to cover not only the craniocaudal view, but also other factors related to image quality. Nevertheless, in the context of mammogram screening, these results constitute a preliminary proof-of-concept that mammogram adequacy may be automatically determined, and that such an assessment, if carried out before the subject leaves the screening centre, may obviate the need for a second visit in case a repeat examination is deemed necessary.

References

1. M. T. Rickard, E. A. Wilson, A. Ferris, and K. H. Blackett, *Mammography Today: Positioning and Quality Control for Radiographers.* Sydney, Australia: Central Sydney Breast X-Ray Programme, 1992.
2. G. W. Eklund, G. Cardenosa, and W. Parsons, "Assessing Adequacy of Mammographic Image Quality," *Radiology*, vol. 190, pp. 297–307, Feb. 1994.
3. G. W. Eklund and G. Cardenosa, "The art of mammographic positioning," *The Radiologic Clinics of North America*, vol. 30, Jan. 1992.
4. L. W. Bassett, I. A. Hirbawi, N. DeBruhl, and M. K. Hayes, "Mammographic positioning: Evaluation from the view box," *Radiology*, vol. 188, pp. 803–806, 1993.
5. S. H. Heywang-Köbrunner, D. D. Dershaw, and I. Schreer, *Diagnostic Breast Imaging: Mammography, Sonography, Magnetic Resonance Imaging, and Interventional Procedures.* Stuttgart, Germany: Georg Thieme Verlag, 2nd, enlarged and revised ed., 2001.
6. S. H. Taplin, C. M. Rutter, C. Finder, M. T. Mandelson, F. Houn, and E. White, "Screening mammography: Clinical image quality and the risk of interval breast cancer," *American Journal of Roentgenology*, vol. 178, pp. 797–803, Apr. 2002.
7. V. F. Andolina, S. Lillé, and K. M. Willison, *Mammographic Imaging: A Practical Guide.* Philadelphia: J B Lippincott Company, 1992.
8. J. Suckling, J. Parker, D. R. Dance, and S. A. et al., "The Mammographic Image Analysis Society Digital Mammogram Database," in *Digital Mammography* (A. G. Gale, S. M. Astley, D. R. Dance, and A. Y. Cairns, eds.), (Amsterdam, The Netherlands), pp. 375–378, Elsevier Science, 1994.
9. R. Chandrasekhar and Y. Attikiouzel, "Automatic breast border segmentation by background modeling and subtraction," in *IWDM 2000: 5th International Workshop on Digital Mammography* (M. J. Yaffe, ed.), pp. 560–565, Madison, WI, USA: Medical Physics Publishing, 2001. Proceedings of the Workshop, June 11–14, 2000, Toronto, Canada.
10. R. Chandrasekhar and Y. Attikiouzel, "A Simple Method for Automatically Locating the Nipple on Mammograms," *IEEE Transactions on Medical Imaging*, vol. 16, pp. 483–494, Oct. 1997.
11. S. M. Kwok, R. Chandrasekhar, and Y. Attikiouzel, "Automatic pectoral muscle segmentation on mammograms by straight line estimation and cliff detection," in *ANZIIS 2001: Proceedings of the Seventh Australian and New Zealand Intelligent Information Systems Conference*, (Perth, Australia), pp. 67–72, ARCME, The University of Western Australia, Nov. 2001.

Peripheral Thickness Correction for Volumetric Breast Density Estimation

D. Rico, J. Yang, B. Augustine, G.E. Mawdsley and M.J. Yaffe

Sunnybrook and Women's College Health Science Centre
Rm. S631 2075 Bayview Avenue, Toronto, Ontario, Canada M4N 3M5
drico@sten.sunnybrook.utoronto.ca

Abstract. The computation of volumetric mammographic density in a breast is based on both image data and knowledge of the thickness at each pixel. Our goal is to compute a thickness map at the periphery of the breast in order to improve the accuracy of measurement of volumetric breast density. Two methods are considered. Using a breast phantom to simulate the thickness changes in an image, we have modelled the radiation profile through the edge of the breast, based on a phantom whose shape approximates a semi-circle. In a second method, direct thickness calibration is performed using a tissue-equivalent triangular attenuator. The phantom thickness map in the peripheral region is then mapped to that of the breast image using a thin-plate spline interpolation algorithm.

1. Introduction

Several investigators have demonstrated a strong association between breast density (the prevalence of fibroglandular tissue) and the risk of breast cancer [1-3]. Byng [3] developed a method that quantifies mammographic density in terms of the fraction of the projected breast area that is occupied by radiographically dense tissue. Limitations of this method include subjectivity, not using information about the thickness of the breast and the variation in appearance of structures due to differing exposure factors. We believe that the risk of breast cancer is more likely related to the volume of dense tissue rather than the projected area.

In previous work, Yang [4], developed a quantitative method for the measurement of the fraction of the breast by volume that is composed of fibroglandular tissue. Using calibration surfaces, analytical equations to describe volumetric % density (D) were developed and at position (i, j) local density is given by the following formula:

$$D(i, j) = [\log(I(I, j)) - C_1 + C_2T - C_3T^2]/(C_4T - C_5T^2)\,. \tag{1}$$

where $I(i, j)$ represents image pixel value, and T is breast thickness (from the readout of the mammography system), while C_1, C_2, C_3, C_4, C_5 are fitting constants.

The total percentage density (TPD) is given by:

$$TPD = [\sum_{breast} A_{pixel} D(i, j)T(i, j)]/[\sum_{breast} A_{pixel} T(i, j)] \text{ x } 100\%\,. \tag{2}$$

where A_{pixel} is the area of a pixel in an image.

The limitation of this method is that thickness is assumed to be constant for all pixels and the rolloff of thickness at the periphery of the breast (up to 25% of whole breast area) is not considered. The estimation of tissue composition in the periphery will be incorrect, contributing to error in *TPD*.

The method described here corrects thickness values in the peripheral region, so that they decrease from the maximum thickness as displayed on the readout of the mammography system to the outer edge of the breast.

2. Materials and Methods

A 4.8 cm thick breast phantom (Fig. 1a), constructed of poly-methyl-methacrylate (PMMA), was machined with a peripheral thickness profile that is semi-circular. Images were taken on a 2000D (GEMS, Milwaukee WI).

The peripheral region (Fig. 1b) of the PMMA phantom was contour segmented according to pixel signal level. The inner edge was found by gradually reducing the outer edge threshold (in steps of 50 intensity units) until the contour lines ceased to be smooth. This condition was determined by comparing the cross-correlation of their second derivative curves, with a value of 0.75 set as threshold.

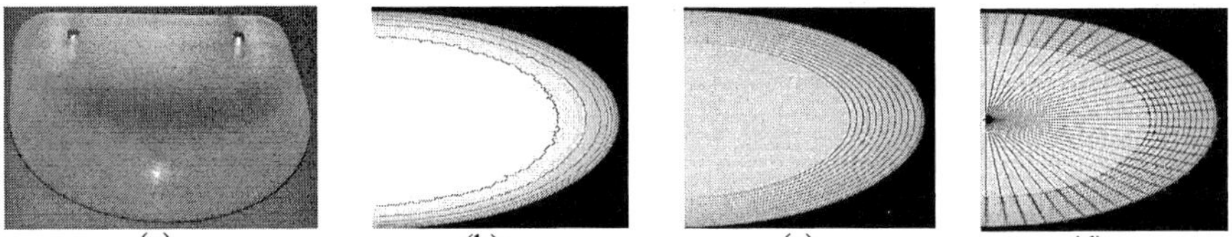

(a) (b) (c) (d)

Fig. 1. (a): PMMA breast phantom, (b) Contour lines in the peripheral region bounded by inner and outer edges, (c) Isothickness curves, (d) Horseshoe grid

To produce different levels of equal thickness in the peripheral region, the outer and inner edges were approximated by ellipses and then, equally-spaced elliptical **isothickness curves** (Fig. 1c) were generated. On the isothickness curves, a horseshoe grid was generated in a radial direction with angular step of 5 degrees (Fig. 1d).

From attenuation measurements on PMMA, we obtained a conversion from detector signal to thickness. Next, a third degree polynomial was generated to fit the previously-computed thickness values along each radial profile.

To compute thickness values for points inside the horseshoe grid, we use a distance minimization technique to calculate a relative distance between the inner and outer edges. From a point P (Fig. 2a) we compute the minimum Euclidian distance to the two ellipses. These two distances are summed to find the total peripheral width. The ratio of the inner distance to total distance is then calculated to give a relative distance value used as input to the polynomial function. The final thickness map is shown in Fig. 2b, where the thickness of the inner region was determined from the readout of the mammography system.

To verify our thickness calculations we used a second technique to produce a phantom thickness map, by using as a calibration device a breast tissue-equivalent

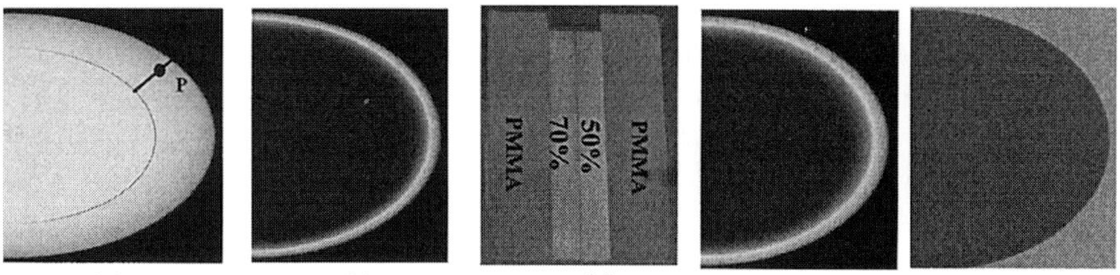

(a) (b) (c) (d) (e)

Fig. 2. (a) Point inside periphery and distances to the outer and inner edge, (b) Thickness map based on relative distance, (c) 3D - triangle phantom, (d) Thickness map based on logarithmic gray pixel value conversion, (e) Density map derived from (d).

triangular attenuator (Fig.2c). The triangle contains slabs of PMMA as well as plastics simulating 50% and 70% fibroglandular tissue. From the profile along the PMMA band (from top (7cm) to base (1mm)) in the triangle phantom, position along the wedge (i.e. thickness) is determined from the logarithm of image pixel signal, L by interpolation using a second-degree polynomial fit. The approximation functions for different materials are shown in Fig. 3a.

The thickness map for the known PMMA phantom, derived from the conversion of L to thickness is shown in Fig. 2d. With a corrected thickness map, using Eqn (1), we compute a density map (Fig. 2e). As expected, it is constant almost everywhere, with small variations around the outer edge. We performed an error analysis between the two models and found an absolute maximum error in thickness of ~3mm in most of the periphery and ~5mm in a narrow band close to the outer edge. In Fig. 3b, we present two horizontal profiles from thickness maps which show the same behavior.

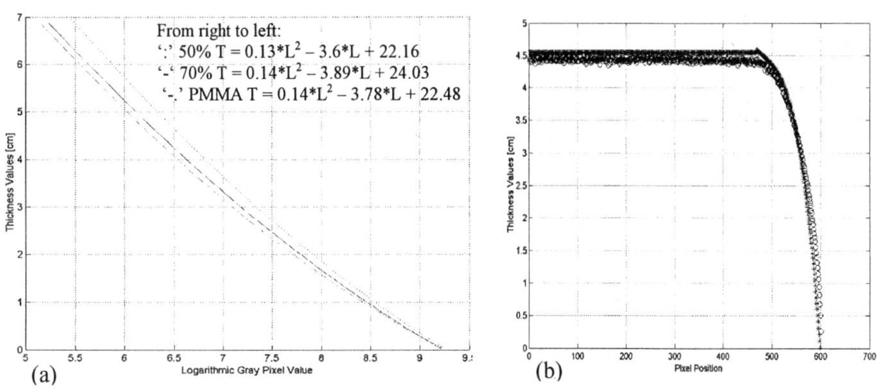

Fig. 3. (a) Thickness calibrations from the triangle phantom, (b) Horizontal profiles from thickness maps: 'o' thickness correction based on distance minimization technique, '*' thickness correction based on direct logarithmic gray pixel value conversion (triangle).

In order to build a thickness map for an individual mammography image, first we rescale the phantom thickness map to the size of the image and then overlay it using a thin-plate spline interpolation algorithm [5], which is efficient at recovering local deformations. With this technique, special care is needed in the selection of the landmarks. Two different sets of landmarks are chosen, both in the phantom thickness map and in the mammography image, from profiles in a radial direction with a step size of 5 degrees (Fig.4 a, b).

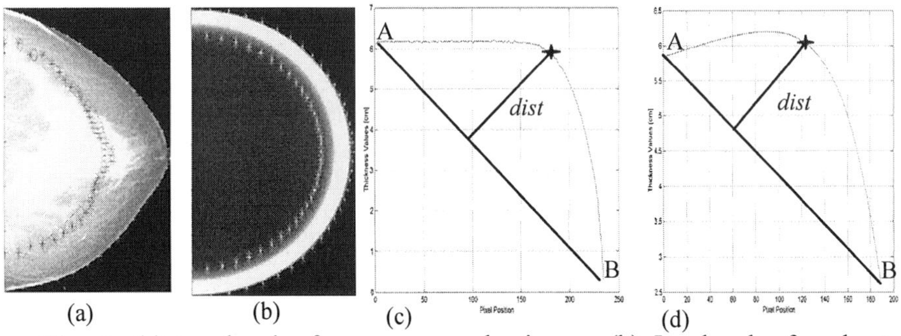

Fig. 4. (a) Landmarks for mammography image, (b) Landmarks for phantom thickness map, (c) Profile from phantom thickness map and landmark, (d) Profile from mammography image converted to thickness using a 50% material equation and landmark.

The first set of landmarks is located on the outer edge of each image. For the inner landmarks, a rough estimate is made of breast thickness, first converting the logarithmic profiles to thickness using a formula for 50% material (Fig. 3a), then the landmarks are chosen from the thickness profiles (Figs. 4c and 4d) as points for which the distance (*dist*) to line AB is maximal. Finally a smoothed version of the landmark coordinates is computed by a second degree polynomial approximation ('o' points from Fig. 4a). The warped thickness template of the mammographic image Fig. 5a is shown in Fig. 5b.

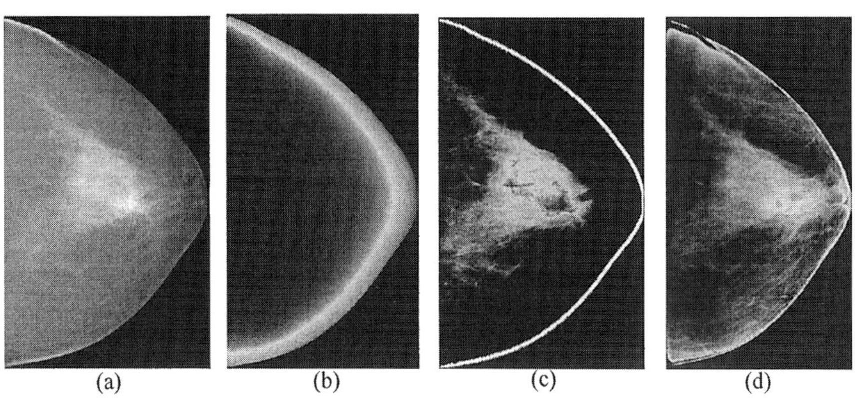

Fig. 5. (a) Original breast image, (b) Corrected warped thickness, (c) Density map computed using constant thickness, (d) Density map computed using corrected thickness map.

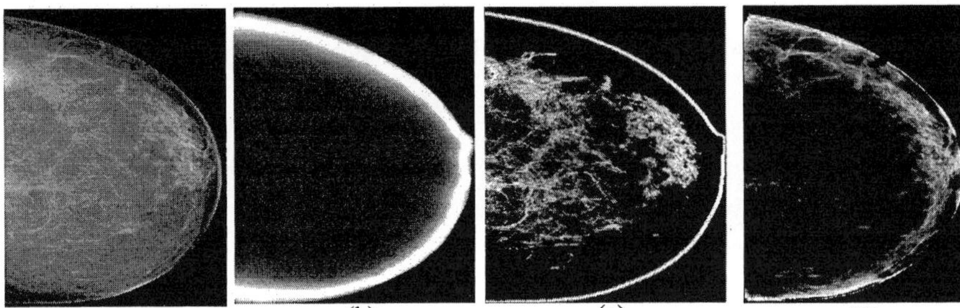
(a) (b) (c) (d)

Fig. 6. (a) Original image of fatty breast, (b) Corrected warped thickness map edge, (c) Density map computed using constant thickness and outer edge, (d) Density map computed using corrected thickness map.

Results

In Figs. 5 and 6 we present the results of density map computation for two digital mammograms using constant and corrected thickness maps. In the first case, the peripheral region added about 42% to the area contributing to the density measurement, *TPD* value for constant thickness increased from 7.33% to 21.73%. In the second case, the peripheral correction added 27% to the area contributing to density and *TPD* increased from 4.22% to 11.44%. The method was applied to a series of 20 images and reasonable ranges of density (10-100%) were obtained in the peripheral region.

Discussion

We have developed a peripheral thickness correction method to improve volumetric breast density estimation. We plan to refine the method by taking into account the deflection of the compression paddle. We expect that the volumetric method will provide a stronger correlation with risk than the current area method.

References

1. Wolfe, J.N., Risk for breast cancer development determined by mammographic parenchymal pattern, Cancer 37, 2486-2492, 1976.
2. Boyd , N.F., Lockwood , G.A., Byng , J.W., Tritchler , D.L., Yaffe, M.J.: Mammographic densities and breast cancer risk, Cancer Epidemiol. Biomark. Prev., 7, 1133-1144, 1998.
3. Byng, J.F., Boyd , N.F., Fishell , E., Jong , R.A., Yaffe , M.J.: The Quantitative Analysis of Mammographic Densities, Physics in Medicine and Biology, 39, 1629-1638, 1994.
4. Yang. J., Rico D., Mawdsley G.E., Yaffe, M.J.: Volumetric Breast Density Estimation Method for Full-Field Digital Mammography, RSNA, 2002.
5. Bookstein, F.L: Principal Warps: Thin-Plate spline and the decomposition of deformations. IEEE Trans. Patt. Anal. Machine Intell., 11, 567-585, 1989

An Adaptive Enhancement Filter For Mammographic Phantom Image

Guis V, Adel M, Rasigni M, Rasigni G, *Seradour B, *Heid P

INTERFACE - PHYSIQUE- BIOLOGIE – MEDECINE, Université d'Aix-Marseille III
Faculté des Sciences et Techniques de Saint-Jérôme Case EC1 13397 Marseille Cedex 20
France
*ARCADES, Hôpital de la Timone Rue Saint-Pierre 13005 Marseille Cedex 5 FRANCE
v.guis@free.fr

Abstract. We evolve an image enhancement method for facilitating further object detection process. For this purpose an adaptive neighbourhood image processing technique with a contrast-enhancement function is used. In order to compare function performance, simulated images containing objects similar to those observed in the phantom, with various relative contrasts and various Signal to Noise Ratio levels, were generated. When using appropriate contrast enhancement functions results show that the process enhances noteworthy features both in simulated images and real phantom images with little noise enhancement.

1. Introduction

To be relevant a diagnosis has to be done from a high quality mammogram. For this purpose a phantom image is used to perform this control. Showing this phantom film to several observers and scoring it by visual observation is now accepted as a standard method to perform quality control evaluation in mammographic facilities. Automating this control by using image processing on a digitised phantom film, will make this control easier and less subjective. Such a project requires first to digitise phantoms films with the adequate spatial resolution, then to enhance features we need to detect and at last to segment and characterize the objects contained in the phantom image. In this paper, we evaluate the performance of an important step in the automating scoring project namely: image enhancement task. For that purpose, an evaluation of a noise reduction and enhancement method is done on simulated images (on which contrast and noise parameters can be modified) and then on real phantom images.

2. Material and methods

2.1 Phantom Description

The phantom used in this study is the MTM 100/R [1] which is used in France for Mammography Accreditation. It is made of tissue equivalent material in which are embedded objects simulating microcalcifications (pentagonal-shaped groups), masses or nodules and fibrils of progressively smaller size and contrast.

2.2 Simulated and real phantom images

Simulated images containing objects similar to those observed in the phantom are generated with different contrast and noise levels. Masses, which are more difficult to detect than the others objects[2], are studied. Contrast level is defined as the difference between the mean grey level of the object and the background divided by the mean grey level of the background. The classical mammographic additive noise model where the noise is signal-dependent is used [3]. Contrast levels were in the range [10%; 60%] with a step size of 10% and the standard deviation σ was chosen so that the signal to noise ratio takes the values 21 and 15 which simulate low and high noise levels respectively. So 12 images were simulated we denote I. The 6 images relative to different contrast levels only (without noise) were denoted I_0.

Phantom films were digitised using a high resolution scanner (Scanmate 1100) with a resolution of 50 μm per pixel (or 508 dpi) and were coded on 256 grey levels.

2.3 Algorithm and method

For taking local features into account the method is based on computation of a local contrast around each pixel using a variable neighborhood whose size (j W) and shape depend on statistical properties around the given pixel[4],[5],[6]. The obtained image C is transformed into another image C' using a mathematical function. At last the inverse contrast transform of the process used to obtain image C from the original image I is applied to image C'. Depending on mathematical functions used the method yields noise reduction or contrast enhancement. So the algorithm consists in applying twice the method, first as a denoising filter[4] and second as an enhancement filter. For this purpose various functions were tested for reducing noise [3] (Step 1) and for enhancing contrast (Step 2). Two threshold parameters, a local one T_l and a global one T_g were used in the adaptive neighborhood process. The local threshold T_l is the standard deviation within the W size window around each pixel and the global threshold T_g is the standard deviation of the whole image. In a first time the best maximal size W_{max} for the neighborhood window was determined from the study of the output contrast level (contrast level in the image I_1 obtained at the end of step 1) versus W. This study was made on image I by using the T_l and T_g values computed from image I after a 3*3 average filtering, and various mathematical functions. The value W_{max} was defined as the mean W value yielding the better output contrast level. Once W_{max} was known, influence of various mathematical functions on noise reduction was then quantitatively evaluated by means of Signal to Noise Ratio (SNR's) parameters. The study concerning the step 1 dealt with a previous paper [3]. Global threshold associated with tangent function turned out to provide valuable results. We denote I_2 the corresponding image obtained concerning the enhancement step (step 2) to which this paper is devoted. The method is the same as in step 1, but T_l and T_g values are now computed from images I_1 after a 3*3 average filtering. W_{max} is evaluated as previously in step 1, by using others mathematical functions. In order to compare enhancement contrast functions namely root square and hyperbolic tangent, and to evaluate performance of the whole method (step 1 + step 2), we used the output contrast level (relative to images I_2 obtained at the end of the step 2) versus the input contrast level (relative to images I_0)

3. Results

The results obtained show similar quantitative performance for the two functions and the two threshold levels whatever noise levels. However, we note an advantage for the trigonometric function associated with the local threshold parameter. The less valuable results were obtained with the trigonometric function associated with the global threshold for each noise level. Visual evaluation of real phantom images processed with the above method show results similar to those obtained from simulated images.

4. Conclusion

In this paper, we presented a contrast enhancement method using contrast parameter and contrast enhancement function. It is the second part of a method whose first part, based on the same principle was devoted to image noise reduction. Simulated images were generated to evaluate its efficiency. In particular, in this second part two contrast enhancement functions were tested. It follows that the whole method provides valuable results when global threshold associated with tangent function and local threshold associated with hyperbolic tangent function are successively used. This method provides also good visual results on real phantom images.

References

1. Computerized Imaging Reference Systems, Inc., 2428 Almeda Avenue suite 212, Norflok, VA 23513, U.S.A.
2. Qian W, Clarke LP, Kallergi M, Clark RA : Tree-Structured Nonlinear Filters in Digital Mammography,. IEEE Trans. Med. Imag. Vol 13, N°1, (1994) 25-36.
3. V. Guis, M. Adel, M. Rasigni, G. Rasigni, B. Seradour, P. Heid : Noise reduction in mammographic phantom images using adaptive neighbourhood contrast enhancement. Advanced Concepts for Intelligent Vision Systems, Proceedings of The Second International Symposium on Intelligent Vision Systems Baden Baden (2001) 106-111
4. Gordon R, Rangayyan RM : Feature enhancement of film mammograms using fixed and adaptative neighborhoods, Appl. Opt.Vol 23, N°4 (1984) 560-564
5. Dhawan AP, G. Buelloni G, Gordon R : Enhancement of mammographic features by optimal adaptative neighborhood image processing, IEEE Trans. Med. Imag.Vol MI-5, N°1, (1986).
6. A. P. Dhawan E. Le Royer: Mammographic feature enhancement by computarized image processing," Computer Methods and Programs in Biomedecine Vol 27 (1988) 23-25.

Analysis and Classification of Breast Masses by Fuzzy-set-based Image Processing

Denise Guliato[1], Rangaraj M. Rangayyan[2], Fabricio Adorno[1], and Mário M. G. Ribeiro[1]

[1] Faculty of Informatics, Federal University of Uberlândia, Uberlândia, Minas Gerais, Brazil, e-mail: guliato@ufu.br
[2] Department of Electrical and Computer Engineering, University of Calgary, Calgary, Alberta, Canada T2N 1N4, e-mail: ranga@enel.ucalgary.ca

Abstract. We propose parameters to characterize breast masses based upon the fuzzy transition present in their boundaries. We have developed an interactive graphical interface that integrates fuzzy-set-based segmentation and classification tools. Using a database of 47 mammograms including 22 benign masses and 25 malignant tumors, the coefficient of variation of the fuzzy membership values in ribbons surrounding mass regions provided a sensitivity of 0.8 and a specificity of 0.91.

1 Introduction

Most benign masses are well-circumscribed with sharp boundaries that delineate them from surrounding tissues, while most malignant tumors possess fuzzy boundaries with slow and extended transition from a dense core region to the surrounding, less-dense tissues. Many works have addressed the problem of segmentation and classification of breast tumors [1], [2]; however, few of them consider the transition information around tumor/mass boundaries [3], [4], [5]. We have recently proposed two segmentation methods that consider the uncertainty present around the boundaries of tumors. The first method determines the boundary of a tumor by region growing after a preprocessing step based on fuzzy sets to enhance the region of interest (ROI) [6]. The second method is a fuzzy region growing method that takes into account the uncertainty present around the boundaries of tumors [7], and results in fuzzy ROIs that include the boundary transition information.

2 Methods

The first segmentation procedure [6] executes a fuzzy-set preprocessing step using a membership function that evaluates the similarity between the pixel being analyzed and pixels in the ROI based upon a feature vector. The result is a preprocessed image that represents pixels with values close to the reference feature vector with high membership degrees. A region growing procedure is then applied to the preprocessed image to obtain a contour. An erosion procedure is applied to the contour so that the core of the ROI is separated from the boundary. A parameter labeled as ΔCV is computed from the fuzzy-set preprocessed image, by taking the difference between the coefficient of variation of the entire ROI and that of the core of the ROI. A high value of ΔCV represents an inhomogeneous ROI, which could be indicative of a malignant tumor.

In the case of the fuzzy ROIs obtained by the second fuzzy region growing method [7], it was observed that the transition regions around malignant tumors are darker (i.e., have lower membership values) than the corresponding regions for benign masses. The pixels in the transition region of a malignant tumor are expected to possess low agreement with the characteristics of the corresponding core tumor region. A fuzzy boundary was defined for each ROI as the connected region whose pixels possess membership degree less than unity and separate the tumor core from its background. We computed the coefficient of variation CV_{fr} of the membership degrees of pixels inside the fuzzy boundary, and the ratio η of the number of pixels with membership degree less than 0.5 to the total number of pixels within the fuzzy boundary. CV_{fr} and η are expected to be higher for malignant tumors than for benign masses.

An interactive graphical interface has been developed in Java, using an object-oriented architecture with controller classes. Some of the features of the interface are fast and easy upgradability, portability, and threads to support parallelism between tasks. The interface is ergonomic and easy to use, and includes on-line support/help. The interface integrates procedures to detect contours using fuzzy preprocessing and region growing, extract fuzzy regions using fuzzy region growing, compute statistical parameters, and classify masses and tumors as benign or malignant. The interface also provides access to basic image processing procedures including zooming in/out, filters, histogram operations, the Bezier method to manipulate contours, and image format conversion.

The methods were tested with 47 mammograms from the Mammographic Image Analysis Society (MIAS, UK) database and local cases from the Alberta Cancer Board, including 22 benign masses and 25 malignant tumors. The classification potential of the proposed parameters was evaluated by simple logistic regression using the statistical package SAS System Release 6.12.

3 Results

Discrimination between benign masses and malignant tumors with the parameter η had no statistical significance ($\alpha > 0.05$). For CV_{fr} and ΔCV, we obtained probability of malignancy curves; the curve for CV_{fr} is illustrated in Figure 1. Several cut points were analyzed for each curve. For CV_{fr}, the cut point of 0.52 resulted in the correct classification of 20/25 malignant tumors and 20/22 benign masses (sensitivity = 0.80 and specificity = 0.91). For ΔCV, the cut point of 0.6 resulted in 16/25 malignant tumors and all 22 benign masses being correctly classified. ΔCV exhibited a low sensitivity of 0.64, but a high specificity of 1.0. Further work on the computation and assessment of the parameters is in progress.

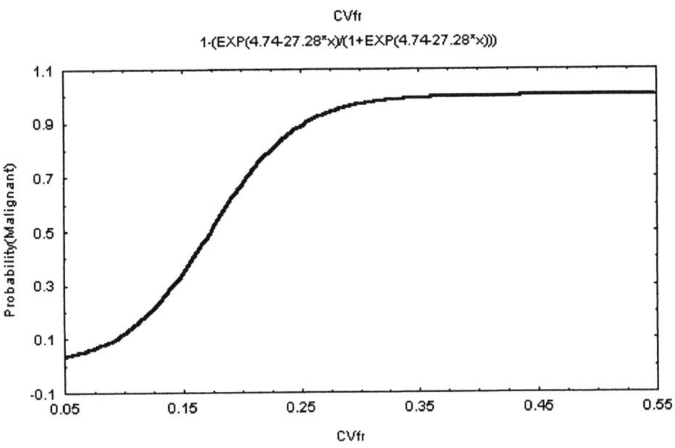

Fig. 1. Probability of malignancy curve for the parameter CV_{fr}.

References

1. L. MILLER and N. RAMSEY. The detection of malignant masses by non-linear multiscale analysis. In K. Doi, M.L. Giger, R.M. Nishikawa, and R.A. Schmidt, editors, *3rd International Workshop on Digital Mammography*, pages 335–340, Chicago, IL, 9-12 June 1996.
2. M. A. KUPINSKI and M. L. GIGER. Automated seeded lesion segmentation on digital mammograms. *IEEE Transactions on Medical Imaging*, 17(4):510–517, August 1998.
3. N.R. MUDIGONDA, R.M. RANGAYYAN, and J.E.L. DESAUTELS. Detection of breast masses in mammograms by density slicing and texture flow-field analysis. *IEEE Transactions on Medical Imaging*, 20(12):1215–1227, December 2001.
4. R.M. RANGAYYAN, N.M. EL-FARAMAWY, J.E.L. DESAUTELS, and O.A. ALIM. Measures of acutance and shape for classification of breast tumors. *IEEE Transactions on Medical Imaging*, 16(6):799–810, 1997.
5. C.H. CHEN and G.G. LEE. On digital mammogram segmentation and microcalcification detection using multiresolution wavelet analysis. *Graphical Models and Image Processing*, 59(5):349–364, September 1997.
6. D. GULIATO, R.M. RANGAYYAN, J.A. ZUFFO, and J.E.L. DESAUTELS. Detection of breast tumor boundaries using iso-intensity contours and dynamic thresholding. In N. Karssemeijer, M. Thijssen, J. Hendriks, and L. van Erning, editors, *4th International Workshop on Digital Mammography*, pages 253–260, Nijmegen, The Netherlands, June 1998. Kluwer Academic, Dordrecht.
7. D. GULIATO, R.M. RANGAYYAN, W.A. CARNIELLI, J.A. ZUFFO, and J.E.L. DESAUTELS. Segmentation of breast tumors in mammograms by fuzzy region growing. In *20th Annual International Conference of the IEEE Engineering in Medicine and Biology Society*, pages II:1002–1004 and four pages in CD–ROM, Hong Kong, 29 October - 1 November 1998.

Acknowledgment: We thank Dr. Heyder D. Silva, for help with statistical analysis, and Dr. Naga Mudigonda for help with tumor detection and analysis.

Three comparative methods for mammograms segmentation: by Master-Slave algorithm and by two parallel fusion algorithms

Carlos Avilés-Cruz, Juan A. Domínguez-López, Mario Reyes-Ayala and Edgar Andrade-González

Universidad Autónoma Metropolitana – Azcapotzalco Departamento de Electrónica Av. San Pablo 180, Col. Reynosa, Del. Azcapotzalco. C.P. 02200, México D. F.
Phone: (+52) 5318-9549, 5318-9037. Fax: 5394-6843
caviles@correo.azc.uam.mx

Abstract. In this paper we compare three different segmentation schemes, in order to segment mammograms (taken from MIAS database): the first one is our proposed Master-Slave method, the second one is the parallel data fusion algorithms such as Bayes formalism and the third one is Dempster-Shafer theory. The Master-Slave algorithm works under the following logic: there are two classifiers (Master or slave), if Master classifier rejects the feature vector (bad classification), then at the same pixel centered-window there are a second features estimation taking a bigger or a smaller window, this second feature vector is now classified by Slave classifier (the decision could be the reject class). Both classifier decisions (Gaussian or KNN) pass to the reconstruction task giving the final mammography segmentation. For the parallel data fusion algorithms we have to estimate at the same time two vector features (one for bigger window and other for smaller window), both feature vector are classified; their decisions could be well or bad classification. From the classifier decisions, we have implemented the Bayes fusion which is based on the Belief function taking the probability to belong a given class. We have implemented also the fusion by Dempster-Shafer theory.

Introduction

At present, mammography associated with clinical breast examination and breast self-examination is the only effective and viable method for mass breast screening. The literature report since last 20 years different methods using statistical features [3][10] but there is not one method that find good segmentation results for all tumor type. There are others approximations like multi scale [8][5], neural network [9], wavelet domain [7][15] and structural analysis [1][2] in order to find shape and tumor area. In the classification and segmentation domain of micro-textures, one feature is not sufficient to segment a very large gamma of micro-textures at 100%. A solution is to build a robust decision process fusing many features [11]. The fusion process has been used in robotic [12][13], in character recognition [14], in texture segmentation [15], etc. Other technique to take into account the decision of one or plus features under one or plus classifiers in data fusion domain is the architecture Master-Slave [15]. This architecture is based under idea of: to do the estimation with only one features, if the estimation is well classified then it's the final decision else we have to estimate the other features and classifier it, the final decision could be the good classification or also the reject class. In the following paragraph those techniques will be described.

1. Theoretical Foundations

The used features are well known [ref]: mean, variance, co-occurrence matrix, Fourier Transform, Cosine transform, third order moments and fourth order moments. For more details, you can refer to the bibliography. We are going to present three fusion technique from theoretical view.

Serial Architecture: the Master-Slave architecture (see figure 1) works under logic that firstly a windows size is taken to estimate second or fourth order moments classified by the Master classifier (could be K-NN o Gaussian classifier) given two decisions: a) the window is well classified and, b) the window is rejected, in b) case, at the same position a window is taken in order to estimate fourth or second order moments , those features are now classifieds by the Slave classifier (could be K-NN o Gaussian classifier). The slave classification could rejection or well classification. For both classifier decisions, the result are used to reconstruct segmented image

Parallel Architecture:

Fusion by Bayes theory: Decision fusion is weighted by the knowledge of error distribution for each classifier ($P(\vec{x} \in w_j / e_k(\vec{x}) = j_k)$ given by the confusion matrix). So the winner class is estimated by a Belief function, meaning the proposition that $\vec{x}$ belongs to class c_i , according to the equation 1

$$Bel(i) = P(\vec{x} \in w_j / e_1(\vec{x}) = j_1, e_2(\vec{x}) = j_2, ..., e_k(\vec{x}) = j_k) \quad (1)$$

The winner class is the argument of the maximum.

Fusion by Theory of Evidence: The theory of Evidence was developed by Dempster and Shafer [10]. Its goal is to combine the propositions or evidences following the *a priori* knowledge given by the matrix confusion. Here the author define a belief function $Bel(A_i)$, where $A_i = \vec{x} \in w_i$. The function is found by the mass function: **Fehler! Es ist nicht möglich, durch die Bearbeitung von Feldfunktionen Objekte zu erstellen.**. The winner class will be the bigger mass function.

Methodology and setup parameters

The segmentation task was the mammography scanning from top to bottom and from left to right, pixel by pixel. The features used were: mean, variance, co-occurrence matrix, Fourier Transform, Cosine transform, third order moments and fourth order moments. The features estimation was done from a window; the window size was optimized in order to get minimal error: 26x26 pixels with an error less than 5% and 13x13 pixels with an error less than 10%, for the Master-Slave architecture (cross-validation method). The tumor characteristics are :(A) Well-defined/circumscribed masses, type fatty-glandular, benign; (B) Well-defined/circumscribed masses, type fatty-glandular, malignant; (C) Well-defined/circumscribed masses, type fatty , benign; and (D) Well-defined/circumscribed masses, type fatty , malignant. As a result, the Master-Slave architecture gives best border segmentation while the parallel data fusion algorithms segment well the principal area. The main advantage for the Master-Slave architecture is less computationally expensive giving good results

5. Results and Conclusions

Figure 1 shows segmentation results for the proposed Master-Salve Architecture (figure 1.a); and for two parallel data fusion schemes: By Bayes formalism (figure 1.b) and for Dempster-Shafer theory. The best segmentation area is obtained by Master-Slave architecture (reaching 90% of tumor area), the fusion algorithms reach 80% and 85% for Bayes formalism and Dempster-Shafer, respectively. For Master-Slave architecture, the window size for master classifier was 25 pixels and for Slave was 13 pixels; those window size was chosen by cross-validation method; both classifiers were KNN.

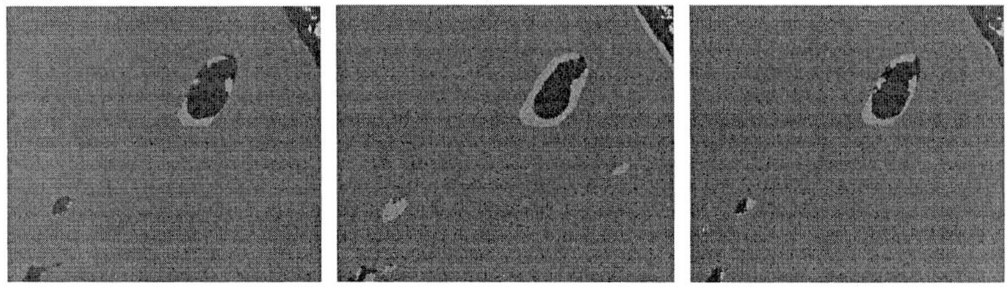

Figure 1: Segmentation results by three techniques: (a) Master-Slave architecture, (b) By Bayes formalism and (c) By Dempster -Shafer theory

In order to find the best window size for the parallel fusion schemes, we have done cross-validation at 50%. To having an error less than 5%, for Bayes formalism, the window size is 24 pixels, and for Dempster-Shafer was 15 pixels. You can see cross-validation results in figure 2.

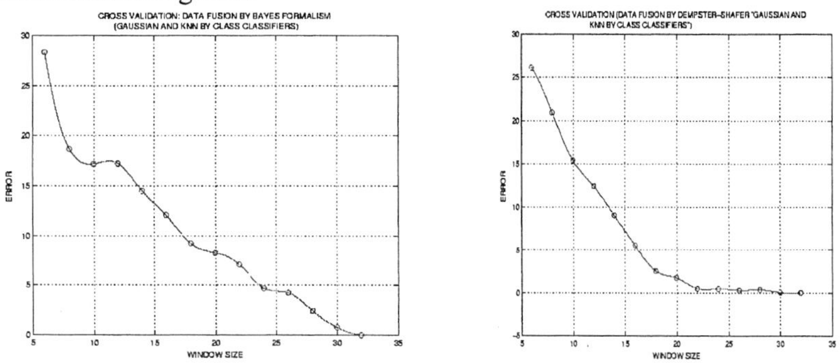

Figure 2: Cross Validation (fusing gaussian and KNN classifiers): (a) By Bayes formalism and (b) By Dempster -Shafer theory

Conclusions: In this paper we have shown the efficiency and significant improvements in accuracy of tumor segmentation by incorporating Master-Slave architecture (serial type) and two parallel schemes. The features combination proposed gives goods results in order to segment fatty-glandular tumor (malignant or benign). The best tumor segmentation was obtained by Master-Slave scheme (90%). The main advantage for the Master-Slave architecture is less computationally expensive giving good results

Acknowledgments

This work was supported by CONACyT grand J31916-A

References

1 N.R. Mudigonda, R.M. Rangayyan, and J.E.L. Desautels, 2000, "Gradient and texture analysis for the classification of mammographic masses", IEEE Transactions on Medical Imaging, 19(10):1032-1043.

2 R.M. Rangayyan, N.R. Mudigonda, and J.E.L. Desautels, 2000, "Boundary modeling and shape analysis methods for classification of mammographic masses", Medical and Biological Engineering and Computing, 38(5):487-496.

3 Dhawan, Christine Kaiser – Banasso and Myron Moskowitz : "Analysis of mammographic micro calcifications using gray–level image structure features", Atom P, Vol. 15, N. 3, June 1996, pp.246-259.(0278-0062/96$05.00).

4 Heng – Da Cheng, Yui Man Lui and Rita I. Freimanis: "A new approach to micro calcification detection in digital mammograms", 1997, pp.1094-1098. (0-7803-3534-1/97 10.00).

5 M. Nafi Gürcan, Yasemin Yardimici, A Enis Cetin and Rashid Ansari : "Automated detection and enhancement of micro calcifications in mammograms using nonlinear sub band decomposition", 1997, pp. 3069-3072. (0-8186-7919-0/97 $10.00)

6 Mark Wilson, Roger Hargrave, Sunanda Mitra, Yao – Yang Shieh and Glenn H. Roberson : "Automated detection of micro calcifications in mammograms through application of image pixel remapping and statistical filter", Eleventh IEEE Symposium on Computer – Based Medical Systems, pp. 270-274.

7 Giussepe Boccignone, Angelo Chianese and Antonio Picariello : "Entropy – based detection of micro calcifications in wavelet space", 1998, pp. 2713 – 2716. (0-7803-4428-6/98 $10.00)

8 Howard C. Choe and Andrew K. Chan : "Micro calcification cluster detection in digitized mammograms using multiscale techniques",1998, pp. 23 –28. (0-7803-4876-1/98/$10.00)

9 Baoyu Zheng, Wei Quian and Laurence P. Clarke : "Digital mammography: mixed feature neural network with spectral entropy decision for detection of micro calcifications", Vol. 15, no. 5, octubre, 1996, pp. 589-597. (0278-0062/96$05.00)

10 Gregory McGarry and Mohamed Deriche: "Modellining mammographic images using fractional brownian motion", 1997 Speech and Image Technologies for Computing and Telecommunications, pp.222.

11 Bloch , Information Combination Operators for Data Fusion: A Comparative Review with Classification, In IEEE Trans. on SMC.-Part A, Jan 1996, Vol. 26

12 J.L. Crowley and Y. Demazeau. Principles and techniques for sensor data fusion. Signal Processing, 32:5{27, 1993

13 R.C. Luo and M.H. Lin, Robot multisensor and integration : optimum estimation of fused sensor data, Ch2555-1/88/0000/1060\$01-00 {IEEE}}, 1988.

14 L. Xu, A. Krzyzak, and C.Y. Suen. Methods of combining multiple classifiers and their applications to handwriting recognition. IEEE Transaction systems, Man. and Cybernetics, 22(3), 1992.

15 C. Avilés-Cruz and A. Guerin-Dugué. Texture Discrimination Enhancement by Fusion with Second end Fourth Order Statistics. In G. Ramponi, editor, Signal Processing VII, Theories and Applications, Trieste, Italy, September 1997. Elsevier

3D Object Localization and Visualization in Breast Tomosynthesis

Lihua Li , Yong Chu, Xiaohua Hu, Maria Kallergi, Jerry A. Thomas*, Robert A. Clark,Jeffrey W. Eberhard**, and Bernhard E. H. Claus**

Department of Radiology, College of Medicine, H. Lee Moffitt Cancer Center & Research Institute
University of South Florida, Tampa, FL 33612
* Uniformed Services University of the Health Science, Bethesda, MD 20814
** General Electric Global Research Center, 1 Research Circle, Niskayuna, NY 12309
lilh@moffit.usf.edu

Abstract. This paper presents a preliminary study of CAD in breast tomosynthesis. The problem addressed is how to discriminate the objects on the in-focus plane from its blurred image superimposed on other planes. Instead of developing a preprocessing module to suppress the tomosynthesis artifacts in the reconstruction, we locate the object by utilizing the inherent 3D information in the reconstructed planar images. This study was done on tomosynthesis data of a stereo breast biopsy phantom (RMI 164A) reconstructed with the simple backprojection (or shift-and-add) method. The experimental results demonstrate the ability of the proposed method to identify the focal plane of objects. It can potentially be applied to remove the blurred out-of-plane structure and improve the clinical application of breast tomosynthesis.

1. Introduction

Breast cancer is the second leading cause of cancer death among American women. In an attempt to improve mammographic imaging and interpretation, digital tomosynthesis has been proposed in recent years as a new breast imaging method [1]. Compared to conventional mammography, tomosynthesis has the following potential advantages: (1) it may be a valuable breast screening tool for women with dense breasts, who have a statistically higher risk of cancer incidence, and therefore improve detection sensitivity; (2) it may improve the confidence level of radiologists in lesion characterization and classification, and therefore increase the specificity of diagnosis; (3) it may reduce the call-back rate because tomosynthesis can provide better discrimination between superimposed structure and real masses; (4) it may be possible to use less compression since blurring of out-of-plane structures actually increases with less compression [2]. However, breast tomosynthesis technology still has several hurdles to overcome in practice to realize its highest potential. For example, the tomosynthesis reconstruction suffers from blurred images of structural detail lying outside of the plane of interest superimposed on the image of the in-focus plane. Several methods have been proposed for suppressing non-relevant planar information and enhancing image quality in tomosynthesis, including optimization of sampling geometry, pre-filtering of projections, and post processing of reconstructed images. As a preliminary study of CAD in breast tomosynthesis, this paper addresses the problem of object localization in tomosynthesis images. Instead of developing a preprocessing module to suppress the tomosynthesis artifacts in the reconstruction, we try to locate the object by utilizing the *a priori* 3D information in the reconstructed planar images.

2. Artifact Analysis in Breast Tomosynthesis

In breast tomosynthesis imaging, projection images were first obtained at discrete X-ray source positions as the tube moved above the breast, as shown in Figure 1. For simplicity, only six X-ray source positions are shown. The tomosynthesis images of any plane in the breast may then be reconstructed by using various reconstruction methods. In simple backprojection reconstruction as shown in Figure 1, for a projection at angle θ, in order to reconstruct a planar image at height z, the projection image has to be shifted by

$$x_o(\theta, z) = L \cdot \sin\theta \cdot z /(D + L \cdot \cos\theta - z), \tag{1}$$

followed by a scaling with factor $1-(z/(D+L\cdot\cos\theta)$ which counteracts the cone-beam magnification in the image acquisition. Here L is the distance between the axis of rotation and the X-ray tube position, D is the distance between axis and the image plane, and the zero degree position of the X-ray tube is assumed to be at $x=0$.

An object $O(x,y,z)$ at (x,y,z), will produce an artifact on each adjacent plane. Their relative positions to the object $O(x,y,z)$ on adjacent planes at $z+\Delta$ and $z-\Delta$ can be represented approximately as

$$\pm\Delta \cdot (L\cdot\sin\theta)/(D + L\cos\theta) \tag{2}$$

The artifacts on planes at $\pm\Delta$ are approximately symmetric with respect to the object on the in-focus plane. The artifact $A(x,y,,z)$ resulting from $O(x,y,z)$ and imposed on the planes at $z\pm\Delta$ can be described as

$$A(x, y, z \pm \Delta) = \sum_{i=0}^{N-1} \alpha_i \cdot O(x \pm \Delta x_i, y, z) \tag{3}$$

where α_i is the out-of plane intensity factor, N is the number of projections, and

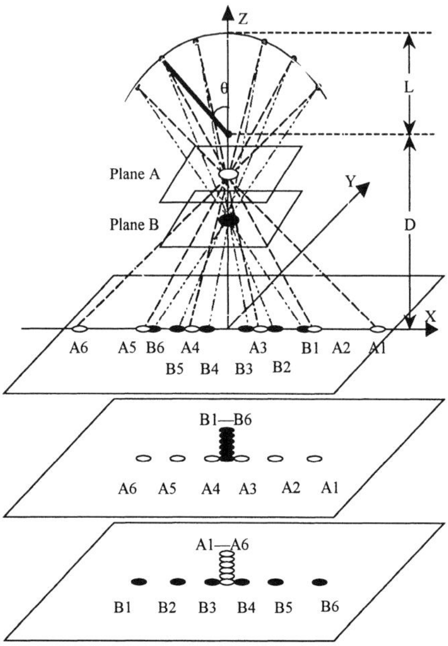

Fig. 1. An illustration of tomosynthesis image reconstruction.

$$\Delta x_i \approx \pm\Delta\cdot\left(L\cdot\sin\theta_i\right)/\left(D+L\cdot\cos\theta_i\right) \tag{4}$$

with θ_i denoting the projection angle.

3. Object Localization Method and Results

The proposed object localization method consists of two steps. First, a clustering based segmentation method was applied to the reconstructed image to extract the breast region. Then a 3D processing method was applied to locate the objects in the tomosynthesis images, using the following steps:(a) a 3D symmetric matching algorithm was applied to the tomosynthesis image slices to detect the symmetry of artifacts; (b) in order to enhance the contrast of the 3D symmetric filtered image, a high pass filter was applied to the filtered tomosynthesis images; (c) with the filtered slice images, a minimal-value image was then generated, in which each pixel takes the minimal value among all the pixels at the given location from different slices; (d) the minimal-value image was then segmented using an adaptive thresholding segmentation method to get regions with lower pixel value; (e) the segmented regions were classified to eliminate the non-object regions. A region with big enough size was classified as a potential object. Each segmented region was then examined to determine the slice from which different pixels in the region originated and to calculate its focus index (defined here as normalized average pixel value of region).

The centroid coordinates of the region and its corresponding slice image number, which has the maximum focus index, are the location of detected object.

The method was evaluated using a set of tomosynthesis images of a stereotactic breast biopsy phantom (RMI 164A). In tomosynthesis imaging, 11 projections were taken over a 50-degree angular range to reconstruct the 43 tomosynthetis images by simple backprojection. Figure 2(a) shows a projection image, in which 10 objects were observed in addition to 15 very subtle objects. A typical tomosynthesized image (slice #29) is shown in Figure 2(b), in which there are one in-focus and several blurred out-of-plane objects. A symmetric filtered slice image is shown in Figure 2(c). Figure 3 shows an example of locating the image plane with the object being in focus as shown in Figure 2(b) by the proposed method. It is presented as a plot of focus index versus slice image number. The detection output in the X-Y plane is shown in Figure 2(d). It is observed that the proposed method can locate the object accurately. To demonstrate the advantage of breast tomosynthesis in depth discrimination, an example of 3D visualization of tomosynthesis segmentation images is shown in Figure 4.

4. Conclusion

An object localization method was presented in this paper to discriminate the objects on the in-focus plane from its blurred image superimposed on other planes. Experimental results on a set of tomosynthesis phantom images demonstrated its effectiveness. Further research work will be aimed at the modification and application of the localization method to tomosynthesis images generated by other reconstruction methods with different artifact characteristics, such as filtered back-projection, order statistics-based back-projection, and order statistics-based filtered back-projection [3].

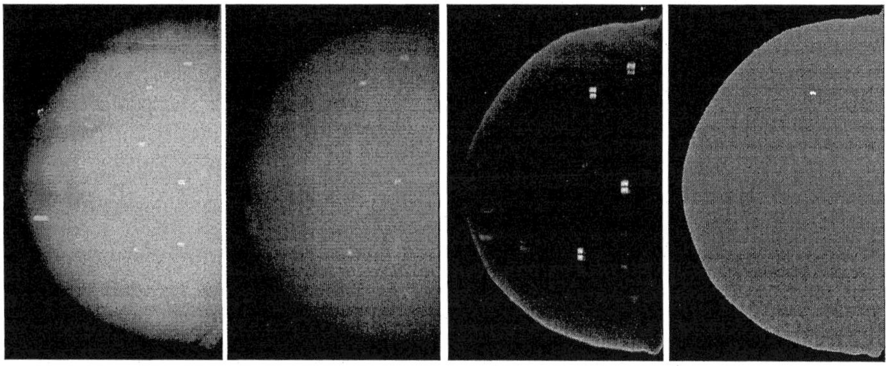

(a) (b) (c) (d)

Fig. 2. (a) a projection image; **(b)** a tomosynthesis image (slice 29) reconstructed by simple backprojection; **(c)** a symmetric filtered image; **(d)** detection output of an in-focus object.

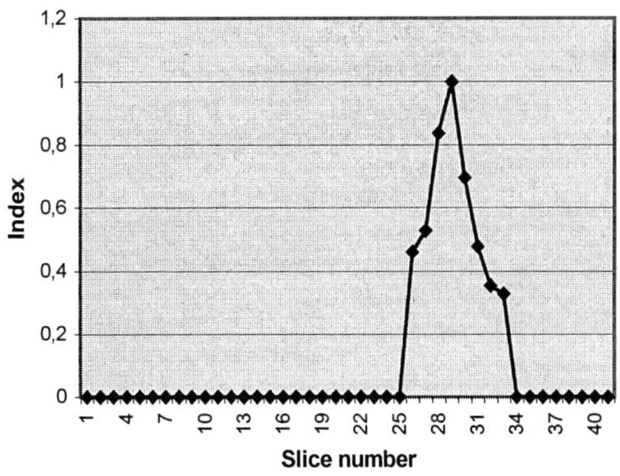

Fig. 3. A plot of focus index versus slice image number. The in-focus object is located on slice #29.

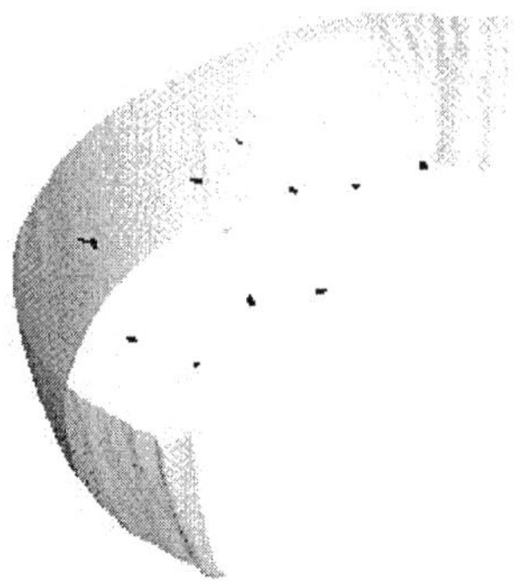

Fig. 4 3D visualization of segmented images.

References:

1. Suryanarayanan, S., Karellas, A., Vedantham, S. et al., "Comparison of tomosynthesis methods used with digital mammography", Academic Radiology 2000; 7:1085-1097.
2. Niklason L.T., Christian, B.T, Niklason L.E. et al., "Digital tomosynthesis in breast imaging," Radiology 1997; 205:339-406.
3. Claus, B.E.H., Eberhard, J.W.: A New Method for 3D Reconstruction in Digital Tomosynthesis, Proc. SPIE Vol. 4684, Medical Imaging 2002 – Image Processing, San Diego, CA, 2002.

Automatic Breast Orientation in Mediolateral Oblique View Mammograms

Martin Masek[1], Christopher J.S. deSilva[1, 2] and Yianni Attikiouzel[1, 2]

[1]Centre for Intelligent Information Processing Systems, Department of Electrical and Electronic Engineering, The University of Western Australia.
[2]Australian Research Centre for Medical Engineering, The University of Western Australia, 35 Stirling Highway, Crawley, Perth 6009, Western Australia
masek-m@ee.uwa.edu.au

Abstract. An algorithm for determining the orientation of mediolateral oblique view mammograms is presented. First, the chest wall is found using the variation in thickness of the breast near its edge. The top of the image is then determined using the asymmetry of the breast around its vertical centroid. The algorithm has been tested on the entire MIAS database, with images successively rotated in 90-degree increments, and flipped horizontally and vertically. Correct orientation was determined for all images.

1. Introduction

Orienting the mammogram in a particular direction is required in several computer aided diagnosis schemes. Some, [1,2], offer a solution that differentiates between left facing and right facing breasts while assuming the image is not upside down, others omit a comprehensive solution.

Since there is no orientation standard for mammogram digitisation, the cases of images rotated onto their side (landscape mode) and upside down images need to be considered. Our aim has been to determine automatically the orientation of mammograms in the mediolateral oblique view.

2. Method

An example of a mediolateral oblique view mammogram from the MIAS database [3] is shown in Figure 1(a). Determining image orientation consists of two steps, locating the chest wall and finding the image top.

Poor compression at the breast edge results in intensity contours forming on the image near the skin-air interface as tissue thickness increases into the breast. This property has previously been used in location of the nipple [4] and estimating the compressed breast thickness [5].

The net direction of tissue thickening is into the image edge containing the chest wall. In [2], Lou et al. use the direction of increasing intensity along a row of pixels to determine the image side closest to the chest wall. This use of horizontal gradients limits the algorithm to images where the chest wall is either on the left or right side. Our algorithm overcomes the problem by extracting the near-skin tissue and determining both horizontal and vertical gradients within it.

After removing labels and bright scanning artefacts [6], the image is segmented into near-skin tissue, Fig 1(b-i), and breast regions, Fig 1 (b-ii). Segmentation is accomplished by determining minimum cross-entropy thresholds [7], first from the original image, obtaining a rough breast mask, then using only pixels of a lower intensity than the first threshold. As only the darker pixels are considered for the second threshold, it will be lower than the first, including more near-skin tissue in the resulting binary mask. Applying the X-OR operator to the two masks isolates the near skin tissue.

Horizontal and vertical derivatives are used to determine the direction of increasing intensity in the near-skin tissue (Figure 1(c)); their net direction is into the chest wall, allowing image rotation to place the chest wall on one side. It remains to be determined if the breast in the image is upside down.

The vertical asymmetry of the breast region is used to determine the image top. The vertical centroid is determined as the row with equal number of 'on' pixels above as below it. Asymmetric pixels are defined as 'on' pixels on one side of the vertical centroid that do not have corresponding 'on' pixels on the opposite side. The vertical centroid and asymmetric regions (iii) are shown in Figure 1(c).

The image top is found by assuming the asymmetric region closest to the right side of the vertical centroid is the tip of the breast and should be located towards the bottom of the image.

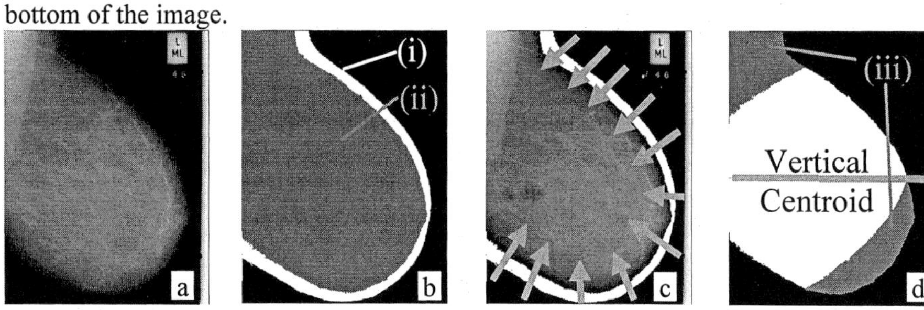

Fig. 1. (a) Original, (b) segmented into (i) near-skin tissue and (ii) breast tissue, (c) direction of intensity gradients in near-skin tissue and (d) breast tissue mask showing vertical centroid and (iii) asymmetric regions.

3. Results and Discussion

The algorithm has been tested on the entire 323-image MIAS database at a resolution of 400 micrometers per pixel. Images were put through all possible 90-degree rotations with upside down and right-side-up images, examples shown in Figure 2. Correct orientation was determined for all cases, even where part of the near-skin tissue, used to locate the chest wall, was cut off. The algorithm demonstrates robustness against: shape variation, incomplete breast image, non-film border, labels and scratches.

4. Conclusion

The algorithm presented provides a solution for determining the orientation of a breast in a mediolateral oblique view mammogram. Two steps are performed to find the orientation. The first determines the location of the chest wall. The subsequent operation uses the chest wall location and asymmetry to determine the image top. Correct orientation was determined for all MIAS database images.

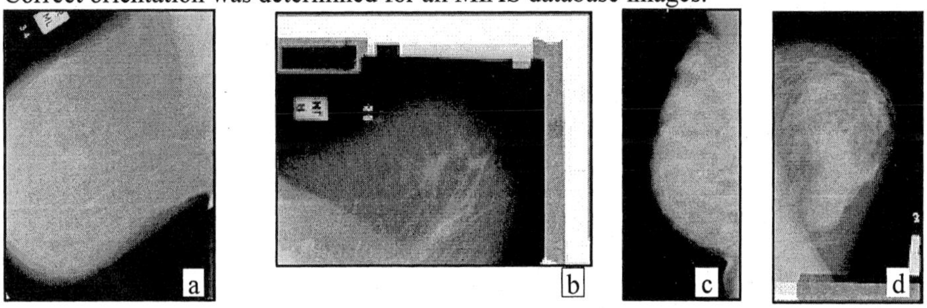

Fig. 2. Examples of images and orientations used to test the algorithm. MIAS database images (a) mdb152r, (b) mdb274r, (c) mdb318r and (d) mdb283l.

References

1. Karssemeijer, N.: Automated Classification of Parenchymal Patterns in Mammograms. Physics in Medicine and Biology 43 (1998) 365-378
2. Lou, S.L., Lin, H.D., Lin, K.P., Hoogstrate D.: Automatic breast region extraction from digital mammograms for PACS and telemammography applications. Computerised Medical Imaging and Graphics. 24 (2000) 205-220
3. Suckling J., Parker, J., Dance, D.R., Astley, S., Hutt, I. et al.: The Mammographic Image Analysis Society Digital Mammogram Database. In: Gale, A.G., Astley, S.M., Dance, D.R., Cairns, A.Y. (eds.): Digital Mammography vol. 1069 of Excerpta Medica International Congress Series, (Amsterdam, The Netherlands) Elsevier Science, (1994) 375-378.
4. Chandrasekhar, R., Attikiouzel, Y.: A Simple Method for Automatically Locating the Nipple on Mammograms. IEEE Transactions on Medical Imaging. 16-5 (1997) 483-494
5. Highnam, R.P., Brady, J.M., Shepstone, B.J.: Estimation of compressed breast thickness during mammography. The British Journal of Radiology, 71 (1998) 646-653
6. Masek, M., Attikiouzel, Y., deSilva, C.J.S.: Automatic Removal of High Intensity Labels and Noise from Mammograms. In: Martin J. Yaffe (ed.): Digital Mammography, IWDM 2000, Proc. 5th Int. Workshop on Digital Mammography, Toronto, Canada, June 2000. Madison, WI: Medical Physics Publishing (2001) 576-581
7. Brink, A.D, Pendock, N.E.: Minimum Cross-Entropy Threshold Selection. Pattern Recognition. 29-1 (1996) 179-188

Enhanced Identification of different types of Microcalcifcations using the wavelet transform Method

B. Oussena[1], A. Griche, K. Bounatiro, A. Henni, R. Alt[2]

[1] National Institute of computing (I.N.I., Algiers) and Research associate at CERIST
LIP6 Laboratory, University Pierre et Marie Curie, Paris6
oussena@wissal.dz

Abstract. Microcalcifications and Clustered microcalcifications are known to be the first sign of a development of an eventual cancer. They appear as small and bright region with irregular shape in the breast. Their diversity in their shape, their directionality, their size and localisation in a dense mammogram confirm the major difficulty of their detection. The aim of our scheme is the development of a method for the detection of all type of microcalcifications. The wavelet transform has recently emerged as a powerful tool for non-stationary signal analysis, its discrete version is closely related to filter banks. Also, multiresolution signal analysis has been used in image processing. This paper uses the relationship between these two techniques to provide a method of enhancing all type of microcalcifications. The digital mammograms are first processed by the wavelet transform with its multiresolution analysis. The enhancement of the microcalcifications is assured for each different type by using for an appropriate wavelet coefficients.

1. Introduction

Breast cancer is a major cause of premature death in women. Treatment is most successful if the tumour is detected early and mammography has been proven to be the most effective primary diagnostic procedure. However an important of cancer cases are known to be missed by radiologists. To assist radiologists in their diagnosis, several techniques have been developed for the automated detection of microcalcifications [1,2]. Recently, there has been some efforts to use the wavelet transform for analysing mammography features. Our study follows the method developed by Yoshida et al [3] using a wavelet transform to enhance the microcalcifications images. In their study, individual microcalcifications were segmented, but the segmentation of clustered microcalcifications need to take in account the diversity of microcalcifications types that exists. This is not performed in their study. Hence, A more positive method of detection is therefore imperative and to this end we have studied the wavelet transform method for all classes of micrcalcifications encountered.

2. Enhancement of the Microcalcification Images : Evaluation and Results

Our approach extends this previous investigations of the wavelet transform method in that we have studied the various classes of microcalcifications which differ in shape, alignment , size and location. Le Gal et al [4] have grouped the observed combinations of attributes of microcalcifications into five basic types which are denoted Type I to Type V. The Type I microcalcifications are annular and rounded in shape, reaching a size of around 1mm across. The microcalcifications of Type II are roughly spherical and large enough to be felt by palpation. Clustered microcalcifications of Type III are the most difficult to observe, and are sometimes confused with noise, since their size does not exceed 3 pixels, and finally, microcalcifications of Types IV and V are slightly bigger than Type III which makes them easier to spot in practice.

To evaluate the performance of the parameters adapted to each of the five microcalcifations type, we used a database consisting of about thirty true regions of interest containing actual microcalcifications and normal regions of interest that were randomly selected from the mammogram database we used. In our experiments, we investigated the effects of the choice of the mother wavelet and its lenght depending on the type of the microcalcifications to be enhanced. Mainly the mother wavelet that has led to the best results was the Daubechies wavelet one called LAD (Least Asymmetric Daubechies) wavelet . We observed that the enhancement of each type of the microcalcifications depends on the length of the wavelet and the applied process.

We experimented Type I microcalcifications first using a LAD4 mother wavelet was decomposed to level 4 with levels 1 and 4 zeroed. Setting level 4 to zero spoils the shape definition of the reconstructed image and setting level 1 to zero reduces the contrast of the fine microcalcifications. We experimented then with a 2D-DWT processing, with LAD8 decomposed up to level 6 and level 5 zeroed in the first operation, and LAD12 decomposed up to level 6 with level 5 zeroed for the second. Over and above the brightness effect that the use of LAD8 produces, the use of LAD12 gave better resolution of the smallest microcalcifications, due to the longer length of the filter. Setting level 5 to zero resulted in a considerable smoothing of the background distribution, thus highlighting the microcalcification structures.

The Type II microcalcifications have been experimented using a simple discrete wavelet transform with LAD12, image decomposition up to level 6 and zeroing of levels 4 and 5. Good background smoothing was achieved, but the microcalcifications contrast and edge definition was impaired to an unsatisfactory level. A histogram equalization performed on the resulting image has improved the microcalcifications definition. An alternative Type-II operation used LAD 8 and decomposition up to level 3 with level 1 zeroed. This process also showed a good enhancement of the microcalcifications.

The Type III microcalcifications were experimented with a simple wavelet transform, using LAD 8 and decomposition up to level 6 with levels 1, 4 and 5 zeroed. Good background smoothing was achieved but the contrast on the microcalcifications image was inadequate. Improved results were obtained with a 2D-DWT using LAD8 and decomposition up to 6 with level 4 and 5 zeroed for P1 and LAD20 with decomposition up to level 6 and levels 4,5 zeroed for P2. LAD8, due to its length gave a bright microcalcifications image and good background smoothing was obtained after zeroing levels 4 and 5. The use of LAD20 resulted in very good spatial resolution of the very fine microcalcifications and in the level 1-3 reconstruction, level 1 was the most important for preservation of the fine detail. Finally, the Type IV and V microcalcifications showed similar response to wavelet transform processing so, we grouped these two types together in the processing. A processing of Type-V image, identical to the operation on a Type-III image described above enhanced the fine microcalcifications structures well but also created false microcalcifactions images. An alternative, simple discrete wavelet transform procedure using LAD8 and decomposition up to level 6 with levels 4 and 5 zeroed of both types IV and V respectively. The histograms resulted from the processed images of type IV and V showed a new and dense repartition of the grey scales; a good enhancement of grey level frequencies situated in the interval [0..130] corresponding to the background and a translation of both histograms toward decreased grey levels hence a good smoothing of the background.

3. Conclusion

A wavelet transform analysis of 30 mammograms has been made to determine optimum procedures for the positive identification of microcalcification structures of Types I-V. Optimisation of the procedure involved the proper choice of one or two-dimensional wavelet transform, mother wavelet and reconstruction level. The quality of the reconstructed images has been evaluated at The Cancer Hospital of Algiers and a user-friendly interface to the image-reconstruction software has been developed using the C++ language. This has been installed on a PC computer for use in routine mammography at the hospital.

References

[1] Nishikawa RM, Jiang Y, Giger ML et al " Performance of Automated CAD schemes for the Detection and Classification of Clustered Microcalcifications." In: Gale AG, Ashley SM, Dance DR, Cairns AY eds. Digital Mammography. Amsterdam, Elsevier Science, 1994; pp. 13-20.

[2] H.Chan, K. Doi, S. Galhotra, CJ. Vyborny, H. MacMahon, PM Jokich " Image feature analysis and computer-aided disgnosis in digital radiography. 1. Automated detection of microcalcifications in mammography" Med Phys 1987; 14:538-548.

[3] H. Yoshida, K. Doi, and R. M. Nishikawa, K. Muto, and M. Tsuda " Application of the wavelet transform to automated detection of clustered microcalcifications in digital mammograms." Acad. Reports of Tokyo Institute of Polytecnics 16: 24-37, 1994.

[4] M.L. Gal, G. Ghavanne, D. Pellier " Valeur diagnostique des microcalcifications groupées découvertes par mammographie (à propos de 227 cas avec vérification histologique et sans tumeur palpable " Cancer (Paris) Masson, 71(1) :57 Bull, 1994.

Non-Rigid Mammogram Registration With Free Boundary Constraints

F. Richard[1] and L. Cohen[2]

[1] MAP5, University Paris V René Descartes, 45 rue des Saints Pères, 75270 Paris Cedex 06, France
Frederic.Richard@math-info.univ-paris5.fr
[2] CEREMADE, University Paris IX Dauphine, Place du Marechal de Lattre de Tassigny, 75775 Paris cedex 16, France
Cohen@ceremade.dauphine.fr

Abstract. In this paper, a new image-matching mathematical model is presented for mammogram registration. In a variational framework, an energy minimization problem is formulated. The model focuses on regions of interest and combines several constraints which are both intensity and segmentation based. A new feature of our model is combining region matching and segmentation by formulation of the energy minimization problem with free boundary conditions. Moreover, the energy has a new registration constraint. Performances of models with and without free boundary conditions are compared on simulated and real mammogram pairs. It is shown that the model with free boundary is more robust to initialization inaccuracies than the one without and also more efficient near contours.

1 Introduction.

In this paper, we deal with the registration of mammogram pairs. Despite the numerous works on Image Registration since the early 80's [3], mammogram registration still remains a challenging problem. Indeed, most of mammogram registration techniques have been only based on breast contours and for that reason have not succeeded in registering accurately breast interiors [2, 9]. In [4, 8], several authors attempted to register breast interiors using Bookstein warping technique with internal control points. However, these authors faced with the difficult problem of reliable internal breast control point extraction and matching. In this paper, we propose a registration approach which is not based on internal control points but instead on image grey-level values. It is more akin to the intensity-based approaches such as the one in [1] than to Bookstein technique. However, it differs significantly from the usual intensity-based approaches. On the one hand, it focuses on the mapping of regions of interest (breasts) rather than the whole image matching. On the other hand, it combines some matching constraints which are intensity-based and segmentation-based. In [5, 7], it was also proposed an approach combining registration constraints. But, in the model designed here, boundary conditions are free and segmentation-based constraints are defined differently. This enables preprocessing inaccuracies to be compensated for during the matching process and relax segmentation-based registration constraints.

In section 2, the previous registration model is reminded and the new one designed. In section 3, it is given some application results and comparisons of both models.

2 Mathematical Problem Formulation.

In [5, 7], we designed a mammogram registration model in the following framework. Let I^0 and I^1 be two mammograms. Let us suppose that these images are segmented and that breast contours are matched. Let us denote by Ω_0 and Ω_1 the coordinate sets of respective breast regions in I^0 and I^1 and by $\mathcal{W}_a$ a space which is composed of smooth functions mapping Ω_1 onto Ω_0. Based on elements of $\mathcal{W}_a$, I^0 can be deformed geometrically as follows: $I^0 \circ \phi$. In [5, 7], the registration problem is stated in terms of the following inverse problem:

Model 1 *Find in $\mathcal{W}_a$ a minimum for an energy J_a which is of the following form:*

$$\frac{1}{2}\int_{\Omega_1} R(\phi)(x)\,dx + \frac{\gamma_1}{2}\int_{\Omega_1} (I^0 \circ \phi(x) - I^1(x))^2\,dx,$$

with Dirichlet boundary conditions defined on breast boundaries of I^1: $\phi = \phi_0$. The function ϕ_0 maps coordinates of breast boundaries of I^1 onto those of I^0.

The energy to be minimized is composed of two terms. The second term is a registration constraint based on image intensities. The more similar the target image I^1 and the deformation $I^0 \circ \phi$ of the source image I^0 are, the lower this term is. The first term is a regularization term which ensures that the problem has a smooth solution. It is design based on an elastic energy [5, 7]. Contrarily to usual registration models [1], this minimization problem is defined on image regions of interest (breasts). Moreover, it combines matching constraints based on intensities with constraints based on image segmentations. These segmentation-based constraints are expressed in boundary conditions. Thanks to combinations of intensity and segmentation-based constraints, registration performances are improved [5, 7]. However, performances of model 1 depend on the quality of preprocessing steps (mammogram segmentations and breast contour matchings). Indeed, since boundary conditions are fixed, preprocessing inaccuracies cannot be compensated for during the matching process and may decrease matching performances. Besides, Dirichlet boundary conditions constrain too strongly the problem and may sometimes disrupt breast registrations near contours.

In order to fixe these drawbacks, we propose another registration model which combines registration constraints differently. Let us denote by $\mathcal{W}$ a space which is composed of smooth functions mapping Ω_1 onto $\mathbb{R}^2$. The inverse problem is stated as follows.

Model 2 *Find in $\mathcal{W}$ a minimum for an energy J which is of the following form:*

$$\frac{1}{2}\int_{\Omega_1} R(\phi)(x)\,dx + \frac{\gamma_1}{2}\int_{\Omega_1} (I^0\phi\phi(x) - I^1(x))^2\,dx + \gamma_2\int_{\Omega-\phi(\Omega_1)} S(|I^0(x)|^2)dx,$$

with free boundary conditions defined on breast boundaries of I^1.

As in model 1, the energy has an intensity-based registration term and a regularization term which are both defined on breast coordinates in I^1. But, boundary conditions are free. The segmentation-based registration constraints are defined via a third energy term (that will be called the segmentation term). This term depends on grey level values

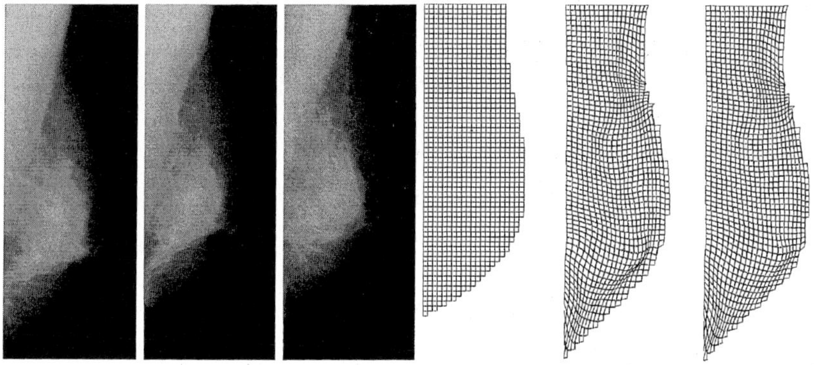

Fig. 1. (a) The source image I^0, (b) the geometric deformation of I^0 after the application of model 2 with γ_2 equal to 1000, (c) the target image I^1, (d) The tessellated breast domain Ω_1 in I^1, the image $\phi(\Omega_1)$ of Ω_1 by the map ϕ obtained by application of (e) model 1, (f) model 2 with γ_2 equal to 1000.

of I^0. It is defined on a region $\Omega - \phi(\Omega_1)$ which is the expected background of I^0. It constrains pixels of the set $\phi(\Omega_1)$ not to be located on the background of I^0 (see [6] for its complete design). In [6], we designed a multigrid gradient descent algorithm for the numerical resolution of problem in model 2. It is expressed in terms of time-dependant partial derivative equations. The initialization of this algorithm is the same as in the one designed for model 1 [5, 7]. This initialization takes into account the breast segmentation and the contour matching.

3 Application to mammogram pairs.

3.1 A simulated case.

Mammograms I^0 and I^1 in figures 1 (a) and (c) were registered using model 1. Based on the obtained solution $\phi^\star$, it was simulated a mammogram pair $(I^0, I^0 \circ \phi^\star)$ for which the registration is known. Model 1 was applied to these simulated image pair with the exact initialization derived from $\phi^\star$. A solution denoted by ϕ_{ref} was obtained. After registration, the image difference was lowered by 80.8 percent. Based on $\phi_\star$, we designed five wrong initializations ϕ_0 (see section 2). Models 1 and 2 were applied to the simulated image pair with the wrong initializations. Registration performances of model 1 were drastically reduced due to initialization errors. The image difference was lowered by only 69.9 percent on average with wrong initializations. Moreover, solution smoothness decreased: the regularization term reached the mean value 344.5 with wrong initializations whereas it was only 117 with the exact initialization. The registration scores of model 2 were better: the image difference were lowered by 74.1 and 76.1 percent in mean when model 1 was applied respectively without and with the segmentation term. The solutions were also much smoother than the ones of model 1.

Besides, as the segmentation term weight γ_2 increased, the registration scores of model 2 became closer to that of the solution ϕ_{ref}. These experiments show that model 2 is more robust than model 1 to initialization errors and its segmentation term is a factor of robustness.

3.2 Application to a real mammogram pair

The bilateral mammogram pair shown in figures 1 (a) and (c) comes from the MIAS database. Comparing both images and observing their absolute differences (figure 2 (a)), it can be noticed that they have a lot of important asymmetries, due in particular to differences in breast shape. On figure 2 (b), it can be observed that asymmetries near breast contours and some inner differences are significantly compensated for after the algorithm initialization. However, due preprocessing step inaccuracies, breast contour asymmetries are not perfectly corrected: in figure 1 (b), it can be observed a small dark border in the upper part of the contour area. Moreover, several important inner differences remain in the corrected image pair. Most of these inner differences can be removed by applying model 1. Indeed, looking at figure 2 (c), it can be seen that this model compensates for many important asymmetries which are due to shape and location differences of bright regions inside breasts. However, several differences still remain in the pair of images corrected by model 1. Since they are caused by breast tissue disparities, some of these differences cannot be corrected by any geometric deformation. However, this registration can be improved. Indeed, in figure 2 (c), we still observe contour differences which remained after the initialization. These differences cannot be compensated for by model 1 due to fixed boundary conditions. Besides, an important difference remains near the nipple position. The algorithm of model 1 is unable to correct it: the difference increases the intensity-based matching term constraint in a way that is opposite to the boundary constraints. As can be noticed in figure 1 (e), this constraint conflict generates a strong compression in the difference area. Further difference corrections are not possible because they would increase the compression and the regularization term value. These results are in sharp contrast with those of model 2. Looking at figures 2 (d) and (e), it can be seen that model 2 succeeds in compensating completely for differences near the nipples. Moreover, comparing figures 1 (e) and (f), it can be seen that deformations are less compressed and smoother than the ones obtained with model 1. As can be observed on figures 2 (d) and (e), model 2 without the segmentation term maps some parts of the breast in I^1 into some parts of the background in I^0 whereas the algorithm with a strong segmentation constraint keeps the mapping inside the breast region of I^0.

4 Conclusion.

It was designed a new mathematical model for the mammogram registration. The model focuses on regions of interest and combines segmentation-based and intensity-based constraints. Moreover, the registration problem is not posed with fixed boundary conditions but with free boundary conditions. On simulated and real mammogram pairs, performances of the model were compared to an equivalent model with fixed boundary

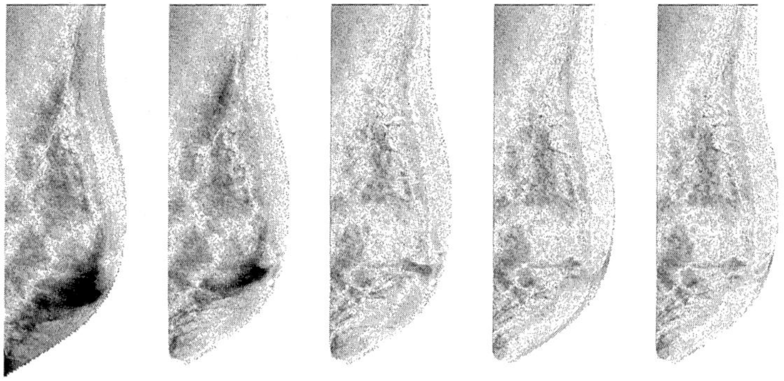

(a) (b) (c) (d) (e)

Fig. 2. The absolute differences between image I^1 and (a) I^0, (b) the deformed image I^0_ϕ after the initialization step, (c) the deformed image I^0_ϕ after the application of model 1, (d) the deformed image I^0_ϕ after the application of model 2 with γ_2 equal to 0, (e) the deformed image I^0_ϕ after the application of model 2 with γ_2 equal to 1000 **[black=high differences, white=low differences]**

conditions. It was shown that the new model is more robust to initialization errors and more efficient near contours.

References

1. Y. Amit. A non-linear variational problem for image matching. *SIAM J. Sci. Comput.*, 15(1):207–224, January 1994.
2. T.K. Lau and W.F. Bischof. Automated detection of breast tumors using the asymmetry approach. *Comput. Biomed. Res.*, 24(3):273–295, 1991.
3. J. Maintz and M.A. Viergever. A survey of medical image registration. *Medical Image Analysis*, 2(1):1–36, 1998.
4. K. Marias and J.M. Brady. Multi-scale landmark selection for improved registration of temporal mammograms. In M. Yaffe, editor, *Proc. IWDM*, pages 580–586, Toronto, Canada, June 2000. Medical Physics Publishing.
5. F. Richard. *Modèles élastiques d'ajustements d'images et applications aux paires bilatérales et temporelles de mammographies.* PhD thesis, University Paris 5, France, dec 2000.
6. F. Richard and L. Cohen. A new image registration technique with free boundary constraints: application to mammography. In *Proc. ECCV*, Copenhaguen, Denmark, 2002. to appear.
7. F. Richard and C. Graffigne. An image-matching model for the registration of temporal or bilateral mammogram pairs. In M. Yaffe, editor, *IWDM*, pages 756–762, Toronto, Canada, June 2000. Medical Physics.
8. M.Y. Sallam and K. Bowyer. Registration and difference analysis of corresponding mammogram images. *Medical Image Analysis*, 3(2):103–118, 1999.
9. J.L. Semmlow, A. Shadagopappan, L.V. Ackerman, et al. A fully automated system for screening Xeromammograms. *Comput. Biomed. Res.*, 13:350–362, 1980.

Comparison of Three Different Mass Segmentation Methods

Sheila Timp, Nico Karssemeijer, Jan Hendriks

Department of Radiology, University Medical Center Nijmegen, Geert Grooteplein 18, 6525 GA Nijmegen, The Netherlands
sheila@radiology.azn.nl

Abstract. Our current study compares a new segmentation method based on dynamic programming with two other automated segmentation methods. Dynamic programming makes it possible to combine several criteria as the notion of a best boundary by using an evaluation function. The segmentation methods are tested on a dataset consisting of 133 masses and evaluated by similarity measures.

1 Introduction

An important step in mass detection is the segmentation and characterization of suspect regions. Based on this segmentation shape and contrast features can be computed providing information to classify the region as normal, benign or malignant. The segmentation methods used can be manual, semi-automated or fully-automated. A large number of automated segmentation methods have been developed in the field of image analysis and many of them have been used to segment masses in mammograms. Dynamic programming was first described by Bellman in 1962. Since that time dynamic programming has been used for different optimization problems in image processing. One of the applications is the segmentation of images [7]. A very popular segmentation method is region growing. Many groups applied region growing to the task of segmenting masses (e.g. [3]). In recent years, deformable models have become popular in the field of medical image analysis ([4], [6], [1]). Only a few studies compare different segmentation methods ([6], [3] and [2]). The first study compares region growing and a discrete dynamic contour model and uses the area overlap measure between the segmented region and the annotated region to assess the quality of segmentation. The second study compares the accuracy of three automated segmentation methods to that of manual segmentation. The last study compares a mass segmentation method based on an active contour model with manual segmentation by two expert radiologists.

2 Segmentation methods

We applied three different segmentation methods to the task of mass segmentation.

Region Growing Region growing takes an image and a set of seeds as inputs. The seeds mark each of the regions to be segmented The algorithm grows the seed regions in an iterative fashion. At each iteration all those pixels that border the growing regions are examined. The pixel that is most similar to a region that it borders is appended to that region. We implemented an extended version of the algorithm developed by Kupinski and Giger based on simple probabilistic models [3]. Region growing gives good results when the mass borders have uniform grey level, as the algorithm is based on finding the best grey level for the contour. On the other hand, when a mass overlaps with other mammographic structures region growing can give poor results.

Deformable Models A snake is an elastic curve placed on an image that deforms itself from an initial shape in order to adjust to the image features [5]. The deformation is the result of the action of external forces that attract the snake towards image features and internal forces that keep smooth the shape of the curve. The solution is given by a minimum of the snake total energy. Our implementation of the deformable model is based on an algorithm developed by Lobregt and Viergever [4][6], the discrete dynamic contour model. Because deformable models are based on gradient differences, they do not always give the best solution when a mass is embedded in a uniform background. In a uniform background, such as in fatty tissue, the boundary preferably should have a uniform grey level.

Dynamic Programming To overcome some of the problems of the former two segmentation methods we implemented a segmentation method based on dynamic programming where flexibility of the use of a cost function allows a combination of criteria. Dynamic programming is a method of finding the global optimum of multistage processes. It is based on Bellman's *principle of optimality*, which states that the optimum path between two given points is also optimum between any two points lying on the path [8]. Thus if C is a point on the optimum path between A and B, then the segment CB is the optimum path from C to B, no matter how one arrives at C. To apply this idea to boundary extraction, one must define an evaluation function that embodies a notion of the *best boundary* [7]. The evaluation function we used is the following:

$$S(\mathbf{x}_1,\ldots,\mathbf{x}_n) = \alpha\sum_{k=1}^{n} s(\mathbf{x}_k) + \gamma\sum_{k=1}^{n-1} d(\mathbf{x}_k) + \mu\sum_{k=1}^{n-1} g(\mathbf{x}_k) + \beta\sum_{k=1}^{n-1} q(\mathbf{x}_k,\mathbf{x}_{k-1})$$

where $\mathbf{x}_k, k = 1,\ldots,N$ represents the nodes in the kth stage of the costmatrix. The components of the evaluation function are:

- Edge strength $s(x_k)$. The edge strength is measured as the gradient magnitude in the direction normal to the initial estimate of the tumor boundary.
- Proximity to the initial approximation. Our CAD program provides us with an initial estimate of the contour. Boundaries near this initial approximation

are favored by adding $\alpha * dist(x_i, B)$ to the costmatrix, where B is the location of the initial boundary.
- Equal grey level $g(\mathbf{x}_i)$: a contour that is embedded in a uniform background is expected to have equal grey level. The grey level of the boundary is expected to be in between the grey level of the region inside the contour and the region outside the contour. To determine which pixels are inside cq outside the contour we use the initial estimate of the contour.
- Curvature $q(\mathbf{x}_k, \mathbf{x}_{k-1})$. The curvature measures the angle between the edge elements at $\mathbf{x}_k$ and $\mathbf{x}_{k-1}$. As low curvature boundaries are desirable, the constant β should be positive.

As starting point for the segmentation program we use the center of gravity of the annotation made by the radiologist. Our CAD program used this starting point to provide us with an initial estimate of the contour with radius R. A circular region with radius 4R is then resampled into a rectangular array of height 4R. For all pixels inside this region the edge strength $s(x_k)$, the proximity to initial approximation $dist(x_i, B)$, and the difference between the expected and measured grey level $g(\mathbf{x}_i)$ are calculated. The resulting matrix is the costmatrix. For each radius r from $r = 0$ till $r = 4R$ the path with the lowest cost is calculated by optimization of the evaluation function. The evaluation function S is optimized in stages [7]. The initial value is specified as:

$$S_0(\mathbf{x}_1) = 0.$$

The recursive step is given by, for $1 \leq k \leq N - 1$,

$$S_k(\mathbf{x}_{k+1}) = \max_{\mathbf{x}_k}[\alpha s(\mathbf{x}_k) + \beta q(\mathbf{x}_k), \mathbf{x}_{k+1} + \gamma d(\mathbf{x}_k) + \mu g(\mathbf{x}_k)],$$

The path with the lowest cumulative cost is taken as the optimal path.

3 Experiments

3.1 Dataset

A set of 133 mammograms was used to test the performance of the segmentation methods. All mammograms come from the Dutch screening programme. The set includes spiculated, circumscribed and vague masses. All mammograms have been digitized at $50\mu m$ and are downsampled to $200\mu m$.

3.2 Similarity measure

The performance of the segmentation methods has been evaluated by an overlap criterion $O = S \cap T / S \cup T$, where S is the segmented area and T is the annotation made by the radiologist. A value close to one means a good match between the two regions. To visualize the performance of the methods, the success rate will be displayed as a function of the overlap.

3.3 Results

The average overlap for dynamic programming is 0.68, for dynamic contouring 0.64 and for region growing 0.66. Robust methods will have a reasonable overlap in a high percentage of cases and will only fail in a few cases. Accuracy of the methods can be judged by the percentage of cases that have a large overlap, for example more than 0.7. This percentage is 54% for dynamic programming, 45 % for region growing and 36% for discrete dynamic contouring. Figure 1 shows results for the three segmentation methods. Horizontally the overlap is shown, vertically the fraction of tumors for which the method achieved at most this overlap. Figure 1 also shows scatterplots for the different segmentation methods. Each point here represents a mass from the dataset and shows the overlap with manual segmentation for two methods. The scatterplots for discrete dynamic contouring and dynamic programming are rather symmetric. The performance of both methods is equal for most masses. The scatterplots for region growing and dynamic programming/dynamic contouring are more asymmetric. The different segmentation methods perform different for a part of the masses.

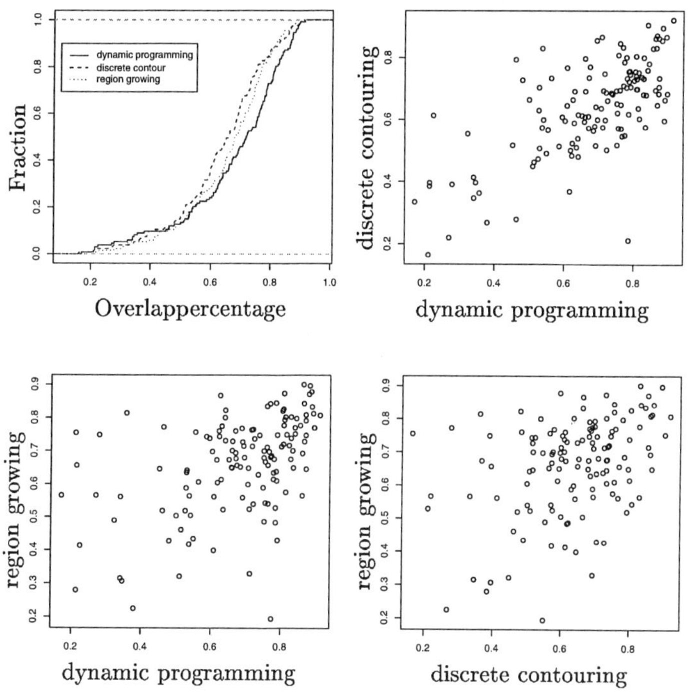

Fig. 1. The figure on the upper left compares the three segmentation methods. The y-axis shows the fraction of tumors for which the method achieved at most this overlap. The other figures show scatterplots of the overlap for the different segmentation methods

4 Discussion

We have quantitatively analyzed the accuracy of three automated mass segmentation algorithms by comparing their performance with manual segmentation by one expert radiologist. The differences between the average performance of the different methods are small. The part of tumors with high overlap (70%) however is much larger for dynamic programming. All three methods rarely achieve more than 85% overlap. One reason for this is that the annotated regions are not always very accurate. Often the annotations are rather large to make sure the whole tumor is inside the annotation. Another reason is that when the annotation and the segmented area are not identical the chosen overlap criterion quickly decreases. A disadvantage of the chosen overlap criterion is that it only measures the overlap and doesn't evaluate how well the segmentation follows the contour. Another way to evaluate the different segmentation methods is comparison of the classification performance. At the moment most of the features we use do not strongly depend on the contour, so only a small difference in classification accuracy is expected for the different segmentation methods. Sahiner et al. investigated the effect of different segmentation methods on classification accuracy [2]. They found that the overall classification accuracy using features extracted based on one of the segmentation methods was nearly identical. Even when the radiologist and the computer had high disagreement, they observed no decrease in classification accuracy. At the moment we are developing features that do depend on the exact location of the contour. We expect these features to be more sensitive for small changes in the segmentation then existing features. The average time to segment one image on a Pentium 1000 MHz computer is for dynamic programming 1.17 seconds, for region growing 1.29 seconds and for discrete dynamic contouring 1.95 seconds.

References

1. Bischof, L. , Adams, R.: Seeded region growing. IEEE Trans Pattern Anal Machine Intell **16** (1994) 641–647.
2. Sahiner B., Petrick N., Chan H., and Hadjiiski,L., Paramagul, C.,Helvie, M.Gurcan, M.: Computer-Aided characterization of mammographic masses: accuracy of mass segmentation and its effects on characterization IEEE Trans. Med Imaging **20** (2001) 1275–1284.
3. Kupinski, M. and Giger, M.: Automated seeded lesion segmentation on digital mammograms. IEEE Trans on Med Imaging **17** (1998) 510–517.
4. Viergever, M., Lobregt,S.: A discrete dynamic contour model. IEEE Trans on Medical Imaging **14** (1995), 12–24.
5. Terzopoulos, D., McInerney, T.: Deformable models in medical image analysis: a survey. Medical Image Analysis (1996).
6. te Brake, G., Stoutjesdijk, M. ,Karssemeijer, N.: A discrete dynamic contour model for mass segmentation in digital mammograms. SPIE Medical Imaging 1999 **3661** (1999) 911–919.
7. Ballard, H., Brown, C.: Computer Vision. Prentice-Hall. Chapter **4** (1982)
8. Jain, A.: Fundamentals of digital image processing. Prentice-Hall. Chapter **9** (1989)

EM Texture Segmentation of Mammographic Images

Reyer Zwiggelaar[1], Pere Planiol[2], Joan Martí[2], Robert Martí[1], Lilian Blot[1], Erika R.E. Denton[3], and Caroline M.E. Rubin[4]

[1] School of Information Systems, University of East Anglia, Norwich, UK
reyer.zwiggelaar@sys.uea.ac.uk
[2] Computer Vision and Robotics Group, University of Girona, Girona, Spain
[3] Department of Breast Imaging, Norfolk and Norwich University Hospital, Norwich, UK
[4] Breast Screening Unit, Royal South Hants Hospital, Southampton, UK

Abstract. We have investigated a combination of statistical modelling and expectation maximisation for a texture based approach to the segmentation of mammographic images. Texture modelling is based on the implicit incorporation of spatial information. Statistical modelling is used for data generalisation and noise removal purposes. Expectation maximisation modelling of the spatial information in combination with the statistical modelling are compared to expectation maximisation modelling based on single grey-level values. The developed segmentation results are used for two specific applications which are registration of mammographic images and mammographic risk assessment.

1 Introduction

Statistical modelling in combination with expectation maximisation (EM) [1] is used for the segmentation of mammographic images. Two variations have been investigated, the first based on basic grey-level information and the second based on information derived from this. Realistic texture modelling is possible as spatial information is implicitly incorporated. Statistical modelling has been used as a pre-processing step to generalise the data whilst at the same time remove some noise aspects. Initial results from this automatic segmentation of mammographic images are promising with a good correlation with annotated regions. This work is done with two main applications in mind. The first is automatic risk assessment [2] whilst the second is the registration of mammographic data [3].

2 Methods

A Gaussian mixture model G with k classes is defined as

$$G(x|\varphi) = \sum_{i=1}^{k} w_i g(x|\theta_i) \tag{1}$$

where φ is a vector with the parameters w_i (weight) and θ_i (mean and covariance) for each class, and $g(x|\theta_i)$ is defined as

$$g(x|m_i, v_i) = \frac{1}{(\sqrt{2\pi})^n(\sqrt{det(v_i)})} e^{-\frac{(x\Gamma m_i)^T v_i^{\Gamma 1} (x\Gamma m_i)}{2}} \tag{2}$$

where m_i is the mean, v_i is the covariance, $()^T$ indicates the transpose of a vector, v_i^{-1} indicates the inverse of v_i and $det(v_i)$ stands for the determinant of v_i.

The *likelihood* function is a function that gives a measure of how well the probability density function defined by the parameters fits the data. If a set of parameter maximises the likelihood, then these parameters will be the optimum set for the given problem. The likelihood function is defined as

$$\mathrm{L}\,(\varphi) = \prod_{x \varepsilon \chi} p(x|\varphi) \tag{3}$$

where χ is the data set and $p(x|\varphi)$ is the density function. Here the assumption of independence for all data χ is made. Usually, the *log-likelihood* function is used, mainly to use a sum instead of a product and to reduce the magnitude of the result.

$$\mathrm{L}\,(\varphi) = \sum_{x \varepsilon \chi} log(p(x|\varphi)) \tag{4}$$

The EM algorithm [1] is a numerical method to estimate a set of parameters that describe a probability distribution, based on data that belongs to this distribution. On each iteration of the algorithm, two steps are performed: first, the E-step evaluates a probability distribution for the data using the parameters of the model estimated on the previous iteration, then the M-step finds the new parameters that maximises the likelihood function. It can be proven mathematically that on each iteration the likelihood increases [1].

One of the problems of the EM algorithm in application to Gaussian Mixture Models is the initialisation [4], with the end results depending on the initial starting point. It is common to select a random point of the data set χ as the centre of the class. We initialise the centre of the class with the result of the *k-means* algorithm [4].

2.1 Towards Automatic Segmentation

Automatic segmentation methods need a realistic estimation of the number of classes that are to be used. To segment mammograms two approaches are possible. A manual approach based on an understanding of the anatomical structures/tissue present in mammograms or an automatic approach based on the mammographic data. Here we have used an information theoretic approach [5, 6] to investigate the automatic approach. Initially the developed approach was validated by using a set of artificial images with well-defined, but not necessarily well-separated Gaussian classes. For the well-separated classes the results clearly indicated the correct number of classes. However, for less well-separated classes this resulted in a smaller number of possible classes. The resulting estimate always has a higher bound equal to the correct number of classes. Subsequent application to mammograms showed similar results as the less well-separated classes in the artificial data. The results indicated that there are about six possible classes, but as many as four could be clustered together.

2.2 Texture Feature

In general the usage of the EM approach for image segmentation is based on the grey-level information at a pixel level with no direct interaction between adjacent pixels. However, it is well known that texture based segmentation should incorporate spatial correlation information. This means that our modelling is not based on a single grey-level value but incorporates spatial information implicitly.

The used feature vector extracts a number of values from a local neighbourhood. The neighbourhood is made up of a reference pixel and a series of four-connected pixels which have been obtained at a number of scales (increasing levels of smoothing are applied at subsequent scales). The values for the feature vector are made up by the grey-level value of the reference and the difference in grey-level values between the reference pixel and the other pixels in the local neighbourhood. A second approach excludes the grey-level value of the reference pixel from the feature vector.

2.3 Statistical Modelling

The texture feature described above is extracted at a pixel level. Combining all the information results in a feature vector which can be used to generate a statistical model. In general such a model is used for noise removal and data generalisation. In this particular case the added bonus of data generalisation is a reduced dimensionality which speeds up the processing. Here we have used principal component analysis [7], but other statistical methods could have been used instead.

3 Results

Segmentation results for an example mammogram are shown in Fig. 1. The original mammogram is shown in Fig. 1a. The EM and statistical modelling process take only the breast area into account whilst excluding the pectoral muscle and the background. For the results shown in Fig. 1b-f six classes were used.

For all three feature vectors that incorporated the grey-level value of the reference pixel (see Fig. 1b-d) the segmentation process produced plausible results which seem to correlate with the original image. However, this seems less the case when the grey-level of the reference pixel is excluded from the feature vector (see Fig. 1e,f).

3.1 Registration

To assess the potential of the developed approach to mammographic registration a small dataset was used and the results can be found in Table 1. The table shows the original (O in Table 1) and the retrieved parameters for an affine transformation [3]. The retrieved parameters are obtained from a mutual information based registration approach using the original grey-level (GL in Table 1) information or the EM (EM in Table 1) based segmentation results. It should be clear that for large deformations the EM segmentation based registration results are more robust with the retrieved parameters close to the original parameter whilst the grey-level based registration results fail to return any relevant parameter information.

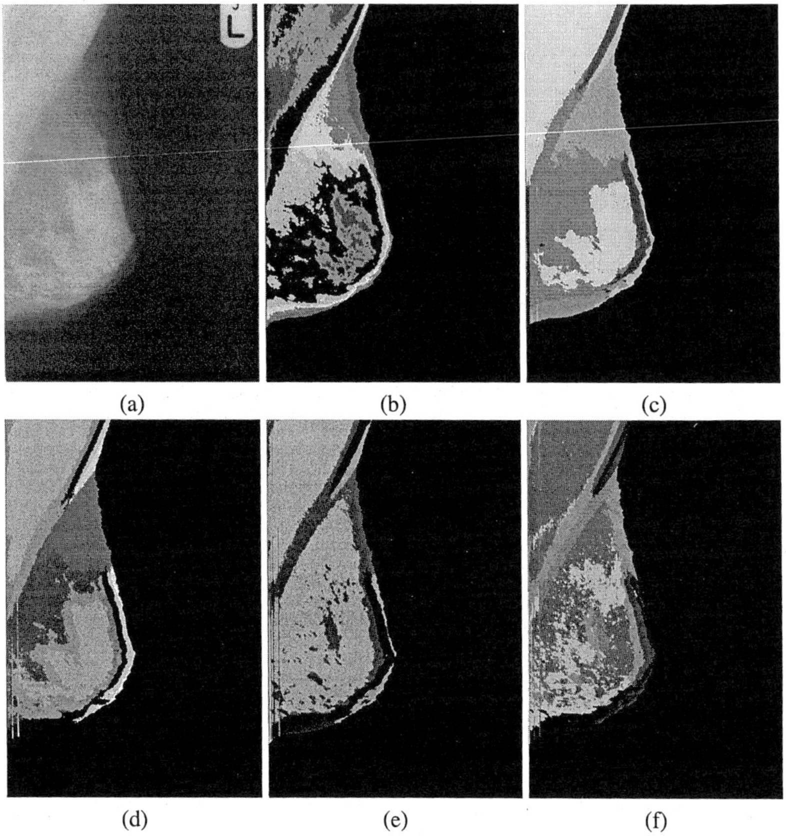

Fig. 1. (a) Original image. Segmentation results where the EM modelling is based on (b) a single grey-level value at the reference pixel, (c) the texture feature vector, (d) statistical modelling of the texture feature vector, (e) the texture feature vector without the reference grey-level value, and (f) statistical modelling of the texture feature vector without the reference grey-level value.

3.2 Risk Assessment

To evaluate the segmentation results for mammographic risk assessment a subset of the MIAS database was used [8, 9]. All the images were assessed by an expert radiologist who provided an estimate of the proportion of dense tissue in each mammogram. The segmentation results, based on EM and statistical modelling incorporating the reference pixel grey-level value, can also be used to obtain an estimate of the proportion of dense tissue. A comparison of both these estimates, when using a kNN classifier on a leave-one-out basis with $k = 3$, can be found in Table 2. This shows an agreement for 67% of the mammograms. This compares well with single grey-level value EM results (50% agreement) and an inter-observer comparison (45% agreement). The intra-observer agreement on the used dataset is 89%.

	t_x	t_y	a_x	b_y	a_y	b_x
O	10.0	10.0	0.995	0.995	-0.105	0.105
GL	10.3	10.6	0.993	0.993	-0.103	0.102
EM	10.5	10.3	0.995	0.996	-0.106	0.100
O	50.0	10.0	0.988	0.988	-0.156	0.156
GL	49.8	10.5	0.988	0.987	-0.155	0.155
EM	49,9	10.3	0.985	0.989	-0.155	0.152
O	150.0	30.0	0.809	0.809	-0.588	0.588
GL	0.9	0.3	0.999	0.997	-0.002	0.004
EM	145.9	36.5	0.865	0.809	-0.588	0.491

Table 1. Registration results (see main text for description).

		Expert Classification				
		1	2	3	4	5
Automatic Classification	1	0.22	0.00	0.11	0.00	0.00
	2	0.00	0.06	0.06	0.11	0.00
	3	0.00	0.00	0.17	0.00	0.00
	4	0.00	0.06	0.00	0.22	0.00
	5	0.00	0.00	0.00	0.00	0.00

Table 2. Comparison of the density estimate as given by an expert radiologist and automatic segmentation.

4 Conclusions

We have shown that a combination of EM and statistical modelling results in a robust approach to the segmentation of mammographic images. It should be noted that some fundamental questions, such as the influence of the size and shape of the local neighbourhood, need further investigation. We have shown that the segmentation results can be used to provide valuable information in mammographic applications such as risk assessment and registration. Extensions into volumetric aspects are currently under investigation, with an emphasis on mammographic MR information.

References

1. P. Demster, N.M. Laird, and D.B. Rubin. Maximum likelihood from incomplete data via the em algorithm. *Journal of the Royal Statistical Society B*, 39:1–38, 1977.
2. J.N Wolfe. Risk for breast cancer development determined by mammographic parenchymal pattern. *Cancer*, 37(5):2486–2492, 1976.
3. R. Marti, R. Zwiggelaar, and C.M.E. Rubin. Automatic point correspondence and registration based on linear structures. *International Journal of Pattern Recognition and Artificial Intelligence*, 16(3):331–340, 2002.
4. P. McKenzie and M.D. Alder. Initialising the em algorithm for use in gaussian mixture modelling. *Proceedings of the International Workshop on Pattern Recognition in Practice IV*, pages 91–105, 1994.
5. J. Rissanen. Modeling by shortest data description. *Automatica*, 14:465–471, 1978.
6. H. Akaike. A new look at the statistical model identification. *IEEE Transactions on Automatic Control*, AC-19(6):716–723, 1974.
7. I.T. Jolliffe. *Principal Component Analysis*. Springer Verlag, 1986.
8. J. Suckling, J. Parker, D. Dance, S. Astley, I. Hutt, C. Boggis, I. Ricketts, E. Stamatakis, N. Cerneaz, S. Kok, P. Taylor, D. Betal, and J. Savage. The mammographic images analysis society digital mammogram database. In Dance Gale, Astley and Cairns, editors, *Digital Mammography*, pages 375–378. Elsevier, 1994.
9. L. Blot, E.R.E. Denton, and R. Zwiggelaar. Risk assessment: the use of background texture in mammographic imaging. 6th *International Workshop on Digital Mammography*, Bremen, Germany:accepted, 2002.

Comparison between JPEG and a New Neural Compression Method for Digitized Mammograms

Anke Meyer-Baese

Florida State University, Tallahassee, FL 32310-6046, USA,
amb@eng.fsu.edu,

Abstract. This paper presents the development and evaluation of a new lossy neural–based compression algorithm for digitized mammograms. The influence of the neural compression method on the mammographic image is not perceptible to a mammogram reader up to a high compression rate. Compared with JPEG the achieved image quality based on the proposed method is much better.

1 Introduction

The research and development of teleradiology and telemedicine systems has progressed through many technical and clinical endeavors. When dealing with large volume image transmission and storage, lossy data compression is an outstanding issue in medical applications to which current technologies were not designed to address.

The goal of this paper is to present and evaluate a new lossy neural–based compression algorithm for digitized mammograms. The described method is an innovative mammographic image compression procedure, which differentiates itself from known systems in several ways. It applies to larger blocks and represents a better probability distribution estimation method. Existing mammographic image compression methods are mostly vector generalizations of the embedded zero–tree wavelet technique [1]. They perform poorly in comparison to sophisticated pattern recognition techniques and involve only operations on small 2×2 pixel blocks.

2 Mammographic Image Compression Scheme

The proposed method shown in Figure 1 combines a PCA–type neural network, based on Oja's learning algorithm [3], with a proposed data compressor ("neural–gas" network) performing vector quantization [2]. The PCA transform is applied to image blocks which are treated like data vectors and performs a projection of the data vector on a lower dimensional space.

Additional data compression can be achieved by using the "neural–gas" network on the coder output to produce its quantized version. The "neural–gas" network uses like Kohonen's feature map a "soft–max" adaptation rule. When applied to vector quantization the network converges quickly to low distortion errors and reaches a distortion error lower than that resulting from Kohonen's feature map and at the same time obeys a gradient descent on an energy surface in contrast to Kohonen's feature map algorithm.

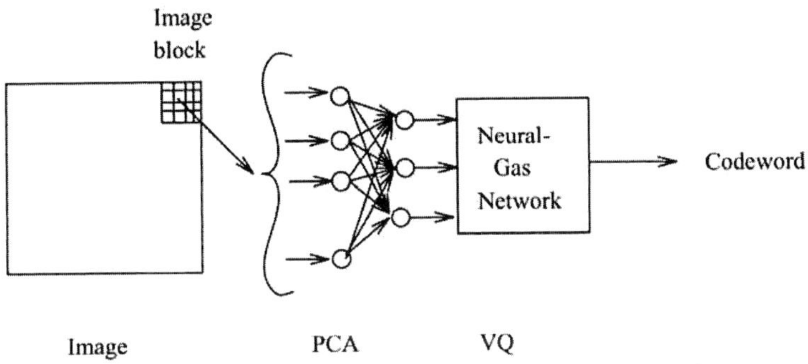

Fig. 1. Architecture of the combined network (OJA and "neural–gas") for compression.

3 Simulation Results

A set of 4 mammograms were selected from the publicly available MIAS database at http://skye.icr.ac.uk/misdb/miasdb.html. All 1024×1024 images are monochrome with 256 graylevels. For the simulations of the whole compression process, we used different blocksizes ranging from 2×2, 4×4, 5×5 and 8×8 pixels.

As an indicator for comparison of information loss due to image compression, we choose the "classical" approach for image quality. Image quality is typically quantified objectively by average distortion or peak signal to noise ratio (PSNR).

In order to achieve higher compression ratios, the principal components are quantized. The quantization will be carried out by forming vectors consisting of the principal components. These vectors are used to train a net which, once converged, represents the codebook for vector lookup. The codebook is trained by using the "neural-gas" algorithm. The size of the codebook is equal to 256.

In order to reduce the blocking effect associated with any transform-based algorithm, we allow for some experiments an overlapping of neighboring image blocks by one pixel. Table (1) shows the compression results with and without overlapping based on OJA's algorithm and vector quantization.

To give an idea of the performance of the proposed method, we compare our results with those obtained with the JPEG standard. Figure 2 shows the difference images between the original image and the reconstructed images. It represents a qualitative measurement for comparing the quality of our method in Figure 2(a) and JPEG in Figure 2(b) at a compression rate=16. Both the PSNR rate and the visual quality of the image is better with our method compared to JPEG. The difference image shows the phantom features more distinctive with JPEG than with our method.

Table 1. Results of the global compression scheme with Oja's symmetric algorithm and vector quantization depending on blocksize, number of principal components, overlapping, compression ratio and PSNR.

Blocksize	Number of PC	Overlap	Comp. Ratio	PSNR
2×2	2	0	4	35.48
4×4	4	1	9	31.61
5×5	8	1	16	37.06
8×8	8	1	48	29.53

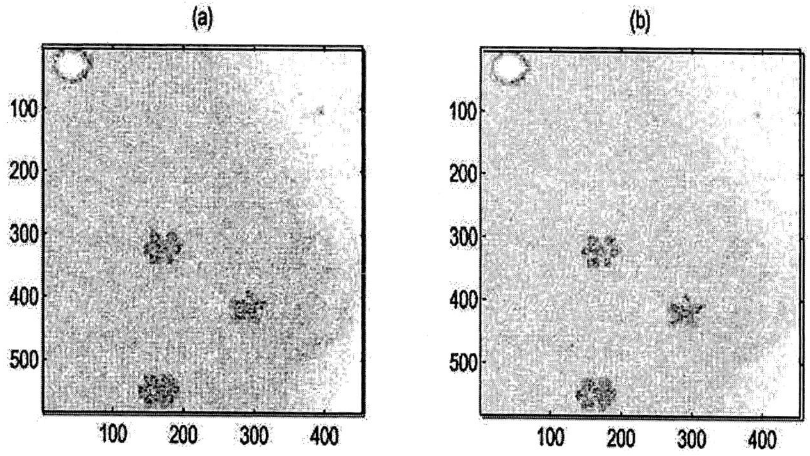

Fig. 2. Difference image of our method with blended mathematical phantom features, PSNR=37.06 (a) and (b) difference image of JPEG, PSNR=36.53 compression rate=16.

References

1. A. Said and W. A.Pearlman: A new fast and efficient image codec based on set partitioning in hierarchical trees. IEEE Transactions on Circuits and Systems for Video Technology **6** (1996) 243-250
2. T. Martinetz, S. Berkovich, and K. Schulten: Neural gas network for vector quantization and its application to time-series prediction. IEEE Transactions on Neural Networks **4** (1993) 558–569
3. E. Oja: Neural networks, principal components, and subspaces. International Journal of Neural Systems **1** (1989) 61-68

Content-based image retrieval in mammography: using texture features for correlation with BI-RADS categories

Marcelo Ossamu Honda, Paulo Mazzoncini de Azevedo Marques and José Antonio Hiesinger Rodrigues

CCIFM – Image Sciences and Medial Physics Center, Medical School of Ribeirão Preto, University of São Paulo, Av. Bandeirantes 3900, 14048-900 – Ribeirão Preto, SP, Brazil
honda@cci.fmrp.usp.br, pmarques@fmrp.usp.br

Abstract. This paper presents a Content-Based Image Retrieval (CBIR) system focused on mammographic images, to aid the diagnosis of breast lesions by visual inspection. The images are classified according to the BI-RADS. Image indexing and retrieving are based on textural features (Haralick's features), automatically extracted from regions of interest (ROIs) previously established in digitized mammograms. We have used the Principal Components Analysis (PCA) to simplify indexing and retrieving processes. The system was evaluated through the quantification of agreements by visual inspection of search and retrieval images. Results obtained with the leave-one-out method, provided Precision values between 22% and 100% for selected ROIs, between 31% and 100% for whole images and between 25% and 100% for classification based on BI-RADS categories. The results indicate that our method can be useful for research, training and aid diagnosis.

1. Introduction

The recent explosion of available information in hospital systems has generated a great increase in the request of multimedia data recording systems into the integrated databases. Particularly in Radiology, with the increased usage of digital image equipment, the search for information in that format has gained importance quickly. The content-based image retrieval (CBIR) is an important alternative and a fundamental complement to traditional systems of search based on text, specially when it refers to the management of data in information systems with image support. One of the great difficulties to be overcome in the development of CBIR systems is the semantic gap between the features automatically extracted by the system (low-level characteristics) and the concepts used on visual human perception (high-level query) [1]. This work presents a CBIR system implemented to aid the diagnosis of breast lesions, and also to be an initial study to overcome the semantic gap between a visual human perception and the textural features automatically extracted from mammographic images.

2. Methods

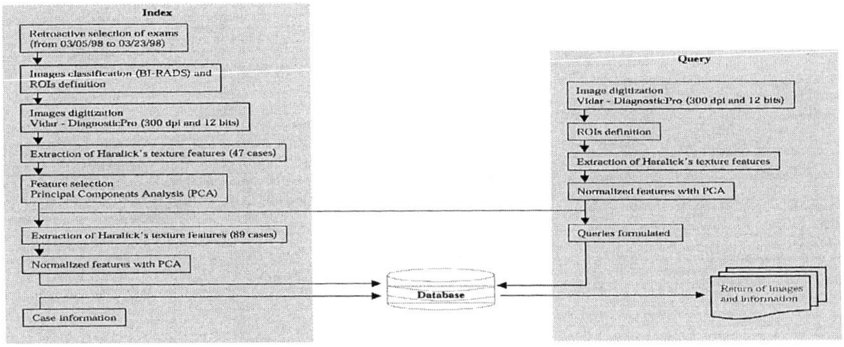

Fig. 1. Scheme describing image index, storage and retrieval.

We have used a total of 136 consecutive clinical cases, from the Radiodiagnosis Facility of Medical School of Ribeirao Preto Hospital (HCFMRP) at University of Sao Paulo (USP), each one containing two mammograms (MLO and CC) of each breast. The images were digitized with a scanner "Vidar" model DiagnosticPro with spatial resolution of 300 dpi and 12 bits of quantization. Each clinical case was classified according the Breast Imaging Reporting and Data System (BI-RADS) by a radiologist physician of the Image Sciences and Medial Physics Center (CCIFM) of Medical School of Ribeirao Preto at USP, whom also identified the regions of interest (ROIs) into the original films. Fourteen texture features (Haralick's features), obtained from the spatial gray level dependence (SGLD) matrices, were used for ROIs characterization and indexing [2]. The method of Principal Components Analysis (PCA) was employed to select the more significant features and to reduce the dimension of the feature vectors [3]. The queries are performed with the presentation of a ROI to the system, which calculates and normalizes the texture features and carries out the searches on database for images with similar characteristic, ranging them in a degree of approximation defined by the user. The images retrieved are then presented to the physician who can compare them, verify the diagnostic of the recovered cases and the BI-RADS classification. Figure 1 shows the principal methods used in this work. The evaluation of the system employing the leave-one-out methodology was performed through the quantification of the specialist subjective responses of the in relation to the degree of similarity between reference and retrieved images based on visual inspection. In such case, the retrieved images of ROIs were presented for radiologist appreciation along with the image used to search. So, images similarities were quantified (1 - Different as well, 2 - Almost different, 3 - Similar, 4 - Almost identical and 5 – Identical as well). After, the complete images of retrieved and reference cases were presented to the specialist, for a new evaluation of similarity. The evaluation just of the ROIs quantifies the similarity between the regions used to images indexing, while the evaluation of the complete clinical case provides us information about the ROIs utilization for clinical cases characterization.

3. Results

The initial results obtained from mammograms indexing and retrieval process provided Precision values between 22% and 100% for selected ROIs, between 31% and 100% for whole images and between 25% and 100% for classification based on BI-RADS categories, considering relevant the retrieved images within the same category or one category above or one category below of the query image category (Table 1).

Table 1. Precision results of ROIs, whole images and BI-RADS categories

ROIs	BI-RADS	Recall	Precision (ROI)	Precision (whole)	Precision (BI-RADS)
5	II	13	0.46	0.31	0.92
13	II	4	0.50	0.50	0.25
23	II	9	0.22	0.44	0.89
33	III	7	0.43	0.57	1.00
40	III	3	1.00	1.00	1.00
59	III	7	0.86	0.71	0.86
108	II	9	0.22	0.33	0.89
129	IV	7	0.71	0.43	0.71
139	IV	10	0.80	0.50	0.70
145	IV	14	0.57	0.36	0.78
152	IV	11	0.45	0.73	0.82
161	III	15	0.40	0.47	1.00
208	III	14	0.36	0.43	1.00

4. Conclusions

Despite the large variation obtained for Precision values, what was probably caused by the limited number of cases in our database, the general results denote that our CBIR system has the potential to aid the radiologist diagnosis. Also, queries based on image content seem to be useful for research and medical training.

References

1. Vailaya, A., Figueiredo, M.A.T., Jain, A.K., Zhang, H-J.: Image Classification for Content Based Indexing. Vol. 10, N. 1 , IEEE Trans. Image Processing (2001) 117-130
2. Haralick, R., Shanmugan, K., Distein, I.: Textural features of images classification., Man and Cibernetics SMC-3, N. 6, IEEE Transactions on Systems (1973) 610-621.
3. Johnson, R.A., Wichern, D.W.: Applied multivariate Statistical Analysis. 4rd Pretice Hall inc., New Jersey (1998)

Contrast enhancement by digital equalization in digital mammography

Walter Huda, Kent Ogden, Ernest Scalzetti, Anthony Sajewicz, Galina Levin

Department of Radiology, SUNY Upstate Medical University
750 E Adams Street, Syracuse NY 13210 USA
hudaw@mail.upstate.edu

Abstract. We evaluated an image processing algorithm based on contrast enhancement by digital equalization (CEDE), which is designed to enhance image contrast by employing digital equalization of digital mammograms. Digital images were obtained on a Digital Mammography imaging system (Lorad). Mammograms were obtained of an anthropomorphic breast phantom (Rachel) with added simulated lesions. A statistical analysis was made of the processed images, and observer compared the visibility of simulated lesions in the processed image with the original image. The display contrast in processed images increased by up to ~40%, which correlated well with a subjective improvement in lesion conspicuity. Our result indicate that the CEDE algorithm has the potential to improve mass lesion visibility in digital mammography.

1. Introduction

Contrast enhancement is useful in mammography because of the inherent low contrast of subtle lesions [1]. Visualization of low contrast features is difficult because mammograms can contain regions of glandular and adipose tissues which have different x-ray attenuation characteristics. The resultant large intensity differences in mammograms dominate the overall contrast of a mammogram, and will therefore reduce local contrast in the vicinity of any abnormal lesion.

The purpose of this study was to evaluate an image processing algorithm based on contrast enhancement by digital equalization (CEDE) [2].

2. Method

The principle idea of CEDE is to decrease the average intensity in the bright regions and increase the brightness in relatively dark regions [3]. The CEDE algorithm operates by subtracting the average brightness over a set of local square regions of a specific size. Digital images were obtained of an anthropomorphic breast phantom (Rachel) on a Lorad Full Field of View Digital Mammography imaging systems. Digital versions of mass lesions were obtained by subtracting images of the Rachel phantom with & without the lesion. The contrast of the lesion was adjusted to the observer detection threshold, and added back to a digital image of the Rachel phantom. In addition, a statistical analysis was made of the image data in the original and processed images.

3. Results

3.1 Region of interest size

The figure below shows the results obtained for processing a digital image of the Rachel phantom using a region of interest (ROI) of 128 (top left), 256 (top right) and 512 (bottom left). The radiograph in the bottom right corner is the original image of the Rachel phantom acquired at 28 kVp and 80 mAs. The smoothing kernel for each of these images was made equal to the ROI size.

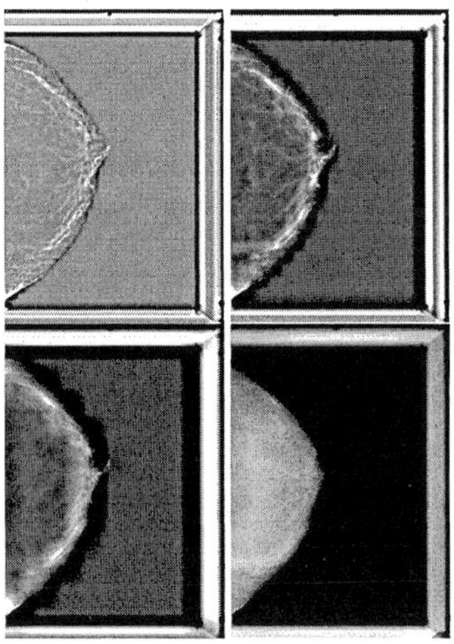

These images illustrate the general characteristics of the CEDE algorithm when used with arbitrary square ROIs to achieve the required equalization. Depending on the size of the ROI used, the resulting image used for subtraction will approximate well the original image in all areas except those where there is a steep gradient in intensity relative to the ROI size. In these areas, there tends to be large differences between adjacent ROI's. These differences lead to the 'blockiness' artifact that is particularly noticeable in the 512x512 ROI image. For digital mammograms, the most prominent area where this gradient exists is the region near the skin line where tissue is not compressed to a uniform thickness by the compression device.

3.2 Size of smoothing kernel

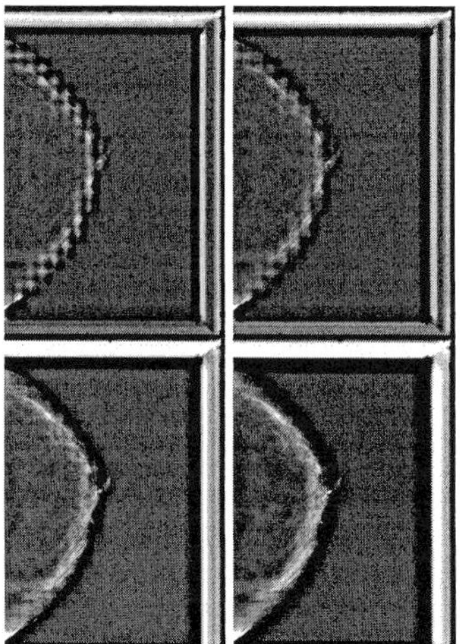

The figure to the left shows the effect of the smoothing kernel on mammograms processed using the CEDE algorithm. All images were processed using an ROI of 256x256 pixels. The smoothing kernel sizes were 128 (upper left), 192 (upper right), 384 (bottom left), and 512 (bottom right). The effect of a kernel size of 256 for an ROI of 256 was given in Section 3.1 (upper right image).

Use of a kernel size that is smaller than the ROI is clearly undesirable as this results in obvious image artifacts at the edge of the kernel size. Increasing the smoothing kernel size beyond the ROI size reduces the effect of the discontinuity at the boundary of adjacent regions. Larger smoothing kernels minimize the effect of processing artifacts, thereby providing a greater visibility of structure.

3.3. Contrast enhancement

The standard deviation of pixel values in the digital mammogram was calculated as a percentage of the data dynamic range. Empirical values of the standard deviation fell monotonically from 22% in the original image, to 3.6% for a 512^2 matrix size, and to 0.9% for the 32^2 matrix size. The average intensity of a lesion ranges linearly from 0% (white) to 100% black. The average lesion intensity value was ~15% in the original image, but this increased to between 50 and 70% in the processed image, so that the lesions had a markedly darker appearance.

The percentage of the display dynamic range that is actually occupied by the lesion (i.e., display contrast) was also investigated. The display contrast in processed images increased by up to ~40%, which correlated well with a subjective improvement in lesion conspicuity. After processing with the CEDE algorithm, small variations in gray levels of a malignant lesion and its nearby background will occupy more gray levels (dynamic range) for display, thereby increasing local contrast.

4. Discussion

Our quantitative data on processed mammograms, together with the subjective improvements of lesion visibility, indicate that the CEDE algorithm has the potential to improve mass lesion visibility in digital mammography. Two initial problems that need to be overcome in the next version of the algorithm are: (a) segmentation of the breast to eliminate artifacts at the skin line and chest wall; (b) development of an alternative to the arbitrary squares used in this study to serve as the template for equalization. Work on overcoming both problems is currently underway.

References

1. A. F. Laine, S. Schuler, J. Fan, and W. Huda, "Mammographic feature enhancement by multiscale analysis," *IEEE Trans. Med. Imag.* **13** (1994) 725-740.

2. D. B. Plewes, "A scanning system for chest radiography with regional exposure control: Theoretical considerations." *Medical Physics* **10** (1983) 646-654. .

3. J. M. Sabol, I. C. Soutar, and D. B. Plewes, "Mammographic scanning equalization radiography." *Medical Physics* **20** (1993) 1505-1515.

Representing clustered microcalcifications by their cluster shape

Pere Planiol, Joan Martí, Josep Español, Elisabet Golobardes, Jordi Gay and Jordi Freixenet

UdG - University of Girona
Computer Vision and Robotics Group
Campus Motilivi, 17071 Girona, Spain
planiol@eia.udg.es

Abstract. The shape and arrangement of clustered microcalcifications help the radiologists to judge the likelihood of cancer being present. In general, malignant calcifications are very numerous, clustered, small, dot-like or elongated, and variable in size, shape, and density. In contrast, benign calcifications are generally larger, less numerous, more rounded, more diffusely distributed, and more homogeneous in size and shape. Starting from a segmentation algorithm that individually identifies the microcalcifications, we have used a bottom-up hierarchical algorithm to group them into clusters for a later characterization. This behavior leads to meaningfully differentiated shapes for both kinds of clusters. A Case-Based Reasoning classifier has been applied to classify the data and validate the cluster composition with promising results (at a false positive fraction of 10%, an 86% true positive fraction has been attained).

1. Introduction

This paper presents the results of analysing the shape of the resulting clusters when grouping the individual microcalcifications. It follows a previous microcalcification analysis work [1], where a statistical model was built-up to issue a diagnosis only attending the shape-based properties of individual microcalcifications.

Following the rules usually applied for grouping individual microcalcifications into sets [2][3], a cluster is defined as a collection of three or more microcalcifications within $1cm^2$. In a great number of malignant diagnosed mammograms, it has been noticed that the solely indicator used to issue the diagnosis was the number of microcalcifications and their distribution inside every cluster. Thus, the relevance of the cluster properties for issuing a diagnosis seems to be clear.

In order to characterize the clusters, we take advantage of the already developed microcalcification detection algorithm, and afterwards the cluster is built-up by adding individual microcalcifications following a hierarchical algorithm. The resulting clusters are then parametrized through their shape. Then, a Case-Based Reasoning algorithm is applied to return the mammogram from the working database with the most similar cluster. Finally, and as a measure of results, a diagnosis comparison of the two mammograms has been made.

2. Cluster Analysis

To detect the clusters, we have used a bottom-up hierarchical algorithm to group the individual microcalcifications. It starts with the initial assumption that each single microcalcification constitutes a cluster, which enables the generation of the distance matrix (a symmetrical matrix which includes all the distances among two clusters). Then, at each step, the two closest clusters are added into a new one, allowing the recalculation of the distance matrix. Obviously, clusters containing less than 3 microcalcifications are discarded.

Once the final set of clusters has been achieved, each cluster is characterised by means of its shape. We have developed a new algorithm to detect the envelope contour, trying to overcome some of the drawbacks of using snakes [4]. This algorithm named the *fit-stamp*, tries to fit different round stamps to the background of the image while preserving the integrity of the microcalcifications. This iterative process starts with an initial 1-pixel radius, which is later increased until only one blob is reached. The shape of the final cluster is extracted by using the Chain codes of the perimeter. The figure 1 shows several steps of the algorithm when applied to a cluster.

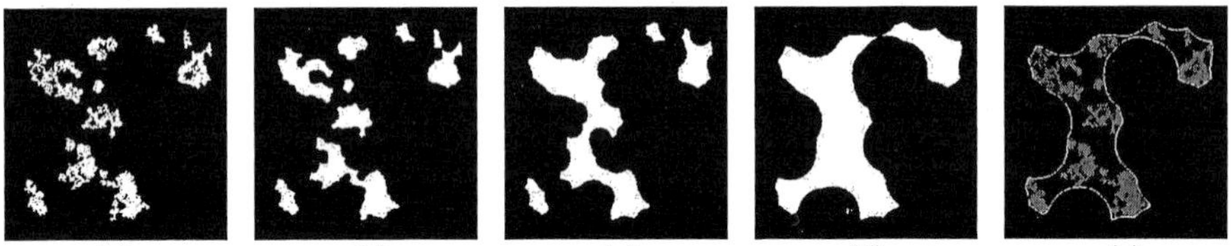

(a) (b) (c) (d) (e)

Fig. 1: Application of the *fit-stamp* algorithm to a cluster of microcalcifications: a) Individual microcalcifications b) Cluster detected using a 5-pixel radius c) Cluster detected using a 15-pixel radius d) Final cluster detected, using a 25-pixel radius e) Envelope of the detected cluster.

Among several possibilities, we have selected the Compactness and the Normalised Fourier Descriptors [5] as features to describe the cluster shape.

3. Results

To evaluate the performance of representing the microcalcifications by their cluster shape, we have used a Case-Based Reasoning technique. Due to the easiness of implementation, we have selected the Minkowski distance and Clark distance [6] as similarity functions during the retrieval step. The former uses Euclidean distance, while the latter employs a previous normalised range of features. These two similarity functions have been tested over a set of 145 cases, where 71 were benign and 71 were malignant. The total number of clusters is 247 where 87 belong to benign mammograms and 160 belong to malignant mammograms. For each cluster, we have searched the most similar cluster, and then the diagnosis has been compared. The table 1 shows the results for the Minkowski distance and the results for the Clark distance.

	Minkowski distance		Clark distance	
Results	Total	Percentage	Total	Percentage
Correct	180	72	186	75
Incorrect	67	28	61	25

Table 1. Minkowski and Clark results

4. Acknowledgments

This work is supported by the grant program 2001FI 00687 UG PG of the Generalitat de Catalunya, and has partially been funded by the *Fondo de Investigación Sanitaria (Ministerio de Sanidad y Consumo)* under the grant FIS-00/0033.

References

1. Martí J, Cufí X, Regincós J, et al. Shaped-base features selection for microcalcification evaluation. In Kenneth M. Hanson ed., Medical Imaging 1998, SPIE vol. 3338, pages 1215–1224. February 1998.
2. Woods K, Automated Image Analysis Techniques for Digital Mammography Ph.D. Dissertation, December 1994. University of South Florida.
3. Shen L, Rangayyan RM, Leo Desautels JE. Detection and Classification of Mammographic Calcifications, World Scientific, State of the Art in Digital Mammographic Image Analysis, volume 9, pages 198–212, June 1994.
4. Kass M, Witkin A, Terzopoulos D. Snake: Active Contour Models, International Journal of Computer Vision, Kluwer Academic Publishers, 1(4): 321-331, 1987.
5. Shen L, Rangayyan RM, Leo Desautels JE. Application of Shape Analysis to Mammographic Calcifications. IEEE Transactions on Medical Imaging, vol. 13, no. 2, pages 263–274, June 1994.
6. Martí J, Español J, Golobardes E, et al. Classification of Microcalcifications in Digital Mammograms using Case-Based Reasoning. Proceedings of the 5th International Workshop on Digital Mammography, pages 285-294. Toronto, Canada, June 2000.

Analysis of Changes in Masses Using Contrast and Size Measures

Sheila Timp, Nico Karssemeijer, Jan Hendriks

Department of Radiology, University Medical Center Nijmegen,
Geert Grooteplein 18, 6525 GA Nijmegen, The Netherlands
sheila@radiology.azn.nl

1 Introduction

One of the techniques used by radiologist to detect developing abnormalities is comparison of the current screening mammogram with previous ones. An observed change from a previous examination may bring attention to subtle signs of malignancy such as a new or growing mass or new or increasing calcifications that may have been overlooked otherwise [1].

The purpose of this study is to retrospectively determine mammographic changes in masses with respect to size and contrast. This information could furthermore be incorporated in CAD programs to improve the detection of masses and reduce the number of false-positives, just as in radiological practice.

2 Materials and Methods

A total of 250 biopsy proven breast cancer cases was taken from the Dutch national screening program. These cases were either screen detected or interval carcinoma. From these cases the mammograms at three different points in time were collected: the diagnostic mammogram, the index round screening mammogram and the previous round screening mammogram (figure 1). The diagnostic mammogram is either a clinical mammogram or a screening mammogram. In every screening round an mediolateral oblique (MLO) image is made. Guidelines exist on when to make an additional craniocaudal (CC) image. When attending to the screening program for the first time CC images are always taken. In subsequent rounds the radiographer decides on these extra views for reasons like notable changes in the mammogram.

The mammograms were digitized at a pixel size of $50 \mu m$. The location of the biopsied mass was identified by an expert radiologist. The radiologist also determined whether the tumor was already visible on the previous mammograms and whether it was clearly visible or minimal sign. All visible masses were selected and analyzed by our CAD program that segmented the regions and calculated size and contrast features.

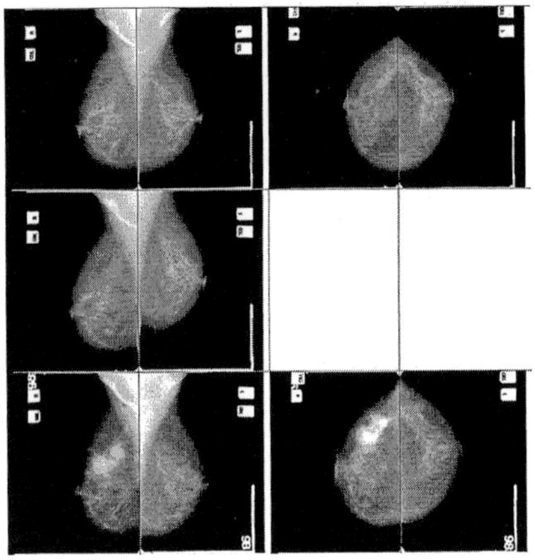

previous round screening mammogram

index round screening mammogram

diagnostic mammogram

Fig. 1. Case

3 Size and Contrast measures

To compare the current mammogram with the previous ones, we used size and contrast measures. To compute features such as contrast, differences between the area inside and outside the contour must be determined. For this purpose, an area outside the contour was defined based on the effective radius R of the segmented region. All pixels within a distance of 0.6*R to the segmented area form the outside region. The outside area is approximately twice the size of the segmented area. The set of pixels in the segmentation is denoted by I, the set of pixels in the outside region by O. $E(X)$ is the mean value of pixels in the set X. The contrast measure we used is the difference in intensity between I and O:

$$Contrast = E(I) - E(O)$$

4 Results

All 250 cases were classified into histological classes. Most tumors were invasive carcinoma (90%). For further study the cases with carcinoma is situ and carcinoma that only consisted of microcalcifications were excluded (total 28 cases). 7 additional cases were excluded for several reasons (lost mammogram etc). The resulting 215 cases have been analysed using size and contrast measures.

In 54% of the cases the tumor was visible in retrospect on the last mammogram and in 25% of the cases the tumor was visible both on the last mammogram and the mammogram one screening round before. This resulted in a total of 547 mammograms with a visible abnormality: 344 diagnostic mammograms and 136 and 67 from the previous two screening rounds. Of all visible abnormalities size and contrast of the lesion were determined. The results are summarized in figure 2. The average size of the lesions at the time of diagnosis was 2.9 cm^2, while the size at the prior two screening round was 1.66 cm^2 and 1.58 cm^2 respectively. We define the growthrate as:

$$\frac{\text{size current screening round - size previous screening round}}{\text{size previous screening round}}$$

The growthrate was calculated for all tumors that were visible on two successive screening rounds. The average growthrate between the previous and index screening round was 109% and between the index and diagnostic round 152%. Figure 3 shows the distribution of growthrates. The average contrast of the lesions at time of diagnosis was 0.720, at the index round 0.502 and at the previous screening round 0.371.

	size	contrast
previous round	395	0.371
index round	414	0.502
diagnostic round	734	0.720

Fig. 2. Size and contrast values of visible lesions at three different time moments

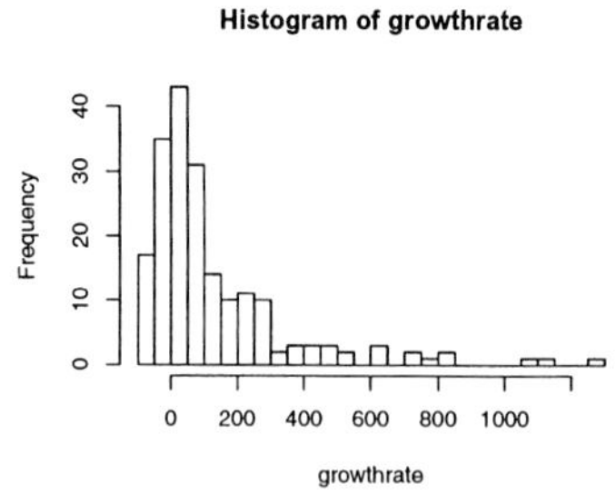

Fig. 3. The x-axis shows the growthrate ∗ 100, the y-axis shows the number of tumors with the specified growthrate

5 Discussion

The data show that on average contrast-features and size-features both increase during time. About 25% of the masses decreased in size or remained the same. Further inspection of these masses showed that the largest part (27%) of these masses were architectural distorsions that contracted to a smaller but denser mass. Other reasons for this decrease in size were segmentation problems (25%), masses that remained the same size (20%), masses that indeed decreased in size (15%), masses situated on the border of the mammogram (8%) and other (8%). This knowledge can be incorporated in CAD systems to increase the specificity of the detection of tumors.

References

1. White, K., Berbaun, K., Smith, W.L.: The role of previous radiographs and reports in the interpretation of current radiographs. Invest Radiol **29** (1994), 263–265.

A model for nonrigid mammogram registration using mutual information

Michael A. Wirth, Jay Narhan and Derek Gray

Department of Computing and Information Science, University of Guelph, Guelph, Ontario, Canada
mwirth@uoguelph.ca

Abstract. This approach to mammogram registration uses a similarity-measure known as mutual information as the cost-function used to determine the degree of similarity between two corresponding mammograms. An initial registration is performed to remove global differences and bring the mammograms into approximate alignment. The mammograms are then partitioned into sub-images and each of the corresponding sub-images is matched independently using normalized mutual information. The centroids of each of the matched sub-images are then used as control-point pairs in association with a radial basis function to produce a global nonrigid registration.

1. Nonrigid Mammogram Registration

Comparative analysis is a process in computerized mammogram analysis whereby mammograms are inspected for characteristic signs of potential abnormalities through the comparison of various corresponding bilateral or temporal mammograms. There are many factors which contribute to spatial differences between corresponding morphological structures in mammograms [1]. Some of these characteristics relate to the fact that the breast is a deformable, mobile, soft-tissue structure which is inhomogeneous, anisotropic, and compressible; others relate to differences in the 3D positioning of the breast, and the amount and geometry of compression applied to it. Such spatial differences can make a pair of mammograms look quite different, thereby significantly complicating the comparative process. The process of *mammogram registration* minimizes spatial differences between corresponding mammograms.

Many previous approaches to the task of nonrigid mammogram registration have relied on matching corresponding control-points derived from anatomical feature points. One of the caveats encountered when using pure point-matching techniques such as radial basis functions is their reliance on accurately extracted anatomical features points. In most cases such features are extracted from the periphery of the mammogram and includes control-points identified from along the breast contour. Identification of such feature-points is made difficult because breasts are, in essence, compressible structures, lacking rigid structures and containing very few distinct morphological features. The underlying rationale for using similarity-measures is their ability to function in an autonomous manner, removing the reliance on accurate control-point extraction.

2. Hierarchical Registration Algorithm

The proposed nonrigid registration algorithm is a *hierarchical model* composed of a global transformation and a series of localized transformations [2]. An initial global registration is performed on the mammograms using *normalized mutual information* [3] to remove rigid differences and bring the mammograms into approximate alignment. This global transformation describes the overall motion of the breast which may include changes in breast positioning. The simplest choice is a rigid transformation which is composed of translations and rotations. To model the localized deformations the mammograms are partitioned into smaller sub-images and each of the corresponding sub-images is matched independently using normalized mutual information. The localized spatial transformations are simple, commonly only translations, restricting the deformations to very small deformations in the x and y directions. Each of the matched sub-image pairs generates a displacement vector, characterizing the spatial difference between the centroids of each of the sub-images. A *displacement vector field* between corresponding mammograms is formed when the individual localized displacement vectors of the sub-images are grouped together. This vector field of local displacements represents corresponding control-point pairs, which when used in association with a Thin-Plate Spline [4] spatial transformation helps generates a smooth global nonrigid transformation. This approach couples the nonrigid properties of radial basis functions, with the a function to calculate a measure of the similarity between the mammograms.

3. Experimental Results

The technique is illustrated by matching mammograms from the MIAS digital mammogram database. Preliminary results show some promise in using this hierarchical model to perform mammogram registration. The example shown in Fig. 1 demonstrates the registration of a pair of bilateral mammograms containing an asymmetry. In the pre-registration difference image, much of the misregistration occurs along the periphery of the breast. After the mammograms have been registered, the asymmetry between the two mammograms is more distinctly delineated. In most cases the global rigid registration successfully removes any globalized rigid deformations present between the corresponding mammograms. The localized component of the registration algorithm proved more challenging due to the effect of objects such as x-ray markers and stripe artifacts.

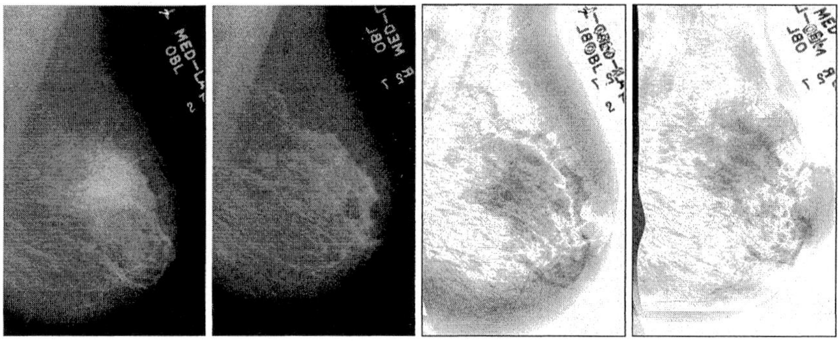

Fig. 1. Hierarchical registration of bilateral mammograms (MIAS image 041) Left and right mammograms; pre-registration and post-registration difference images.

4. Discussion & Conclusion

We have presented a method for nonrigid mammogram registration which investigates the combination of normalized mutual information and a nonrigid spatial transformation. The results obtained were in no way definitive. One of the principal benefits of this approach is its ability to function in an autonomous manner, removing the reliance on accurate control-point extraction. One of the major limitations results from intensity variations between similar morphological structures in different mammograms. This is partly due to the fact that mammograms are 2D projections of 3D structures, and slight variations in positioning between screenings may result in differential tissue overlap and subsequent changes in intensity values. There are often differences in intensity distributions between temporal mammograms caused by inconsistencies in the imaging protocol used in acquiring the mammograms, or natural changes in the composition and distribution of breast tissue between screenings. Bilateral mammograms suffer additional problems in that contralateral breasts may not necessarily contain the same morphological structures.

References

1. Wirth, M.A., "Characterizing spatial deformation in breast images: A rationale for registration", Technical Report, University of Guelph, (2002).
2. Wirth, M.A., Narhan, J., and Gray, D., "Nonrigid mammogram registration using mutual information", SPIE: Medical Imaging: Image Processing, San Diego, CA, Vol. 4684 (2002).
3. Rueckert, D., Sonoda, L.I., Denton, E., Rankin, S., Hayes, C., Leach, M.O., Hill, D. and Hawkes, D.J., "Comparison and evaluation of rigid and non-rigid registration of breast MR images," SPIE Medical Imaging: Image Processing, San Diego, CA, Vol.3661, (1999) 78-88
4. Bookstein, F.L., "Principal Warps:Thin-Plate Splines and the decomposition of deformations". IEEE Transactions on Pattern Analysis and Machine Intelligence, Vol. 11(6): (1989) 567-585

Computer Aided Diagnosis

Evaluation of Breast Ductal Networks Using Ramification Matrices

Predrag R. Bakic, Michael Albert, and Andrew D.A. Maidment

Thomas Jefferson University, 111 S 11th St., Philadelphia, PA, 19107, USA
pbakic@esther.rad.tju.edu

Abstract. We evaluated the use of ramification (R-) matrices in analysis and modeling of breast ducts. The elements of an R-matrix are the branching probabilities at different tree levels. The analysis was performed on 10 normal and 13 benign galactograms. The ductal trees were manually segmented from the galactograms and corresponding R-matrices were inferred. Effects of segmentation were tested by successively removing each of the terminal branches and computing the corresponding matrices on the clinical galactograms and a large number of synthetically generated ductal trees. We also examined a classification scheme to distinguish between normal and benign galactograms based upon the matrix coefficients. The classification using the $r_{3,3}$ coefficient performed correctly for 90% of normal and 62% of benign cases (p=0.027).

1. Introduction

About 90% of breast cancers originate in the ductal epithelium [1]. Some of these are revealed by nipple discharge alone, with no palpable or mammographic lesions. Galactography, indicated mostly in cases with nipple discharge, is a procedure for imaging the contrast-enhanced ductal network. Unfortunately, galactography lacks specificity, thus a large number of benign and normal biopsies result. An improved radiographic classification scheme for galactograms would help significantly to reduce the psychological and economic burden of a large percentage of negative biopsies.

There have been a few attempts to reconstruct the breast ductal network, e.g., by tracing the points of duct entrance to and exit from a series of subgross histologic slices [2]. However, providing a description of the normal ductal network is a very complex task due to anatomical variability and low radiographic contrast. Statistical analysis of ductal networks for breast modeling has also been reported in the literature [3], [4].

We have analyzed ductal networks based upon ramification (R-) matrices, which describe the topological shape of a tree. The R-matrix elements represent branching probabilities at various levels of a ductal tree and are inferred, e.g., using the algorithm by Viennot et al. [5]. Due to their probabilistic nature, a variety of synthetic trees can be generated using the same matrix, matching statistically the branching properties of the original tree. The R-matrix representation of ductal networks has been used in breast modeling for mammography simulation [4].

2. Materials and Methods

We have evaluated the classification of normal and benign pathologies based upon R-matrices. Ductal trees were manually segmented from galactograms and the corresponding matrices were inferred. The robustness of the R-matrix representation was tested by analysis of pruned trees. The probability of correct classification with the R-matrix elements was computed, in order to identify the combination of elements with the best performance.

2.1 Ductal tree identification from clinical galactograms

We have analyzed 23 clinical galactograms (15 CC and 8 ML/O). Ten (7 CC and 3 ML/O) corresponded to normal and 13 (8 CC and 5 ML/O) to benign pathologies; no malignant cases were included in this set. We traced the network of larger ducts from galactograms in order to reconstruct their topological structure. The branching pattern was identified manually by placing a tracing pad over the galactogram on a light box and marking the points where ducts branch or overlap. These were distinguished by assuming that the points of overlap look brighter than branching points, due to superposition of the x-ray attenuation of two ducts on top of each other. Large ducts were reconstructed by connecting the marked points. This procedure is illustrated in Fig. 1.

In each of the segmented ductal trees, the root, internal and terminal nodes, and the branches were labeled and the R-matrix elements computed as described by Viennot et al. [5]. We used matrices with at most nine nonzero elements arranged into three rows (see Fig. 1) corresponding to a maximum of four branching levels. The elements in each row sum to one, representing the probability of branching into any possible combination of children nodes.

2.2 Test of robustness

We performed a preliminary test of robustness by analyzing pruned ductal trees, derived from an original tree after removing a single terminal branch. The R-matrix of a pruned tree was computed and the procedure repeated for each of the terminal branches in the original tree. The R-matrix elements, averaged over all pruned versions of the original tree, were compared with the original matrix elements. This test was proposed based upon the observed ambiguity in tracing terminal branches, which can be easily confused due to their small size and low contrast. Consequently, some of the terminal branches could have been omitted, resulting in a pruned version of the original tree.

2.3 Automated classification of galactograms

The values of the R-matrix elements inferred from clinical galactograms and averaged over all benign and all normal cases are plotted in Fig. 2. Some of the matrix elements show a noticeable difference between the 2 classes, e.g., $r_{3,2}$ and $r_{3,3}$, suggesting the possibility of classifying galactographic findings based upon R-matrices. We evaluated a classification scheme using either a single or a pair of matrix elements and a linear Bayesian decision rule, in order to avoid overspecification by the small number of samples. Evaluation was performed in a round-robin fashion and the probability of correct classification estimated.

3. Results and Discussion

The analysis of the pruned versions of the clinical galactograms showed an average RMS fractional difference between the original R-matrix elements and the elements averaged over all pruned trees of 6.7% for the normal cases and 11% for the benign cases. In addition, we repeated the test on 1000 synthetic random binary trees, and obtained an average RMS fractional difference of 6.8%. The RMS differences are small compared to the sample standard deviations, shown in Fig. 2, confirming the robustness of the R-matrix representation of ductal networks.

The best classification performance of a single R-matrix element was observed for $r_{3,3}$ with the probability of correct classification of 90% for the normal cases and 62% for the benign cases. In a combination of two elements, $r_{3,2}$ and $r_{3,3}$ showed the best performance being correct for 80% of normal cases and 77% of benign cases.

In order to estimate the statistical significance of the classification results, an additional experiment using random numbers as description parameters was performed. Six numbers, corresponding to the linearly independent elements of the R-matrix with nine elements, were randomly generated for each sample. Two classes, with a total of 10000 samples, were randomly generated and classified based upon a single or a pair of parameters (out of the six random numbers). In 2.7% of trials one of the parameters showed a classification power of at least 89% for one class and at least 60% for the other, comparable with the performance of the element $r_{3,3}$ on the clinical galactograms. Thus, if the classification result observed on the clinical galactograms were by chance alone, it would be encountered in 2.7% of repeated experiments, which represents a statistical significance of $p=0.027$ for the classification using $r_{3,3}$. In a similar manner, the classification results using the ($r_{3,2}$; $r_{3,3}$) pair of R-matrix elements was not found to be statistically significant ($p=0.25$).

This preliminary analysis indicates that it might be possible to distinguish between benign and normal findings using R-matrices. Further experiments should use a larger number of galactograms and a more sophisticated decision rule.

Acknowledgements

This work was funded by U.S. Department of Defense, Grant DAMD-17-98-1-8169.

References

1. Kopans, D.B.: Breast Imaging. 2nd edn. Lippincott-Raven, Philadelphia (1998)
2. Ohtake, T., et al: Intraductal Extension of Primary Invasive Breast Carcinoma Treated by Breast-Conservative Surgery: Computer Graphic Tree-Dimensional Reconstruction of the Mammary Duct-Lobular Systems. Cancer. 76 (1996) 32-45
3. Taylor, P., Owens, R., and Ingram, D.: Simulated Mammography Using Synthetic 3D Breasts. In: N. Karssemeijer, et al. (eds.): Digital Mammography Nijmegen, 1998. Kluwer Academic, Dordrecht (1998)
4. P.R. Bakic: Breast Tissue Description and Modeling in Mammography. Ph.D. Dissertation, Lehigh University, Bethlehem, PA (2000)
5. Viennot, X.G., et al: Combinatorial Analysis of Ramified Patterns and Computer Imagery of Trees. Computer Graphics. 23 (1989) 31-40

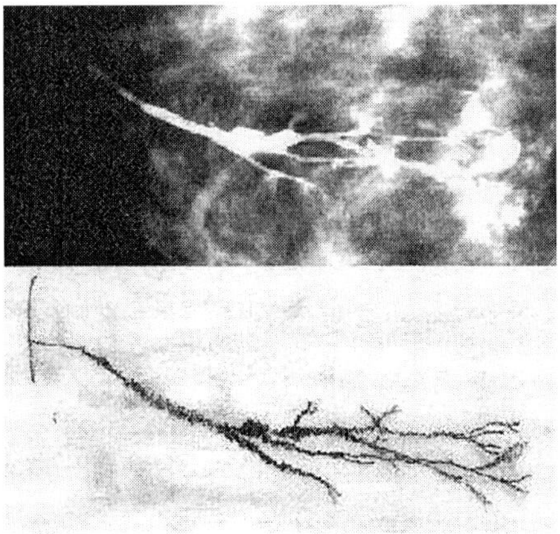

$$R=\begin{bmatrix} r_{2,1} & r_{2,2} & . & . \\ r_{3,1} & r_{3,2} & r_{3,3} & . \\ r_{4,1} & r_{4,2} & r_{4,3} & r_{4,4} \end{bmatrix} = \begin{bmatrix} 0.43 & 0.57 & . & . \\ 0.00 & 0.33 & 0.67 & . \\ 0 & 0.75 & 0 & 0.25 \end{bmatrix}$$

Fig1. Segmentation of a ductal tree, showing a part of galactogram with an enhanced ductal network (*top*), the manually traced enhanced portion of the ductal network (*center*), and the elements of the R-matrix, inferred from the segmented ductal tree (*bottom*).

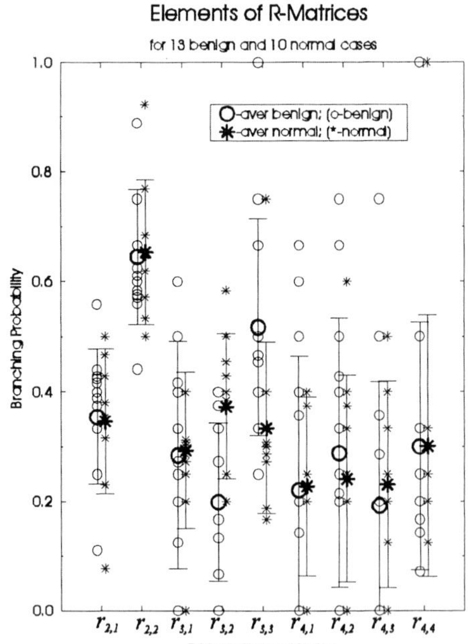

Fig. 2. Values of the R-matrix elements. The bold symbols (*circles = benign, stars = normal*) represent the element values averaged over all benign and all normal cases, while the regular symbols represent all the individual cases. The error bars correspond to the sample standard deviations.

Computer aided detection (CAD) in direct digital full field mammography

Baum Friedemann, Fischer Uwe, Benali Karim, Muller Serge, Obenauer Silivia, Grabbe Eckhardt

Department of Radiology, Georg-August-Universität Göttingen, Germany
Baumfried@web.de

Abstract. Introduction: For the first time, FFDM allows CAD analysis of directly acquired digital image data. The purpose of this study was to evaluate a CAD system in patients with histologically correlated breast cancer depicted with FFDM. Methods 61 cases of histologically proven breast cancer detected with FFDM (Senographe 2000D, GE Medical Systems) were analyzed using a CAD system (Image Checker V2.3, R2 Technology). 14 of these malignancies were characterised by microcalcifications, 36 by masses and 12 by both. The mammographic findings were categorized to BI-RADS 3 (n=5), BI-RADS 4 (n=17), and BI-RADS 5 (n=40). The sensitivity for malignant lesions and the rate of false positive marks per image were calculated. The sensitivity and its 95% confidence interval (IC) was estimated. Results: The sensitivity of the CAD R2 system in breast cancer seen on FFDM was 89% for microcalcifications (CI95%=[70%; 98%]) and 81% for masses (CI95%=[67%; 91%]). As expected the detection rate was higher in lesions categorized as BI-RADS 5 (37 of 40) compared to lesions categorized as BI-RADS 4 (11 of 17). In the group categorized as BI-RADS 3 the detection rate was 4 of 5 lesions, however this group was very small. The rate of false positive marks was 0.35 microcalcification marks/image and 0.26 mass marks/image. The overall rate of false positive marks was 0.61 per image. The PPV for malignant microcalcifications was 0.26 and for malignant masses was 0.45. Conclusions: CAD based on FFDM provides an optimized workflow. Results are equivalent to the results reported for CAD analysis of secondarily digitized image data. Sensitivity for microcalcifications is acceptable and for masses is low. The PPV for masses should be improved and the number of false positive marks per image should be reduced.

Introduction

In the last few years, computer aided diagnosis (CAD) systems have become available for use with conventional film-screen images. These systems require a digitizer that converts the analog image to a digital image prior to implementation of the CAD algorithms (1-3). Now a CAD system is available, that processes primary digital images and can be used directly on digital mammography images (4-6). The goal of this study was the evaluation of such a CAD system developed for digital mammography. The system accuracy and usefulness were evaluated.

Material and Methods

The application of the primary digital CAD technique (Image Checker V2.3; R2 Technology, Los Altos, CA, USA) was done retrospectively on a select group of 61 patients with 63 histologically verified carcinomas, which had full-field digital mammography (FFDM) (Senographe 2000D, GE Medical Systems, Buc, France) images made before surgery. One of the patients had a multicentric and another one a bilateral carcinoma. Digital mammograms were available in two views for 46 cases and in a single view in 15 cases. Images of the opposite side that did not have a pathologic result were available in 30 cases in two views and 20 cases in one view. Thus a total of 189 mammographic images were analyzed.

Fourteen cases of the 63 breast carcinomas showed microcalcifications without additional masses, in 37 cases the carcinomas were masses without microcalcifications and in 12 patients the carcinomas were masses with microcalcifications. BI-RADS™ classification was done by 2 reviewers in consensus with the results: BI-RADS 3 (n=5), BI-RADS 4 (n=18) and BI-RADS 5 (n=40). In order to exclude a multifocal, multicentric, or bilateral tumor a presurgical MR mammography was done with all patients.

CAD marks, that were consistent with the histology result of a carcinoma, were counted as a true positive (tp) while CAD marks in other parenchyma areas were counted as a false positive (fp). Carcinomas not marked were considered as false negative (fn) and areas with no suspicion of carcinoma and no CAD mark were counted as a true negative (tn). The sensitivity (tp/ tp+ fn) and the positive predictive value (PPV = tp/ tp+fp) for malignant lesions as well as the false positive marks per image were evaluated. Additionally the confidence interval for the mean sensitivity was calculated taking into account the size of the sample.

Results

The CAD system marked in the primary digital images all 14 breast carcinomas, that presented with only microcalcifications (sensitivity 100%). Of the 37 carcinomas that had a breast carcinoma mass without microcalcifications, 30 were marked correctly and 7 not correctly (sensitivity 81%). In the group of carcinomas, that showed a suspicious mass and microcalcifications, the CAD system marked both components in 8 out of 12, only the mass in 2 of 12, only the calcification in 1 of 12 and none of the two components in 1 of 12 cases, respectively (sensitivity 92%). Considering microcalcifications with or without masses the sensitivity was 89%. The confidence interval of the mean sensitivity was $CI_{95\%}$ = (70 – 98%), for microcalcifications associated with a carcinoma and $CI_{95\%}$ =(67% - 91%) for breast carcinoma masses. The PPV for malignant microcalcifications was 0.26 and for malignant masses was 0.45.

CAD detected 37 of 40 lesions of the category BI-RADS™ 5. BI-RADS™ category 4 was correctly recognized in 14 of 18 cases and carcinomas that were classified BI-RADS™ category 3 were marked in 4 of 5 cases. Including the mammograms with no pathologic result the number of false positive marks per image was 0.35 for microcalcifications (marks per image) and 0.26 for masses. The total rate of false positive marks per image was 0.61. Beyound the two cases detected with FFDM there were no aditional multifocal, multicentric or bilateral carcinomas detected by MR mammography.

Discussion

Primary digital CAD software has a number of advantages compared to CAD systems using analog images. The major advantage is that the primary digital CAD system does not require a digitizer and allows display of the CAD markers very rapidly after the image acquisition. A digitizer adds noise during the digitization of analog images and adds a large delay in the availability of the images making it difficult to use the CAD software without a significant time delay.

The primary digital CAD software tested in this study identified 55 out of 63 breast cancers for a sensitivity of 87.3%. This compares to a large trial using conventional analog images which were digitized, for these analog images the CAD software found 906 out of 1083 cancers for a sensitivity of 83.6% (7). Both CAD software systems were from the same company, one starting with digital mammograms and the other with analog mammograms. In addition, the primary digital CAD system had 0.61 false positives per image, this compares to 1.02 false positives per image with the system using analog images (7). The system presented well in the detection of microcalcifications (sensitivity 89%), however the PPV for microcalcifications (0,26) should be improved. To evaluate the profit for the reader in the detection of masses without microcalcifications (sensitivity 81%, PPV 0,45) further studies are required. Although the current study is preliminary and of limited size, the primary digital CAD software preformed very well and the results compare favorably with current systems based on analog images.

References

1 Vyborny CJ. Can computers help radiologists read mammogramms? Radiology (1994) 191: 315 – 317
2 Doi K, MacMahon H, Katsuragawa S, Nishikawa RM, Jiang Y. Computer-aided diagnosis in radiology: potential and pitfalls. Eur J Radiol (1999) 31: 97 -109
3 Funovics M, Schamp S, Helbich T.H, Lackner B, Wunderbaldinger P, Fuchsjäger M, Lechner G, Wof G. Evaluierung eines computerassistierten Diagnosesystems in der Erkennung des Mammakarzinoms. Fortschr Röntgenstr (2001) 173: 218-223
4 Muller S. Full field digital mammography designed as a complete system. Eur J Radiol (1999) 31: 25 –34.

5 Bick U. Digitale Vollfeldmammographie. Fortschr Röntgenstr (2000) 173: 957 – 964
6 Fischer U, Baum F, Vosshenrich R, Obenauer S, Grabbe E. Detektion von Mikroverkalkungen in der direkten Vollfeldmammographie. Fortschr Röntgenstr (2000) 172: 41
7 Warren Burhenne LJ, Wood SA, D'Orsi CJ, Feig SA, Kopans DB, O'Shaughnessy KF, Sickles EA, Tabar L, Vyborny CJ, Castellino RA. Potential contribution of computer-aided detection to the sensitivity of screening mammography. Radiology (2000) 215(2):554-62.
8 Tabar I, Fagerberg CJ, Gad A, Baldetrop I, Holmberg LH, Grontoft O, Ljinquist U, Lundstrøm B, Manson JC, Eklund G. Reduction in mortality from breast cancer after mass screening with mammography. Lancet (1985) 1: 829-883.
9 Fracheboud J, de Koenig HJ, Beemsterboier PMM. Nationalwide breast cancer screening in the Netherlands: results of initial and subsequent screening 1990- 1995. Int J Cancer (1998) 75: 694-698.
10 Thurfjell EL, Lerneval KA, Taube AA Benefit of independent double reading in a population-based mammography screening programm. Radiology (1994) 191: 241-244.

A new method for optimising and evaluating mammographic detection algorithms

Michael Board and Sue Astley

Division of Imaging Science and Biomedical Engineering, The University of Manchester, M13 9PT, UK
michael.board@stud.man.ac.uk

Abstract. We have developed and evaluated a new technique for measuring the performance of mammographic feature detection algorithms, with the aim of overcoming some of the limitations of ROC analysis. The method outputs a cost derived from the transportation algorithm to give a smoothly varying measure of detector performance that can be used both for comparison and optimisation of algorithms. The method has been used to optimise a morphological microcalcification detection algorithm. A transportation cost curve was generated by applying the detection method over a range of parameters. The minimum cost point is compared with an operating point drawn from an ROC curve. Our new technique deals well with a variety of cases. It quantifies performance in terms of both proximity and extent, and gives an appropriate cost for detections around the borders of lesions.

1. Introduction

In computer-aided detection systems for mammography, algorithms detect potentially abnormal areas in the images, and thus generate prompts to attract the attention of the radiologist to the most suspicious areas of the original films. There is evidence that, provided the prompts are sufficiently accurate, this approach can improve human detection performance [1]. The method by which these systems are evaluated has become increasingly important. Studies of reader performance with and without prompting are costly and time-consuming; it would not be feasible to repeat such studies each time an algorithm is updated. It would thus be advantageous to have a measure expressing both the likelihood of a prompt attracting attention to an abnormality and the distracting effect of any falsely positioned markers.

The most common method of evaluation is by Receiver Operating Characteristic (ROC) analysis [2]. Performance is indicated by the area under the ROC curve, or by the proximity of the curve to the top left corner of the graph. Adaptations such as free response ROC (FROC) deal with cases in which the detection of a number of lesions is addressed. One limitation of FROC analysis is that every prompt must be categorised either as a true positive (hit) or a false positive. In general, a prompt is only recorded as a hit if it overlaps the truth region by some degree (Figure 1(a)). However, the degree of overlap required may vary; in some cases a very large detection may be considered to be a hit, even though it is clearly not a useful prompt

(Figure 1(b)). In addition, algorithms that generate multiple detections around the edge of the truth region (Figure 1(c)) will record multiple false positives even though such a prompt image would clearly draw the radiologist's attention to the area in question.

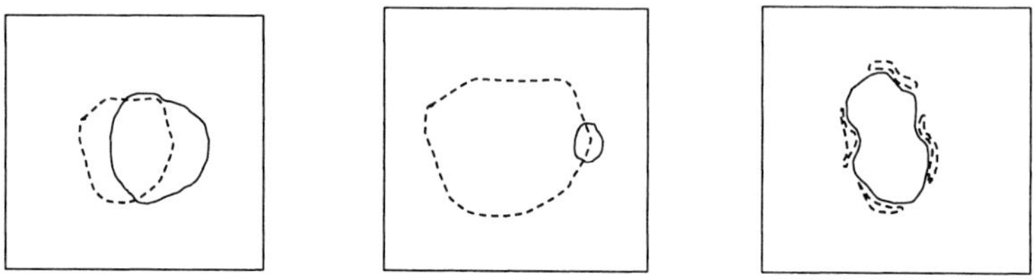

(a) (b) (c)

Fig. 1. Three diagrammatic examples of prompt and truth regions; dotted lines enclose the prompt regions and solid lines surround the truth regions

The aim of our research is to develop an alternative method of evaluating different types of detection algorithms that will overcome these difficulties, and provide a quantitative measure of the accuracy of each hit. We have used the transportation algorithm [3] as a basis for this.

2. Transportation-based performance measurement

The transportation problem is the problem of distributing goods from warehouses to markets at minimum cost. It can be solved using linear programming to output a total minimum cost [4]. Applied to images, we are treating the detection image as a map of warehouse locations, with pixel intensities representing the goods. The truth image (in which truth regions are assigned a positive value, and the background is zero) is our image of markets; the cost of moving a unit of intensity is the distance it must travel to satisfy the demand. Thus the total cost of efficiently distributing the pixel intensities from the detection image to the truth image gives us a measure of similarity [5]. Here we use the standard linear programming formulation of the transportation algorithm. To equalise supply and demand, the total brightness of the detection image pixels is normalised to equal that of the truth. Ideally, we want the cost to be zero for a perfect hit, and to increase for less useful prompts. The cost should also be independent of the size of the truth region; a prompt occupying 50% of a 1cm truth region should score similarly to a prompt occupying the same proportion of a 2cm truth region. Our final cost is thus normalised to the size of the truth region.

Where there are no truth regions, all detector responses are false positive and we must adopt a different approach. One method we have investigated involves calculating a cost by inverting both truth and detection images. This is computationally intensive, but a region-based approach using both ROC analysis and costing overcomes this problem. An alternative is to cost each miss as a false positive some distance from the truth.

In the case where an image contains both an accurately detected truth region and a distant false positive, the overall cost may be high despite the accurate detection. In some respects this is intuitive, since the more distant the false positive, the more the attention will be drawn from the real target. However, in the case where there is both an accurate detection and a distant truth which has been missed, the high cost associated with the miss could mask the fact that a target has been detected. For this reason, we have implemented a solution in which the costs are only calculated in the vicinity of truth regions, and sensitivity and specificity are also measured by counting regions.

3. Evaluation

To test the basic transportation method of assessing the performance of detection algorithms, we have used as an exemplar is the detection of microcalcifications in mammograms. These appear in the images as small bright blobs superimposed on the underlying glandular pattern. A simple morphological detection algorithm was developed. Firstly, the image is opened, this image is then subtracted from the original image to leave only objects the size of microcalcifications or smaller. A further opening is performed to remove very small scale objects and noise before thresholding to obtain a binary prompt image. The objective of our evaluation was to determine the most appropriate size of structuring element for this algorithm, firstly by looking for a suitable operating point based on ROC analysis, and secondly, by finding the value which results in the lowest transportation cost.

Regions of interest 300 pixels square and 50 microns per pixel were taken from 6 images containing malignant microcalcifications in the DDSM database [6]. Truth images were generated using the DDSM annotations as a guide. An example of a region of interest and its associated truth and detection images is shown in Figure 2.

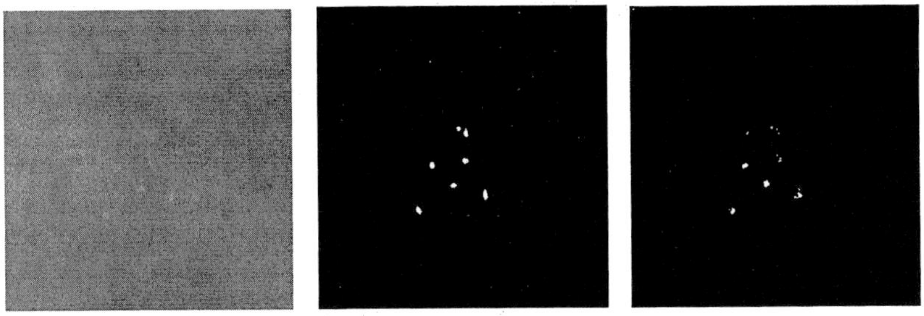

(a) (b) (c)

Fig. 2. Mammographic microcalcifications (a), with the associated truth image (b) and the output from the morphological detection method (c)

The detection algorithm was run at a range of structuring element sizes over all the images. A plot of the average transportation cost against structuring element size is shown in Figure 3; the cost curve reaches a minimum at a structuring element size of

5 pixels. The cost curve is at first high when the detection image is sparse and consists only of a few small dots, then reaches a minimum where the detection image most closely matches the detection image, before increasing as more false positives appear. A conventional ROC curve corresponding to the same experiment is also shown in Figure 3. Each pixel is classified as being either on or off target. The optimum cost threshold corresponds to the third data point from the left. The point closest to the top left of the ROC curve corresponds to the noisy detection image in Figure 3(d) – i.e. a structuring element size of 7 pixels.

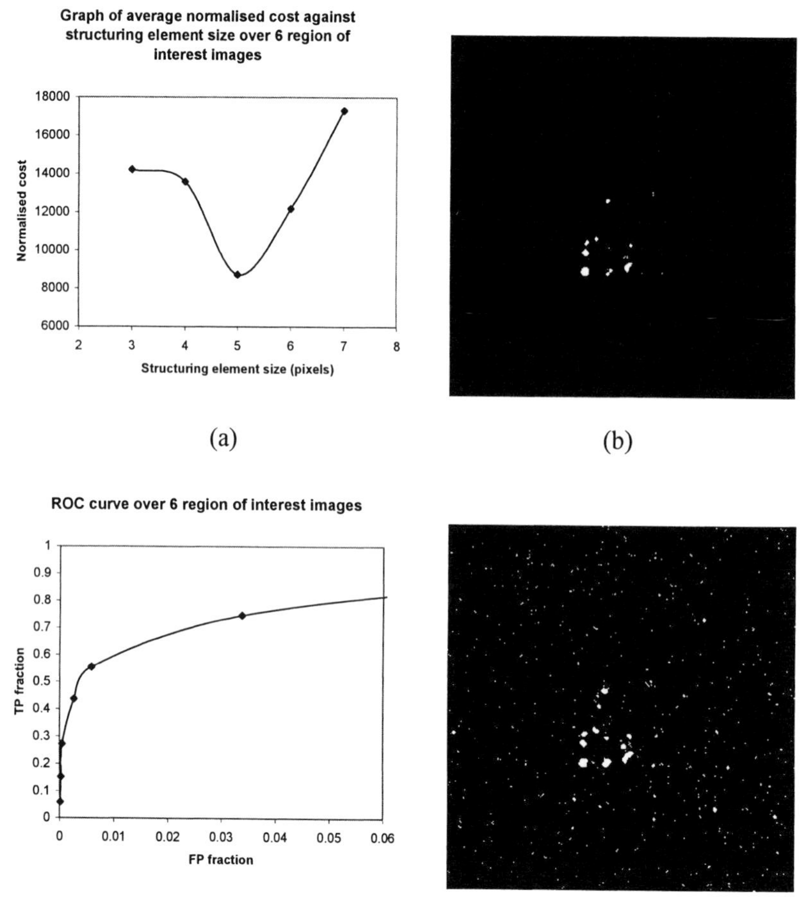

Fig. 3. (a) Cost curve (b) An example of a detection image at cost curve minimum (c) ROC curve (d) Detection image corresponding to the upper-left most point of ROC curve

4. Discussion

Over the regions of interest used in the above experiment, the basic costing method works well, reaching a minimum cost at what appears intuitively to be a good compromise between sensitivity and specificity. The low cost reflects the fact that all the detection information is concentrated in the area of the truth blobs. Every microcalcification is detected and there is little noise. The basic method deals equally well with multiple detections within the truth region and multiple edge detections outside it. It gives a fair cost for these cases instead of generating multiple false positives as FROC analysis may do. It deals less well with false positives and missed truths, and this could be problematic for larger, more complex images. It does not distinguish between a single distant false positive detection, and multiple closer ones.

The most appropriate evaluation method may be a hybrid of FROC and cost analysis, which records both quality of detection (cost) and a count of false positives and misses. We are now investigating the feasibility of calculating the cost only in the vicinity of truth regions, and displaying these local costs alongside FROC data to provide a measure of the quality of detection.

Acknowledgements

We are grateful for support from the EPSRC for Michael Board's PhD studentship.

References

1. Astley, S., Zwiggelaar, R., Parr, T.C. et al.: Prompting in mammography: how good must prompt generators be? In 4th International Workshop on Digital Mammography (1998)
2. Metz, C.E.: Evaluation of digital mammography by ROC analysis. In 3rd International Workshop on Digital Mammography (1996) 61-68
3. Hitchcock, F.L. The distribution of a product from several sources to numerous localities. Journal of Mathematical Physics 20 (1941) 224-230
4. Ravindram, A., Philips, D.T. & Solberg, J.J.: Operations research: principles and practice John Wiley & Sons, 2nd Edition (1987)
5. Miller, P. & Astley, S.: Automated detection of breast assymmetries. In British Machine Vision Conference (1993) 519-528
6. Heath, M., Bowyer, K.W., Kopans, D. et al.: Current status of the Digital Database for Screening Mammography. In Digital Mammography, Kluwer Academic Publishers (1998) 457-460

Invasive lobular carcinoma: Detection of cases occult at screening

Murk J. Bottema and John P. Slavotinek

School of Informatics and Engineering, IST Building Flinders University of South Australia, PO Box 2100, Adelaide SA 5001, Australia

murkb@infoeng.flinders.edu.au

Abstract. Invasive lobular carcinoma is missed at screening at least twice as often as other forms of breast cancer. We used simple structural texture features to search for signs of invasive lobular carcinoma in cases that were missed at screening and in which cancer could not be seen by radiologists with expertise in mammography in retrospect. The study comprised 24 positive images and 24 normal images. The algorithm detected cancer in 12 of the 24 positive images with zero false positive detections among the 24 normals. The locations within the breast of features used for classification were recorded and found to correspond to the locations of the tumors as indicated by histopathology reports.

1. Introduction

Invasive lobular carcinoma is a type of breast cancer that is more difficult to detect at screening than other invasive breast cancers. These cancers are infrequently associated with suspicious clusters of microcalcifications and often have opacity similar to normal breast parenchyma [1],[2]. As a result, invasive lobular carcinoma is at least twice as likely as other forms of breast cancer to be assigned as benign or normal at screening based on visual inspection of film mammograms [3]. For the same reason, this form of breast cancer is difficult to detect using computer algorithms in which initial detection relies on recognizing regions of high contrast.

Here we present an algorithm for detecting invasive lobular carcinoma in screening mammograms based on structural texture measures [4]. The use of texture in computer-aided detection is certainly not new [5],[6],[7], but in most cases, texture is used to generate features after initial detection which relies on recognizing anomalous regions of high contrast. Here classification is based solely on texture features and hence does involve identifying masses, clustered microcalcifications, or stellate patterns.

2. Methods and materials

2.1 Data

A total of 24 mammographic images were obtained representing 12 cases of invasive lobular carcinoma. In each of these cases, no evidence of cancer was found at screening, but invasive lobular carcinoma was detected and verified by histopathology within 2.5 years after screening (range: 4 to 28 months, median; 14 months). The sizes of the tumors were recorded at histopathology for all but three of the cases. The recorded sizes ranged from 15 mm to 100 mm with median diameter 35 mm. As part of normal policy, these missed cancers were reviewed and, in each case, the carcinoma could not be detected in the screening mammogram in retrospect by experienced mammographers. In addition, 24 normal images from 12 subjects were obtained for comparison. Normal images were included in the study only if no evidence of cancer was found within three years after the date of image acquisition.

All images were digitized using a Lumisys Lumiscan 150 laser digitizer at 20 pixels per mm spatial resolution and 12 bit depth.

2.2 Preprocessing

Images were cropped to remove patient information and restrict the image to the smallest rectangle containing the entire breast. The combined film and digitizing system was found not to be entirely linear in the range of interesting intensity values. Accordingly, the intensity response curve was measured using a step wedge and a standard correction curve was established for the system. Image intensity values were corrected according to this curve, stretched linearly to fill the range 0 to 4095.

A template of the breast region was determined automatically using subsampling, thresholding, region growing, upsampling and morphology.

2.3 Image features

Every local minimum of the image intensity surface was identified by comparing each pixel value to its eight immediate neighbors. Four parameters were recorded for each local image minimum: the background value, B, the height, H, the radius, R, and the symmetry, S.

The distributions of the features H, R, S, and B were examined in five normal images and five lobular carcinoma images selected randomly from the 48 images in the data set. Visual inspection of distributions suggested that anomalous high H values were slightly more common in carcinoma images than in normal images within certain regions of the H, R, S, B feature space. Based on this observation, the feature space was restricted to the set

$$F = F_1 + F_2 + F_3 \quad (1)$$

where

$$F_1 = \{(H,R,S,B) : R = 1, H > 19, S < 150, B > 2100\} \quad (2)$$

$$F_2 = \{(H,R,S,B) : R = 2, H > 38, S < 200, B > 2100\}$$

$$F_3 = \{(H,R,S,B) : R = 3, H > 76, S < 300, B > 2100\}$$

The features H, R, S, and B are local features in that they specify properties of individual local minima. They were used to generate the following six image features.

$$N_k = |F_k|/N, \qquad A_k = \text{mean}\{H(p) : p \text{ in } F_k\}, \quad k = 1,2,3, \quad (3)$$

Here, N represents the total number of local minima in the image.

Since the number of images in the study was small, attention was restricted to one and two-dimensional subspaces of the 6 dimensional image feature space. For each of these 21 feature spaces, the Az score (area under the ROC curve) and the number of true detections at the operating point of zero false positive detections were recorded.

3. Results

The best results were obtained for feature spaces that included feature N_1 (Fig. 1).

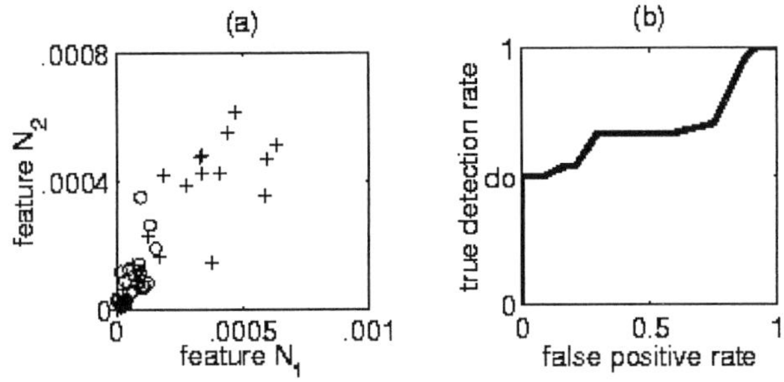

Fig. 1. (a) The scatter plot for features 1 and 2. ``+" indicates lobular carcinoma image and ``o" indicates normal image. (b) ROC curve for the features in (a). Although some combinations of features provided higher Az scores and some provided higher detection rates at zero false positive detections, a realistic summary of the performance is that approximately half of the cancers were detected at zero false detections.

As a check to see that the structural texture features used for classifying the images could plausibly be related to the presence of invasive lobular carcinoma, the locations in the breast image of these features were recorded and compared to the locations specified in the histopathology reports. In all cases where the algorithm detected the cancer, the location of the features matched the true location of the cancer (Fig. 2).

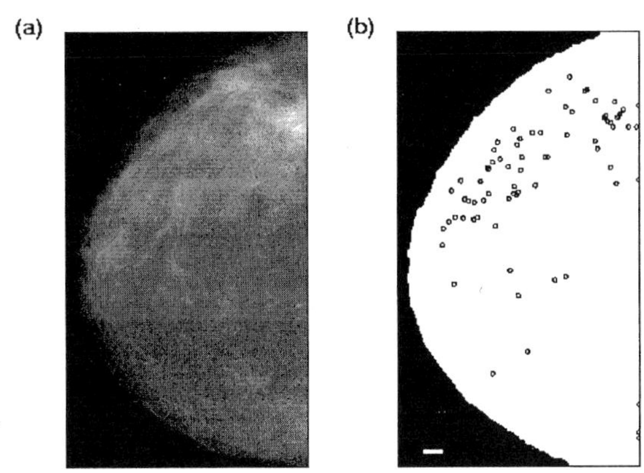

Fig. 2. (a) A representative invasive lobular carcinoma image from the data set. The bright region near the top of the image is consistent with normal tissue and at screening, this image was judged to demonstrate no evidence of cancer. Four months later, a 45 mm carcinoma was found. In retrospect, radiologists with expertise in mammography could not find evidence of cancer when the entire screening mammogram was reviewed. (b) The binary image showing the breast region of (a) with the locations of anomalous structural texture used to classify the image as cancerous. The region of the image with high concentration of anomalous structural textures is consistent with the location of the carcinoma recorded in the histopathology report. The scale bar indicates 1 cm.

4. Discussion

An algorithm for detecting an adverse medical condition is useful only if positive action can be taken in consequence of output from the algorithm. Since the presence of lobular carcinoma is difficult to ascertain otherwise, the decision for further intervention must be based solely on the report of the algorithm. This is in contrast to algorithms for finding evidence of breast cancer such as masses or clustered microcalcifications where the results of the algorithms are intended to alert the radiologist who then re-evaluates the mammogram. Accordingly, an algorithm for detecting invasive lobular carcinoma must find a significant number of true cancers at an extremely low false alarm rate. For this reason, the detection rate of 50 percent at zero false positive detections is more important in this study than the Az score.

The Az scores and the ROC curves (Fig. 1) indicate that minor changes in the process are not likely to increase the number of true detections at zero false positive detections significantly. While this may seem discouraging, the algorithm presented can also be viewed as a first, and perhaps simplistic, attempt to detect breast cancer based on structural texture features. The structures used, namely local intensity minima, and the features derived from these structures were the only ones tested and their selection was not based on a model for the appearance of cancer in mammograms. So unless these choices were extremely fortunate, it is likely that other structural texture measures can provide better discriminatory power.

References

1. D. J. Hilleren, I. T. Andersson, K. Lindholm, and F. S. Linnell. Invasive lobular carcinoma: Mammographic findings in 10 year experience. Radiology, 178:149-154, 1991.
2. K. N. Krecke and J. J. Gisvold. Invasive lobular carcinoma of the breast: Mammographic findings and extent of disease at diagnosis in 184 patients. American Journal of Roentgenology, 161:957-960, 1993.
3. M. Le Gal, L. Olliver, B. Asselain, M. Meunier, M. Laurent, P. Vielh, and S. Neuenschwander. Mammographic features of 455 invasive lobular carcinomas. Radiology, 185:705-708, 1992.
4. R. C. Dubes and A. K. Jain. Random field models in image analysis. Journal of Applied Statistics, 16(2):131-164, 1989.
5. G. M. te Brake, N. Karssemeijer and Jan H. C. L. Hendriks. An automated method to discriminate malignant masses from normal tissue in digital mammograms. Phys. Med. Biol. 45:2843-2857, 2000.
6. N. R. Mudigonda, R. M. Rangayyan, and J. E. Leo Desautels. Gradient and texture analysis for the classification of mammographic masses. IEEE Trans. Medical Image Analysis, 19(10):1032-1043, 2000.

7. B. Sahiner, H-P Chan, Computerized characterization of masses on mammograms: The rubber band straightening transform and texture analysis. Medical Physics, 25(4):516-526, 1998.

A test to evaluate the impact of the CAD tools in mammographic diagnosis

U. Bottigli[1], P. Delogu[2], M.E. Fantacci[2], F. Fauci[3], B. Golosio[1], P.L. Indovina[4], A. Lauria[4], R. Magro[3], R. Palmiero[4], G. Raso[3], S. Stumbo[1], S. Tangaro[1]

[1]INFN of Cagliari and University of Sassari, Italy
[2]INFN and University of Pisa, Italy
[3]Dipartimento di Fisica e Tecnologie Relative, University of Palermo, Italy
[4]University "Federico II" of Napoli, Italy

Abstract. In this work we present the results of a study about the impact of CAD tools on Sensitivity and Specificity in mammographic diagnosis. The approach is aimed to evaluate the statistical significance through the comparison of these figures of merit obtained in different situations.
For this purpose two different CAD tools, the CALMA station (INFN project) and the SecondLook^{TM} station (by CADx) have been used as a support for radiologists.

1. Introduction

Breast cancer is the main cause of death among women in the world [1]. Early diagnosis, as achieved through screening programs [2], seems to be the best "cure" to reduce mortality. Mammography is the best tool for early detection [3][4]. Two figures of merits, namely, Sensitivity and Specificity, are often used to evaluate the reliability of the results of this diagnostic tool. The Sensitivity is defined as the true positives fraction, and the Specificity as the true negatives fraction.

It is customary, for a good radiologist, to regard values of these parameters of the order of 80% as reliable. Personal diagnostic skill, as well as the quality of the images, and the experimental conditions, are important factors in making a reliable diagnosis. Although better results can be achieved through independent readings by different radiologists [5][6][7], this is unpractical for several reasons (e.g., a large number of records resulting from screening, cost and logistic reasons). Computer Aided Detection (CAD)[8][9], as a substitute computerised "second reader", may offer a viable solution.

2. Materials and Methods

The goal of a CAD system is to emphasise any Region Of Interest (ROI), where a pathology is likely.

The evaluation of the effect of CAD upon Sensitivity and Specificity is paramount. Therefore, standard criteria to compare these parameters in the cases “man÷man” and “man÷man+CAD” are needed. In order to obtain a statistical significance in a comparison, the errors by which the measured parameters are affected must be determined. With p the Sensitivity, the error σ_p (binomial) is:

$$\sigma_p = \sqrt{\frac{p\cdot(1-p)}{N_p}}$$

where N_p is the number of pathological images in the sample. Thus σ_p will decrease as N_p increases [10][11]. When comparing Sensitivities p and p' in the cases ”radiologist” and “radiologist + CAD” respectively, it is necessary to establish the confidence level [12]. With a Confidence Level of 95%, for $\Delta p = p' - p$ µ 5%, at least 250 pathological images are necessary. Fig.1 shows N_p vs. Δp for two values of p.

In any comparison between different modalities of a diagnostic test it is important that different values of Sensitivity be obtained at the same value of Specificity. It is therefore important to take into account also the Specificity (k) when comparing Sensitivities. As a consequence, the sample must contain a minimum number N_h of images of healthy patients [12], where

$$N_h \geq \frac{N_p\cdot(1-p)}{k}\left[\sqrt{\frac{N_p\cdot(1-p)}{p}}-1\right]$$

In the present work, 250 more images of healthy patients (with at least three years of follow up) have been added to the sample.

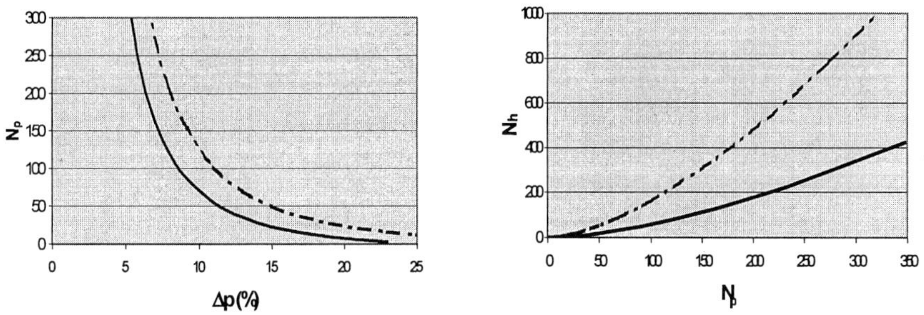

Fig. 1. a) Minimum number N_p of pathological images vs. Δp. b) Minimum number N_h of non-pathological images vs. N_p. In both figures, dashed lines correspond to p=75%, and solid lines to p= 85%.

Two different CAD systems were considered. The first is a commercial one, SecondLook™ (CADx, Medical Systems) produced in Canada, and the second is the CALMA system, developed in an Italian research program sponsored by INFN (Istituto Nazionale di Fisica Nucleare)[13][14][15].

Two radiologists (A, B) of different experience in mammography (5 and 3 years respectively) were considered. The same images were viewed a first time independently by the radiologists, and their isolated diagnoses recorded. After a month the images were viewed again, but this time with the clues provided by CADx. With the readings taken in the same conditions (e.g., isolated or with the assistance of CAD) the diagnosis of each radiologist were compared with the true diagnosis (Gold Standard), and counted as true positive, false positive, true negative, false negative.

A further test was to confront "CADx" and "CALMA" performances concerning Sensitivities to microcalcifications. In this case, a different sample has been used for each CAD. In particular, for CALMA, 865 images ($N_p = 370$, $N_h = 495$) have been used, while for CADx the sample was 500 images long ($N_p = N_h = 250$).

3. Results

The results obtained by the two radiologists, isolated and with the help of CAD, are summarised in Table I.

Radiologist	Sensitivity (%)	Specificity (%)
A	82	92
A+CAD	88	86
B	86	85
B+CAD	89	84

In both cases ("man" and "man+CAD") an increase of Sensitivity and a decrease of Specificity is observed. For radiologist A, however, a meaningful discrepancy results, while, for radiologist B the performance is almost unaffected by the use of CAD. A decrease of Specificity is expected, since CAD's tendency to false positives leads to a reduced Specificity. Our findings agree with others studies[16,17] showing that the CAD systems in mammography increase the Sensitivity and decrease the Specificity.

Fig. 2 shows the result of the comparison between CALMA and CADx.

As a conclusion, CAD systems may actually offer a valid help to the radiologist particularly in those programs involving massive mammographic screening.

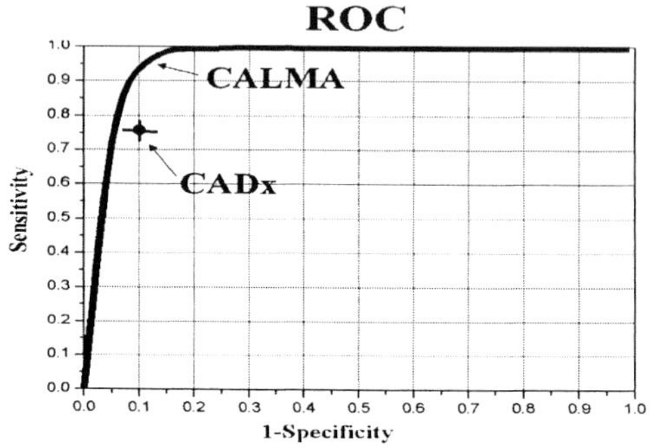

Fig. 2 The ROC Curve for CALMA. The CADx point is also reported.

References

1. R.A. Smith, "*Epidemiology of breast cancer*", "*A categorical course in physics. Imaging considerations and medical physics responsibilities*", Madison, Wisconsin, 1991, Medical Physics Publishing.
2. Blanks, *British Medical Journal* 321, 655-659, 2000.
3. S.A. Feig, M.Yaffe, "*Digital mammography, computer aided diagnosis and telemammography*", *Radiol. Clin. N. Am.* 33, 1205-1230, 1995.
4. R.A. Scmidt, R.M.Nishikawa, "*Clinical use of digital mammography: the presents and the prospects*", *Digit. Imaging* 8/1 suppl. 74-79, 1995.
5. S.A. Feig and M.Yaffe, Radiologic Clinics of North America, Vol.33 n.6, 1205, 1995.
6. R.E. Bird, "*Professional quality assurance for mammographic programs*", *Radiology* 177, 587-592, 1990.
7. E.L. Thurfjell, K.A. Lernevall, A.A.S. Taube, "*Benefit of independent double reading in a population based mammography screening program*" *Radiology* 191, 241-244, 1994.
8. C.J. Viborny "*Can computer help radiologists read mammograms?*" *Radiology* 191, 315-317, 1994.
9. C.J. Viborny, M.L. Giger, R.M. Nishikawa, "*Computer aided detection and diagnosis of breast cancer*", *Radiol. Clin. N. Am.* 38(4), 725-740, 2000.
10. Reid MC, MS Lachs, AR Feinstein. " Use of methodological standard in diagnostic test research. Getting better but still not good." JAMA 1995; 274:645-51.
11. Altman DG. "Pratical Statistics for Medical Reserch" Chapman & Hall, 1991.
12. F. Fauci and G.Raso, " *A statistical method to compare diagnostic tests*", in press.
13. R. Palmiero, *"The search for spiculated lesions in the CALMA project: status and perspectives"* in "Neural Nets WIRN, Vietri-99", Springer 1999.
14. S.R. Amendolia et al., *"The CALMA mammographs database: image collection and CAD tools for spiculated lesions detection and texture classification"* presented at TORONTO IWDM 2000 Conference.
15. M. Bazzocchi et al. "*Application of a computer-aided detection (CAD) system to digitalized mammograms for identifying microcalcifications*" *Radiol. Med.* 101**:** 334-340, 2001.
16. Burhenne L, Wood S, D'Orsi C e Coll., "*Potential contribution of computer-aided detection to the sensitivity of screening mammography*". Radiology 215: 554-562, 2000.
17. Freer TW, Ulissey MJ., "*Computer-aided detection (CAD) in screening mammography: a prospective study of 21860 patients in a community breast center*", LXXXV Annual Meeting Radiological Society of North America. Chicago IL (USA) pag. 400; 2 November - 1 December, 2000.

Detection of very subtle microcalcification clusters in high resolution full field X-ray mammograms

Michel Bruynooghe and Christiane Messainguiral

University Louis Pasteur of Strasbourg, Boulevard Sébastien Brant 67100 Illkirch, France
and C. Messainguiral, Yorckstrasse 49, 76185 Karlsruhe, Germany [1]
Michel.Bruynooghe@t-online.de

Abstract. Concerning the detection of microcalcification clusters, CAD methods or commercial systems generally announce sensitivity scores ranging between 92 and 98%. But the sensitivity is almost never dispatched according to the class of difficulty of analyzed images. A recent evaluation of two well known detection algorithms has shown that they only detect 25% to 50% of very subtle clusters from the USF/DDSM database. We have developed a CAD method proving a higher sensitivity level for the very subtle cases as found in the class 1 from the USF mammography database, without resulting in a large amount of false positives. We present the validation of our detection method using 43 very subtle images from the USF/DDSM database.

1. Introduction

Comparing objectively the performance of different algorithms for the detection of clustered microcalcifications requires the use of a common mammography image database. Yarlagadda et al. [11] have implemented and evaluated the two well known detection algorithms of Davies and Dance [4] and Karssemeyer [7] using the Digital Database for Screening Mammography (DDSM) distributed by the University of South Florida (USF) (Heath et al. [6]). The measured performances obtained by Yarlagadda et al. are below those reported by Davies and Karssemeyer. This is likely because the DDSM data set is harder than previous data sets. According to the Yarlagadda experiments, the best performance is achieved by the Karssemeyer algorithm at 69.5% True Positive (TP) with 2.11 False Positive (FP) per image. This result has been obtained using a testing subset of 50 cases of various rated subtlety, ranging from obvious to very subtle.

Lee et al. [8] have implemented and evaluated the four well known detection algorithms of Guillemet [5], Karssemeyer [7], Strickland [9], and Wallet [10], using thirty pairs of mediolateral oblique images from the USF/DDSM database, containing 34 microcalcification clusters. According to Lee et al., the poor FP rate of the four evaluated algorithms compared to their performance as reported by their authors is disappointing. It should be observed that the performance of the same algorithms on the Nijmegen database used by Karssemeyer is considerably superior [8]. Once more,

---

[1] On sabbatical leave from Commissariat à l'Energie Atomique, CEA-Cadarache, France

this is likely because the DDSM data set is harder than other data sets. The algorithms of Karssemeyer and Strickland respectively achieve a sensitivity level of 81% and 84% for cases with various cluster subtlety (from obvious to very subtle). However, these two algorithms only detect 25% and 50% of the most subtle clusters (subtlety rated as 1 in DDSM) [8].

In this paper, we present a comparison of a new CAD algorithm with the five well known detection algorithms that were evaluated by Yarlagadda et al. [11] and Lee et al. [8]. The evaluation of our CAD algorithm has been performed using images of the highest subtlety from DDSM.

2. Methods and materials

Algorithms : A novel CAD method has been developed to detect clustered microcalcifications, using non-linear image enhancement, image segmentation by multidimensional clustering [1], and statistical clustering rules. The first step of our approach is to enhance the mammography image by unsharp masking using a multi-resolution approach. The second step is to characterize the texture of 3 mm x 3 mm zones by granulometric spectra and to select regions of interest (ROI) which could contain individual microcalcifications [3]. The third step is to confirm the presence or the absence of significant individual microcalcifications in each region of interest, using a detection algorithm [2] that segments the enhanced mammography image by multidimensional clustering of local gray level histograms. Clustering rules are then used to determine if a cluster of microcalcifications exists.

Data : The data set used in our experiments is from the Digital Database for Screening Mammography (DDSM) (Heath et al. [6]). Twenty two very subtle cases representing 43 images were selected and analyzed, each digitized on a Howtek MultiRAD scanner and having one confirmed malignant microcalcification cluster. The training set and the test set are each composed of 11 cases, representing respectively 22 and 21 images. The spatial resolution of the DDSM images is 43.5 microns, with 12 bits per pixel. The ground truth information about each cluster location is given in DDSM. The counting of true cluster detections and false cluster detections is made fully automatic and objective according to the following matching criteria: a region of interest is considered as a true positive if and only if it contains at least 3 significant individual microcalcifications belonging to the annotated region defined in the publicly available ground truth file.

3. Results

In this work, clustering rules are inferred from the training image data and then used to detect microcalcification clusters in test images. We have first performed a comparison of our CAD algorithm with the four well known algorithms of Guillemet [5], Karssemeyer [7], Strickland [9], and Wallet [10], which have been implemented and evaluated by Lee et al. [8] using DDSM images.

Sensitivity scores reported in Table 1 are related to images. For our evaluations, an image is considered as true positive, if it contains at least one true positive cluster candidate.

A second comparison of our CAD algorithm has been performed with the two well known algorithms of David and Dance [4] and Karssemeyer [7], which have been implemented and evaluated by Yarlagadda et al. [11] using DDSM images. The FROC curve for our results obtained on the 11 very subtle DDSM test cases (21 images) is given in figure 1. In this figure, the scores are related to cases and not to images. A case is considered as true positive, when the right view or the left view of the same breast side is a true positive image.

Table 1. Sensitivity from Lee et al. [8] together with our results. The percentages are sensitivity scores on a subset of the USF database. Subtlety rating cover very difficult images (subtlety 1) to obvious ones (subtlety 5) for Lee et al. evaluations. Our results only concern very subtle test cases, representing 21 images.

Sensitivity by class of difficulty					
Subtlety rating	1	2	3	4	5
Number of images (analysis of ref. [4])	4	5	6	6	13
CAD Algorithms (evaluated in ref. [4])					
Wallet	25%	75%	29%	67%	85%
Guillemet	25%	0%	57%	33%	85%
Strickland	50%	50%	71%	67%	92%
Karssemeijer	25%	75%	86%	50%	92%
Number of images (present analysis)	21				
Algorithm Bruynooghe/Messainguiral	76%				

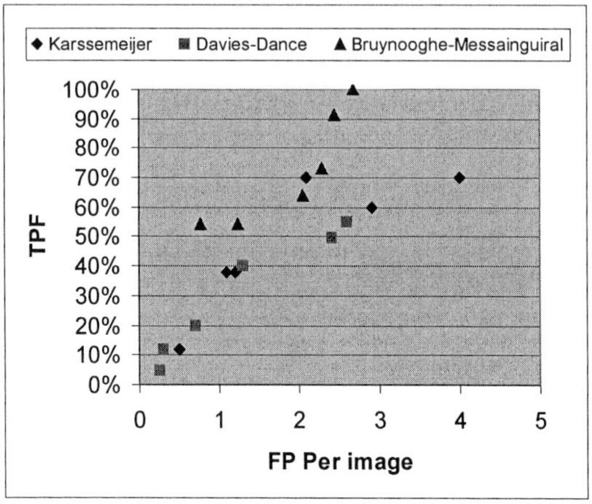

Fig.1 shows the FROC curve of our CAD method compared to two other well known algorithms, that were tested on the 100 cases of the "Training" and "Testing" subset of the USF Database (roughly 200 malignant images, ref.[11]). As indicated above our results however concern 11 test cases of the maximal subtlety level and hence are related to more difficult cases.

Fig. 1. FROC curves from [11] together with our results

3. Discussion and conclusion

Comparing the performance of different CAD algorithms is generally problematic. According to Yarlagadda [11], this is because researchers almost always use their own image database for evaluation. The consequence is that it is difficult to demonstrate that a new CAD algorithm makes a practical advance in the state-of-art. In this work, to allow such a comparison, we have used the publicly available USF/DDSM image database. It is the objective of sceening campaigns to provide an early detection of breast cancer. In this frame CAD systems should be able to cope with very subtle cases, allowing breast cancer detection at a very early stage. Our CAD method has been able to improve cluster detection sensitivity for very subtle cases selected from the testing subset of the USF public database.

References

1. Bruynooghe, M: "Maximal Theoretical Complexity of Fast Hierarchical Clustering Algorithms Based on the Reducibility Property". International Journal of Pattern Recognition and Artificial Intelligence, 7(3), pp. 541-571, 1993.
2. Bruynooghe, M: "Detection of Fine and Subtle Microcalcifications in Very High Resolution Mammography Images". First International Workshop on Computer-Aided Diagnosis, Chicago, Illinois, USA, September 20-23, 1998.
3. Bruynooghe, M: "High Resolution Granulometric Analysis for Early Detection of Small Microcalcification Clusters in X-ray Mammograms". 5th International Workshop on Digital Mammography, pp. 154-160, Toronto, Canada, June 11-14 2000.
4. Davies, D. H., and D. H. Dance. "Automatic computer detection of clustered calcifications in digital mammograms". Phys. Med. Biol. 35(8): pp. 1111-1118, 1990.
5. Guillemet,H., H. Benali, E. Kahn, and R. Di Paola. "Detection and Characterization of Microcalcifications in Digital Mammography " Digital Mammography. 3th International Workshop on Digital Mammography, pp. 225-230, Chicago, Illinois, June 1996.
6. Heath M., K. Bowyer, D. Kopans, R. Moore, P. Kegelmeyer : "The Digital Database for Screening Mammography". 5th International Workshop on Digital Mammography, pp. 212-218, Toronto, Canada, June 11-14 2000.
7. Karssemeyer, N. (1993). "Adaptive noise equalization and recognition of microcalcification clusters in mammograms". Int. J. Pattern Recog. Artif. Intel. 7(6): pp. 1403-1416.
8. Lee, R., E. Alberdi, P. Taylor : "A Comparative Study of Four Techniques for Calcification Detection". 5th International Workshop on Digital Mammography, pp. 264-271, Toronto, Canada, June 11-14 2000.
9. Strickland, R.N. (1996). "Wavelet transforms for detecting microcalcifications in mammograms". IEEE Trans. Med. Imag. 15: pp. 218-229.
10. Wallet, B. C., J.L. Solka, and C.E. Priebe (1997). "A method for detecting microcalcifications in digital mammograms". J. Digital Imaging. 10: pp. 136-139.
11. Yarlagadda, N., K. Bowyer, R. Li : "Baseline Comparison of Microcalcification Detection Algorithms". 5th International Workshop on Digital Mammography, pp. 414-420, Toronto, Canada, June 11-14 2000.

Impact of computer-placed prompts on sensitivity and specificity with different groups of mammographic film readers

Jo Champness[1], Paul Taylor[1] and Ros Given-Wilson[2]

Centre for Health Informatics and Multiprofessional Education, University College London[1]
Duchess of Kent Breast Screening Unit, 205 Blackshaw Road, London[2]
j.champness@chime.ucl.ac.uk

Abstract. The UK NHS Breast Screening Programme is facing a manpower crisis. The existing demand for radiologists is not being met and alternative film readers are being considered. The main professional group under consideration is film-reading radiographers.

A number of studies have examined the impact of CAD systems on cancer detection rates by radiologists but none have assessed the effect on radiographers. Manufacturers of CAD systems have generally resisted the idea that their systems could enable non-radiologists to act as film readers. One concern is that the negative impact of false positive prompts would be greater on less qualified staff.

Our study examined the effect of computer-placed prompts on recall rates in 15 radiographers and 30 radiologists. Readers viewed 3 test rollers both with and without computer placed prompts. There was no difference in sensitivity, specificity or time taken to read films with CAD prompts or between different groups of reader.

1. Introduction

The UK NHS Breast Screening Programme was set up by the Department of Health in 1987 following the recommendations of the Forrest Report[1]. 1.69 million women, aged between 50 and 64 are invited each year and 1.3 million attend for screening[2]. There are over 90 breast screening units across the UK, each serving an average population of around 45,000 women. The NHS Cancer Plan, published by the Department of Health in September 2000, set out a number of mandatory changes to existing system. The programme is being extended so that by 2004, women up to and including the age of 70 will receive routine invitations for screening. By 2003 all women will have two views of the breast taken at each attendance instead of just at the first screen as is presently required[3]. It has been suggested that the changes to the programme will lead to a 40% increase in workload[2]

A recent survey by Field found that 61% of units are staffed by no more than one or two consultants [4]. Field found a 50% failure rate in the recruitment of consultants to screening posts, with no applications at all received for four posts advertised in the BMJ. Only a small number of specialist registrars were reported to have indicated an interest in breast imaging. It is, therefore, clearly essential that alternative working practices be introduced. A new skill mix arrangement is being developed and tested at four NHSBSP sites. A 4-tier model is being evaluated in which radiographers can opt to train as film readers. All radiographers complete a 3-year degree course and film reading radiographers go on to complete a further year's film reading course.

Computer-Aided Detection (CAD) systems have also been put forward as an answer to the current manpower crisis. Some studies have suggested that the combination of computer plus human reader can produce better results than a human reader alone and have concluded that CAD systems can be used to prompt human readers[5,6,7]. Most studies of CAD in mammography have focused on the sensitivity of the algorithms. For example, Sittek et al. report a prospective study of 300 patients[8].The system correctly marked 82% of 39 cancers. The authors note the high proportion of false positive prompts (94%) and remarked that readers must have experience to use this system. A few studies have looked at the impact of CADon radiologists' decision-making. Most of these studies have involved only small numbers of radiologists. On a prospective study of 12,860 patients in a US community breast center, Freer & Ulissey found a 19.5% increase in cancers detected. However, only 2 readers took part in the study[9].We have found only one study assessing the impact of CAD on different categories of film-reader. Thurfjell et al. compared the performances of an expert screener, a screening radiologist and a clinical radiologist with and without the system[10]. The expert's sensitivity of 86% was unchanged, the others improved from 80 to 84% and 67 to 75%. The specificities of the expert and of the clinical radiologist were unchanged, while that of the screening radiologist fell from 83 to 80%.

The authors are currently completing an NHS funded project to fully evaluate the impact of computer-placed prompts on sensitivity and specificity with different groups of mammographic film readers in a screening setting. Results from this trial will be available at the end of the year. This paper is concerned specifically with the impact of CAD on film-reading radiographers working within the NHSBSP.

It may therefore be that CAD systems may have a greater impact on less experienced readers. As a professional group, radiographers are new to film reading and it may be that CAD systems are of greatest benefit to radiographers in reading screening mammograms. Our study plans to evaluate the hypothesis that CAD will increase radiographer's sensitivity without adversely affecting specificity.

2. Materials and Methods

2.1 The R2 Imagechecker

The CAD system used in this study was the R2 Imagechecker M1000. This is the only system currently being marketed in the UK.

2.2 Test Films

180 sets of mammograms were used in the study. These were taken from the screening programme, and in each case the outcome had been proven, either by biopsy or by a clear result at a subsequent round of screening. The mammograms were divided into three sets of 60 cases, each to be interpreted at a single sitting. The ratio of cancer to non-cancer cases was different in each set. An additional set of 60 cases was used as a training set to accustom film readers to using the CAD system.

there were 60 cancers in the three test sets:. 40 cancers detected through routine screening and 20 cases that presented in the interval between screening rounds. The interval cancers had been reviewed by a panel of radiologists and classified as false negatives. The control films were unselected cases with a subsequent normal screen. The films were randomly ordered within the rollers.

2.3 Film readers

Fifty film readers, all actively working in the NHSBSP, participated in the study. They included 30 consultant radiologists, 5 breast clinicians and 15 trained radiographers. All of the film-readers were asked to read each of three test rollers in both the prompted and unprompted conditions. The order in which each reader viewed the test sets was randomised, as was the order in which readers completed the two conditions, with and without CAD.

At each reading session the reader was asked to read the films displayed on a light box and to complete a report form for each case. The reader was required to pinpoint any area of abnormality, assess their degree of suspicion for each abnormality and finally give an overall decision on whether to recall the patient for further assessment or not. Readers were asked to make their decision on recall as if they were viewing the films as single readers in the screening programme. The time taken to read each set was also recorded.

The results obtained with the different film-readers were then put together to determine what the decision would have been for each image under the various possible permutations – single and double reader, with and without support – for various categories of film reader.

3. Results and Discussion

Reader's responses were analysed in terms of the overall decision for each case (recall *versus* not recall). The sensitivity and specificity of each reader on each roller under each condition was calculated. Sensitivity is defined as the number of correctly recalled cancer cases divided by the total number of cancer cases. Specificity is the number of correctly identified normal cases divided by the total number of normal cases.

Table 1 shows that there is no significant difference in readers sensitivity in the prompted and unprompted conditions. There is a difference in sensitivity between the rollers and this is probably due the different proportions of cancer cases within the sets and the reader's presumption of the likely number of cases in each set.

Table 1. Mean sensitivity of readers in prompted & unprompted conditions

Sensitivity	Unprompted	Prompted
Roller 1	0.80 (0.76, 0.83)	0.79 (0.76, 0.81)
Roller 2	0.83 (0.81, 0.84)	0.82 (0.80, 0.84)
Roller 3	0.71 (0.67, 0.74)	0.74 (0.70, 0.77)

Table 2 shows that there is no significant difference in readers' specificity in the prompted and unprompted conditions.

Table 2. Mean specificity of readers in prompted & unprompted conditions

Specificity	Unprompted	Prompted
Roller 1	0.83 (0.80, 0.86)	0.85 (0.82, 0.88)
Roller 2	0.82 (0.79, 0.85)	0.81 (0.77, 0.85)
Roller 3	0.85 (0.81, 0.88)	0.85 (0.81, 0.88)

We found no significant difference in recall rate between different professional groups of reader ($p = 0.2$). This in consistent with the findings of Cowley and Gale's study of the comparative performance of different professional groups 11]. Their results show that trained radiographers performed as well as radiologists. They also found that the performance of breast clinicians was similar or slightly better than that of radiologists . Pauli et al. found that radiologist/radiographer double reading gave similar sensitivities to double reading by radiologists[12].

We divided the readers into two groups based on their average sensitivity scores, to see if CAD had a greater effect on readers with lower sensitivities. Neither sensitivity nor specificity was altered in the prompted condition. We found no evidence that use of R2 affects good and poor readers' sensitivities or specificities differently.

Cowley and Gale reported that both breast clinicians and radiographers are slower than radiologists at reporting films. However, we found no significant difference in time taken to read films in either the prompted or the unprompted conditions ($p = 0.6$) or between the different professional groups.

4. Conclusions

We conclude from our study that computer-placed prompts have no impact on sensitivity and specificity with different groups of film reader working within the NHSBSP. Furthermore, there is no difference in time taken to read films between different professional groups of reader and again, this is not affected by the use of computer-placed prompts. Our hypothesis that CAD would be of greater use to radiographers is not supported.

We are considering a new test set of cases that are subtle but prompted by CAD. In these cases there is more scope for detecting improvements due to the computer prompts. It may be that this test set will also reveal some differences in performance between the professional groups.

References

1. Forrest A, P, M, Breast Cancer Screening: Report to the Health Ministers of England, Wales, Scotland and Northern Ireland. HMSO, London, 1986.
2. NHSBSP. http://www.cancerscreening.nhs.uk/breastscreen/research.html (accessed on 12/4/2002)
3. Department of Health. http://www.doh.gov.uk/cancer/cancerplan.htm (accessed on 12/4/2002)
4. Field S. UK Radiologist Workforce Survey - Breast Imaging Service. *Royal College of Radiologists Newsletter* 1998; 54: 12-4
5. Chan H, Doi K, Vyborny C et al. Improvements in radiologists' detection of clustered microcalcifications in mammograms. The potential of computer-aided diagnosis. *Invest Radiol* 1990 25: 1102.
6. Hutt I, Astley S and Boggis C Prompting as an aid to diagnosis in mammography. In Gale A, Astley S, Dance D and Cairns A(eds.) *Digital Mammography* Elsevier, 1994 pp: 389
7. Nishikawa R N, Wolverton D E, Schmidt R A et al. Radiologists' ability to discriminate computer–detected true and false positives from an automated scheme for the detection of clustered micro-calcifications on digital mammograms in Kundel H (ed). *Medical Imaging 1997: Image Perception*, Proceedings of SPIE 3036. 1997; pp. 198-204.
8. Sittek H, Perlet C, Helmberger R et al. Computer-assisted analysis of mammograms in routine clinical diagnosis. *Radiologe* 1998; 38:848-52
9. Freer TW & Ulissey MJ. Screening Mammography with computer-aided detection: prospective study of 12,860 patients in a community breast centre. *Radiol.* 2001; 220(3):781-6
10. Thurfjell E, Thurfjell G, Egge E, Bjurstam N. Sensitivity and specificity of computer-assisted breast cancer detection in mammography screening. *Acta Radiol.* 1998; 39: 384-388
11. Cowley H and Gale A, PERFORMS and Mammographic Film Reading Performance: Radiographers, Breast Physicians and Radiologists. Report for the Workforce Issues in the Breast Screening Programme Meeting. Inst of Behavioural Sciences, Univ of Derby, 1999.
12. Pauli R, Hammond S and Ansell J. Comparison of radiographer/radiologist double film reading with single reading in breast cancer screening. *J Med Screen* 1996; 3:18-22

Breast Density Estimation: Correlation of Mammographic Density and MR Volumetric Density

Heang-Ping Chan, Lubomir M. Hadjiiski, Marilyn A. Roubidoux, Mark A. Helvie, Sophie Paquerault, Berkman Sahiner, Jun Wei, Chuan Zhou, Thomas Chenevert, Mitchell M. Goodsitt

Department of Radiology, University of Michigan, Ann Arbor, MI 48109
Chanhp@umich.edu

Abstract. Studies have demonstrated a strong correlation between mammographic breast density and breast cancer risk. Mammographic breast density may therefore be used as a surrogate marker for monitoring the response to treatment in studies of breast cancer prevention or intervention methods. In this study, we evaluated the accuracy of using mammograms for estimating breast density by analyzing the correlation between the percent mammographic dense area and the percent glandular tissue volume as estimated from MR images. A data set of 37 patients who had corresponding MR images and mammograms was collected. The glandular tissue regions in the MR slices were segmented by a semi-automatic method and the percent glandular tissue volume calculated. Mammographic breast density was estimated by an automated image analysis program. It was found that the correlation between the percent dense area of the CC and MLO views and the percent volumetric fibroglandular tissue on MR images was 0.93 and 0.91, respectively, with a mean bias of 4.4%. The high correlation indicates the usefulness of mammographic density as a surrogate for breast density estimation.

1. Introduction

Previous studies have shown that there is a strong positive correlation between breast parenchymal density on mammograms and breast cancer risk [1-3]. The relative risk is estimated to be about 4 to 6 times higher for women whose mammograms have parenchymal densities over 60% of the breast area, as compared to women with less than 5% of parenchymal densities. The change in mammographic breast density is therefore often used as an indicator for monitoring the effects of preventive or interventional treatment of breast cancer.

Breast cancer risk is expected to depend on the volume of glandular tissue in the breast. Mammographic density is a projection of the volume of glandular tissue onto the two-dimensional image plane. To better understand the correlation between mammographic density and breast cancer risk, it is important to investigate the relationship between the projected areal density on mammograms and the volume of glandular tissue in the breast. In this study, we investigate this relationship by analyzing the percent volumetric glandular tissue in magnetic resonance (MR) images and the percent dense area in corresponding mammograms for the same breasts.

2. Materials and Methods

Our data set consisted of corresponding MR breast images and mammograms from 37 patients acquired between detection and biopsy. The MR image series used in this study, which included coronal 3D T_1-weighted pre-contrast images (coronal sections 2-5 mm thick, 32 slices; 3D Spoiled Gradient-Recalled Echo (SPGR); TE=3.3ms; TR=10ms, Flip=40°, matrix=256x128, FOV=28-32cm right/left, 14-16cm superior/inferior, scan time=2 min 38 sec) was part of a dynamic breast MRI study. This 3D SPGR sequence produced full volume coverage of both breasts with contiguous image slices. An example of images from one breast is shown in Fig. 1. Although this is not the optimal pulse sequence for separating water and fat, the fibroglandular parenchyma (~water) and fatty tissue are well separated with this heavily T_1-weighted acquisition and therefore the series was chosen for this study.

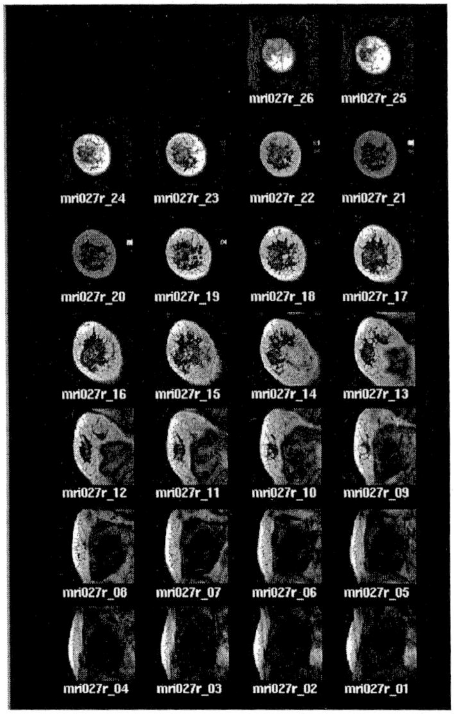

Fig. 1. MR images of the right breast of a patient. The two-view mammogram of the same breast is shown in Fig. 2.

We have developed a graphical user interface that displays the MR series and the corresponding mammogram of each breast. The interface allows the user to perform a combination of manual and automatic operations to segment the MR images. Each MR slice is first thresholded to separate the breast from the surrounding region. For slices close to the chest wall where no clear boundary can be seen, the boundary is manually drawn and evaluated by radiologists. Background correction [4] using the voxel values around the segmented breast region is employed to correct for the nonuniformity across the breast area due to the breast coil. The histogram of the voxel values in the breast region is then formed and interactive thresholding is used to segment the fibroglandular tissue from the fatty tissue. A morphological erosion operation along the breast boundary then excludes the skin voxels from the calculation of the fibroglandular tissue area in each slice. Finally, an integration of the fibroglandular voxels in all slices relative to the breast volume provides the percent volumetric fibroglandular tissue in the breast.

We have previously developed an automated image analysis tool (Mammographic Density ESTimator) to assist radiologists in estimating mammographic breast density [5]. MDEST performs dynamic range compression, breast boundary tracking, pectoral muscle segmentation for the MLO view, automatic thresholding based on gray level histogram analysis, and calculates the percent dense area on a mammogram. We found that the correlation between the computer-estimated percent dense area and radiologists' manual segmentation was 0.94 and 0.91, respectively, for CC and MLO views, with a mean bias of less than 2%. An example of a mammogram segmented by MDEST is shown in Fig. 2.

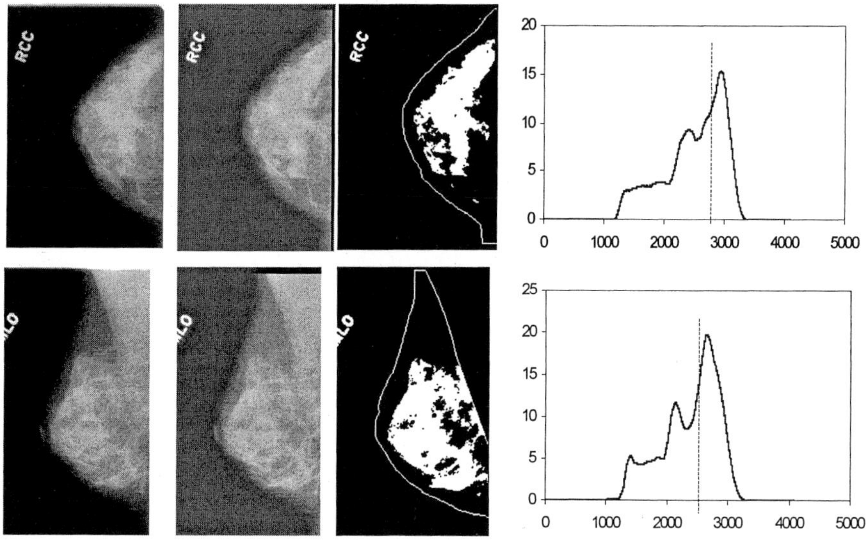

Fig. 2. Automated breast density segmentation from mammograms. Upper row: CC view. Lower row: MLO view.

3. Results

Scatter plots of the percent volumetric fibroglandular tissue versus the percent dense area on mammograms are shown in Fig. 3(a) and 3(b) for the CC- and MLO-view mammograms, respectively. The correlation of percent dense area of the CC and MLO views with the percent volumetric fibroglandular tissue on MR images was found to be 0.93 and 0.91, respectively, with a mean bias of 4.4%.

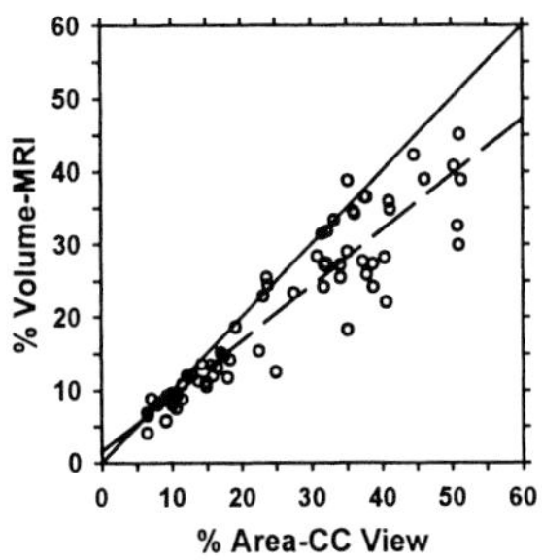

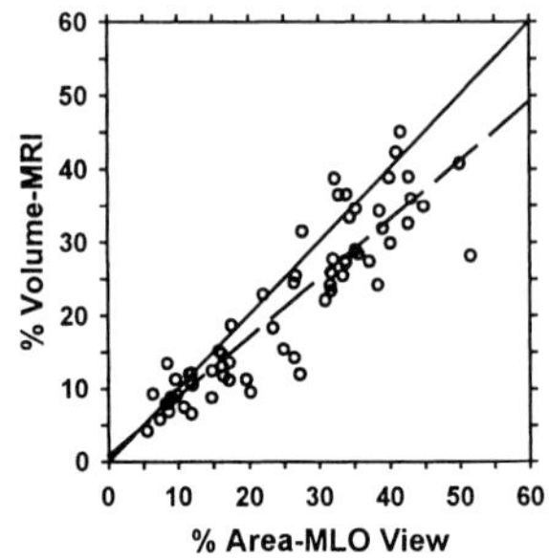

Fig. 3. Correlation of % volumetric fibroglandular tissue on MR images with % dense area on mammograms for 37 patients. The left and right breasts are plotted as separate data points on each graph. The dash lines are linear least squares fits to the data points.

4. Conclusion

Mammographic density is highly correlated with the volumetric fibroglandular tissue in the breast, indicating its usefulness as a surrogate for breast density estimation. The computerized image analysis tool, MDEST, is useful for estimation of mammographic density. The automated analysis is expected to contribute to the understanding of the relationship of mammographic density to breast cancer risk, detection, and prognosis, and to the prevention and treatment of breast cancer.

Acknowledgements

This work is supported by U. S. Army Medical Research and Materiel Command grants DAMD 17-01-1-0326 and DAMD 17-99-1-9294. The content of this paper does not necessarily reflect the position of the government and no official endorsement of any equipment and product of any companies mentioned should be inferred.

References

1. J. Brisson, R. Verreault, A. S. Morrison, D. Tennina and F. Meyer, "Diet, mammographic features of breast tissue, and breast cancer risk," Am. J. Epidemiology 130, 14-24 (1989).
2. A. F. Saftlas, R. N. Hoover, L. A. Brinton, M. Szklo, D. R. Olson, M. Salane and J. N. Wolfe, "Mammographic densities and risk of breast cancer," Cancer 67, 2833-2838 (1991).
3. N. F. Boyd, G. A. Lockwood, J. W. Byng, D. L. Tritchler and M. J. Yaffe, "Mammographic densities and breast cancer risk," Cancer Epidemiology Biomarkers & Prevention 7, 1133-1144 (1998).
4. B. Sahiner, H. P. Chan, N. Petrick, D. Wei, M. A. Helvie, D. D. Adler and M. M. Goodsitt, "Classification of mass and normal breast tissue: A convolution neural network classifier with spatial domain and texture images," IEEE Trans Med Imag 15, 598-610 (1996).
5. C. Zhou, H. P. Chan, N. Petrick, M. A. Helvie, M. M. Goodsitt, B. Sahiner and L. M. Hadjiiski, "Computerized image analysis: Estimation of breast density on mammograms," Med Phys 28, 1056-1069 (2001).

Statistical Characterization of Normal Curvilinear Structures in Mammograms

Carolyn Evans, Keith Yates and Michael Brady

Medical Vision Laboratory, Department of Engineering Science, University of Oxford, OX1 3PJ, UK. - {cje,jmb}@robots.ox.ac.uk
Department of Computing and Mathematics, Manchester Metropolitan University, Chester Street Manchester M1 5GD - K.Yates@mmu.ac.uk

Abstract. Curvilinear structures (CLS) in mammograms physically correspond to milk ducts, blood vessels, Cooper's ligaments and spicules in the breast. All of these structures, bar spicules, are features of normal breast tissue. Spiculres are highly indicative of breast cancer when found near the boundary of a mammographic density.
In this paper we develop a statistical characterization of normal CLS, to be used to identify any normal CLS near the boundary of a mammographic density and avoid mis-diagnosis. Six shape features, were calculated from each CLS description to form a data set. Principal component analysis of the six-dimennsional data set revealed that the majority of information was concentrated in the first two dimensions - the first two principal components. The distribution of normal CLS shape data in these first two dimensions was modeled using a Gaussian Mixture Model (GMM)

1 Introduction

The aim of our work is to obtain a model of the multivariate distribution of shape of CLS found in normal breast tissue so it can be used to diagnose how 'normal' a linear structure appears. We aim to model the shape distribution of normal CLS, rather than the spicules, because we can guarantee that a CLS which does not intersect a known abnormal region is (by definition) normal. We can make no such claim for CLS that intersect abnormal regions; they may be normal, but they may be spicules. We know the positions of all abnormal regions in the mammograms used in this study because they are provided as part of the University of South Florida's database [1].

2 Method

In order to characterize statistically normal CLS, we must perform the following series of tasks in order to gather the CLS shape information.

2.1 Detecting CLS in Mammograms

We have previously reported a method of automatically detecting CLS in digitized mammograms [2]. The method is based on Kovesi's measure of phase congruency [3] and aims to detect locally bright, ridge structures over a specific range of scales. The result of the automatic detection method is a binary image showing all pixels considered to belong to a CLS.

Fig. 1. (a) Original mammogram. (b) Binary image of detected CLS using the method described in [Yates *et al* 2002].

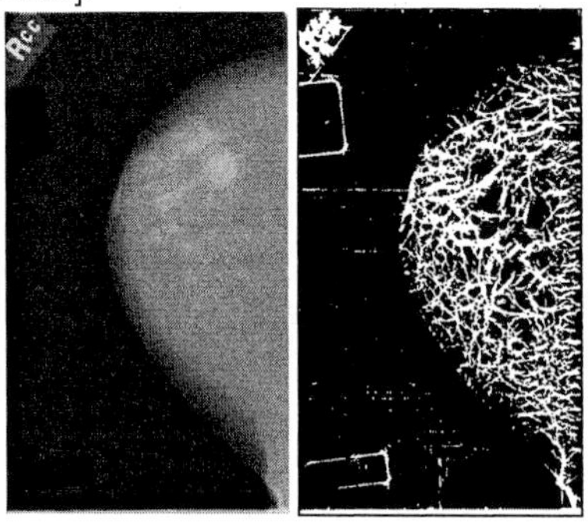

(a) (b)

2.2 Separating CLS into Non-intersecting Line Segments

Ultimately we want to obtain a description of each CLS, comprising the pixels belonging to its central spine, as well as the local width of the CLS measured at each of these pixels. For this reason, we separate the network of detect CLS into non-intersecting line segments in the following way, [4]:

1. Skeletonize the binary image of CLS.
2. Compute the Euclidean distance transform (DT) of the binary image of CLS and retain the DT values at skeleton pixels as measurements of local width.
3. Remove branch points from the skeleton.
4. Remove line segments that do not correspond to the central spine of a CLS or are only 1 pixel long.

The effects of each of these steps on a phantom image of intersecting CLS is illustrated in Fig. 2. The skeleton of the phantom image, figure 2b, was calculated using an approach discussed in [4, 5]. This algorithm was used because it produces a skeleton located along the center spine of binary objects whilst preserving the homotopy ('connectedness') of the original image. This means that no CLS will be split into two disjoint regions by the skeletonization algorithm.

Fig. 2. (a) The original image. (b) Skeleton of (a). (c) Euclidean distance transform of (a). (d) Branch points removed from (b). (e) Result of removing spurious line segments, including ones that are 1 pixel long, from (d). (f) Linked CLS strands. (Each strand has been assigned a unique grey-value.)

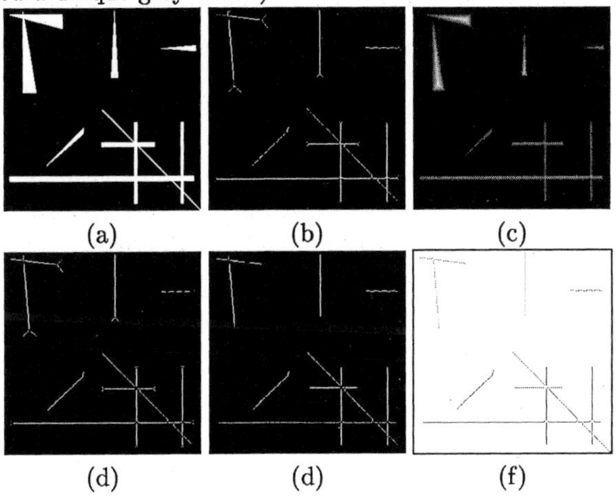

2.3 Reconnect Non-intersecting Line Segments into Individual CLS

Our method of linking non-intersecting line segments into individual CLS is based on the method first proposed in [6].

1. Calculate the local orientation of the line segment, $o_{i,j}$ at each end point $ep_{i,j}$.
2. For each end point, $ep_{i,j}$, construct a list of all end points, $ep_{p,q}$ $(i \neq p)$ within a distance $4w_{i,j}$ of point $e_{i,j}$ and have an absolute angular difference $(\pi - |o_{i,j} - o_{p,q}|) \leq \pi/4$. These are a list of end points that could possibly be linked to $ep_{i,j}$.
3. For each end point, $ep_{i,j}$, list of possible links in increasing order of the absolute angular difference $(\pi - |o_{i,j} - o_{p,q}|)$, and the distance separating the end points.
4. If there are two or more links sharing the same angular difference and distance separation, these links are placed in increasing order of the width difference $\min(|w_{i,j} - w_{p,q}|, |\bar{w_i} - \bar{w_p}|)$.
5. Two end points $ep_{i,j}$ and $ep_{p,q}$ are linked if and only the link is considered mutually optimal for $ep_{i,j}$ and $ep_{p,q}$.

3 Calculating CLS Shape Features

From the description of each CLS, which contains a list of all pixels along its center spine, as well as the local width measurement at each of those pixels, we calculate the following shape features:

1. The average width (W),
2. The Euclidean length (L),
3. The spatial linearity (S),
4. The absolute average rate of change of width along its length (calculated via linear regression) (T),
5. The absolute, average deviation of width variation from the average rate of change (TD),
6. The average curvature (C).

Before collating the CLS shape statistics from a given mammogram, we determined whether each CLS intersects a region known to contain an abnormality, eg. spiculated mass, or whether is was outside all abnormal regions. Only if the CLS was outside the abnormal region, was it considered to be a normal CLS. Its shape features were then used to form the multivariate shape distribution.

Table 1. Table of the eigenvalues of the CLS data correlation matrix, and their percentage of the total data variance.

Eigenvalue	Value	$\lambda_i / \sum_{j=1}^{6} \lambda_j \times 100\%$	$\sum_1^i \lambda_i / \sum_{j=1}^{6} \lambda_j \times 100\%$
λ_1	0.5840	54.72%	54.72%
λ_2	0.3509	32.88%	87.60%
λ_3	0.0673	6.31%	93.91%
λ_4	0.0418	3.92%	97.83%
λ_5	0.0232	2.17%	100.0%
λ_6	0.0000	0.00%	100.0%

4 Results on Mammographic Images

We automatically detected CLS in mammograms taken from the 'Cancer_01' directory of the University of South Florida's database [1], and analyzed these CLS as described in Sections 2 and 3. These mammograms were first reduced in resolution to $200\mu m$ per pixel.

Each mammogram was found to have of the order of 2000 normal CLS (CLS located outside any abnormal regions). We gathered normal CLS from 23 digitized mammograms to work with a dataset of 56873 CLS structures. From this data, we calculated the mean and standard deviation of each of the shape features mentioned in Section 3. The results are given in Table 2.

Knowing the mean and standard deviation of each of the shape features for normal CLS, we now standardized each to have a mean of zero and standard deviation of unity using the following:

$$F_s = \frac{F - \bar{F}}{\sigma_F}. \tag{1}$$

The variables L_s, S_s, etc, in this paper now refer to the standardized version of the shape features defined in Section 3.

From PCA we found the eigenvalues and eigenvectors of the normalized multivariate dataset. Table 3 specifies the eigenvectors in order of their associated eigenvalues, given in Table 1.

Table 2. Average values of shape features for normal CLS.

Shape Property	Mean	Standard Deviation
Length (L) (1 pixel = $200\mu m$)	20.77 pixels	33.39 pixels
Average Width (W) (1 pixel = $200\mu m$)	2.592 pixels	0.7612 pixels
Spatial Linearity (S)	0.1629	0.1516
Taper (T)	0.0533	0.0831
Taper Deviation (TD)	0.0571	0.0571
Average Curvature (C)	-0.7586	0.2544

Table 3. Table of eigenvectors of the standardised shape features of normal CLS.

Eigenvector	Components
$\boldsymbol{e_1}$	$-0.0032L_s + 0.3258W_s - 0.4941S_s + 0.4186T_s + 0.3998TD_s - 0.5609C_s$
$\boldsymbol{e_2}$	$0.6426L_s + 0.3925W_s - 0.2474S_s - 0.5045T_s - 0.3065TD_s - 0.1528C_s$
$\boldsymbol{e_3}$	$-0.5705L_s + 0.7716W_s + 0.0686S_s - 0.1286T_s - 0.1466TD_s + 0.1906C_s$
$\boldsymbol{e_4}$	$0.0949L_s + 0.1351W_s + 0.5220S_s - 0.4063T_s + 0.7091TD_s - 0.1797C_s$
$\boldsymbol{e_5}$	$-0.0060L_s + 0.0515W_s + 0.5726S_s + 0.2254T_s - 0.4627TD_s - 0.6361C_s$
$\boldsymbol{e_6}$	$-0.5025L_s - 0.3513W_s - 0.2993S_s - 0.5812T_s - 0.0886TD_s - 0.4346C_s$

Table 4. Mean vectors associated with the three Gaussians forming the two-dimensional GMM of the CLS shape data.

Mean Vector	(e_1, e_2) Components
$\boldsymbol{\mu_1}$	(-0.7064, 0.0906)
$\boldsymbol{\mu_2}$	(0.7736, -0.2892)
$\boldsymbol{\mu_3}$	(-0.5454, 0.4486)

The second column of Table 1 specifies the percentage each eigenvalue contributes to the total sum of the eigenvalues, ie. the total variance. This percentage indicates the fraction of data variation explained by the associated eigenvector.

Table 5. Covariance matrices associated with the three Gaussians forming the two-dimensional GMM of the CLS shape data.

Σ_1	$\begin{bmatrix} 1.4978 & 0.5205 \\ 0.5205 & 0.1863 \end{bmatrix}$
Σ_2	$\begin{bmatrix} 0.7504 & -0.5659 \\ -0.5659 & 1.2617 \end{bmatrix}$
Σ_3	$\begin{bmatrix} 1.7356 & 1.1483 \\ 1.1483 & 2.7270 \end{bmatrix}$

For example, over half (54.72%) of the variation in our dataset is accounted for by the first eigenvector specified in Table 3. Another 32.88% of the variation in our dataset is accounted for by the second eigenvector (Table 3). The last column of Table 1 shows that 87.6% of the data variation can be accounted for using only the first two PCs. We choose to simplify our 6-dimensional shape feature space to two dimensions, and are able to do so without loosing much information by ensuring the two dimensions correspond to those represented by the first two PCs.

To model the multivariate distribution of normal CLS shape data, we fitted a Gaussian Mixture Model (GMM). The best fitting GMM in two dimensions for the normal CLS shape data was,

$$\begin{aligned} GMM_{2D} &= 0.3203G_1(\boldsymbol{\mu_1}, \Sigma_1) \\ &+ 0.4526G_2(\boldsymbol{\mu_2}, \Sigma_2) \\ &+ 0.2271G_3(\boldsymbol{\mu_3}, \Sigma_3), \end{aligned} \tag{2}$$

where G_1, G_2 and G_3 are bivariate Gaussians, with means $\boldsymbol{\mu_1}, \boldsymbol{\mu_2}, \boldsymbol{\mu_3}$ respectively, and covariance matrices, $\Sigma_1, \Sigma_2, \Sigma_3$, as specified in Tables 4 and 5.

The function in Eq. 2 yielded a negative log-likelihood error value of 1.5664×10^5 when fitted to the first two PCs of the normal CLS shape data.

5 Conclusion

The purpose of this paper was to statistically characterize the shape of curvilinear structures (CLS) found in normal breast tissue. To this end, we automatically detected CLS in a set of mammograms and obtained shape information about each individual CLS. For each CLS located in normal breast tissue, we calculated 6 shape features including average width, Euclidean length, taper, average curvature and straightness. The average values of each of these parameters for normal CLS are specified in Section 4.

We found, through principal component analysis, that the six-dimensional shape data could be condensed into two principal components with relatively little loss of information.

This work quantitatively characterizes the shape of normal CLS detected in real mammograms. Our future goal is to use this characterization to distinguish normal CLS located at the boundary of mammographic masses to improve the false positive rate in mass classification.

References

1. M. Heath and K.W. Bowyer and D. Kopan Current status of the Digital Database for Screening Mammography - Digital Mammography 457-46 (1998)
2. K. Yates and C.J. Evans and J.M. Brady Improving te Brake's mammographic mass detection algorithm using phase congruency Proceedings of Digital Image Computing: Techniques and Applications, DICTA 2002
3. P. Kovesi Image Features from Phase Congruency Journal of Computer Vision Research Vol 1 no 3
4. P. Soille Morphological Image Analysis Springer-Verlag 1999
5. L. Vincent Efficient Computation of Various Types of Skeletons Medical Imaging V: Image Processing p 297-311 1991 Vol SPIE-1445
6. N. J. Cerneaz Phd Thesis Model-based Analysis of Mammograms (1994) Department of Engineering Science, University of Oxford
7. T. Parr and S. Astley and C. Boggis The Detection of Stellate Lesions in Digital Mammography Digital Mammography. Proceedings of the 2nd International Workshop on Digital Mammography p 231-239 (1994)
8. L. da-Fontour-Costa and R. Marcondes-Cesar Shape Analysis and Classification. Theory and Practice CRC Press (2001)

Improved mammographic accuracy with CAD assisted classification of lesions

Fields S[1], M.D. Lederman R, M.D.[1] , Buchbinder S, M.D.[2] , , Novak B, Ph.D.[3] , Sklair-Levy M, M.D[1].Bamberger P, Ph.D.[4] Leichter I, Ph.D. [5],

1. Department of Radiology, Hadassah Hospital, Jerusalem, Israel
2. Department of Radiology, The Montefiore Medical Center, NY
3. Department of Mathematics, Jerusalem College of Technology
4. Department of Electronics, Jerusalem College of Technology, Israel
5. Department of Electro-Optics, Jerusalem College of Technology

scott@hadassah.org.il

Abstract. We evaluate a CAD device with detection and classification capabilities and compare conventional to computerized analysis. 243 cases (126 malignant, 117 benign) were analysed using BI-RADS and digitized (600 DPI, 12 bits). Lesions were detected, classified by likelihood of malignancy, and stratified into BI-RADS categories 2-5 by the CAD device. The falsely detected findings scored by CAD as low probability of malignancy were discarded to evaluate the true false positive rate. The CAD device sensitivity was 96% for masses and 95% for clusters of MCs. Malignancies were correctly classified by CAD in 95%. 67% of the false positive detected masses and 76% of the false positive clusters were classified benign by the CAD device, reducing the false positive rate per view from 0.59 to 0.20 for masses and from 0.30 to 0.07 for clusters. Conventional interpretation yielded a ROC Az of 0.76. CAD improved the Az to 0.88 ($p<0.001$).

Introduction

With increased prevalence of breast cancer and the use of mammography for early detection, there are efforts to improve accuracy. BI-RADS [1] creates a uniform system for interpretation of mammography and appropriate course of action. Mammography has a low specificity, which leads to further evaluation of suspicious findings[2]. One method to improve mammography is the use of CAD analysis [3].

Materials and Methods

243 retrospective cases of mammographically detected lesions, with proven pathologies (126 malignant, 117 benign) were examined. Consecutive cases with malignant pathology results were selected for the study if a mammogram identifying a lesion was performed within two months prior to the biopsy or with benign pathology

results if a mammogram identifying a lesion was performed within one year prior to the biopsy.

Following the retrospective conventional BI-RADS interpretation of the 243 cases, the films were digitized at 600 dpi by a prototype CAD system [4] and displayed for computerized analysis. The CAD system detection algorithms search for suspicious lesions and automatically demarcate the detected lesions with a solid ellipse (mass) or dotted ellipse (clusters of MCs). These lesions were then analyzed by a radiologist, using the classification algorithms of the CAD system. After the region encompassing the mammographic lesion was interactively defined on the digital images, by the radiologist, the CAD system automatically extracted quantitative features that characterized the lesion. In cases that the suspicious finding was not detected by the CAD system, the radiologist manually defined the region of the lesion and subsequently the lesion was classified by the CAD system.

For the analysis of mass lesions, the CAD device extracted 50 features that characterized the findings by their spiculation, shape and margins. All the extracted features, for each lesion, were provided to a Stepwise Discriminant Analysis (SDA) procedure, along with the pathology result and the power of each feature to discriminate benign from malignant lesions was analyzed. The SDA procedure selected only the features that contributed to the discrimination model most significantly, to be included in the classification scheme. The features which characterize the spiculation associated with the mass lesions [5] were selected by the SDA procedure with the highest weighting factors.

For the analysis of clusters of micro-calcifications, the radiologist defined on the digital images the region encompassing the cluster, and the CAD device automatically indicated an initial selection above a preset threshold as candidates, by highlighting in red. The radiologist was then allowed to alter target selection by modifying the threshold, so that only appropriate spots, which represent calcifications, would be included in the quantitative analysis. Once the radiologist was satisfied with the selection of targets, the algorithm proceeded with automated extraction of 49 features characterizing the cluster. The SDA procedure analyzed the features related to the shape and brightness of the individual MCs and to the cluster geometry [6]. that best discriminated malignant from benign clusters.

A pattern recognition scheme based on the Discriminant Analysis method was constructed in order to classify each lesion by a single score derived from a combination of the features extracted by the CAD system and selected by the SDA procedure. For constructing the classification scheme the device utilized a training procedure on a database of cases, for which the extracted features were provided along with the pathology result, for each lesion. Based on this training procedure, the classification scheme, embedded in the software, assigned an unknown lesion a single score, or a classifier; the higher the score, the higher the probability of the lesion to be malignant.

The Jack-knife analysis [7] was applied to a database of 541 proven pathology cases (309 malignant, 232 benign) in order to score the mammographic lesions by the classification scheme. Following the scoring of the lesions by their likelihood of malignancy, limit values for the score were calculated in order stratify the cases into groups. The first limit value assessed up to which score no malignant cases were found. The second included 10% of the malignant cases. The third limit assessed above which score, 90% of the malignant cases were found. Based on these three limit values, the CAD device automatically stratified the 243 cases, with the retrospective conventional interpretation, according to their score, into BI-RADS categories 2 -5.

The performances of the conventional interpretation and of the computerized interpretation were evaluated by receiver operating characteristic (ROC) analysis [8,9].

Results

96% of the malignant masses were detected by the CAD system. 95% of the malignant clusters of MCs cases were detected. The detected lesions were correctly classified by using the CAD system in 95% of the cases. The malignant mass lesions were both detected and correctly classified in 88% of the cases, while malignant clusters were both detected and correctly classified in 84%. The false(+) rate of detection per image was 0.59 for mass lesions and 0.30 for clusters of MCs. Of all false positive detected lesions, 67% of the false positive detected mass lesions and 76% of the false positive detected clusters were classified benign by using the CAD system. Thus, of the false positive findings, only 0.20 mass lesions per view and only 0.07 clusters per view remained suspicious after classification. Figure 1 shows the ROC curve describing the performance of the classification scheme used by the CAD device. This curve is based on the Jack-knife analysis of the score assigned to by the device to each of the 541 lesions with proven pathology. The Az value for this curve was 0.91 and the point corresponding to 95% sensitivity on this curve yielded a specificity value of 53% and PPV value of 73%.Figure 2 shows the ROC curves describing the performance that was obtained for the retrospective conventional BI-RADS interpretation of the 243 cases by the 3 radiologists and the computerized analysis of these cases. The Az value for the conventional analysis was 0.76. The ROC curve for the computerized analysis of these cases, based again on BI-RADS categories, but this time these categories were allocated automatically by the CAD device, according to the likelihood of malignancy scores that were assigned to the cases by the device, had an Az value of 0.88.

Table 1 displays the results of the conventional interpretation versus the pathology outcome. For the test performance analysis cases which were assigned BI-RADS categories 2 and 3 were considered as "test negative" (denoted by a minus symbol), while cases which were assigned categories 4 and 5 were considered as "test positive" (denoted by a plus symbol). Cases with malignant pathology results were considered "true positive", while cases with benign pathology results were considered "true negative". The conventional mammographic interpretation correctly identified 119 of the 126 malignant cases (94.4% sensitivity) and 40 of the 117 benign cases (34.2% specificity). The PPV value was 60.7%, and the overall accuracy 65.4%.

Table 2 shows that the computerized analysis of the CAD correctly identified 124 of the 126 malignant cases (98.4% sensitivity) and 80 of the 117 benign cases (68.4% specificity). The PPV value for the computerized analysis was 77%, and the overall accuracy 84%.

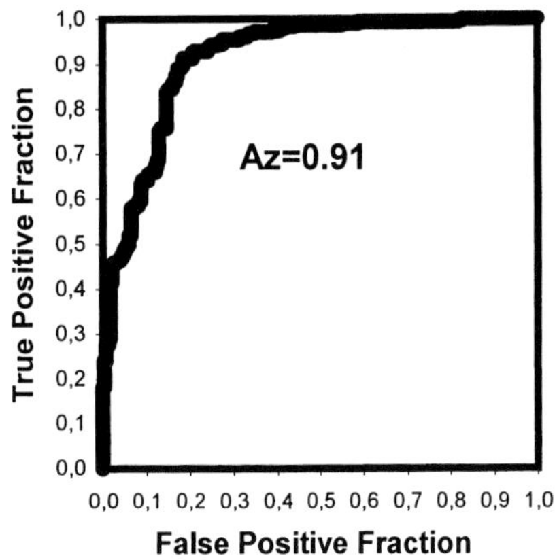

Figure 1: ROC curve describing the performance of the computerized score assigned by the CAD device.

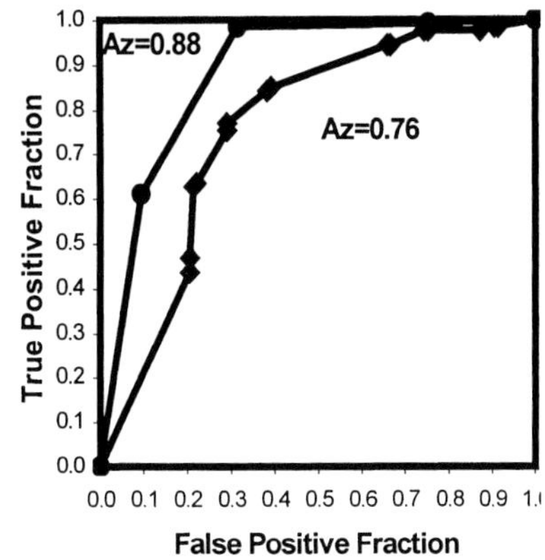

Figure 2: ROC curves results of the conventional (A_z=0.76) and the CAD device computerized interpretation (Az=0.88) by BI-RADS categories.

Table 1: Results of conventional interpretation (BI-RADS categories) vs. the pathology outcome.

		Conventional Interpretation +	-	
Path	+	119	7	126
	–	77	40	117
		196	47	243

Table 2: Computerized analysis versus the pathology outcome.

		Comp. Analysis Interpretation +	-	
Path	+	124	2	126
	–	37	80	117
		161	82	243

Discussion

The detection sensitivity of the CAD device was 96% for mass lesions and 95% for clusters of MCs. The false positive rate of detection per view was 0.59 for mass lesions and 0.30 for clusters of MCs. Sixty seven percent of the false positive detected mass lesions and 76% of the false positive detected clusters were classified benign by using the CAD device, reducing the false positive rate per view to 0.20 for mass lesions and to 0.07 for clusters.

The conventional interpretation of the mammographic lesions yielded a ROC curve with an Az of 0.76, indicating a specificity of 34.2% and a PPV of 61% for 95% sensitivity. The computerized classification of lesions significantly improved the Az to 0.88 ($p<0.001$). The specificity and the PPV values of the computerized analysis were significantly improved to 68.4% and 77%, respectively ($p<0.001$), for 98% sensitivity. The device described in this study was not intended to replace the radiologist, and indeed only 86% of the lesions were correctly detected and classified by the system alone. Moreover, the sensitivity obtained when all the lesions, detected both by the system and the radiologist were analysed reached a value of 98%. The results of this study demonstrate marked improvement in the performance of the CAD device when classification of the findings is applied in addition to automatic detection of the findings. Therefore, it will be critical for the next generation of CAD systems for mammography to include ranking of lesions to optimize the use of the system in clinical practice

References

1. Breast imaging reporting and data system American College of Radiology, Reston Virginia(1993).
2. Liberman L, Abramson AF, Squires FB, et al. The breast imaging reporting and data system: Positive predictive value of mammographic features and final assessment categories. Am. J. Roentgenol. 1998 171:35-40.
3. Huo Z, Giger M.L, Vybrony CJ, Wolverton DE, Schmidt RA, Doi K. Automated computerized classification of malignant and benign masses on digitized mammograms. Acad. Radiol. 1998; 5: 155-168.
4. Fields S, Leichter I, Bamberger P, et al. Clinical evaluation of computerized enhancement and analysis of mammographic findings. In: Doi K, Giger ML, Nishikawa RM, Schmidt RA (eds.) Digital mammography '96. Amsterdam, Holland: Elsevier, 1996; pp 81-86.

5. Leichter I., Bamberger P., Novak B., Fields S., Buchbinder S., Lederman R. Quantitative Characterization of Mass Lesions on Digitized Mammograms for Computer Assisted Diagnosis. Investigative Radiology 2000; 35: 366-372.
6. Leichter I, Lederman R, Bamberger P, et al. The use of an interactive software program for quantitative characterization of microcalcifications on digitized film-screen mammograms. Invest. Radiol. 1999 34:394-400.
7. Efron B. The jackknife, the bootstrap and other resampling plans. Philadelphia PA: Society for Industrial and applied Mathematics (SIAM), 1982.
8. Metz CE. ROC methodology in radiologic imaging. Invest. Radiol. 1986; 21: 720-732.
9. Hanley JA, McNeil BJ. A method of comparing the areas under receiver operating characteristic curves derived from the same cases. Radiology 1983; 148: 839-843.

Results of an Observer Study with an Intelligent Mammographic Workstation for CAD

Maryellen L. Giger, Zhimin Huo, Carl J. Vyborny, Li Lan,
Robert M. Nishikawa, Ingrid Rosenbourgh

The University of Chicago, Department of Radiology, MC2026
5841 South Maryland Avenue Chicago, Illinois 60637
m-giger@uchicago.edu

Abstract. We have investigated the usefulness of an intelligent search workstation for computer-aided diagnosis as an aid to radiologists in the classification of lesions in mammography. Upon presentation of an unknown mammographic case, the workstation shows the computer output in terms of (a) computer-estimated likelihoods of malignancy, (b) images of lesions with known diagnoses from an on-line lesion atlas, and (c) graphics illustrating the characteristics of the unknown lesion relative to characteristics of lesions in the known reference atlas. These images are retrieved automatically from a similarity search of lesions in the known mammographic atlas. In an observer study, five radiologists interpreted 100 cases (that were unknown both to the computer and to the human observer) before and after presentation of the computer output. On average, the radiologists' improved in terms of Az value (area under the ROC curve) from 0.86 to 0.90 with a p-value < 0.02, in the task of distinguishing between malignant and benign mammographic mass lesion cases. .

1. Introduction

Early detection of breast cancer through screening mammography is the most effective way to reduce the mortality rate resulting from breast cancer [1,2]. However, radiologists are unable to classify correctly all lesions detected at mammography as being benign or malignant. Computer-aided diagnosis (CAD) is being investigated as a means to provide radiologists with objective information, such as estimates of likelihood of malignancy, to aid in the classification of abnormalities detected at screening [3-5]. In addition various observers studies have been performed [6-8] to evaluate and demonstrate the improvement in radiologists' performance due to the effect of computerized classification schemes as an aid to radiologists in differentiating between benign and malignant breast lesions.

2. Computerized Classification of Mammographic Masses

Our mass classification method includes three components: 1) automated segmentation of mass regions, 2) automated feature-extraction, and 3) automated classification [8-14]. The scheme was initially trained with 95 mammograms containing masses occurring in 65 patients. Features related to the margin, shape, and density of each mass are extracted automatically from the image data and merged into an estimate of the likelihood of malignancy using artificial neural networks. In a round-robin analysis, the computer classification scheme yielded an A_z value of 0.94, similar to that of an experienced mammographer (A_z=0.91) and statistically significantly higher than the average performance of five radiologists with less mammographic experience (A_z=0.81). [9,10].

The computerized mass classification method was also independently evaluated on a 110-case clinical database containing 50 malignant and 60 benign mass cases. The effects of variations in both case mix and in film digitization technique on the performance of the method were assessed. In the task of distinguishing between malignant and benign lesions, the computer achieved an A_z value (area under the ROC curve) of 0.90 on the prior training database (Fuji scanner digitization) in a round-robin evaluation, and A_z values of 0.82 and 0.81 on the independent database for Konica and Lumisys digitization formats, respectively. However, in the statistical comparison of these performances, we failed to show a statistical significant difference between the performance on the training database and that on the independent validation database (p-values > 0.10). Thus, our computer-based method for the classification of lesions on mammograms is robust to variations in case mix and film digitization technique [11].

In order to evaluate the effectiveness of our computerized classification method as an aid to radiologists in differentiating between benign and malignant mammographic mass lesions, we conducted an observer study [8,14]. Six mammographers and 6 community radiologists participated in an observer study in which the computer aid was the computer-estimated likelihood of malignancy for each lesion. The radiologists interpreted, without and with the computer aid, 110 cases that were unknown to both the radiologist observers and the trained computer classification scheme. The radiologists' performances in differentiating between benign and malignant masses without and with the computer aid were evaluated using ROC analysis. When the computer aid was used, the average performance of the radiologists improved as indicated by an increase in A_Z of 0.93 to 0.96 (p=0.0002) by an increase in partial A_z of 0.56 to 0.72 (p=0.0002), and by an increase in sensitivity from 94% to 98% (p=0.022). No statistically significant difference in specificity was found between readings with and without computer aid (p=0.44). When we analyzed results from the mammographers and community radiologists as separate groups, a larger improvement was demonstrated for the general radiologists. This study indicated that computer-aided diagnosis can potentially help radiologists improve their diagnostic accuracy in the task of differentiating between benign and malignant masses seen on mammograms.

3. Intelligent Workstation based on Similarity Search with a Known Mammographic Atlas

We previously developed an intelligent workstation based on similarity to a known atlas of breast images [15], and have since incorporated our mammographic and sonographic computerized mass classification methods into this workstation [16]. Upon viewing an unknown case, the display shows both the computer classification output as well as images of lesions with known diagnoses (e.g., malignant vs. benign) and a graphical representation of the unknown lesion relative to all the cases in the known databases (the atlases). The similarity index used in the search can be selected by the radiologist and can be based on a single lesion feature, multiple features, or on the computer estimate of the likelihood of malignancy. The output of a computer-aided diagnostic scheme can take a variety of forms such as the estimated likelihood that a lesion is malignant either in terms of probabilities or along a standardized rating scale. This computer-determined information is then available for use by the radiologist when making decisions regarding patient management.

4. Observer Study

The database used in the observer study consisted of 50 biopsy-proven malignant masses, and 50 biopsy-proven benign masses. An IRB-approved protocol for retrospective use of the mammograms and clinical data was employed. For each case, all four standard views and one special view (e.g., a spot-compression view or a spot-compression magnification view selected by an experienced mammographer) were collected. All the mammograms were digitized using a Lumisys laser scanner (Lumiscan 100, Lumisys, Sunnyvale, CA) at a 0.1-mm pixel size and 12-bit quantization (subsequently scaled to 10-bit quantization).

Both the unknown database of images for the observer study and the known atlas images were loaded onto the intelligent search workstation. For this particular observer study, upon presentation of an unknown mammographic case, the workstation displayed the results of the computer analyses in three manners: (a) computer-estimated likelihood of malignancy, (b) images of lesions with known diagnoses from an on-line lesion atlas, and (c) graphics illustrating the characteristics of the unknown lesion relative to characteristics of lesions in the known reference library.

For each clinical case, radiologists were shown the four standard mammographic views on a 17" x 17" video monitor, with arrows indicating the locations of the mass lesion. The monitor also displayed ROIs containing the mass lesion in question from the CC, MLO and/or special views. Figure 1 shows the computer interface for the observer study for (a) the condition without the computer aid and (b) the conidition with the computer aid. The radiologists were able to zoom the ROIs to full resolution (0.1 mm/pixel) and were able to interactively change the contrast and brightness of the displayed images according to their preference.

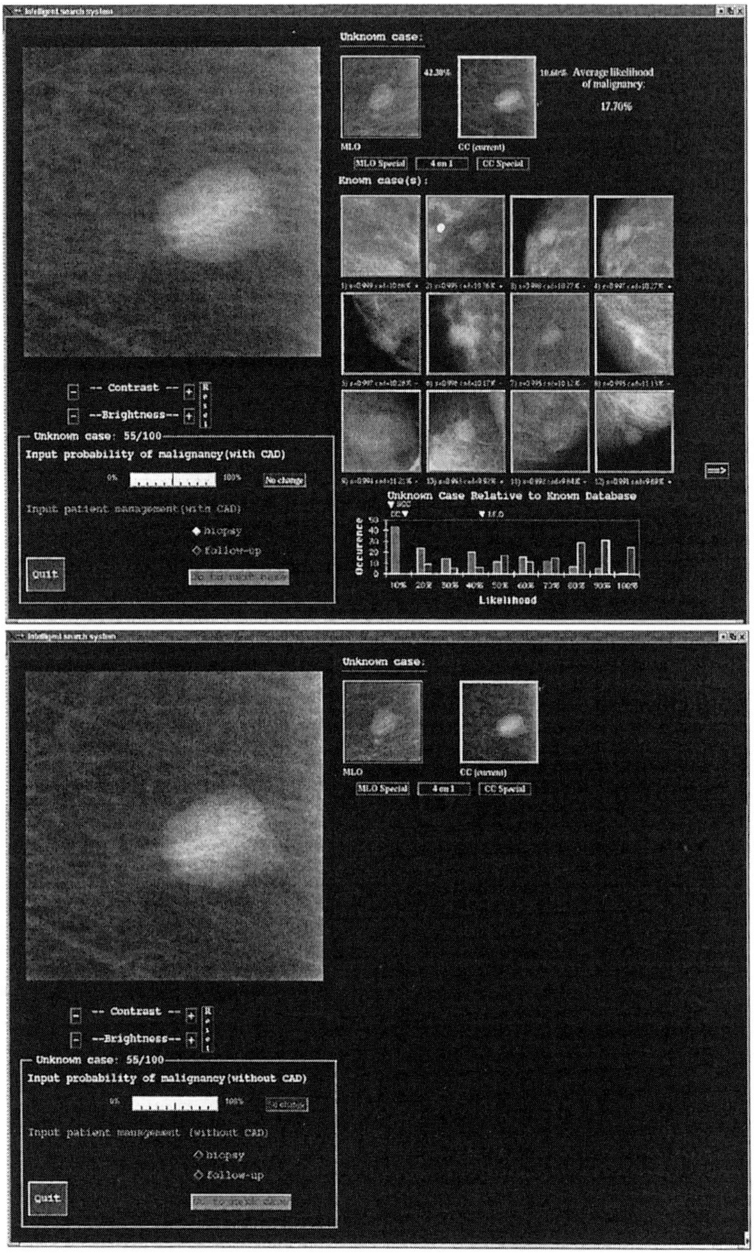

Fig. 1. The computer interface used in our observer study: a) without the computer output and b) with the computer output in terms of computer-estimated likelihoods of malignancy, images of lesions with known diagnoses from an on-line lesion atlas, and graphics illustrating the characteristics of the unknown lesion relative to characteristics of lesions in the known reference atlas.

In order to acquaint radiologists to the computer output, each observer read 25 training cases with feedback on the actual pathology in the case. The true diagnosis was given immediately after each training case. The order of the training cases was the same for all the observers.

During the actual observer study, each observer interpreted the 100 cases that were unknown both to the computer and to the human observer. For the interpretation, each radiologist was asked two questions under each of the two conditions. First, "what is your confidence that a lesion is malignant on a continuous scale ranging from 0% to 100%" and second, "what is your recommendation for patient management – i.e., long-term/short-term follow-up or core/surgical biopsy." After seeing the computer output, the observer could modify his/her confidence rating and biopsy recommendation if needed. It should be noted that this sequential reading order is appropriate for this evaluation since such reading order mimics that which would be used clinically [17]. In our situation, the stand-alone imaging modality, i.e., the mammograms themselves, is being compared to a combination of that modality and a supplemental one, i.e., the computer output. In addition, the stand-alone modality, i.e., the mammograms themselves, is expected to be read first before the combination in clinical practice. The order of the 10 independent test cases was randomized differently for each observer. No time limit was imposed on observers, and each observer decided when the computer output would be shown.

The confidence ratings (that a lesion is malignant) from each observer were analyzed using ROC analysis [18,19]. The area under the ROC curve (A_Z) was calculated to summarize the overall performance of each observer in the task of differentiating between benign and malignant mass lesions. Student's t-test for paired data [20] was employed to assess the significance of differences between the performances with and without computer aid for the group of radiologists.

5. Results

On average, the radiologists' improved in terms of Az value (area under the ROC curve) from 0.86 to 0.90 with a p-value < 0.02, in the task of distinguishing between malignant and benign mammographic mass lesion cases. The ROC curves indicating the average performance of the five radiologists is shown in Figure 2. It is interesting to note the performance of the computer alone in the task of distinguishing between malignant and benign mammographic lesions. On the known and unknown databases the computer achieved Az values of 0.85 and 0.76, respectively.

6. Summary

We have shown the usefulness of a workstation that allows a radiologist to use either numerical, pictorial, and/or graphical aids in the classification of unknown mammographic mass lesions. The additional presentation of the computer output is performed based on a similarity search of a known image atlas. Information generated by our automatic computerized classification method improved the

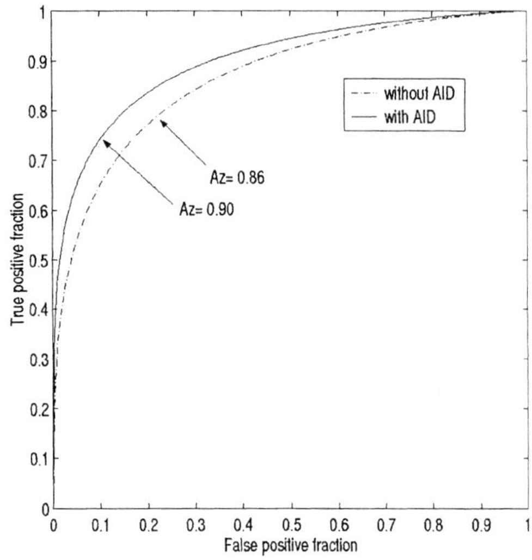

Fig. 2. ROC curves of the 5 radiologists with and without the computer aid.

performances of radiologists in the task of differentiating between benign and malignant disease.

Acknowledgements:

The authors are grateful to the five radiologists who participated in the observer study. This work was supported in parts by an USPHS grant CA89452 and a grant from the US Army Medical Research and Materiel Command (DAMD 97-2445).

Z. Huo, M. L. Giger, R. M. Nishikawa, and C. J. Vyborny are shareholders in R2 Technology, Inc. (Los Altos, CA). It is the policy of the University of Chicago that investigators disclose publicly actual or potential significant financial interests that may appear to be affected by the research activities.

References:

1 Smith RA. Screening women aged 40-49: where are we today? JNCI 1995; 87:1198-1199.

2. Tabar L, Fagerberg G and Chen RH. Efficacy of breast screening by age: new results from the Swedish two county trial. Cancer 1995; 75:1412-1419.

3. Giger ML: "Computer-aided diagnosis". In: AAPM/RSNA Categorical Course in Diagnostic Radiology Physics: Physical Aspects of Breast Imaging -- Current and Future Considerations, (Haus A. and Yaffe M., eds.) pp. 249-272, 1999.

4. Giger ML, Huo Z, Kupinski MA, Vyborny CJ: "Computer-aided diagnosis in mammography", In: Handbook of Medical Imaging, Volume 2. Medical Imaging Processing and Analysis, (Sonka M, Fitzpatrick MJ, eds) SPIE, pp. 915-1004, 2000.
5. Vyborny CJ, Giger ML, Nishikawa RM: Computer-aided detection and diagnosis. Radiologic Clinics of North America 38:725-740, 2000.
6. Jiang Y, Nishikawa RM, Schmidt RA, Metz CE, Giger ML, Doi K: Improving breast cancer diagnosis with computer-aided diagnosis. Academic Radiology 6: 22-33, 1999
7. Chan H-P, Sahiner B, Helvie MA, et al. Improvement of radiologists' characterization of mammographic masses by using computer-aided diagnosis: An ROC study. Radiology 1999; 212:817-827.
8. Huo Z, Giger ML, Vyborny CJ, Metz CE: Effectiveness of CAD in the diagnosis of breast cancer: An observer study on an independent database of mammograms. Radiology (in press) 2002.
9. Huo Z, Giger ML, Vyborny CJ, Bick U, Lu P, Wolverton DE and Schmidt RA. Analysis of spiculation in the computerized classification of mammographic masses. Med Phys 1995; 22:1569-1579.
10. Huo Z, Giger ML, Vyborny CJ, Wolverton DE, Schmidt RA and Doi K. Automated computerized classification of malignant and benign masses on digitized mammograms. Academic Radiology 1998; 5:155-168.
11. Huo Z, Giger ML, Vyborny CJ, Wolverton DE and Metz CE. Computerized classification of benign and malignant masses on digitized mammograms: a study of robustness. Academic Radiology 2000; 7:1077-1084.
12. Huo Z, Giger ML, Metz CE: Effect of dominant features on neural network performance in the classification of mammographic lesions. PMB 44: 2579-2595, 1999.
13. Huo Z, Giger ML, Vyborny CJ: Computerized analysis of multiple-mammographic views: Potential usefulness of special view mammograms in computer-aided diagnosis. IEEE Transactions on Medical Imaging 20: 1285-1292, 2001.
14. Huo Z, Giger ML, Vyborny C, Jiang Y, Nishikawa R, Engelmann R: Effectiveness of computer aid for radiologist's classification of mammographic mass lesions. Radiology 213: 200, 1999.
15. Giger ML, Huo Z, Lan L, Vyborny CJ: Intelligent search workstation for computer-aided diagnosis. Proc. of Computer Assisted Radiology and Surgery (CARS'2000), pp. 822-827, 2000.
16. Giger ML, Huo Z, Vyborny CJ, Lan L, Bonta I, Horsch K, Nishikawa RM, Rosenbourgh I: Intelligent CAD workstation for breast imaging using similarity to known lesions and multiple visual prompt aids. Proc. SPIE 2002 (in press).
17. Metz C. Fundamental ROC analysis. In Beutel J, Metter R and Kundel H (eds) : Handbook of Medical Imaging, Volume 1, Washington, SPIE Press, 2000:751-764.
18. Metz CE. ROC methodology in radiologic imaging. Invest Radiol 1986; 21:720-733.
19. Metz CE. Some practical issues of experimental design and data analysis in radiological ROC studies. Invest Radiol 1989; 24:234-245.
20. Hays WL. Statistics. Philadelphia, Harcourt Brace College, 1994.

An Adaptive Similarity Measure for Automated Identification of Breast Lesions in Temporal Pairs of Mammograms for Interval Change Analysis

Lubomir Hadjiiski, Berkman Sahiner, Heang-Ping Chan, Nicholas Petrick, Mark A. Helvie,

Department of Radiology, University of Michigan, Ann Arbor, MI 48109
lhadjisk@umich.edu

Abstract. An adaptive similarity measure (ASM) is designed to improve automated identification of corresponding lesions on prior mammograms. It combines adaptive filtering to enhance the lesion and a similarity measure (SM) as a figure-of-merit (FOM) measure. The filters are designed with a training set to maximize and minimize the FOM for the similar and dissimilar image pairs, respectively, by using a gradient optimization technique. The ASM was applied to the final stage of our multistage regional registration technique for identification of the mass on the prior mammogram. A search for the best match between the lesion template from the current mammogram and a structure on the prior mammogram was carried out within a search region, guided by the ASM. This new approach was evaluated by using 179 temporal pairs of mammograms containing biopsy-proven masses. 86% of the estimated lesion locations resulted in an area overlap of at least 50% with the true lesion locations. The average distance between the estimated and the true lesion centroids on the prior mammogram was 4.5 ± 6.7 mm. In comparison, the correct localization and the average distance using a conventional correlation SM were 84% and 4.9 ± 7.0 mm, respectively. The ASM improved the identification of the corresponding lesions on temporal pairs of mammograms.

1. Introduction

Mammography is currently the most effective method for early breast cancer detection [1, 2]. Analysis of interval changes is an important method used by radiologists to detect developing malignancy in mammographic interpretation [3, 4]. A variety of computer-aided diagnosis (CAD) techniques have been developed to detect mammographic abnormalities and to distinguish between malignant and benign lesions. We are studying the use of CAD techniques to assist radiologists in interval change analysis.

A number of methods for lesion registration between current and prior mammogram have been developed. Some of the methods depend on the identification of control points [5-7]. However, because the breast is mainly composed of soft tissue that can change over time, there are no obvious landmarks on mammograms. The crossing line structures are often fibrous tissue from different depths of the breast which overlap in a projection image. These crossing points are not invariant landmarks on the serial mammograms. Because of the elasticity of the breast tissue, there is large variability in the positioning and compression used in mammographic examination. As a result, the relative positions of the breast tissues projected onto a mammogram vary from one examination to the other. Techniques that depend on identification of control points may not be generally applicable to registration of breast images.

Gopal *et al.* [8, 9] and Hadjiiski *et al.* [10-12] have developed a multistage technique that defines a transformation to locally map the position of the mass on a current mammogram to that on the prior mammogram. A local search for the mass is then performed on the prior mammogram. Good *et al.* [13] also have developed a technique that defines a transformation to map all points from the current mammogram onto a prior mammogram. The current mammogram is then subtracted from the prior mammogram.

The goal of our research is to develop a technique for computerized analysis of temporal differences between a lesion on the most recent mammogram and a prior mammogram of the same view. The computer algorithm will assist radiologists in quantifying interval changes and thus distinguishing between benign and malignant masses for CAD. The local search is an important step in our registration technique. It compensates for the inaccuracies due to variability in the positioning and compression between the current and prior mammograms. A successful detection at that step depends to high extent on the similarity measure. In this study, we designed an adaptive similarity measure (ASM) to improve automated identification of corresponding lesions on prior mammograms.

2. Materials and Methods

2.1 Registration Technique

A multistage regional registration technique was developed for identifying corresponding masses on temporal pairs of mammograms. In the first stage, an initial fan-shaped search region was defined on the prior mammogram based on the mass location on the current mammogram. In the second local alignment stage, the location of the search region on the prior mammograms was first refined by maximizing a correlation similarity measure (CSM) between a template of the fan-shaped region centered at the mass extracted from the current mammogram and the breast structures on the prior mammogram [12]. The affine transformation in combination with simplex optimization was then employed to warp this local region and further improve the correlation. In the final stage, a search for the best match between the lesion template from the current mammogram and a structure on the prior mammogram was carried out within the refined search region by maximizing the CSM (Fig 1.). In this study we investigated the effect of replacing the CSM at the final stage with an adaptive similarity measure (ASM).

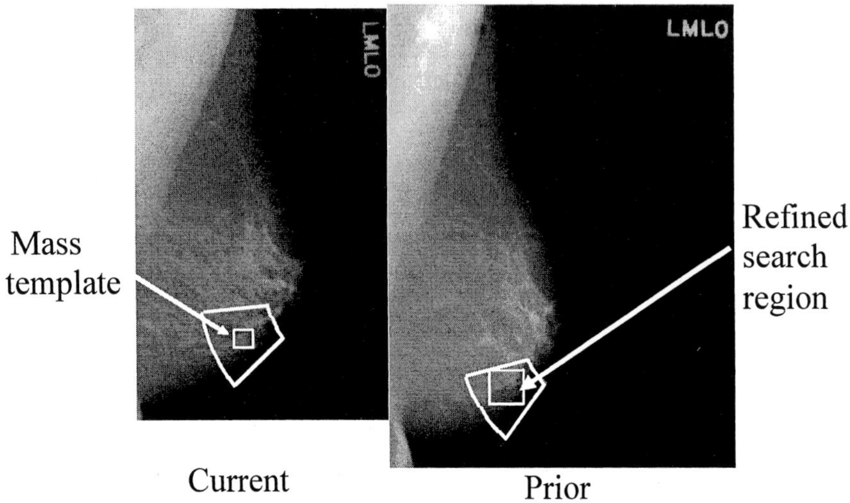

Fig. 1. A search for the best match between the mass template from the current mammogram and a structure on the prior mammogram was carried out within the refined search region.

2.2 Adaptive Similarity Measure

We are developing a new class of similarity measures (SM) for the registration of masses on the current and prior mammograms. It combines adaptive filtering to enhance the lesion and a SM as a figure-of-merit (FOM) measure. The filters are designed with a training set to maximize and minimize the FOM for the similar and dissimilar image pairs, respectively, by using a gradient optimization technique. The filter kernel sizes are fixed and scaling and interpolation are used in order to match the sizes of the image template when it is applied to a given mass. The filter is a part of the similarity measure scheme and its kernel is optimized by training in such a way that the particular SM will be maximized at the objects of interest. If a different SM is chosen, the filter kernel will have different optimal values.

The ASM was applied to the final stage of our multistage regional registration technique for identification of the mass on the prior mammogram. A search for the best match between the lesion template from the current mammogram and a structure on the prior mammogram was carried out within a search region, guided by the ASM.

2.3 Data Set

A set of 179 temporal pairs of mammograms containing biopsy-proven masses on the current mammograms was used to examine the performance of this approach. A total of 308 mammograms from 74 cases were digitized. Thirty five of the mammograms were digitized with a LUMISYS DIS-1000 laser scanner at a pixel resolution of $100\mu m \times 100\mu m$ and 4096 gray levels. The digitizer was calibrated so that gray level values were linearly proportional to the optical density (OD) within the range of 0.1 to 2.8 OD units, with a slope of 0.001 OD/pixel value. Outside this range, the slope of the calibration curve decreased gradually. The OD range of the digitizer was 0 to 3.5. The remaining 273 mammograms were digitized with a LUMISCAN 85 laser scanner at a pixel resolution of $50\mu m \times 50\mu m$ and 4096 gray levels. The digitizer was calibrated so that gray level values were linearly proportional to the OD within the range of 0 to 4 OD units, with a slope of 0.001 OD/pixel value. Output from both digitizers was linearly converted so that a large pixel value corresponded to a low optical density. In order to process the mammograms digitized with these two different digitizers, the images digitized with LUMISCAN 85 digitizer were averaged with a 16×16 box filter, resulting in $800\mu m$ images. The images digitized with LUMISYS DIS-1000 digitizer were averaged with a 8×8 box filter, resulting in $800\mu m$ images. The true lesion locations were identified by an experienced MQSA radiologist on all mammograms. The 308 mammograms contained 306 biopsy-proven and 2 follow-up masses. The 179 temporal pairs of mammograms included 90 CC-view pairs, 76 MLO-view pairs, and 13 lateral-view pairs.

2.4 Evaluation Methods

The accuracy of the multistage regional registration was analyzed in terms of two measures. The first measure is the overlap area between the estimated and the true lesions on the prior mammogram. The fractions of registered temporal pairs that could provide an accuracy of over 50% area overlap were examined. The second measure is the average Euclidean distance between the centroids of the estimated and true lesion locations.

3. Results

The ASM used in this study combined a 9×9 filter kernel with the CSM. When the ASM was applied to the final stage of our multistage registration technique, 86% of the estimated lesion locations resulted in an area overlap of at least 50% with the true lesion locations. The average distance between the estimated and the true lesion centroids on the prior mammogram was 4.5 ± 6.7 mm. In comparison, the correct localization and the average distance using a conventional CSM were 84% and 4.9 ± 7.0 mm, respectively.

4. Conclusion

The ASM improved the identification of the corresponding lesions on temporal pairs of mammograms. Further studies are underway to improve the technique, expand it to different types of SM, and evaluate its performance on a larger data set.

Acknowledgements

This work is supported by U. S. Army Medical Research and Materiel Command grant DAMD17-98-1-8211. The content of this publication does not necessarily reflect the position of the government and no official endorsement of any equipment and product of any companies mentioned in the publication should be inferred.

References

1. Zuckerman, H.C., *The role of mammography in the diagnosis of breast cancer*, in *Breast Cancer, Diagnosis and Treatment*, I.M. Ariel and J.B. Cleary, Editors. 1987, McGraw-Hill: New York. p. 152-172.
2. Tabar, L. and P.B. Dean, *The Control of Breast Cancer through Mammography Screening.* Radiologic Clincs of North America, 1987. **25**: p. 961.
3. Bassett, L.W., B. Shayestehfar, and I. Hirbawi, *Obtaining previous mammograms for comparison: usefullness and costs.* Amer. J. Roentgenology, 1994. **163**(5): p. 1083-1086.
4. Sickles, E.A., *Periodic mammographic follow-up of probably benign lesions: results in 3183 consecutive cases.* Radiology, 1991. **179**: p. 463-468.
5. Sallam, M. and K. Bowyer, *Detecting abnormal densities in mammograms by comparison with previous screenings*, in *Digital Mammography '96*, K. Doi, et al., Editors. 1996, Elsevier: Amsterdam. p. 417-420.
6. Brzakovic, D., et al., *Mammogram Analysis by Comparison with Previous Screenings*, in *Digital Mammography*, A.G. Gale, et al., Editors. 1994, Elsevier: Amsterdam. p. 131-140.
7. Vujovic, N. and D. Brzakovic, *Establishing the correspondence between control points in pairs of mammographic images.* IEEE Transactions on Medical Imaging, 1997. **6**: p. 1388-1399.
8. Gopal, S.S., et al., *A regional registration technique for automated analysis of interval changes of breast lesions.* Proc. SPIE, 1998. **3338**: p. 118-131.
9. Gopal, S.S., et al., *A regional registration technique for automated interval change analysis of breast lesions on mammograms.* Medical Physics, 1999. **26**: p. 2669-2679.
10. Hadjiiski, L.M., et al., *Automated identification of breast lesions in temporal pairs of mammograms for interval change analysis.* Radiology, 1999. **213(P)**: p. 229-230.
11. Hadjiiski, L.M., et al., *Interval change analysis in temporal pairs of mammograms using a local affine transformation.* Proc. SPIE, 2000. **3979**: p. 847-853.
12. Hadjiiski, L.M., et al., *Automated registration of breast lesions in temporal pairs of mammograms for interval change analysis - local affine transformation for improved localization.* Medical Physics, 2001. **28**(6): p. 1070-1079.
13. Good, W.F., et al., *Generalized procrustean image deformation for substraction of mammograms.* Proc. SPIE, 1999. **3661**: p. 1562-1573.

An indexed atlas of digital mammograms

Hilary Alto[a], Rangaraj M. Rangayyan[a,b], and J.E.Leo Desautels[a,c]

[a]Department of Electrical and Computer Engineering, [b]Department of Radiology, University of Calgary, 2500 University Dr. N.W., Calgary, Alberta, Canada T2N 1N4
[c]Alberta Cancer Board, 120, 1040-7th Ave. S.W., Calgary, Alberta, Canada T2P 3G9
ranga@enel.ucalgary.ca

Abstract. The improvements made to mammography equipment and x-ray film techniques have not significantly altered the fact that between 10 and 25% of invasive cancers are missed in mammography of women over the age of 50 and women aged 40 to 49 years, respectively. To address this issue, image processing methods for the detection and analysis of mammographic features have been developed by many research groups to improve the detection capabilities and diagnostic confidence of radiologists in breast cancer screening or diagnosis. We are constructing an indexed atlas of mammograms for use in the development and testing of image processing algorithms, training, and design of decision-making support tools related to diagnosis and treatment planning. The atlas should serve as an important database, information resource, and reference tool in computer-aided detection of breast cancer.

Introduction

Image processing methods for the detection and analysis of mammographic features have been developed by many research groups to improve the detection capabilities and diagnostic confidence of radiologists in breast cancer screening or diagnosis. Discussions on the design of mammographic databases were facilitated by a panel of digital mammography experts at the first conference on digital mammography [1]. A well-balanced, comprehensive database of digital mammographic images is key to the development of image-processing algorithms, teaching and training tools for radiologists, and decision-support related to diagnosis and treatment planning. The Digital Database for Screening Mammography (DDSM) and the Mammographic Image Analysis Society (MIAS) databases were developed to specifically address the needs of the digital mammography community by providing access to 2,620 and 161 cases, respectively. These databases, and others developed over the past ten years, contain limited information with which to make decisions and evaluate image processing algorithms [2]. Although the DDSM and MIAS databases are well-balanced datasets that are easily accessible to researchers, they contain minimal detail related to the mammograms and pathology reports, and at most two or four images per case (where a case is one screening exam of either one or two views per breast).

Methods

The continually increasing demand for more information to make better informed and more confident diagnoses has motivated us to construct a comprehensive database or indexed atlas of digitized mammograms with complete patient information for each case.
Eighty-five percent of the data for the database has been acquired. The data include 170 cases of screening examinations obtained through Screen Test: Alberta Program for the Early Detection of Breast Cancer, established in 1990 [3]. Each case contains all views taken in all the exams over all the years that the woman participated in the screening program. As a result, we have between four and 28 high-resolution digitized mammograms in a given case, depending upon when the woman entered the screening program. A full patient history, mammography report, and pathology report if a biopsy or surgery was performed are also included in each case. To date, 100 malignant, 45 (of the proposed 50) benign, and 25 (of the proposed 50) normal cases have been acquired and digitized. Films were digitized at 50 μm spatial and 12 bits per pixel gray-scale resolution, resulting in very large uncompressed raw images of between 40 and 60 MB each. A TeraByte server is being used to store the images and the associated patient information. Ethics approval was obtained from the Conjoint Health Research Ethics Board and the Research & Development Committee of the Calgary Regional Health Authority. All data and images have been anonymized to comply with the Freedom of Information Protection of Privacy Act which was applied to post-secondary educational institutions in Alberta on September 1, 1999.

Discussion

A requirements engineering study was carried out to determine how best to design the atlas for optimal usability and integration in a radiology clinic. It was determined that a case-base approach to storing and retrieving the information closely resembles the current clinical workflow process. The three radiologists consulted for the present study indicated the importance of easy access and flexible querying of information in the atlas. They also highlighted the desirability of viewing image processing results by selecting an image and then an icon corresponding to the desired image processing operation. The image processing algorithms to be used in the atlas include: 1) Contrast enhancement, 2) Detection of calcifications, 3) Analysis of calcifications, 4) Detection of masses and tumors, 5) Shape analysis of tumors, 6) Texture flow-field analysis, 7) Texture analysis of tumors, 8) Pattern classification and diagnostic decision. Providing these capabilities requires the development of a user interface that can utilize data indexed in a vector-like structure designed to facilitate the retrieval process. Therefore, to create the index structure, each case must be described by a set of parameters representing clinical, pathological, and image-based features such as: ID = 165; Age = 58; Status = malignant, benign, or normal; Tumor = present or not present; Shape factors = values computed to represent shape roughness [4]. An example of an index vector: Index vector = [165 58 malignant present 0.8 0.7 1.2].

Initially, the boundaries of tumors and masses will be drawn by an experienced radiologist for one set of images from cases with these mammographic features. Shape factors will be computed for the boundaries and stored as part of the corresponding case information. Use of the atlas for content-based retrieval may proceed as follows. Given a difficult or ambiguous case, a user (radiologist) can search for similar cases by drawing the outline of a suspicious mammographic feature (mass or tumor) on the image. Shape factors are then computed for the feature in question, and compared with the corresponding values in the index vectors of all the cases with tumors or masses in the atlas. A similarity measure is then used to select the closest matches to the query image. The cases retrieved and their associated information should assist the radiologist in reaching an improved diagnosis.

The integration of several pieces of equipment and image processing algorithms will pose a challenge to making the proposed atlas a viable reference tool in computer-aided detection and diagnosis of breast cancer. However, once assembled, the image processing algorithms and content-based retrieval methods may be used in a variety of application areas of mammography such as clinical image interpretation, medical decision making, distance learning/training, radiology training, and tele-radiology.

Acknowledgments

We gratefully acknowledge financial support of this project from the Alberta Heritage Foundation for Medical Research (AHFMR) and the Natural Sciences and Engineering Research Council (NSERC) of Canada.

We thank Dr. Heather Bryant, Director of Epidemiology, Alberta Cancer Board, for her advice and assistance; Mrs. Zeva Mah and Mrs. Caroline Resner of Screen Test for their efforts in acquiring the case files; Dr. J. H. MacGregor, Diagnostic Imaging, Foothills Medical Care Centre, Calgary, and Dr. J. Quintero, ENST-Bretagne, Brest, France for their input to the requirements engineering study, and Mr. Steven Leikeim for systems analysis and maintenance services.

References

1. Rangayyan, R.M.: A database for mammographic image research. In: Proceedings of SPIE, Vol. 1905 (1993) 550-551
2. Karssemeijer, N., Thijssen, M., Hendriks, J., and van Erning, L.(eds): Fourth International Workshop on Digital mammography. Kluwer Academic, Dordrecht, The Netherlands (1998)
3. Alberta Cancer Board, Division of Epidemiology, Prevention and Screening: 1997/99 Biennial Report. Screen Test: Alberta Program for the Early Detection of Breast Cancer. Calgary, Alberta, Canada (1999)
4. Alto, H., Rangayyan, R.M., Solaiman, B., Desautels, J.E.L., MacGregor, J.H.: Image processing, radiological and clinical information fusion in breast cancer detection. In: Proceedings of SPIE, Vol. 4731 (2002) 134-144

Segmentation of Suspicious Clustered Microcalcifications in Digital Mammography: Using Fuzzy Logic on Wavelet Coefficients

J.Nasehi.Tehrani,N.Riahi,A.Ahmadian,M.Guiti

Tehran University of Medical Science , School of Medicine , Medical Physics and Biomedical Engineering Dept.
Tehran-Iran
Joubin_nasehi@yahoo.com

Abstract. We proposed an automated detection and segmentation of suspicious clustered microcalcifications in digital mammography. The algorithm consists of three main processing steps. In the first step , high-frequency content of breast was enhanced using wavelet atrous . In the second step , individual microcalcifications were segmented using wavelet histogram analysis on overlapping subplanes. For this step, extracted histogram features for each subplane used as input to a fuzzy rule-based classifier that identified subimages containing microcalcifications. In the third step , subtractive clustering were applied to assign individual microcalcifications to the closest cluster. Features of each cluster were used as input to another fuzzy rule-based classifier to identify suspicious clusters. The results of 80 images containing one or more clusters showed a sensitivity of 90% and average of 0.5 false positive clusters per image.

Key words: Computer-aided diagnosis, Clustered microcalcifications, Segmentation, Fuzzy rule, Digital mammography, Wavelet

1. Introduction

Breast radiographs are used for presence of malignant masses and indirect signs of malignancy, such as the presence of microcalcifications and skin thickening[1]. Between 1990 and 1994 mortality rates in women decreased about 1.8% per year for breast cancer and mammography has significantly contributed to this outcome[2], however clinical studies have shown that 10% to 30% of breast cancers visible on mammograms in retrospective studies were initially missed by radiologists[3]and only 15% to 30% of the patients who have under gone biopsy due to a suspicious finding on mammograms are found to have breast cancer[4]. Computer-aided diagnosis(CAD) programs are being developed in order to increase diagnostic accuracy. These programs work as a second reader and final decision depends on radiologist's observation[5]. For the feature extraction several techniques have been developed such as morphological filtering[6], wavelet transform based methods [7], methods to reduce false positive detection include rule-based methods[8]and artificial neural networks[9]. In this study an automated multistage technique is used for segmentation of suspicious microcalcifications clusters in digital mammograms.

2. Materials and Methods

We studied a database of 80 single-view mammograms collected over a period of one year by two experienced radiologists for the development of our method. The images were digitized at 100μm and 12 bits per pixel. It contained 52 images with biopsy proven malignant microcalcification clusters and 14 images with benign clusters. The set of images was divided into a training set consisting of 20 images and a testing set of 60 images.

2.1 Unsharp Masking

At first, high frequency content of images were enhanced using unsharp masking, implemented by smoothing the image with a median filter of size 11*11 pixels and then subtracting the smooth image from the original. we applied wavelet atrous[10]which caused high separation between the image histogram lobes.

2.2 Segmentation of Individual Microcalcifications

After enhancement, individual microcalcifications were segmented using local thresholding and fuzzy logic. The size of the subplane was chosen to be 16*16 pixels based on clinical information about the size of microcalcifications. All subplane were allowed to overlap by 75% in each dimension in order to minimize the risk of missing any microcalcifications. The wavelet histogram analysis is used to identify the subplanes containing microcalcifications. The following features such as; Area of the main lobe of histogram (a_1); Area of the outer lobes of histogram (a_2); Ratio of the standard deviations of the main lobe and the outers ($\sigma_{1,2}$); Mean contrast of the outer lobes relative to the main lobe($con_{1,2}$)were utilized in fuzzy rules to segment individual microcalcifications. The fuzzy membership function $s(\alpha,\beta)$ was used in this study which had been applied in a similar case to build a fuzzy binary decision tree[11]and fuzzy intervals were adjusted to increase the sensitivity or reduce the number of false signals as illustrated in Table.1. By this method subplanes classified into two classes; the subplanes contain no microcalcifications named class 1. And those which contain microcalcifications known as class 2. At first, if the value of a_1 was smaller than 0.9 , the following fuzzy rule was examined .

$$[1-\mu_1(\sigma_{1,2})]+\mu_2(con_{1,2})>1 \qquad \textbf{(1)}$$

Those satisfying(1)were classified as class 2. Since there was a 75% overlap, a pixel could be selected up to 16 times by overlapping subplanes. The value of the overlap threshold was initially set to 12. Labeling algorithm is used on the detected microcalcifications to label individual ones. After labeling, area of microcalcifications were checked in order to decrease false positive detection .

Table 1. Fuzzy intervals used in decision rules

Fuzzy Intervals	Features	Y_{min}	Y_{max}
1	$con_{1,2}$	0.7	1
2	$\sigma_{1,2}$	0	0.5
3	numc	3	10
4	Avedist	0.5	1.5

2.3 Clustering

The last step of our algorithm is clustering of individual microcalcifications. Subtractive Clustering[12], has been applied to assign individual microcalcifications to the closest cluster (the area of each cluster is 1 cm^2). In each cluster the following features were extracted: a) number of microcalcifications per cluster (numc), according to a clinical study[13]. b) Average distance between microcalcifications within the cluster (avedist) then clusters were tested using the following fuzzy rule:

$$[1-\mu_3(\text{avedist})]+\mu_4(\text{numc})>1 \qquad \textbf{(2)}$$

The intervals were adjusted to enable the accurate removal of false positives without eliminating real suspicious clusters (Table1). Clusters that not satisfied(2)were removed and others that survived were left on the final output image .

3. Results and Discussion

After optimizing all above parameters, the algorithm was implemented to images. As a sample, the original mammographic image, containing a cluster of low contrast microcalcifications is shown in fig 2a, the enhanced image after segmentation of individual microcalcifications is shown in fig 2b. At the end the clustering scheme removed isolated small objects in the image that could merge with a true cluster(fig 3). The performance of the algorithm on the training set was a TP rate of 92% with 0.4 FP per image. The algorithm was tested using a set of 60 images, consisting of 32 malignant cases and 6 benign cases. Performance of the algorithm on the testing set was a TP rate of 90% and average of 0.5 false clusters per image. The FROC curve correspond to increasing values of the density threshold is plotted in fig 1.

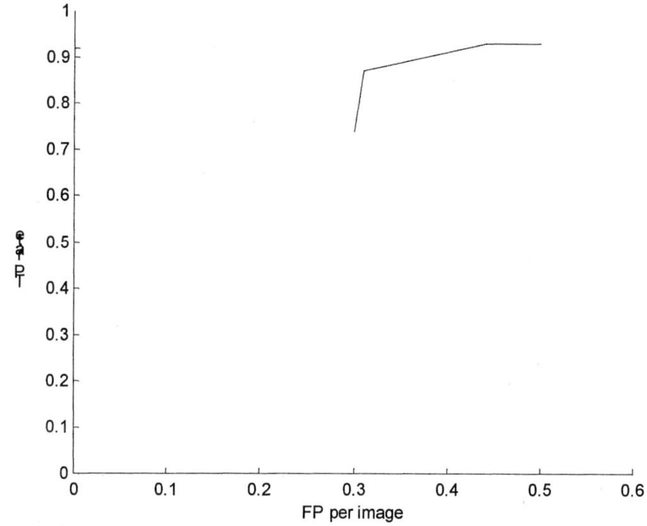

Fig. 1. The FROC curve by varying the value of density

3. Conclusion

We designed a method for segmentation of suspicious microcalcifications cluster in digital mammograms using fuzzy logic on wavelet coefficients . Using fuzzy rule-based methods on different features can lead to diagnosis of breast cancer more accurate and efficient.

Fig. 2a. Original Image

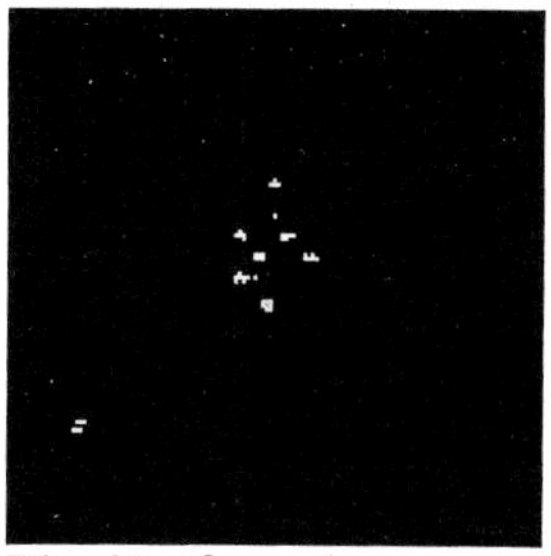

Fig. 2b after enhancement

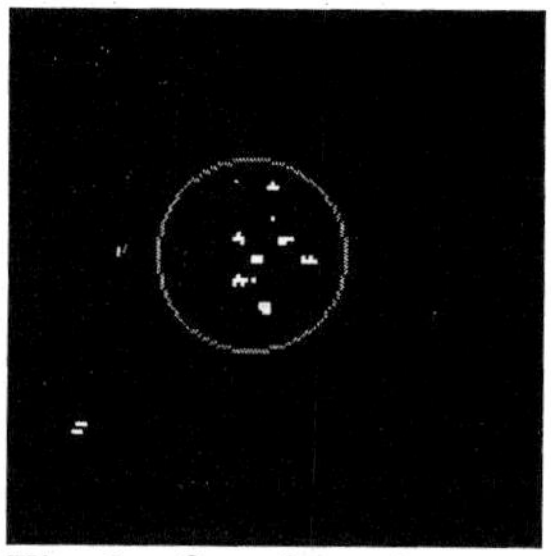

Fig. 3. after clustering

References

1. Ted C.Wang and Nicolaos. B " detection of microcalcifications in digital mammograms using wavelets "IEEE 498-509(1998).
2. S.H.Landis , T. Murray , S.Bolden and P.wingo"cancer statistic 1998"CA-cancer clinicians 48,6-30(1998).
3. R.E.Bird ,T.W.wallance ,and B.C. yankaskas" Analysis of cancers missed at screening mammography " Radiology 184,613-617(1992)
4. D.B.Kopans , "the positive predictive value of mammography"Am.J.Radiol.158,521-526(1991)
5. H.P.Chan , K.Doi , G.Simranjit , C. J. Vyborny , H. MacMahon , and P . M . Jokich "Image feature analysis and computer-aided diagnosis on digital Radiography.1.Automated detection of microcalcifications in mammography"Med.Phys.14.538-548(1987)
6. J.Dengler , S. Behrens , and J. F . Desaga "segmentation of microcalcifications in mammograms "IEEE trans .Med .Imaging 12,634-642(1993)
7. J.J.Heine , S.R.Deans , D.K , Cullers , R.stauduhar and L. Pclarke " multiresolution statistical analysis of high resolution digital mammograms" IEEE trans.med Imaging 16,503-515(1997)
8. D.H.Davies and D.R . Dance "Automatic computer detection of clustered calcifications in digital mammograms "Phys.Med , Biol 35.1111-1118(1990)
9. H.P.Chan , S.C.Lo ,B.Sahiner , K.L.Lam , and M.A.Helvie "computer-aided detection of mammographic microcalcifications :pattern recognition with an artificial neural network "Med Phys 22-1555-1567(1995)
10. J.C.Olivo "Automatic detection of spots in biological Images by a wavelet based selective filtering technique "IEEE 311-314(1996)
11. H.D.Li , M.Kallergi , L.P.Clarke , V.K.Jain , and R.A.Clark "Markov random field for tumor detection in digital mammography " IEEE trans Med Imaging 14-565-576(1995).
12. S.L.Chiu . Fuzzy Model identification based on cluster estimation Journal of intelligent and fuzzy systems 2(3).1994.
13. I . M.Freundlich , T.B. Hunter , G. W.seeley , C.J.Dorsi and N.L. Sadowsky "computer assisted analysis of mammographic clustered calcifications " clin.Radiol,40,295-298(1989)

Comparison of BI-RADS Lesion Descriptors and Computer-Extracted Image Features for Automated Classification of Malignant and Benign Breast Lesions

Yulei Jiang, Robert M. Nishikawa, Robert A. Schmidt, Carl J. D'Orsi*, Carl J. Vyborny, Maryellen L. Giger, Li Lan, Zhimin Huo, and Alexander V. Edwards

Department of Radiology, The University of Chicago, Chicago, Illinois
*Department of Radiology, Emery University, Atlanta, Georgia
y-jiang@uchicago.edu

Abstract. We compared Breast Imaging Report and Data System (BI-RADS) lesion descriptors provided by radiologists and image features extracted by a computer for computer classification of breast lesions as malignant or benign. Our results indicate that combining the BI-RADS lesion descriptors provided by radiologists and the computer-extracted image features produced the best computer classification performance.

1. Introduction

We are developing computer-aided diagnosis (CAD) techniques to help radiologists more accurately diagnose suspicious malignant and benign breast lesions. Using only computer-extracted image features that we have developed previously, we have shown that our computer techniques can classify breast lesions as malignant or benign as accurately as or more accurately than radiologists [1, 2]. Another approach to computer classification of malignant and benign breast lesions is to use lesion descriptions provided by radiologists in terms of the standard lexicon of the Breast Imaging Report and Data System (BI-RADS) [3, 4]. The purpose of our present study was to compare these two approaches and to investigate whether it is beneficial to combine BI-RADS lesion descriptors provided by radiologists and computer-extracted image features for computer classification of malignant and benign breast lesions.

2. Materials and Methods

The computer-extracted image features of suspicious breast lesions that we have developed previously are described in detail elsewhere. For masses, the computer-extracted image features include two features that characterize spiculations of a mass, margin sharpness of the mass, the density of the mass (average gray level), and texture [5]. For clustered microcalcifications, the computer-extracted image features include the number of microcalcifications within a cluster, the area of the cluster, the circularity of the cluster, the average area of the individual microcalcifications, the average volume of the individual microcalcifications where volume is defined as the product of area and contrast with contrast expressed in terms of a measurement of effective thickness, the relative standard deviation in microcalcification volume, the relative standard deviation in microcalcification effective thickness, and a microcalcification shape irregularity measure [6].

We used the lexicon of lesion descriptions defined in the 3rd edition of BI-RADS (1998) [4]. For masses, the BI-RADS contains mass size (we implemented this descriptor into six categorical measurements from < 1 cm to > 5 cm in 1 cm intervals), 4 descriptors of mass shape, 5 descriptors of mass margin, and 4 descriptors of mass density. Because it is often difficult to select one descriptor to represent accurately the entire margin of a mass, we instructed the radiologists to select up to two margin descriptors for each mass. For clustered microcalcifications, there are 5 descriptors for the distribution of microcalcifications, and 14 descriptors for the morphology of microcalcifications. Similar to the analysis of masses, because it is often difficult to select one morphology descriptor to represent accurately all microcalcifications in a cluster, we instructed the radiologists to select up to two morphological descriptors for each microcalcification cluster. In addition, we added 4 categorical descriptors for the number of microcalcifications in a cluster: <5, 5-10, 10-30, and >30.

We used a database of 92 cases of mass lesions and 127 cases of clustered microcalcifications lesions in this study. The following analysis is on a subset of cases: 67 mass lesions (33 malignant) and 99 microcalcification lesions (42 malignant). In all cases, 4 standard-view mammograms and magnification or spot-compression views of the lesion were available to the radiologists. The standard-view mammograms were digitized to a 100-micron pixel size and analyzed by the computer that extracted the image features. The computer did not analyze the magnification and spot-compression views. Two expert mammographers who are familiar with the BI-RADS standard participated in the study and each of them interpreted all the cases.

The radiologists reviewed the mammograms in a similar fashion as in typical clinical practice where all mammograms of a given case were interpreted together based on which the radiologist reported an overall interpretation. The cases were presented in random order and no time limit was imposed on reading of the mammograms. The radiologists reported their impression either via a laptop computer or verbally to an assistant who recorded the data on the laptop computer. For each case, the radiologists reported on all relevant BI-RADS lesion descriptors for either a mass or a cluster of microcalcifications, the BI-RADS final assessment category, and a quasi-continuous estimate of the likelihood of malignancy.

For the classification of masses, we used a Bayesian artificial neural network [7]. For the classification of clustered microcalcifications, we used the standard feed-forward error back propagation artificial neural network. These classifiers were designed to differentiate between malignant and benign breast lesions. Separate classifiers were designed that used the following as input: (1) the computer-extracted image features only, (2) the BI-RADS lesion descriptors provided by a radiologist only, and (3) the computer-extracted image features *plus* the BI-RADS lesion descriptors provided by a radiologist. In addition, separate classifiers were designed to use as input the BI-RADS lesion descriptors provided by each radiologist. Finally, separate classifiers were designed to classify masses and clustered microcalcifications as malignant or benign. Each classifier was trained and evaluated using the leave-one-out method. Area under the receiver operating characteristic (ROC) curve, A_z, was used as a measure of the performance of the classifiers.

3. Results

Table 1 shows a comparison of the A_z values of the various computer classifiers described above and the A_z values achieved by the radiologists based on their own assessment of the lesions.

Table 1. Summary A_z values of computer classification of malignant and benign breast masses or clustered microcalcifications in comparison to radiologists' assessment of the same lesions.

	Masses		Microcalcifications	
Reader	Reader A	Reader B	Reader A	Reader B
Computer-extracted image features only	0.73	0.73	0.73	0.73
BI-RADS descriptors only	0.88	0.87	0.48	0.72
Computer-extracted image features *plus* BI-RADS descriptors	0.96	0.89	0.75	0.81
BI-RADS final assessment	0.88	0.92	0.60	0.61
Estimate of likelihood of malignancy	0.88	0.91	0.62	0.66

4. Discussion

Computer classification of masses achieved higher A_z values based on the BI-RADS descriptors provided by radiologists than based on the computer-extracted image features. The opposite was true for computer classification of clustered microcalcifications: higher A_z values were obtained based on the computer-extracted image features. The results do not show clearly whether computer classification based on the BI-RADS lesion descriptors provided by radiologists performed better than the radiologists' own assessments in terms of the BI-RADS final assessment categories. In general, the A_z values associated with the classification of masses by either the computer or the radiologists were higher than the corresponding A_z values for the classification of clustered microcalcifications.

The results indicate that combining the computer-extracted image features and the BI-RADS lesion descriptors provided by the radiologists produced the highest A_z values in the classification of both masses and clustered microcalcifications. The combined results were better than results from the computer-extracted image features alone and from the BI-RADS lesion descriptors provided by the radiologists alone.

There is considerable amount of variability in the A_z values based on the BI-RADS lesion descriptors provided by each of the two radiologists. This variability is not unexpected [8, 9]. However, given this variability, we need to collect BI-RADS data from additional expert radiologists and to investigate the effect of this variability on the computer classification of malignant and benign breast lesions.

Acknowledgements

This work was funded in part by NIH through grant R01 CA92361, the US Army Breast Cancer Research Program through grant DAMD17-00-1-0197, and the Illinois Department of Public Health Penny Severns Breast and Cervical Cancer Research Fund. RM Nishikawa, RA Schmidt, CJ Vyborny, ML Giger, and Z Huo are shareholders of R2 Technology Inc., Los Altos, CA. It is the University of Chicago Conflict of Interest Policy that investigators disclose publicly actual or potential significant financial interests that would reasonably appear to be directly and significantly affected by the research activities.

References

1. Jiang, Y., Nishikawa, R.M., Schmidt, R.A., Metz, C.E., Giger, M.L. and Doi, K.: Improving Breast Cancer Diagnosis with Computer-Aided Diagnosis. Acad. Radiol. 6 (1999) 22-33
2. Huo, Z., Giger, M.L., Vyborny, C.J. and Metz, C.E.: Effectiveness of CAD in the Diagnosis of Breast Cancer: An Observer Study on an Independent Database of Mammograms. Radiology (in press)
3. Baker, J.A., Kornguth, P.J., Lo, J.Y. and Floyd, C.E.J.: Artificial Neural Network: Improving the Quality of Breast Biopsy Recommendations. Radiology 198 (1996) 131-135
4. American College of Radiology (ACR): Breast Imaging Reporting and Data System (BI-RADS^{tm}). 3rd ed. American College of Radiology, Reston, VA, (1998)
5. Huo, Z., Giger, M.L., Vyborny, C.J., Wolverton, D.E., Schmidt, R.A. and Doi, K.: Automated Computerized Classification of Malignant and Benign Masses on Digitized Mammograms. Acad. Radiol. 5 (1998) 155-168
6. Jiang, Y., Nishikawa, R.M., Wolverton, D.E., Metz, C.E., Giger, M.L., Schmidt, R.A., Vyborny, C.J. and Doi, K.: Malignant and Benign Clustered Microcalcifications: Automated Feature Analysis and Classification. Radiology 198 (1996) 671-678

7. Kupinski, M.A., Edwards, D.C., Giger, M.L. and Metz, C.E.: Ideal Observer Approximation Using Bayesian Classification Neural Networks. IEEE Trans. Med. Imaging 20 (2001) 886-899
8. Baker, J.A., Kornguth, P.J. and Floyd, C.E., Jr.: Breast Imaging Reporting and Data System Standardized Mammography Lexicon: Observer Variability in Lesion Description. AJR Am. J. Roentgenol. 166 (1996) 773-778
9. Berg, W.A., Campassi, C., Langenberg, P. and Sexton, M.J.: Breast Imaging Reporting and Data System: Inter- and Intraobserver Variability in Feature Analysis and Final Assessment. AJR Am. J. Roentgenol. 174 (2000) 1769-1777

CAD of Breast Cancer on Current and Prior Mammograms

R A Jong, ES Tu, RS Shumak, JE Glazier, LJ Justynski MJ Yaffe

PhDDepartment of Medical Imaging, Sunnybrook & Women's Health Sciences Centre, University of Toronto
2075 Bayview Avenue, Toronto, Ontario, Canada M4N 3M5
roberta.jong@swchsc.on.ca

Abstract. The mammograms of 123 patients with 124 biopsy-proven malignant lesions were retrospectively analyzed by two versions of a CAD System. The features of the cancers that were false negative on CAD were analysed. On the current mammograms, 82% of the malignancies were marked on at least one view by the CAD system. Performance was better for calcifications than for masses. The CAD system marked signs of cancer on the prior examination for more than half of the cancers subsequently detected with mammography. The new system detected 14 out of 31 previously missed malignancies.

Introduction

The recent decrease in breast cancer mortality may be attributed to earlier diagnosis due to screening mammography and better treatment. However, there is room for improvement, because false negative mammograms occur in up to 20% of cases, particularly when the breasts are mammographically dense [1], [2]. Studies have shown that double reading of mammograms by two different radiologists increases cancer detection up to 15% [3]. There are multiple factors that can contribute to a missed diagnosis of breast cancer, such as poor positioning or sub-optimal technique. Another is the radiologist's failure to perceive the abnormality. This problem may be corrected by employing computer-aided detection (CAD) as a second reader to flag significant findings on the images [2], [4]. The objective was to evaluate the accuracy of CAD of breast cancers on current mammograms and on those obtained at a time prior to the detection of cancer and to analyze the features of the cancers not found by CAD.

Method and Materials

A retrospective study was done of the screen-film mammograms of 224 women identified from a logbook of core biopsies performed with imaging guidance. In 123 women there were 124 breast cancers diagnosed between March 1998 and March 2001. The remainder of the women had benign diagnoses. The women with cancer were aged 36 to 85 years. Seventy-three of the examinations were for screening and fifty were for diagnostic purposes. These included women with prior lumpectomy and radiation therapy for breast cancer.

From the mammogram, the lesions were categorized as a mass, cluster of calcifications or a combination of both and the size was measured. The pathological diagnosis was made by 14-gauge core needle biopsy or surgical excision. Since mammographically dense fibroglandular tissue may obscure signs of cancer, the breast density was recorded. This was classified using the American College of Radiology BI-RADS™ categories. Since the appearance of a scar can simulate cancer, note was made of whether there was prior surgery and radiation therapy to the affected breast.

Prior mammograms were available for eighty of the women. Although these ranged from 4 months to 5 years earlier, two thirds were from 11 to 25 months before the time of diagnosis. These previous mammograms were also tested with CAD to determine if CAD could have identified the abnormality earlier.

The mammogram at the time of diagnosis and the most recent previous study were analyzed using Second Look™ (CADx Medical Systems, Laval, Quebec). The film was digitized using a pixel size of 43.5 microns at 12 bits/pixel. The image was cropped and image processing performed. Details of the CAD algorithms have been provided elsewhere [5]. The information was evaluated in the context of the patient with not more than the seven most significant areas marked. A paper copy of the images was produced with rectangles to mark clusters of calcifications and ovals to mark masses. A true positive CAD finding occurred when the lesion was correctly marked on at least one view. Each case required about 6-8 minutes to process.

When the new software (4.0) became available, 31/36 cancers that were missed by the earlier version were re-analyzed. Five cases including 4 masses and 1 calcification cluster could not be reanalyzed. The sensitivity was then calculated for the two versions.

Results

Of the 124 cancers, 75 presented as masses, 41 as microcalcifications and 8 as a mass with calcifications. The average size of the masses was 14.7 mm and the average diameter of the cluster of calcifications was 17.9 mm. The average number of false marks was 3.7 masses and 0.7 calcifications per examination. CAD correctly marked 51/75 (68%) of the masses, 31/41 (76%) of the clusters and 6/8 (75%) of the combined lesions. Overall the initial CAD sensitivity for cancer was 71%.

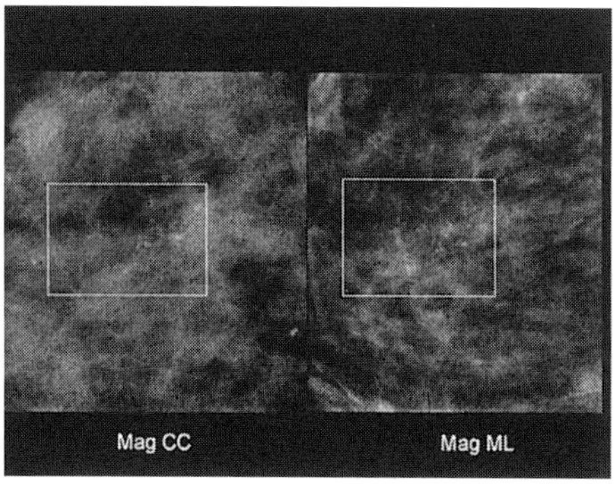

Figure 1 Calcifications of DCIS detected

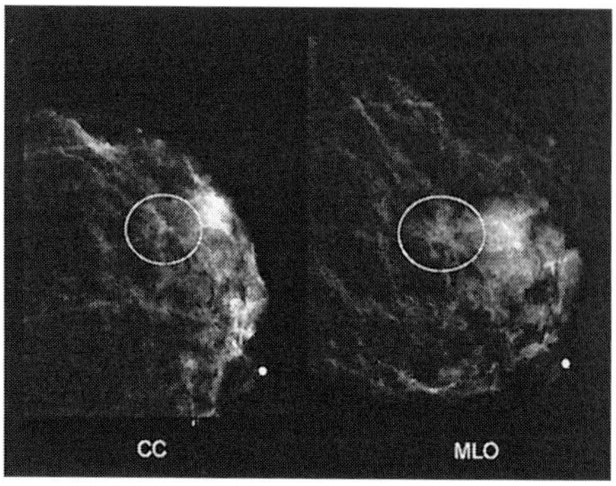

Figure 2 Mass of ILC not detected

The breast composition of the women with cancers missed by CAD and for the entire group of 224 women is shown in Table 1. The proportion of heterogeneously dense and dense breasts was similar in those with cancers missed by CAD as in the total population studied. The pathological diagnoses are shown in Table 2. Although invasive lobular carcinomas are known to be more difficult to diagnose on mammography, the proportion of cancers missed by CAD with this diagnosis was similar to that normally expected. Table 3 shows the number and percentage of women with prior ipsilateral breast surgery with benign and malignant diagnoses. The frequency of surgery was similar in those whose cancers were not detected on CAD as in the entire group.

Table 1. The breast composition categories of the women whose cancers were missed by CAD are similar to that of all the women.

Composition	Missed		All
Fatty	5/36	14%	15%
Scattered FG	10/36	28%	24%
Hetero Dense	15/36	42%	48%
Dense	6/36	17%	13%

Table 2. Pathology of false negatives on CAD, DCIS - ductal carcinoma in-situ, IDC - infiltrating ductal carcinoma, ILC - infiltrating lobular carcinoma

DCIS	9	25%
IDC	16	44%
IDC+DCIS	4	11%
IDC+ILC	2	5%
ILC	5	14%

When the 80 prior mammograms were analyzed, the original CAD algorithm found 28/80 (35%) of the cancers that were eventually diagnosed. Only 49 of these 80 cancers were considered visible in retrospect by the radiologist. Of these 49, 30 were masses and 19 were clusters of calcifications. CAD correctly marked 26/49 (53%) of these visible cancers. Of these, 15 were masses and 11 were clusters of calcifications. The 31 remaining examinations were considered negative by the radiologist. However CAD correctly marked the location of 2 cancers from this group (1 mass and 1 calcification cluster). Pathologically, of the visible cancers 9 were ductal carcinoma-in-situ (DCIS), 16 were invasive ductal carcinomas (IDC) and 1 was invasive lobular carcinoma. One of the 2 occult lesions was DCIS; the other was IDC.

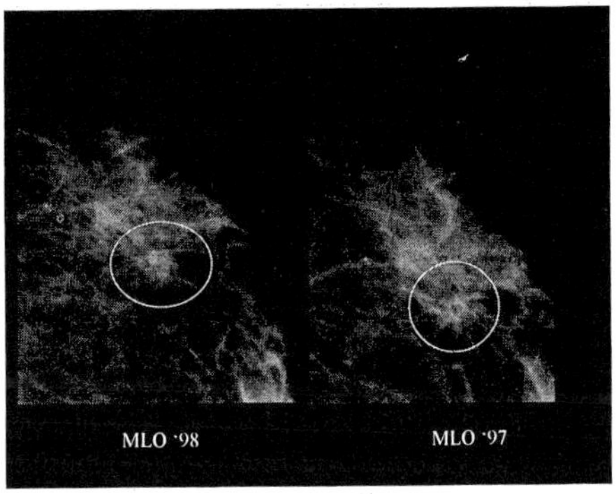

Figure 3 CAD detected IDC as mass 1 year earlier

	Benign	Malignant	Total
Misses	3/36 (8%)	6/36 (17%)	9/36 (25%)
All	26/224 (12%)	31/224 (14%)	57/224 (25%)

Table 3. Prevalence of previous surgery

With the new version Second Look^{TM} 4.0, 14/31 cancers that were originally missed were marked. Of these, 4 cancers were masses, 8 were clusters of calcifications and 2 were both. Assuming, conservatively, that those not re-analyzed would not have been found, and that all the originally detected cases would have again been marked with the new system, the sensitivity for masses became 73%. For calcifications it was 95% and when both were present in the lesion, it was 100%. As seen in Table 4, the overall sensitivity was 82%. It should be noted that CAD detected 2 masses not evident to the radiologists on the mammograms.

The characteristics of the cancers undetected on the newest software were evaluated. In the one case of missed calcifications, they were fine and low contrast. Of the 16 missed masses, 4 were considered mammographically occult by the radiologist. These had been detected by virtue of being palpable and seen on ultrasound or being seen on MRI. The masses varied in size from 4 mm to 4 cm but 7/12 had obscured or indistinct margins and 9/12 were isodense. Two of the three that were hyperdense were also large, with diameters of 3.5 and 4.0 cm.

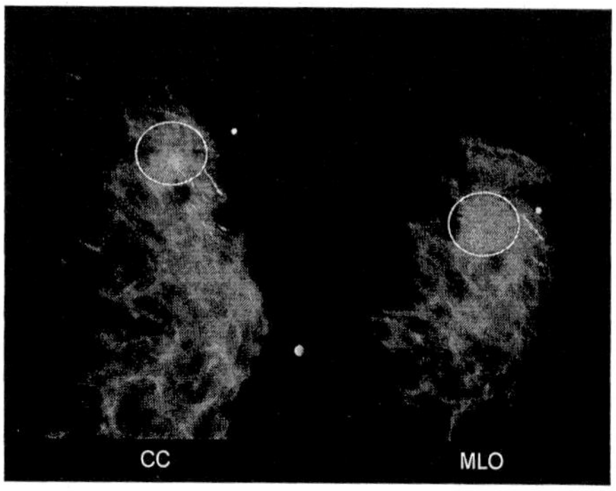

Figure 4 New version of CAD detected missed IDC

CAD SENSITIVITY

	3.4e	4.0
Mass	68%	73%
Calcs	76%	95%
Mass+calcs	75%	100%
Total	71%	82%

Table 4. Sensitivity of CAD versions

Discussion

CAD can find most breast cancers. However its role remains that of a second reader. Some lesions obvious to the radiologist were not identified, while other clearly benign findings were marked. Nevertheless, CAD did find abnormalities that the radiologist had overlooked on the previous mammogram and, therefore potentially could have led to an earlier diagnosis. For the radiologist to have confidence in the findings, there must be as few false marks as possible. A further reduction is desirable. The CAD system needs to be consistent with the same marks placed each time the image is analyzed. In a few cases, inconsistent marking was observed. There was improvement with the upgrade, which has an algorithm to recognize lesions overlying the pectoralis muscle. It also uses the combination of mass and calcifications at the same site to weight the area as being more suspicious.

Conclusion

Computer aided detection systems can help the radiologist increase breast cancer detection by marking lesions that have been overlooked. Performance on the system tested was better with calcifications than masses. The masses most difficult to find were isodense with obscured or indistinct margins. The technology continues to improve and evolve.

References

1. Bird, R., Wallace, T., Yankaskas, B.: Analysis of Cancers Missed At Screening Mammography. Radiology 1992; 184:613-617

2. Warren Burhenne, L., Wood, S., D'Orsi, C., Feig, S., Kopans, D., O'Shaughnessy, K., Sickles, E., Tabar, L., Vyborny, C., Costellino, R.: Potential Contribution of Computer-aided Detection to Sensitivity of Screening Mammography. Radiology 2000; 215:554-562
3. Thurfjell, E., Lernevall, K., Taube, A.: Benefit of Independent Double Reading in a Population-based Mammography Screening Program. Radiology 1994; 191:241-244
4. Birdwell, R., Ikeda, D., O'Shaughnessy, K., Sickles, E.: Mammographic Characteristics of 115 Missed Cancers Later Detected with Screening Mammography and the Potential Utility of Computer-aided Detection. Radiology 2000; 219:192-202
5. Worrell, S., Mitchell, R., Collins, M., Desimio, M., Rogers, S., Bauer, K., and Kabrisky, M.: Plug & Play CAD: A Proof of Concept. In: Yaffe, M.J. IWDM 2000 - Proceedings of the 5th International Workshop on Digital Mammography. Medical Physics Publishing, Madison WI (2001) 408-413

Optimal feature set for the detection of breast tumors on mammograms --- preliminary study ---

Jun WEI, Sachiko FURUYA, Mitsutaka NEMOTO, Yoshihiro HAGIHARA, Akinobu SHIMIZU, Hidefumi KOBATAKE, Shigeru NAWANO*

Tokyo University of Agriculture and Technology
Koganei, Tokyo 184-8588, Japan
{nemo-m, hhag, simiz, kobatake}@cc.tuat.ac.jp
* National Cancer Center Hospital East, Kashiwa, Chiba, Japan

Abstract. The feature set used in a computer-aided diagnosis system is the most important factor which influences its performance. Components of the optimal feature set depend on a classifier. This paper shows the results of image feature selection experiments using a forward stepwise selection approach. We evaluated 39 features using three classifiers. The performance of each classifier and the analysis of the optimally selected feature sets are given.

1. Introduction

Numerous systems were reported for detecting breast tumors on mammograms. The performance of the classifier depends directly on the ability of characterization of candidate regions by the adopted features. There have been, however, a few researches on comparing the effectiveness of features proposed hitherto[1]-[3].

The purpose of our research is to find the optimal feature set from many kinds of features and to enable a CAD system for breast cancer screening to take large step toward a practical application. Components of the optimal feature set depend on a classifier which distinguishes tumors from normal tissues and the comparison of the performance of various classifiers working with their own optimal feature sets is also necessary. This paper shows the results of the preliminary experiments under our large-scale research project. Three kinds of classifiers were examined. The analysis of their sub-optimal feature sets is given.

2. Feature Selection

2.1 Features

The number of features evaluated in this paper is 39. They are categorized into 4 groups.

(1) First-order Statistical Features : Seven first-order statistical features are calculated from each of two histograms of the gray-scale values which are obtained from the candidate region and its boundary region.

(2) Second-order Statistical Features : Thirteen features are extracted from the so-called Haralick transformation of the co-occurrence matrix obtained from the distribution image of contour points of the optimal mask of the iris filter[4].
(3) Density Features : Nine kinds of features proposed in [5] are calculated from the candidate region.
(4) Shape Features : The fourth group consists of three feature parameters; the area, the spreadness and the circularity.

2.2 Classifiers and Feature Selection Method

We have adopted three kinds of classifiers; a classifier based on the Mahalanobis distance measure, the maximum likelihood method and the nearest neighbor method. In this work, we adopted the forward stepwise selection method and the leave-one-out method to evaluate various feature set. In the case of the nearest neighbor method, the average correct classification rate was used as the criterion to evaluate the performance of feature sets. For the other two methods, the area under ROC curve, Az, was adopted as the criterion.

3. Experiments

The number of tumor candidate regions used in the following experiments is 1458 detected from 231 digital mammograms by the CAD system[4], [6]. Among them, 258 regions correspond to malignant tumors and the others are false positives.
Fig. 1 shows the relationship between the number of features and the area Az where the Mahalanobis distance measure was used. The area Az becomes the maximum (Az=0.932) in the case where the number of combined features is 19. If we set the system parameters so that the true positive detection rate is 90.3%, the average number of false positives per image is 1.06.

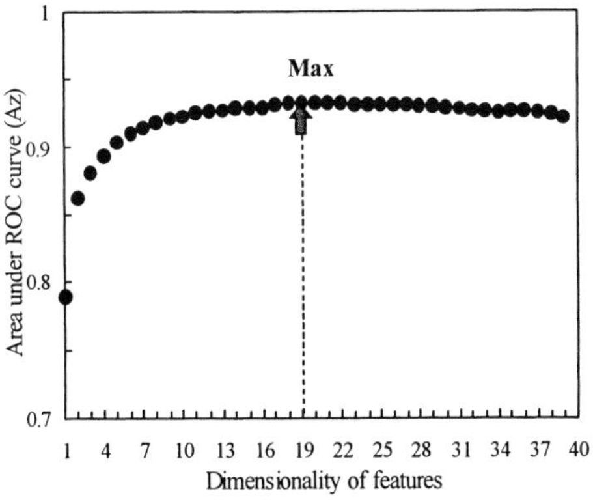

Fig. 1 The relationship between the area under the ROC curve and the number of features.

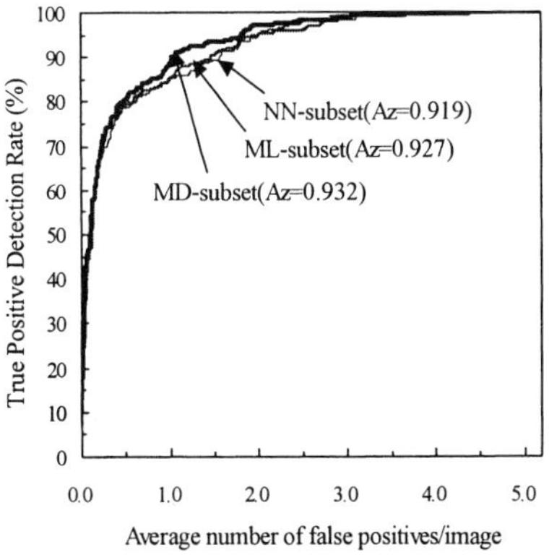

Fig. 2 Comparison of FROC curves

The numbers of features consisting of the sub-optimal feature sets for the maximum likelihood classifier and the nearest neighbor one were 19 and 25, respectively. Three sub-optimal feature sets selected by the three classifiers were analyzed. Ten features are common to the three sub-optimal feature sets and five and four of them belong to the first-order statistical feature group and the density feature one, respectively. It has been confirmed that the difference of Az's of the sub-optimal feature sets obtained by the Mahalanobis distance measure and the maximum likelihood method is not statistically significant at the 5% significance level. It has also shown that the performance of the sub-optimal feature set selected by the nearest neighbor classifier is lower than that of the others. Fig. 2 shows the comparison of ROC curves of the classifiers based on the Mahalanobis distance measure in which three sub-optimal feature sets are installed.

4. Conclusion

Feature selection for the computerized detection of mass lesions in digital mammography has been performed. Three classifiers have been examined and their sub-optimal feature sets were analyzed. Experimental results showed that ten features were common to the three sub-optimal feature sets.

This is the work in progress and a large scale experiments using much more features and experimental materials are now being performed. Their results will be shown in a near future.

This work was supported in part by the Grant-in-Aid for scientific research from the Ministry of Education, Culture, Sports, Science and Technology, Japan and the Grant-in-Aid for Cancer Research from the Ministry of Health, Labor and Welfare, Japan.

References

1. Sahiner, B., Chan, H.P., et al.: mage feature selection by a genetic algorithm: Application to classification of mass and normal breast tissue. Med. Phys. 23 (1996) 1671-1683
2. Kupinski, M.A., Giger, M.L.: Feature selection and Classifiers for the Computerized Detection of Mass Lesions in Digital Mammography. Proceedings of IEEE International Congress on Neural Networks (1997) 2460-2463
3. Tourassi, G.D., et al.: Application of the mutual information criterion for feature selection in computer-aided diagnosis. Med. Phys. 28 (2001) 2394-2402
4. Kobatake, H., Murakami, M., et al.: Computerized detection of malignant tumors on digital mammograms. IEEE Trans. on Medical Imaging 18(1999) 369-378
5. Brake, G.M., Karssemeijer, N., et al.: An automatic method to discriminate malignant masses from normal tissue in digital mammograms. Phys. Med. Biol. 45 (2000) 2843-2857
6. Wei, J., Hagihara, Y., Kobatake, H.: Detection of Cancerous Tumors on Chest X-ray Images - Candidate Detection Filter and Its Application -. Proc. of ICIP (1999) Paper No. 27AP4.2

CAD methodology transfer from 2D to 3D digital mammography for calcification enhancement and segmentation: A feasibility study

Maria Kallergi,[1] Wei Qian,[1] Jerry A. Thomas,[2] Jeffrey W. Eberhard,[3] Bernhard E.H. Claus,[3] and Robert A. Clark[1]

[1] College of Medicine and H. Lee Moffitt Cancer Center & Research Institute, University of South Florida, Tampa, Florida
kallergi@moffitt.usf.edu
[2] Uniformed Services University of the Health Sciences, Bethesda, Maryland.
[3] General Electric Global Research Center, 1 Research Circle, Niskayuna, New York.

1. Introduction

Mammography is currently the best imaging method for breast cancer screening with demonstrated reduction in mortality. Mammography, however, can be improved because 10%-30% of the cancers may be missed or not detected early enough particularly in dense breasts. New technological developments in three-dimensional (3D) x-ray imaging of the breast may offer significant improvements over the standard two-dimensional (2D) mammography by reducing the problem of superimposed tissue structures and/or by providing more details on the morphology and distribution of abnormalities. Computer aided diagnosis (CAD) algorithms developed for digitized screen/film mammography and recently expanded to 2D digital mammography are expected to face an entirely new challenge in 3D mammography, the image characteristics of which may impact CAD design and performance significantly. In this work, we examined the properties of 3D tomosynthesis phantom images and studied the potential impact of different reconstruction methodologies on CAD algorithm performance. Algorithms developed for the enhancement, segmentation, and detection of calcification clusters in 2D digital mammography were evaluated.

2. Materials and Methods

Phantom data were acquired with a full field digital mammography tomosynthesis prototype system, based on a Senographe DMR (GE Medical Systems, Milwaukee, WI) film/screen mammography system retrofitted with an amorphous silicon flat panel x-ray detector and an x-ray tube motion drive. Eleven projections were acquired with this system with effective projection angles between ±17° from the perpendicular to the digital detector. The images have a resolution of 100 μm and 12 bits per pixel, and are reconstructed to slices parallel to the detector with 100 μm in-plane resolution and 1 mm slice separation [1],[2],[3].

Reconstructed tomosynthesis slices and standard 2D projections of the CIRS Model 11A were evaluated in this work. This is a tissue equivalent phantom for mammography. It is made of an uncompressable resin material, 4.5 cm thick, with an average glandular tissue composition (50/50). The CIRS 11A contains calcification-like specks, mass-like objects of various sizes, fibers, a line pair target, and a step wedge. We focused on the analysis and evaluation of a region that contained five groups of specks from 0.196 to 0.4 mm in size. Seven reconstruction methods were used that are combinations of simple backprojection (BP), or order statistics-based backprojection (OSBP)[3] with different 1D or 2D pre-filtering steps, and are summarized in Table 1. Our interest in this paper was to evaluate the potential impact of the various reconstruction schemes on the CAD design, application, and performance for breast calcification clusters.

Table 1. Algorithm characteristics of the seven reconstructed datasets evaluated in this study.

Set #	Method	Filtering	Operation on the projections
1	BP	None	BP with bilinear interpolation
2	OSBP	None	OSBP with bilinear interpolation
3	OSBP	None	OSBP with nearest neighbour (NN) interpolation
4	Filtered BP	1D low-pass cosine	BP with bilinear interpolation
5	Filtered OSBP	1D low-pass cosine	OSBP with NN interpolation
6	Filtered OSBP	2D rotationally symm. Shepp_Logan	OSBP with NN interpolation
7	Filtered OSBP	2D rotationally symm. scale enhancing filter	OSBP with NN interpolation

All images were processed with a CAD technique recently developed for the enhancement, segmentation, and detection of calcifications from FFDM data. The FFDM CAD method evolved from a CAD algorithm for digitized screen/film mammography and, hence, a more detailed description can be found in Ref. [4]. The algorithm consists of the following modules: (a) breast area segmentation and artifact elimination, (b) multiresolution nonlinear filter bank for calcification-specific enhancement, (c) adaptive segmentation of calcification-like structures, and (d) feature extraction and neural network classification of identified clusters. The same algorithm, optimized for 2D CAD, was applied to all reconstructed slices and all cases. No modifications were done in the methodology in this study.

3. Results and Discussion

Both the enhancement and the detection algorithms generally seem to perform better on the unfiltered reconstructions (sets 1-3 in Table 1) than on the filtered reconstructions (sets 4-7), which is not consistent with the visual rating of the data. A possible explanation is that the slices in the unfiltered datasets retain the appearance of the 2D standard projections, for which the current CAD algorithms are optimized.

The enhancement stage of the algorithm performed relatively well on sets #2, 3, 4, and 5 and increased speck contrast by 3% to 10%. Performance was not consistent, however, and the algorithm generated very noisy and grainy images in sets #6 and 7. The detection algorithm showed greater variability in performance both among slices of the same set and among reconstruction methods. Note that the enhancement module in this case includes adaptive parameter selection to optimize performance. Unfiltered backprojection data (sets 1-3 in Table 1) yielded higher true positive detections and lower false positive signals than the filtered backprojection data (sets 4-7 in Table 1). Speck groups in the latter sets were only partially segmented and false speck-like signals were numerous and diffused in the entire image area.

4. Conclusions

Tomosynthesis imaging and the various reconstruction approaches generate images that differ significantly from the 2D data and from one reconstruction to the other. Application of 2D CAD algorithms to tomosynthesis datasets generally performed best for cases where the reconstructed slices resemble 2D projection data, which is inconsistent with the visual rating of the reconstructions. An entire new generation of CAD algorithms seems necessary that will be designed specifically for 3D. True 3D CAD should consider the entire data set as a whole and not individual slices alone and possibly include adaptive and standardization mechanisms to boost performance.

Acknowledgments

This study was sponsored by The Naval Medical Research and Development Command, contract nb. # 42952, funds managed by The Henry M. Jackson Foundation. Development of the tomosynthesis prototype was supported by the U.S. Army Medical Research and Materiel Command under grant DAMD 17-98-8309.

References

1. Niklason LT, Christian BT, Niklason LE, Kopans DB, Castleberry DE, Opsahl-Ong BH, et al. Digital tomosynthesis in breast imaging. Radiology 1997; 205:399-406.
2. Suryanarayanan S, Karellas A, Vedantham S, Glick SJ, D'Orsi CJ, Baker SP, and Webber RL. Comparison of tomosynthesis methods used with digital mammography. Acad. Radiol. 2000; 7:1085-1097.
3. Claus, B.E.H., Eberhard, J.W.: A New Method for 3D Reconstruction in Digital Tomosynthesis, Proc. SPIE Vol. 4684, Medical Imaging 2002 – Image Processing, San Diego, CA, 2002.
4. Qian, W., Clarke, L.P., Zheng, B., Kallergi, M and Clark, R.A.: Computer Assisted Diagnosis for Digital Mammography. IEEE Eng. Med. Biol. Magazine, 14 (1995) 561-569.

Mass detection algorithm for digital mammograms based on an adaptive thresholding technique utilizing multi-resolution processing

Satoshi Kasai [1], Daisuke Kaji [1], Akiko Kano [1],
Hiroshi Fujita [2], Takeshi Hara [2] and Tokiko Endo [3]

[1] MI Solution Group, Medical & Graphic Company, Konica Corporation, No.1 Sakura-machi, Hino-shi, Tokyo 191-8511, Japan
{Satoshi.K, D.Kaji, A.Kano}@konica.co.jp
http://www.konica.co.jp
[2] Department of Information Science, Faculty of Engineering, Gifu University, 1-1 Yanagido, Gifu-shi, Gifu 501-1193, Japan
{fujita, hara}@fjt.info.gifu-u.ac.jp
http://www.fjt.info.gifu-u.ac.jp
[3] Department of Radiology, National Hospital of Nagoya, 4-1-1 Sannomaru, Naka-ku, Nagoya-shi, Aichi 460-0001, Japan

Abstract. While developing an automated detection scheme for mass candidates in digital mammograms, the authors desired better detection of masses adjacent to skin lines from the algorithm involved, which was based on an adaptive thresholding technique, and further desired more accurate segmentation between extremely low-contrast masses and surrounding mammary-gland tissues. This study, undertaken to raise the detection rate with such masses and thus overall performance, resulted in a new detection algorithm based on multi-resolution processing, adaptive thresholding, and discriminant analysis. The algorithm provided a sensitivity of 87.7%, with 1.5 false-positive detections per image from a database of 626 digitized clinical mammograms. Eighteen masses were detected of 23 masses that had previously gone undetected. These results demonstrate the effectiveness of the proposed method.

1. Introduction

The increasing prevalence of breast cancer stresses the significance of mammography in the early detection of breast abnormalities. Breast cancer is commonly evident in the presence of masses, and a number of research groups have been developing CAD systems for their detection in digital mammograms. We have been developing an automated detection scheme based on a thresholding

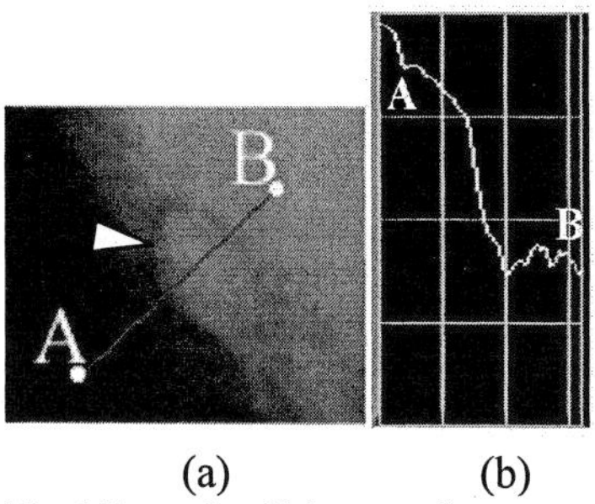

(a) (b)

Fig. 1 Example of (*a*) mass adjacent to skin line (*triangle points to mass*) and (*b*) profile of pixel values between A and B technique for mass candidates [1, 2]. In our previous method, digital mammograms were classified according to glandular conditions into four categories, and thresholds for each category were established. Candidate areas were then extracted and classified by feature analyses. However, the algorithm involved obtained a relatively low detection rate for masses adjacent to skin lines because of steep density gradients in the background trends. Figure 1(a) is an example of a mass adjacent to the skin line, while Figure 1(b) presents the pixel value profile between points A and B. The influence of the background trend on the profile is obvious here. The technique also presented difficulty in discriminating masses from surrounding normal tissue when only a slight difference of density existed between them. This study aimed at developing a new detection algorithm which would both raise the mass detection rate and provide clearer discrimination between masses and surrounding normal tissue.

2. Materials and Methods

Our algorithm has four steps: 1) multi-resolution pre-processing, 2) candidate area determination, 3) nine-parameter multivariate analyses, and 4) false-positive candidate elimination.

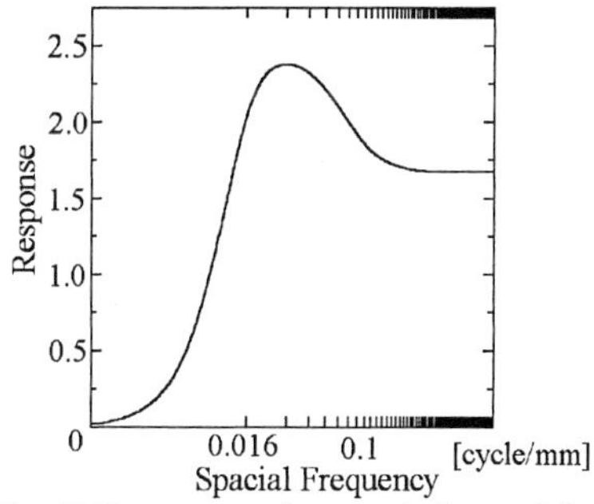

Fig. 2 Frequency characteristic used in multi-resolution pre-processing

2.1 New multi-resolution pre-processing

Pre-processing via multi-resolution processing decomposes images into plural frequency bands and enhances each frequency band independently. The algorithm enhances masses while simultaneously suppressing low-frequency components such as background trend and high-frequency components such as mammary glands. Masses targeted for detection were delineated to be from 5mm to 30mm in size, and a continuous frequency characteristic selectively enhances these masses, as illustrated in Figure 2. The lowest frequency band, corresponding to background trend, has nearly zero response. The frequency bands between 0.016 and 0.1 cycle/mm that involve potential mass candidates are enhanced so as to have a peak enhancement frequency with a response of nearly 2.5. Frequency bands below 0.016 cycle/mm and above 0.1 cycle/mm are relatively suppressed.

Multi-resolution pre-processing is presented schematically in Figure 3. In the decomposition stage, multiple unsharp images are created from the original image using a binomial filter [3], a fast filtering technique utilizing binomial

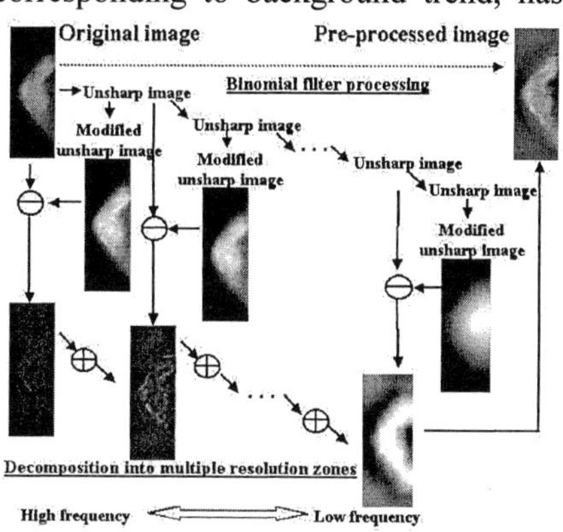

Fig. 3 Multi-resolution pre-processing

distribution characteristics. Image data are subjected to repetitive 2x2 simple averagings to obtain results equivalent to a Gaussian weighting filter. Moreover, an enhancement characteristic for each unsharp image is established based on a compensation function determined by the density and contrast of the unsharp image. Based on these smooth functions, as illustrated in Figure 4, compensation values are calculated, and the unsharp image is modified by adding those compensation values to their corresponding pixel values. A subtraction image from the modified unsharp image and the unsharp image of the adjoining frequency band is then obtained. The resulting pre-processed image is reconstructed as a summation of the subtraction images.

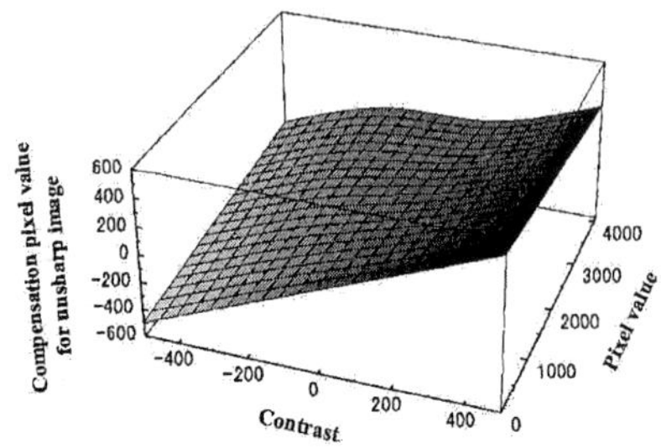

Fig. 4 Compensation function for unsharp image

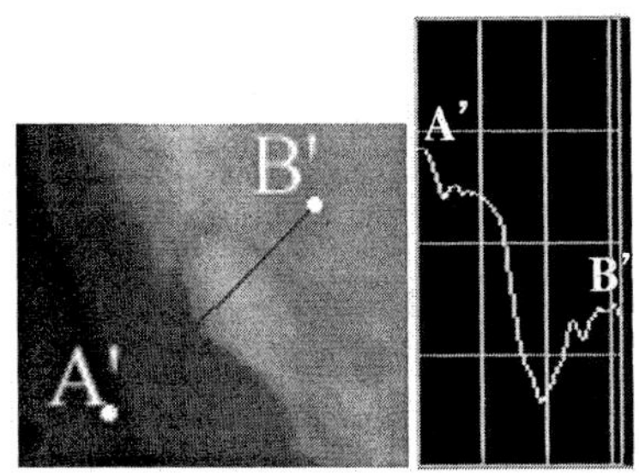

(a) (b)

Fig. 5 From original image in Fig. 1, (*a*) multi-resolution pre-processed image and (*b*) profile between A' and B'.

The enhancement characteristics employed in the proposed method enable the selective suppression of the enhancement of tissues which have high contrast and low density. Consequently, artifacts due to overshoot and undershoot are prevented along with excessive granularity in low-density regions. This process also improves the later step of false-positive candidate elimination based on feature analyses. There are differences between the features of masses with and without microcalcifications, and the process reduces differences which can produce misclassifications in multivariate analyses.

The pre-processed image in Figure 5(a) is obtained from the original image in Figure 1(a), while the profile between points A' and B' in Figure 5(b) correspond to points A and B in Figure 1(b). Compared, these images and profiles demonstrate the effective suppression of the background trend and the enhancement of the mass.

2.2 Determination of candidate areas

Binary images are created from different threshold values corresponding to the pixel values of possible masses in the pre-processed image obtained through multi-resolution pre-processing. To minimize false-negatives, the threshold values vary between 10% and 60% of the pixel value distribution within the entire breast region. To identify mass contours with precision, the steps between the thresholds are narrow. However, when there is little density difference between a mass and its surrounding normal tissue, it is often difficult for a thresholding technique to distinguish between the two. To compensate, morphological opening processing with a structure factor of 1.2 mm (radius) is used to discriminate masses from linear mammary glands.

2.3 Multivariate analysis using nine parameters

Each candidate area in a multi-resolution processed image is labeled, and multivariate feature analyses is applied using nine parameters: size, contrast, two kinds of circularity (one based on comparison with a circle, and the other based on the candidate's contour length), standard deviation, normalized average value, concentration, volume (a summation of the differences between the threshold and every pixel value within a candidate area), and representative pixel value of the candidate area (defined as a normalized threshold between the minimum and the maximum pixel values within the breast region). An appropriate threshold is determined for each parameter with a rule-based method to distinguish masses from other tissues. For instance, when a candidate's circularity value is greater than the threshold, it is classified as a mass candidate. For further false-positive elimination, discriminant analysis is applied to the nine parameters.

Seventy-nine masses and 3,066 normal tissues selected from 63 images were used to create each variance-covariance matrix. The ratio of Mahalanobis distances was modified to provide a true-positive rate of 83.8% at an average number of 1.1 false positives per image with the training data set.

2.4 Elimination of False-Positive Candidates

To eliminate false-positive candidates, co-occurrence and gray level difference matrices, with angles of 0°, 45°, 90°, and 135°, are used. Angular second moment, inverse difference moment, and entropy are calculated from the co-occurrence matrix, while contrast is calculated from the gray level difference matrix. The averaged feature over the angles is used to discriminate mass candidates from other structures.

3. Results

The sensitivity of our improved detec-tion algorithm was 87.7% (64/73), with 1.5 false-positive detections per image out of 626 digitized clinical mammograms, which included extremely subtle masses in terms of density as well as masses adjacent to skin lines. We detected 18 of 23 masses that had not been detected through our previous method. Figure 6 shows the result of an FROC analysis using the ratio of Mahalanobis distance as a parameter. It is apparent that the new algorithm outperforms the previous algorithm. Most abnormalities missed with this new algorithm are either partial-loss masses locating near chest-wall regions or architectural distortions not forming masses. System performance should rise with an already

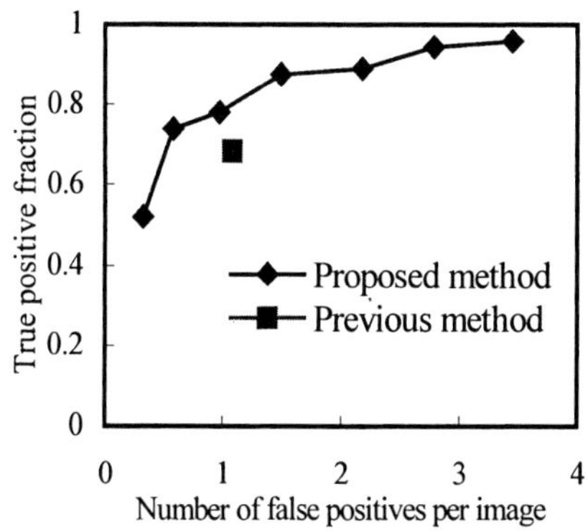

Fig. 6 Result of FROC analysis

developed algorithm dedicated to partial-loss masses locating near chest-wall regions [4, 5].

4. Conclusion

A new technique for detecting masses using an adaptive thresholding technique with multi-resolution processing was proposed. A new algorithm enabled detection of 18 of 23 masses undetected through our previous method. A pre-processing technique using newly developed multi-resolution processing is especially effective with this thresholding technique, and the new technique shows promise in such processing as template matching and filtering because background trends and high frequency components such as mammary glands also undesirably influence such processing. Finally, morphological processing enabled detection of mass candidates whose densities differ only slightly from surrounding normal tissues. In total, these results have significantly improved the overall performance of our CAD system.

Acknowledgments

This work was supported by the Ministry of Health, Labor, and Welfare of Japan under a grant-in-aid for cancer research and by the Ministry of Education, Culture, Sports, Science, and Technology of Japan under a grant-in-aid for scientific research.

References

1. Matsubara, T., Fujita, H., Endo, T., Horita, K., Kido, C., Ikeda, M., Ishigaki, T.: Development of mass detection algorithm based on adaptive thresholding technique in digital mammograms. Proc. of 3rd International Workshop on Digital Mammography, in Digital Mammography '96, Elsevier Science, Amsterdam (1996) 391-396
2. Hatanaka, Y., Hara, T., Fujita, H., Kasai, S., Endo, T., Iwase, T.: Development of an automated method for detecting mammographic masses with a partial loss of region. IEEE Trans. on Med. Imag., Vol. 20 No.12 (2001) 1209-1214
3. Jahne, B.: Digital Image Processing Concepts, Algorithms, and Scientific Applications. Springer-Verlag, Berlin (1991) 77-131
4. Kasai, S., Fujita, H., Hara, T., Endo, T., Yoshimura, H.: Development of a detection algorithm for masses around thick mammary gland on mammograms. Proc. of the 12th International Symposium and Exhibition on Computer Assisted Radiology and Surgery CAR '98 (1998) 213-218
5. Hatanaka, Y., Hara, T., Fujita, H., Kasai, S., Endo, T., Iwase, T.: An automated detection method of mammograph thick mammary gland and near chest-wall regions. Proc. of the 15th International Congress and Exhibition CARS 2001, Elsevier Science, Amsterdam (2001) 527-532

A Non-Parametric Approach to Detecting Microcalcifications

Marius George Linguraru and J. Michael Brady

University of Oxford, Medical Vision Laboratory,
Ewert House, Ewert Place, Summertown, Oxford OX2 7BZ, UK
mglin@robots.ox.ac.uk

Abstract. Microcalcifications are the first and smallest signs of breast cancer and some of the most predominant non-palpable breast lesions. We are developing an automated detection method to assist the clinician in the diagnosis process. Our method is based on processed normalised h_{int} images [2] and uses filters based on Gaussian derivative and anisotropic diffusion [4] to differentiate microcalcifications from breast tissue. Tests are performed on samples of real Standard Mammogram Format (SMF) images by a single-scale non-parametric algorithm with encouraging results. We detect 91.3% of the individual calcifications, whether isolated or clustered, which draws the attention of the radiologist to all the clusters.

1. Background

We have previously presented a new approach for mammographic image normalisation offering a quantitative representation of the breast tissue, the h_{int} [2]. There is a drawback however, the extremely noisy appearance of these images that makes their analysis very difficult. Although the signal-to-noise ratio (SNR) of the mammogram is slightly improved by the generation of h_{int} (without glare removed), by glare removal, to reduce the number of false positives (FPs), the SNR decreases drastically due to the amplification of high frequency noise. Yam *et al.* [5] introduce a de-noising algorithm, which attempts to remove radiographic mottle, a source of false positives in detecting microcalcifications. The SNR is increased and the overall appearance of the h_{int} image improved.

In our previous work, we used the scale-space and edge detection characteristics of anisotropic diffusion [4] to filter h_{int} images and highlight microcalcifications and shot-noise [3]. We used the difference in shape of a microcalcification (hill-shape with slightly blurred edges) versus noise (spikes with sharp edges) as the major property in the detection algorithm. The parametric format of anisotropic diffusion makes this process highly dependent on the fine-tuning of its input parameters. There are three parameters to be considered when attempting to blur an image using anisotropic diffusion: k - the contrast, t - the time or number of iterations and σ - the standard deviation or scale. In our previous work, we adopted a multi-scale approach in which we varied a single parameter, namely the number of iterations [3]. This is undesirable in clinical practice.

2. Method and Results

Since t is not an image characteristic, we choose to vary k, which is image dependent Now we can iterate the blurring filter for a constant number of iterations over the image, but this raises the question: how do we choose the right contrast parameter to determine the values of the eigenvalues? [3].

To solve this, we have designed an adaptive Gaussian derivative filter. The result of applying this filter to a de-noised, glare-removed, h_{int} image results in a gradient-map that highlights suspicious regions as regards microcalcification detection. Furthermore, the same filter outputs the value of k for the subsequent diffusion. We apply the anisotropic diffusion filter [3] to the h_{int} image with the corresponding value of k for a fixed number of iterations. Note the emphasised outline of the microcalcifications, while most of the background is seriously blurred. A new filtering step is introduced at this stage to actually depict the microcalcifications in the processed image. It is based on the same computation as the anisotropic diffusion, but also incorporates some adaptive thresholding suited to the image characteristics and the properties of microcalcifications. This last filtering process concludes with a black-and-white map of detection (BWMD), as in Fig.1.

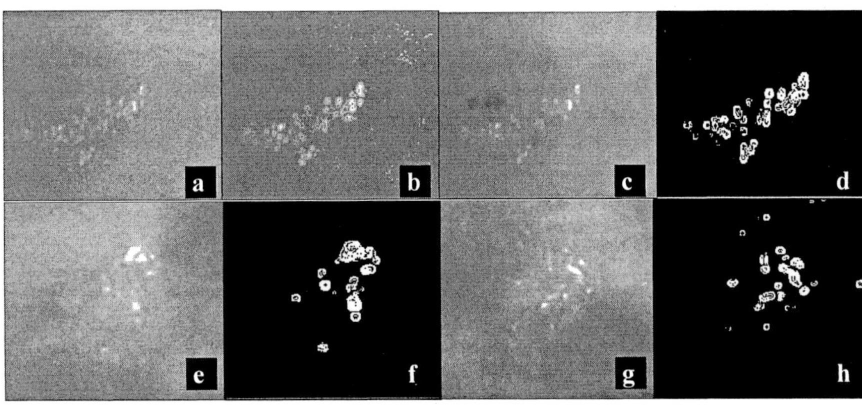

Fig. 1. (a) The h_{int} image (contrast enhanced) of a microcalcification cluster; (b) the corresponding gradient map of the image; (c) the diffused image of (a) after using the computed value of k; (d) the corresponding BWDM of the image; (e), (f), (g) and (h) show two more examples of detection.

We applied the method to a database comprising 35 samples of digital mammograms at a resolution of 50μm with the size of 500x500 pixels. The h_{int} images were in a 32-float format and contained a total of 23 isolated microcalcifications previously labeled by an experienced radiologist. The overall ratio of detection is 91.3% true positives (TPs) for a number of 0.32 FPs per image.

One source of FPs in our detection algorithm is the curvilinear structures, due to the relatively high contrast they have against the average background. In Fig.2. we show an image where our algorithm detected an FP. To avoid these erroneous results, we removed the CLS from the images with FPs [1] and then applied the algorithm again on the CLS-free h_{int} images. The number of FPs/image was reduced to 0.2.

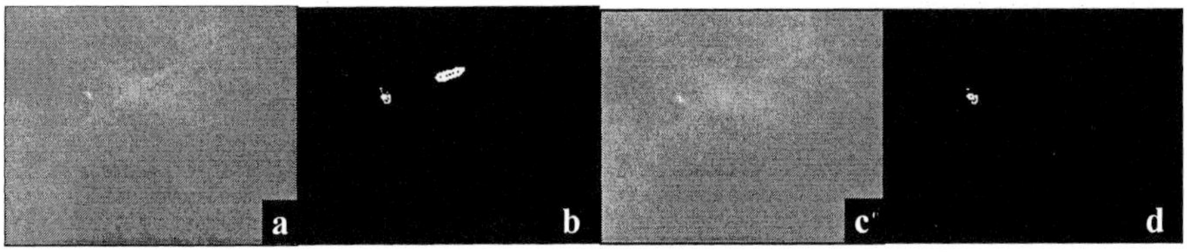

Fig. 2. (a) An h_{int} image (contrast enhanced) containing one subtle microcalcifications and a prominent CLS; (b) the BWMD of image (a) showing an FP; (c) the image (a) after CLS removal; (d) the BWMD of image (b) with the correct detection of the microcalcification.

4. Discussions and Conclusion

The spread of the detected clusters is well defined in the BWMD, although some of the subtle calcifications are missed. We must therefore refine the algorithm so that will be more sensitive to local rather than global variability. A major source of errors can be the breast edge and the shot-noise. The solution would be the breast edge correction together with bringing the background to a h_{int} value similar to that of the average breast tissue and the local interpolation at shot-noise location. Although we have not tested any image of a breast during HRT treatment, we expect similar difficulties in such cases.

We presented an automated method to detect microcalcifications in digital mammography based on a series of subsequent filters and computations designed to output for the user a map of detection showing the regions where salts of calcium are detected. The method uses the facilities and improvements in medical image normalisation offered by the h_{int} image representations. The results we showed are generated by a single-scale non-parametric algorithm. A multi-scale approach would obviously improve our results considerably, but the scope of our work is to develop a robust detection method that could be easily used in clinical conditions. This requires minimal or no intervention from the clinician in the algorithm settings.

References

1. Evans, C.J.: Detecting and Removing Curvilinear Structures from Mammograms. Internal Report, Department of Engineering Science, University of Oxford (2001)
2. Highnam, R.P. Brady, J.M.: Mammographic Image Analysis. Kluwer Academic Publishers, Dordrecht Boston London (1999)
3. Linguraru, M.G. Brady, J.M. Yam, M.: Filtering hint Images for the Detection of Microcalcifications. In Niessen, W. Viergever, M. (eds.): Medical Image Computing and Computer-Assisted Intervention 2001, Lecture Notes in Computer Science, Vol. 2208. Springer-Verlag, Berlin Heidelberg New York (2001) 629-636
4. Weickert, J.: Anisotropic Diffusion in Image Processing. B.G. Teubner, Stuttgart (1998)
5. Yam, M. Brady, J.M. Highnam, R.P. English, R.: Denoising h_{int} Surfaces: a Physics-based Approach. In Medical Image Computing and Computer-Assisted Intervention 1999, Springer-Verlag, Berlin Heidelberg New York (1999) 227-234

Detection of Microcalcifications using SMF

Marius George Linguraru, Michael Brady and Margaret Yam[1]

University of Oxford, Medical Vision Laboratory,
Ewert House, Ewert Place, Summertown, Oxford OX2 7BZ, UK
{mglin,jmb}@robots.ox.ac.uk

Abstract. We have reported previously [10,6] two algorithms for detecting microcalcifications that operate either on Highnam and Brady's [3] h_{int} representation or the latter's presentation as an image: SMF = Standardised Mammogram Form. We introduce a third such method that applies to SMF a model of human foveal image processing. Comparative analysis with [10,6] shows significantly enhanced results for the new method.

1. Introduction

The h_{int} model developed by Highnam and Brady [3] assumes that the attenuation coefficients of normal and cancerous tissue are very similar but that they are both significantly different from fat. The h_{int} generation algorithm then produces a quantitative representation of the amount (in millimetres) of non-fatty tissue at each pixel. It assumes that the percentage of calcifications in a mammogram is insignificantly small. Highnam and Brady [3] show that the h_{int} representation eliminates the specific image acquisition parameters (e.g. exposure time). If "standard" parameters are chosen, the h_{int} representation can be displayed as an image, which is called the Standard Mammogram Form (SMF) of the mammogram. This article compares three algorithms that operate upon the h_{int} representation (or the SMF) to detect microcalcifications. Two of these algorithms have been developed previously in our group [8,10,6]; the third is a refinement of [6] and is introduced here. Using ROC analysis, we demonstrate the superiority of this latter algorithm. First, however, we recall the main features of the two previously published algorithms.

Yam *et al.*'s algorithm [10] aims to find image locations where the assumption of no calcification appears not to hold. It does this by exploiting two ideas: (a) calcifications have an x-ray attenuation that is about 26 times higher than that of normal tissue; so in the h_{int} representation, microcalcifications (interpreted initially as normal tissue) tower above the surrounding landscape; and (b) the estimated volume of the interesting tissue corresponding to the region where a calcification is detected must exceed the estimated volume of the 3-D model of that region. The h_{int} representation is relatively noisy, and so Yam's algorithm incorporates a Wiener filter that smooths the representation as it attempts to assign pixels to noise or calcification.

---

[1] Mirada Solutions Ltd, Mill Street, Oxford OX2 0JX, UK http://www.mirada-solutions.com

See [10] for details of the algorithm. Yam *et al.* [8,10] initially tested their method on isolated macrocalcifications and microcalcifications. They obtained a detection rate of 95% TPs with 0.38 FPs per image for a set of 93 mammogram samples digitised at 50 microns containing 92 isolated microcalcifications. Further tests lead to a rate of 93% TPs with 0.16 FP cluster per image for a set of 83 mammograms with a total of 95 microcalcification clusters.

Of course, the Wiener filter [9] may cause both small spots of noise and very fine microcalcifications to be overlooked. An alternative filtering method should be expected to outperform the existing one. To this end, in our previous work [5,6], we studied filtering the SMF using anisotropic diffusion [7]. In summary, our previous method used three filters in sequence: (i) an adaptive Gaussian derivative filter, which generates a gradient map and, more important, the value of contrast needed for anisotropic diffusion; (ii) an anisotropic diffusion filter, which will enhance certain suspicious regions based on the previously computed contrast value; and (iii) additional statistical analysis to discriminate between microcalcifications and the rest of the image. These three logical steps are in fact integrated into a single computational process. We applied initially the method to a database comprising 35 samples of digital mammograms at a resolution of 50μm with the size of 500x500 pixels. The h_{int} images were in a 32-float format and contained a total of 23 isolated microcalcifications previously labelled by an experienced radiologist. The collection of images was designed to cover a wide range of possible cases of microcalcifications, some subtle, some obvious, some large, and some small. Initially, the overall ratio of detection was 91.3% TPs for a number of 0.32 FPs per image. We noted that a few regions of noise or dense breast tissue were incorrectly detected as microcalcifications. Interestingly, one source of FPs in our detection algorithm are overlaps in CLS. When we removed the CLS from the images with FPs [1] and then applied the algorithm again on the CLS-free h_{int} images. The number of FPs was reduced from the initial number of 0.32 per image to 0.2. Note that in this form, the algorithm does not exploit knowledge of the attenuation characteristics of calcium.

2. "Foveal" Segmentation

In our most recent development, the detection of microcalcifications is completed by a foveal segmentation based on the algorithm of Heucke *et al.* [2]. We initially remove the glare, shot-noise [4] and CLSs [1] from the SMF image. Having the SMF_{noCLS} image, we compute a set of mean values using masks for the inner area, its neighbourhood and background. The histogram of the inner surface provides a mean of the object (μ_O), while the histogram of the entire image gives the mean of the background (μ_B). The mean in a neighbourhood (μ_N) is defined as the weighted sum of intensities depending on the scale of the mask. The perceivable contrast C is:

$$C = \frac{|\mu_o - \mu_N|}{\mu_N} \tag{1}$$

Based on [2] we compute C_{min} (2), where μ_A=0.923· μ_N + 0.077· μ_B [2]. The segmentation parameters are set-up automatically based on the value of k, which is image-adapted. We found that $c_w = \sqrt{k}/200$ gave stable results. SMF regions whose contrast $C > C_{min}$ an adaptable threshold are marked as microcalcifications:

$$C_{\min} = \begin{cases} \frac{c_w}{\mu_N}\left(0.0808 + \sqrt{\mu_A}\right)^2, & \mu_A \ge \mu_N \\ \frac{c_w}{\mu_N}\left(0.808 + \sqrt{\frac{\mu_N^2}{\mu_A}}\right)^2, & \mu_N > \mu_A \end{cases} \tag{2}$$

The overall process flow (k is the contrast for anisotropic diffusion) is:

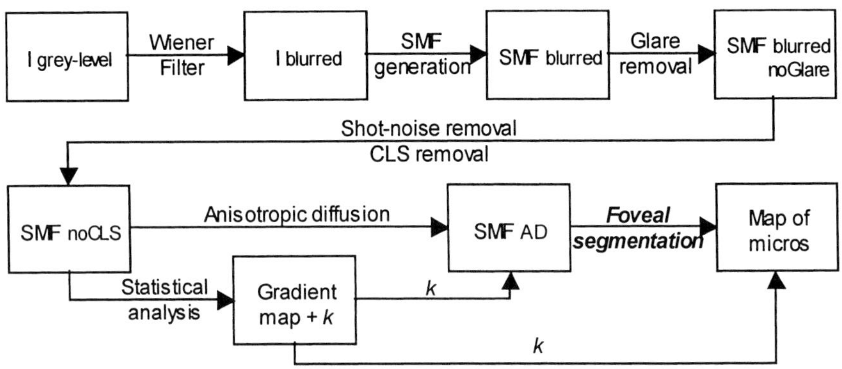

Fig. 1. Process flow to detect microcalcification in Standard Mammogram Format images.

3. Comparative Results

Figure 2 shows a typical result on some mammogram samples containing microcalcification clusters. We present, along the original contrast-enhanced SMF sample, the detection maps of the Physics-based Approach, Statistical Analysis and Foveal Approach. We used a database of 102 samples of digital SMF images, 78 of them contain 1 to 3 clusters per image, while 24 are normal mammogram samples. There are a total of 98 clusters of microcalcification. All images were digitised at a resolution of 50μm and have sizes under 1500x1500. Figure 3 shows the comparative Receiver Operating Characteristic (ROC) curves of the tested detection methods.

4. Conclusion

Adding adaptive contrast segmentation based on human foveal processing significantly enhances the detection of microcalcifications. We continue to develop the algorithm, incorporating additional knowledge of x-ray attenuation.

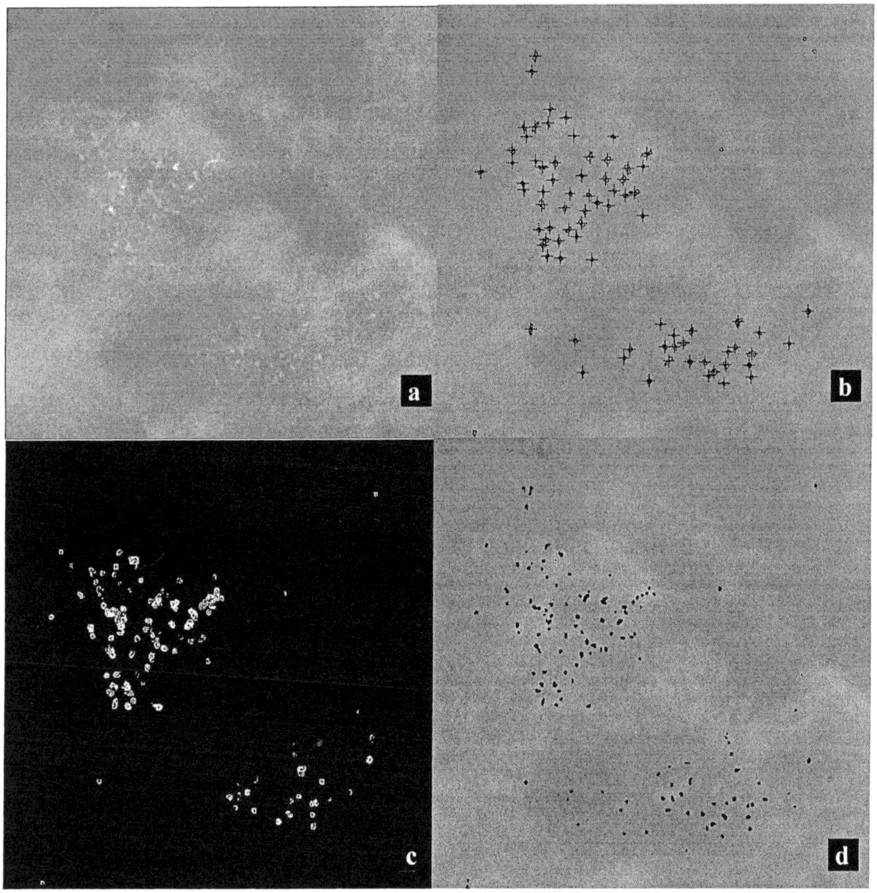

Fig. 2. (a) The original SMF; (b) the detection map of the Physics-based Approach; (c) the BWMD of the Statistical Analysis; (c) the detection map of the Foveal Approach.

References

1. Evans, C.J.: Detecting and Removing Curvilinear Structures from Mammograms. Internal Report, Department of Engineering Science, University of Oxford (2001)
2. Heucke, L. Knaak, M. Orglmeister, R.: A New Image Segmentation Method Based on Human Brightness Perception and Foveal Adaptation. In: IEEE Signal Processing Letters, Vol. 7, No. 6 (2000) 129-131
3. Highnam, R.P. Brady, J.M.: Mammographic Image Analysis. Kluwer Academic Publishers, Dordrecht Boston London (1999)
4. Highnam, R.P. Brady, J.M. English, R.: Detecting Film-Screen Artifacts in Mammography using a Model-Based Approach. In: IEEE Transactions in Medical Imaging, Vol. 18 (1999) 1016-1024

5. Linguraru, M.G. Brady, J.M. Yam, M.: Filtering hint Images for the Detection of Microcalcifications. In Niessen, W. Viergever, M. (eds.): Medical Image Computing and Computer-Assisted Intervention 2001, Lecture Notes in Computer Science, Vol. 2208. Springer-Verlag, Berlin Heidelberg New York (2001) 629-636
6. Linguraru, M.G. Brady, J.M.: A Non-Parametric Approach to Detecting Microcalcifications. In International Workshop on Digital Mammography, Lecture Notes in Computer Science, Springer-Verlag, Berlin Heidelberg New York (2002), to be published
7. Weickert, J.: Anisotropic Diffusion in Image Processing. B.G. Teubner, Stuttgart (1998)
8. Yam, M. Brady, J.M. Highnam, R.P. English, R.: Detecting Calcifications in Mammograms using the h_{int} Representation. In: Computer Assisted Radiology and Surgery, Elsevier (1999) 373-377
9. Yam, M. Brady, J.M. Highnam, R.P. English, R.: Denoising h_{int} Surfaces: a Physics-based Approach. In Medical Image Computing and Computer-Assisted Intervention 1999, Springer-Verlag, Berlin Heidelberg New York (1999) 227-234
10. Yam, M., Brady, J.M. Highnam, R.P. Behrenbruch, C.P. English, R. Kita, Y.: Three-dimensional Reconstruction of Microcalcification Clusters from Two Mammographic Views. In IEEE Trans Med Imaging, Vol. 20 No. 6 (2001) 479-489

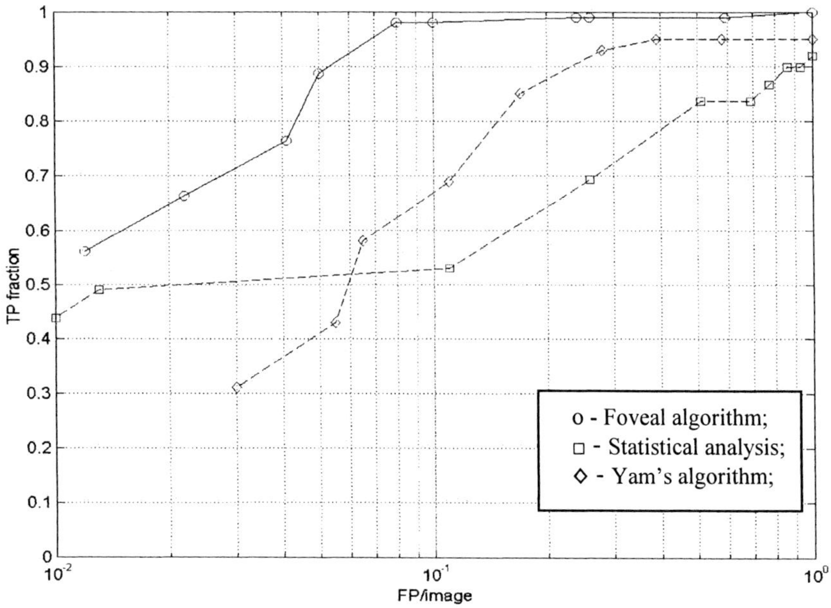

Fig. 3. The ROC curves of the three microcalcification-detection methods, where we notice the better performance of the Foveal Approach.

Temporal Mass Detection

Marius George Linguraru, Konstantinos Marias and Michael Brady

University of Oxford, Medical Vision Laboratory,
Ewert House, Ewert Place, Summertown, Oxford OX2 7BZ, UK
mglin@robots.ox.ac.uk

Abstract. We present a method to prompt a clinician to "suspicious" dense regions in temporal mammogram sequences. The particular context that we envisage is mammogram screening, when the clinician compares the most recent mammogram to previous ones in order to detect significant changes. The method uses anisotropic filtering as a pre-processing step in order to significantly reduce the number of candidate masses, while preserving the important anatomical information about each mass. The method has already been tested on 15 temporal pairs, where pathology has been diagnosed in the most recent image.

1 Method

The method we propose comprises two steps that pre-process the original mammogram prior to the detection of dense regions: mammogram registration and anisotropic diffusion of the registered mammograms. The basic assumption in our work is that masses appear as regions of slightly enhanced brightness. First, the temporal pair is registered using a mammogram registration method developed in our laboratory [2]. Briefly, it is a three-stage process: (i) the images are aligned based on their boundaries using thin-plate spline interpolation; (ii) internal regions of dense tissue are located using a wavelet-based segmentation algorithm and these refine the registration; (iii) a regulariser is used to account for possible inaccuracies in the selection of the internal landmarks. In this work, registration aims to aid mass detection by comparing “suspicious” regions in the registered mammogram sequence, where false positives can be reduced by visually inspecting the correspondence of “temporal prompts”. In order to detect only the most important features of the mammogram, the images are processed using an adaptive anisotropic diffusion-based filter, which enhances the suspicious features in mammograms [1]. The parameters of the filter are computed from a statistical analysis of the image gradient and the mammogram is anisotropically blurred. We find that a large number of suspicious areas become insignificant for subsequent texture classification.

Finally, a texture-based classifier segments the image in different tissue types and the “denser” class is used to automatically prompt to “suspicious” regions. Currently, we detect 4 classes corresponding to: (A) very dense tissue (pectoral muscle and some regions of breast parenchyma); (B) dense tissue, includes all the remaining parts of the dense parenchymal cone (fibrotic stromal tissue and glandular tissue); (C) fatty tissue, represents the fatty background of the mammogram (Wolfe’s “normal” involuted breast patterns [4]); (D) fatty breast edge, a homogenous, low-intensity region near the breast edge. A candidate mass is expected to appear either as a "very dense" or "dense" tissue region according to the above classification depending on the presence of the pectoral muscle and on the local density variations. Density variations around an iso-dense contour in the denser classes indicate the presence of abnormalities, namely tumours. These classes are shown in more detail in the results session.

2 Results

Figures 1 and 2 show typical results on both the original and the diffused mammogram pair. Diffusion significantly reduces the very dense regions Where Figure 1 prompts numerous density variations in the image, Figure 2 shows more homogenous regions and reduces dramatically the number of candidate tumours. Table 1 shows preliminary results in mass detection (true positives and false positives for the "suspicious" regions detected) in 15 temporal pairs. We first show the improvement in detection by including anisotropic diffusion as a pre-processing step. In addition the same Table shows the potential improvement in mass detection by visually inspecting the generated prompts in the mammogram sequence (a prompt in the current mammogram is classified as a mass if there is no similar region in the previous one). However, this further improvement is based only on the visual inspection of temporal "prompts". We aim to incorporate this automatic comparison as an automatic step in future work.

Table 1. True positives and false positives in 15 pairs of mammograms (a mass has previously been diagnosed in each pair).

Temporal comparison of "prompts" (visual)	Anisotropic diffusion pre-processing	True positives	False positives
No	No	15	59
No	Yes	15	13
Yes	No	15	17
Yes	Yes	15	6

3 Conclusion

Anisotropic diffusion can reduce significantly the number of FPs in mass detection based on registered temporal mammogram. Visual inspection of prompts in mammogram sequences (Table 1) indicates that a further improvement can be achieved. Future work will concentrate in developing an automatic method that would enable the temporal comparison of prompts detected in any mammogram of a particular registered patient-sequence.

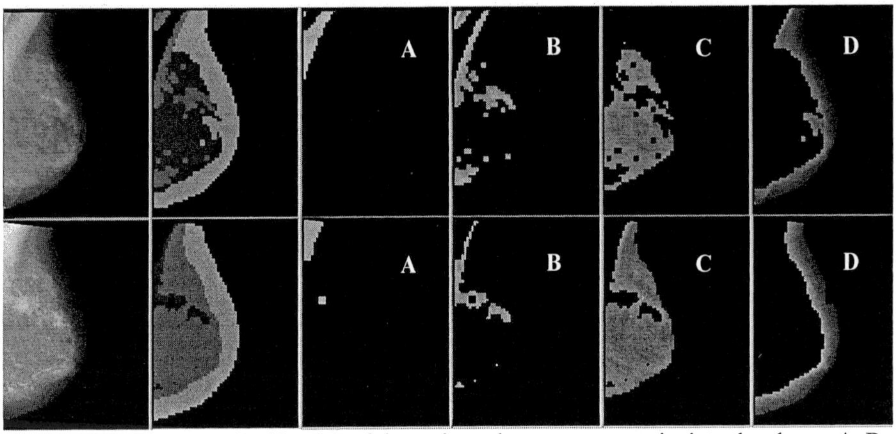

Fig. 1. and 2. Texture classification of the registered mammogram pairs into the classes A, B, C, D. The above set of images show the results before the anisotropic filtering, while the next set of images show the same but after diffusion. The number of candidate masses is reduced.

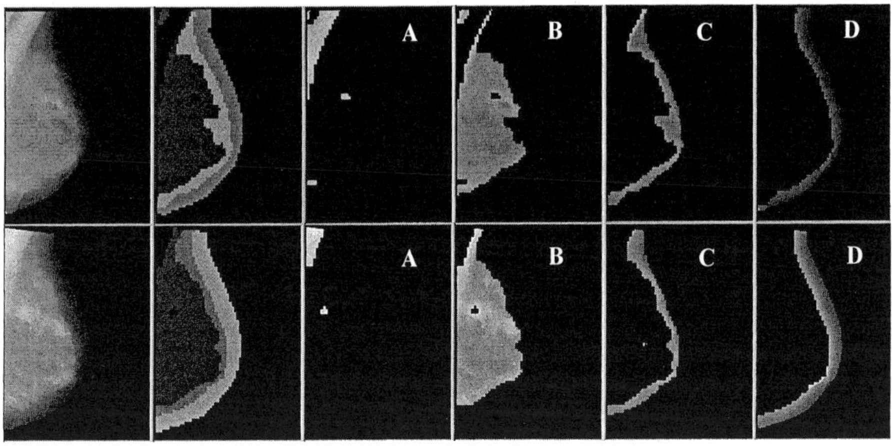

References

1. Linguraru, M.G. Brady, J.M. Yam, M.: Filtering h_{int} Images for the Detection of Microcalcifications. In Niessen, W. Viergever, M. (eds.): Medical Image Computing and Computer-Assited Intervention 2001, Lecture Notes in Computer Science, Vol. 2208. Springer-Verlag, Berlin Heidelberg New York (2001) 629-636
2. Marias, K. Behrenbruch, C.P. Brady, M. Parbhoo, S. Seifalian, A.: Multi-Scale Landmark Selection for Improved Registration of Temporal Mammograms. In Yaffe, M.J. (ed.): International Workshop on Digital Mammography 2000, Medical Physics Publishing, Madison (2000) 580-586
3. Weickert, J.: Anisotropic Diffusion in Image Processing. B.G. Teubner, Stuttgart (1998)
4. Wolfe, J.N.: Breast Patterns as an Index of Risk for Developing Breast Cancer. American Journal of Roentgenology, 126 (1976) 1130-1139

Automated detection of architectural distortions on mammograms

Tomoko Matsubara [a], Daisuke Yamazaki [b], Takeshi Hara [b], Hiroshi Fujita [b]
Satoshi Kasai [c], Tokiko Endo [d] and Takuji Iwase [e]

[a] Nagoya Bunri University, 365 Maeda, Inazawa-cho, Inazawa-shi 492-8520, Japan
tomoko@nagoya-bunri.ac.jp
[b] Gifu University, 1-1 Yanagido, Gifu-shi 501-1193, Japan
[c] Konica Corporation, 1 Sakura-machi, Hino-shi 191-8511, Japan
[d] National Hospital of Nagoya, 4-1-1 Sannomaru, Naka-ku, Nagoya-shi 460-0001, Japan
[e] Aichi Cancer Center Hospital, 1-1 Kanokoden Chikusa-ku, Nagoya-shi 464-8681, Japan

Abstract. The architectural distortion is a very important finding in interpreting breast cancers as well as microcalcification and mass on mammograms. In despite of the importance for detecting architectural distortions, no algorithms for detecting them have been reported. The purpose of this study is to develop a new detection method for focal retraction that is one of architectural distortions around skinline. In order to extract the thick mammary gland regions, binarization technique is performed. The top-hat processing based on morphological operators is applied to determine the suspect depressed regions around skinline. The false positives are eliminated by the features of their sizes and positions. After applying this technique to 51 digitized mammograms, the detection sensitivity was 92% with 3.8 false positives per image. It is concluded that this technique is effective to detect the architectural distortion.

1. Introduction

The architectural distortion is a very important finding in interpreting breast cancers as well as microcalcification and mass on mammograms. In addition, it sometimes appears at the previous stage of obvious mass shadow. It is more difficult for physicians to detect architectural distortion than microcalcification and mass[1]. In despite of the necessity of computer-aided diagnosis system to detect architectural distortions, few algorithms for detecting them have been reported.

The distorted areas can be classified into two typical types existing around skinline and within mammary glandular tissues. The purpose of this study is to develop a new detection method for the area of architectural distortion existing

This research was supported in part by a grant from Research Foundation for the Electrotechnology of Chubu, in part by the Ministry of Health, Labour, and Welfare under a Grand-In-Aid for Cancer Research and in part by the Ministry of Education, Culture, Sports, Science and Technology under a Grand-In-Aid for Scientific Research.

around skinline in order to detect breast cancer at the early stage.

2. Methods

The contours of normal mammary glandular tissue around skinline are tend to be smooth lines, on the other hand, those of distorted ones are depressed (Fig. 1).

Figure 2 shows an automated extraction flow diagram for architectural distortions existing around skinline. Each step in this scheme is explained below.

Firstly, the skinline and the border of pectoral muscle on the digital mammogram are automatically extracted. The dynamic-range compression technique is carried out within the breast regions in order to remove the background density from the breast thickness. Secondly, the thick mammary gland regions are extracted by using binarization technique and local discriminant analysis. The threshold at this process is

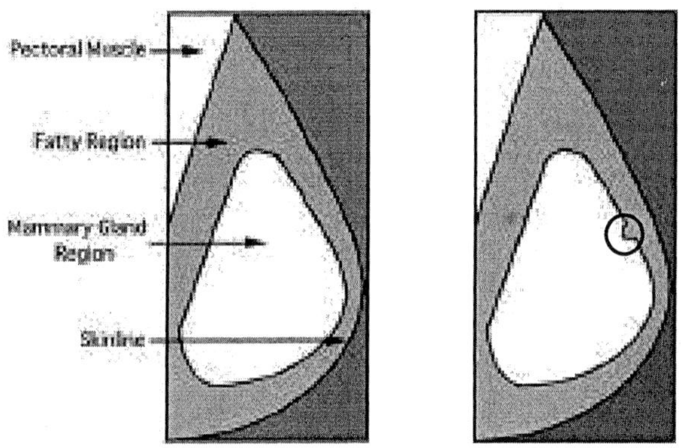

(a) (b)

Fig. 1. Simplified illustrations of (a) normal image and (b) abnormal image with architectural distortion (focal retraction) around skinline indicated by a circle.

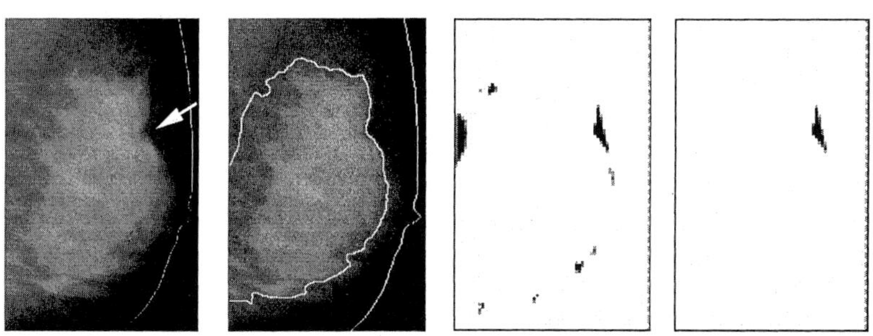

(a) (b) (c) (d)

Fig. 2. Extraction flow diagram for architectural distortion existing around skinline. (a) An original image with distorted area indicated by an arrow. (b) Outline of thick mammary gland region. (c) Candidates extracted by top-hat processing (black region). (d) Elimination of false positives by the features of their sizes and positions. The residual area is true positive.

determined by referring to the density of pectoral muscle to avoid the mis-configuration of the threshold caused by the density difference of radiographed conditions on mammograms[2]. Thirdly, the top-hat processing based on morphological operators[3] is applied to determine the suspect depressed areas. The smoothed image is obtained by the closing of the binary image by structuring elements. In our experiments, we have chosen linear structures in seven direction whose angles are 45, 60, 75, 90, 105, 120 and 135 degrees to fit to the shape of outlines. The difference image of smoothed and binary ones contains the candidates of distorted areas. Finally, the candidates whose sizes are small or which exist out of skinline are eliminated as false positives. The thresholds for sizes depend on the amount of fibroglandular breast tissue because the size of retracted area in dense image is smaller than one in fatty image.

The residuals are indicated by circles as "true" candidates of architectural distortions.

3. Result

Our image database with architectural distortions consisted of 51 cases. As a result, the sensitivity was 92% with 3.8 false-positive detections per image by our proposed method.

The sensitivity by using one linear structure whose angle was 90 degrees was 82%. However, it improved 92% by using linear structures in seven directions. It is possible to detect independence of the angles of retractions by using them.

4. Conclusions

We have developed the automated detection methods of architectural distortions on mammograms based on the top-hat processing. It is concluded that our approach is effective because the performance shows high sensitivity. For the future work, it is necessary to decrease the number of false positives and to add the detection algorithm for architectural distortions within mammary glandular tissues.

References

1. Hatanaka, Y., Matsubara, T., Hara, T., Shinohara, N., Fukuoka, D., Fujita, H., Endo, T.: A comparison between physicians' interpretation and a CAD system's cancer detection by using a mammogram database in a physicians' self-learning course. Jpn. J. Radiol. Technol. 58 (2002) 375-382 [in Japanese]
2. Matsubara, T., Yamazaki, D., Fujita, H., Hara, T., Iwase, T. Endo Y.: An automated classification method for mammograms based on evaluation of fibroglandular breast tissue density. In: Yaffe, J. (ed.): Proceedings of IWDM 2000 -5th International Workshop on Digital Mammography, Medical Physics Publishing (2000) 737-741
3. Kobatake, H.: Morphology, Corona Publishing, Tokyo (1996) [in Japanese]

Detection of Microcalcification Clusters in Digital Mammogram Images

Kristin J. McLoughlin, Philip J. Bones and Peter D. Kovesi

Department of Electrical and Computer Engineering, University of Canterbury,
Private Bag 4800, Christchurch, New Zealand
p.bones@elec.canterbury.ac.nz

Abstract: Microcalcification clusters appear as an early sign of breast cancer and play an important role in interpreting mammograms. Progress is reported towards an automated computer aided detection (CAD) system for clustered microcalcifications utilizing two image feature parameters: local contrast and shape. The use of a shape parameter is necessary to distinguish thin patches of connective tissue from microcalcifications. A deterministic relaxation scheme segments the mammogram into calcification, connective tissue and background. Line connectivity is introduced to reduce the detection of false positive microcalcifications within connective tissue regions. The CAD system presented is compared to one reported by Karssemeijer in 1992. Results show similar true positive detection rates with an improvement in the false positive detection rate from 1.125 to 0.3 false positives per image.

1. Introduction

The identification of microcalcifications is an important early radiological sign of breast cancer. Computer aided methods for detecting clustered microcalcifications have been investigated using a variety of techniques [1], [2], [3], [4]. The CAD scheme presented in this paper uses three different features for representing mammogram data: a shape parameter and the local contrast at two different spatial resolutions. A distinction between faint microcalcifications and connective tissue can only be made on the basis of shape, as these two structures have similar contrast. Karssemeijer's [5] noise equalization technique provides the two local contrast images for this system and a method of 'phase congruency' [6] is used for the shape parameter. These feature parameters are input to a deterministic relaxation scheme, which segments the mammograms into three categories: connective tissue, calcification and background. A random field model represents the contextual relations between pixel labels. Long range interaction is introduced to express the fact that calcifications occur in clusters, and a connectivity parameter is included to reduce the incidence of false microcalcification detections within connective tissue features.

Section 2 outlines the phase congruency shape parameter technique and section 3 describes the deterministic relaxation scheme. Segmentation results for the CAD system described in this paper and a CAD system proposed by Karssemeijer [7] are compared in section 4. Finally, conclusions are drawn in section 5.

2. Phase Congruency Shape Parameter

Wavelet filters are employed to obtain frequency information local to a point in an image. Calculation of the phase congruency shape parameter requires that the local frequency and phase information of the image is preserved. In this case linear-phase log Gabor filters are used [8]. The 1-D log Gabor filters are extended to 2-D by applying a Gaussian spreading function with respect to the polar angle. To detect features at all orientations the filter bank is designed to tile the frequency plane uniformly with six orientations and five scales [9].

Convolving an image with even and odd symmetric log Gabor filters produces an array of response vectors, $R_{i,s,o}$ that are a function of the pixel position i, scale s, and orientation o. The response vectors are summed over all scales to estimate a local energy $E_{i,o}$ and phase $\phi_{i,o}$. The combination over scale ensures there is no bias towards features of a particular size.

The purpose of the shape parameter is to distinguish linear features (connective tissue) from blob-like structures (microcalcifications). $E_{i,o}$ and $\phi_{i,o}$ are combined using

$$U_{i,o} = \Re(E_{i,o}) - \left|\Im(E_{i,o})\right|, \tag{1}$$

which highlights pixels that are indicative of a positive pulse in the current orientation, corresponding to the cross section of a linear or blob-like feature.

Various other parameters are calculated using the results from Equation 1,

$$X_i = \underset{o}{\sigma}(U_{i,o}), \quad M_i = \max_o(U_{i,o}), \quad OM_i = \arg\max_o(U_{i,o}) \,. \tag{2}$$

Orientation OM_i is perpendicular to the major axis of a linear feature. The value of $U_{i,o}$ perpendicular to OM_i is a distinguishing factor between linear and blob-like structures. Let us call this parameter P_i.

The phase congruency shape parameter is calculated as,

$$L_i = (M_i - P_i)X_i, \tag{3}$$

which utilizes the results from Equations 1 and 2 to highlight connective tissue regions while suppressing microcalcifications.

3. Deterministic Relaxation Scheme

The deterministic relaxation scheme for the detection of microcalcifications in digital mammogram images is based on the use of Bayesian techniques and the application of a Markov random field model. Starting from an initial segmentation, the labeling is optimized by applying an iterative rule for updating pixel labels. The image data is represented by three different features: a shape parameter and the local contrast at two different spatial resolutions. Each feature is thought to be important in distinguishing microcalcifications from other structures. A principal advantage of this approach is that all information available, i.e., the image data, the current labeling, and prior beliefs, is exploited simultaneously.

The digital mammogram images are segmented into three categories: connective tissue, calcification and background. A Markov random field model represents the contextual relations between pixel labels. An Iterated Conditional Modes (ICM) algorithm updates the labels by choosing the most probable label given the current estimate of the rest of the labeling and the data. Visiting each site at random the iterative process converges to a local maximum. The ICM method can only be applied when a good initial estimate of the segmentation is available. Such an estimate is obtained by maximum likelihood (ML) of the data without considering neighborhood pixels labels. Once the initial labeling is calculated a nearest neighbor term is included, which is restricted to the class of pairwise interaction models (8 nearest neighbors). The parameter modeling the interaction between calcification and connective tissue labels is chosen high to disallow patches consisting of a mixture of these two classes. Interaction with the background class is chosen small to allow calcifications consisting of only a few pixels to survive if they are bright enough.

Apart from the nearest neighbour term of the model, a long range interaction term is introduced to permit the fact that calcifications occur in clusters. Faint isolated spots should not be interpreted as microcalcifications. For the long range interaction model all sites within a distance of 60 pixels (2.5mm) are considered.

The final parameter in the random field model is connectivity, which is introduced in conjunction with the shape parameter to reduce the false positive microcalcification detections. This parameter utilizes the fact that pixels classified as connective tissue are likely to occur along connected lines within the image. For each pixel i a linear region of orientation P_i and length $2l$ is determined. The fraction of connective tissue labels within the linear region provides a likelihood for the current pixel being within a connective tissue feature. The value of l is set to 20 pixels (0.8mm).

4. Results

A database was constructed by selecting cases from the Digital Database for Screening Mammography (DDSM) [10]. The data set chosen consists of 48 digitized mammograms with 38 microcalcification clusters. All mammograms were scanned at Massachusetts General Hospital on a DBA digitizer at 42 micron sampling resolution and 16 bits per pixel. A subimage (500 x 500 pixels) from each digitized mammogram was used to obtain the results presented.

A well known CAD scheme developed by Karssemeijer [7] for the detection of microcalcification clusters was compared to the scheme presented in this paper. Both techniques have been applied to all mammogram images in the data set. Figure 1 shows two mammogram subimages along with the calcification segmented images resulting from both CAD schemes. In all instances the individual true calcifications within the clusters were detected correctly however for Karssemeijer's technique many more false positive detections occurred.

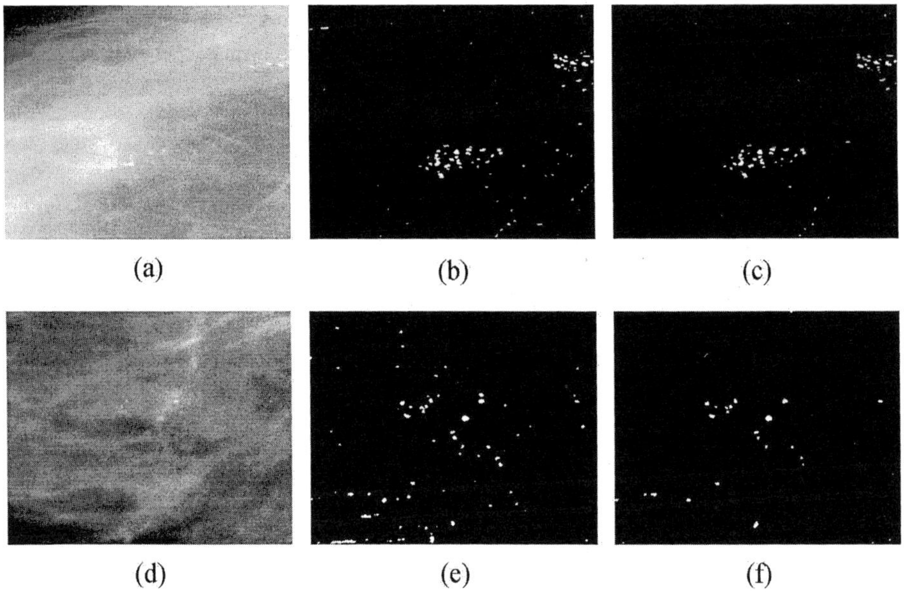

Fig. 1. Digital mammogram images containing (a) two microcalcification clusters, (d) one microcalcification cluster. Binary calcification segmented images using (b,e) Karssemeijer's CAD scheme and (c,f) the CAD scheme described in this paper.

To provide quantitative results the calcification segmented images were clustered using mode analysis [11]. A preprocessing stage minimized the influence of noise by eliminating any calcifications that are of size two pixels or less. True positive clusters were defined as a group of three or more microcalcifications with a convex hull completely enclosed within the ground truth marked by an expert radiologist.

Table 1 summarizes the overall number of true positive (TP) and false positive (FP) clusters obtained when applying the CAD schemes to all images in the data set. Karssemeijer's technique produced a true positive rate of 84% with 1.125 false positive clusters per image. The CAD scheme presented in this paper achieved a true positive rate of 79% with 0.3 false positive clusters per image. The individual calcifications in all mammogram images were detected however the clustering algorithm was not able to find all clusters due to the varied distribution of the microcalcifications. Optimizing the clustering algorithm would improve the true positive detection rates for both techniques.

Table 1. True positive (TP) and false positive (FP) results for all images in the mammogram data set, comparing Karssemeijer's CAD scheme with that presented in this paper

	Karssemeijer CAD	McLoughlin CAD
TP	32	30
FP	54	14

5. Conclusion

Progress is reported towards a computer aided detection system for microcalcification clusters. The detection scheme utilizes two image feature parameters: local contrast and shape. A shape parameter has been developed to highlight connective tissue regions, using phase information in the Fourier domain. Log Gabor filters of multiple scales/frequency and orientations ensure the process is adaptive to features of varying size.

A deterministic relaxation scheme segments the mammogram images into three categories: connective tissue, calcification and background. Pixel labels are updated by a modified version of the ICM algorithm. To increase the likelihood of calcifications being detected in clusters, long range interaction between pixel labels is modelled, in addition to nearest neighbour interaction representing the expectation of spatial continuity. A connectivity parameter is introduced to reduce false positives associated with connective tissue regions.

A comparison with Karssemeijer's [7] CAD scheme on 48 digital mammograms showed similar true positive detection rates and a reduction in the false positive detection rate. Future work on microcalcification detection will include optimizing the execution time of the CAD scheme and further testing of the connectivity parameter.

References

1. S. Yu and L. Guan: A CAD system for the automatic detection of clustered microcalcifications in digitized mammogram films. IEEE Trans. Medical Imaging, Vol 19, No 2, pp. 115-125, 2000.
2. R.N. Strickland and H.I. Hahn: Wavelet transform for detecting microcalcifications in mammograms. IEEE Trans. Medical Imaging, Vol 15, pp 218-229, 1996.
3. T. Netch and H.O. Peitgen: Scale-space signatures for the detection of clustered microcalcifications in digital mammograms. IEEE Trans. Medical Imaging, Vol 18, No 9, pp. 774-786, 1999.
4. H. Cheng, Y.M. Lui and R.I. Feiimanis: A novel approach to microcalcification detection using fuzzy logic techniques. IEEE Trans. Medical Imaging, Vol 17, pp. 442-450, 1998.
5. N. Karssemeijer and W.J.H. Veldkamp: Normalization of local contrast in mammograms. IEEE Trans. Medical Imaging, Vol 19, No 7, pp. 731-738, 2000.
6. P. Kovesi: Image features from phase congruency: Videre: A Journal of Computer Vision Research. MIT Press, Vol 1, No 3, pp.1-26, 1999.
7. N. Karssemeijer: Stochastic model for automated detection of calcifications in digital mammograms. Image and Vision Computing, Vol 10, No 6, pp. 369-375, 1992.
8. D.J. Field: Relations between the statistics of natural images and the response properties of cortical cells. Optical Society of America, Vol 4, No 12, pp. 2379-2394, 1987.
9. K.J. McLoughlin, P.J. Bones, P.D. Kovesi: Connective tissue representation for detection of microcalcifications in digital mammograms. Proceedings of SPIE Medical Imaging 2002.
10. D. Kopans, M. Heath and K.W. Bowyer: Current Status of the digital database for screening mammography. Digital Mammography – IEE Colloquium, pp. 457-460, 1998.
11. B.S. Everitt: Cluster Analysis, Edward Arnold, 338 Euston Road, London, 1993.

The use of joint two-view information for improving computerized microcalcification detection accuracy

Berkman Sahiner, Lubomir M. Hadjiiski, Heang-Ping Chan, Nicholas Petrick, Mark A. Helvie

Department of Radiology, University of Michigan, Ann Arbor, MI 48109
berki@umich.edu

Abstract. We investigated the use of joint CC and MLO view information to improve computerized detection of microcalcifications. Microcalcification cluster candidates were located using our previously developed single-view detection algorithm. Object pairs from the CC and MLO views were formed by using their radial distances from the nipple. The pairs were classified using a correspondence classifier, which analyzed feature similarity measures of the members in a pair. The scores from the correspondence classifier were fused with the single-view detection scores. The algorithm was trained using 109 mammogram pairs from the University of Michigan, and tested using an independent public data set from the University of South Florida (USF). The test set included 124 two-view mammograms containing 272 microcalcification clusters. The false-positive (FP) rate was determined by applying the algorithm to 89 normal mammogram pairs from the USF data set. The two-view detection algorithm had a film-based sensitivity of 80% at 0.22 FPs/image. At the same sensitivity, the single-view detection algorithm produced 0.33 FPs/image. Our results indicate that the use of joint two-view information can improve the accuracy of our computerized microcalcification detection algorithm.

1. Introduction

Clinical studies have demonstrated that imaging the breast in two views increases the cancer detection sensitivity [1]. In this study, we investigated whether the computer can also be trained to jointly use the information from two mammographic views, namely, the mediolateral oblique (MLO) view and the craniocaudal (CC) view. Previously, Paquerault *et al.* [2, 3] and Sahiner *et al.* [4] demonstrated how the geometric, morphological, and texture features from lesion candidates on two different views of the same breast can be combined to increase the accuracy of computerized mass detection on mammograms. In this study, we focused on the detection of microcalcifications using the joint two-view information.

2. Methods

Microcalcification clusters detected by the computer on the two views are expected to exhibit similarities in their geometric, morphological and textural features. On the other hand, a false-positive (FP) detection on the CC view will exhibit a lesser degree of similarity with the true cluster or other FPs on the MLO view, and vice-versa. Our joint two-view detection algorithm uses the high degree of similarity between TP-TP pairs to reduce false positives. The block diagram of the joint two-view detection method is shown in Figure 1.

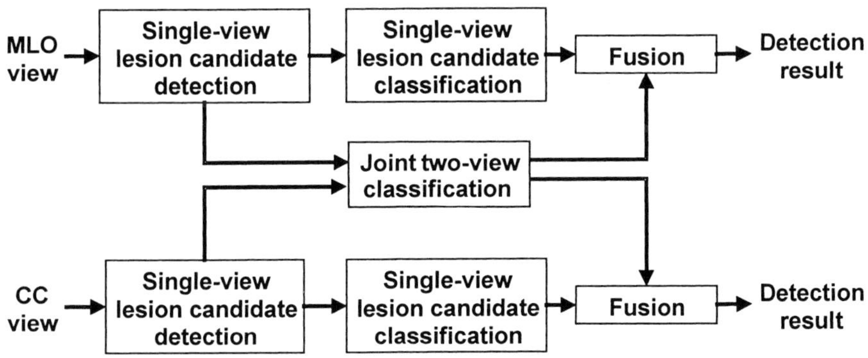

Fig. 1. The block diagram of the computerized two-view microcalcification detection method.

2.1 Single-View Lesion Candidate Detection

The single-view lesion candidate detection technique used in this study has previously been described in the literature [5]. First, the image is processed using a difference-image technique to enhance the signal-to-noise ratio of the microcalcifications [6], and potential signals are segmented from the image background. Next, false-positives are reduced using rule-based classification and convolution neural network (CNN). Finally, regional clustering [5] was used to identify clustered microcalcifications.

2.2 Single-View Lesion Candidate Classification

The parameters of our single-view lesion candidate detection algorithm were adjusted to provide high-sensitivity, at the cost of a relatively large number of false-positives. The single-view lesion candidate classification step aimed at reducing the false-positives while maintaining a high sensitivity. The classifier was designed using stepwise feature selection and linear discriminant analysis (LDA) trained on an independent training set. The feature space used in stepwise selection included the texture and morphological features of the microcalcification clusters, as well as the number of microcalcifications in a cluster and the CNN scores.

2.3 Joint Two-View Classification of True and False Pairs

Joint two-view pair classification distinguishes between true (TP-TP) pairs and false pairs (TP-FP, FP-TP, and FP-FP) by using the similarities between the two objects that constitute the pair. The initial step in this task is to define the object pairs. As described in our previous studies [3] [4], we defined the pairs based on the difference between the nipple-to-object distances (NODs) on the CC and MLO views. For each nodule candidate C_{ci} detected on the CC view, the NOD, D_{ci}, was computed, and an annular region of width $2\Delta R$, centered at the nipple and enclosed between the radii $D_{ci} \pm \Delta R$ was defined on the MLO view. If the centroid of an object C_{Mj} on the MLO view was found inside this annular region, then an object pair (C_{ci}, C_{Mj}) was defined. The width of the annular region, $2\Delta R$, is determined using training data.

A correspondence classifier, based on stepwise feature selection and LDA, was used to estimate the likelihood that the defined pair was a true pair. The feature space used in stepwise selection included the similarity measures of the features that were used in single-view lesion candidate classification.

2.4 Fusion

The correspondence classifier produced a correspondence score for each object pair. This score was converted into a two-view object score before being combined with the single-view object score. The fusion score for an object was defined as the average of its single- and two-view object scores.

2.5 Data Set

Our training data set consisted of 109 pairs of biopsy-proven CC and MLO mammograms containing microcalcification clusters, collected with Institutional Review Board approval at the University of Michigan (UM). The mammograms were digitized with a LUMISYS 85 laser scanner at a pixel size of 50 μm x 50 μm and 4096 gray levels. The digitizer was calibrated so that the gray level values were linearly proportional to the optical density (OD) within the range of 0.1 to 4.0 OD units. The mammograms were filtered with a 2x2 box filter and subsampled by a factor of 2 to produce a 0.1 mm x 0.1 mm images prior to processing.

Our independent test set consisted of 124 pairs of mammograms, selected from the University of South Florida (USF) public mammogram database [7]. The digitization characteristics of these mammograms were similar to those of the UM database, with the difference that a Lumisys 200 laser scanner was used. The test data set contained 272 microcalcification clusters on 248 mammograms, of which 253 were biopsy-proven malignant. The FP rate was determined by applying the algorithm to an additional 89 normal mammogram pairs from the USF data set.

3. Results

The detection accuracy was evaluated using film-based free-response receiver operating characteristic (FROC) curves. In film-based analysis, a microcalcification cluster detected on one view but missed on the other view is considered as one TP and one false-negative (FN). This method provides a more conservative sensitivity estimate than a case-based analysis, in which a cluster detected on one view but missed on the other view would be counted as one FP and zero FN.

The single-view lesion candidate detection algorithm correctly detected 86% (233/272) of the microcalcification clusters, at an average FP rate of 1.1 FPs/image, in the test set. Based on the geometric locations of the microcalcification clusters in the training set, a radial width of 2ΔR=6 cm was used for geometric pairing. Of a total of 18973 possible pairs in the test set, 10159 object pairs were defined using the two-view geometric registration method described in Section 2.3. The object pairs were classified by the correspondence classifier designed using the training set. The pair scores were converted into object scores and were fused with single-view scores as described in Section 2.4. The final FROC curve obtained by the fusion of single-view and two-view scores is compared to the single-view FROC curve in Figure 2 and Table 1.

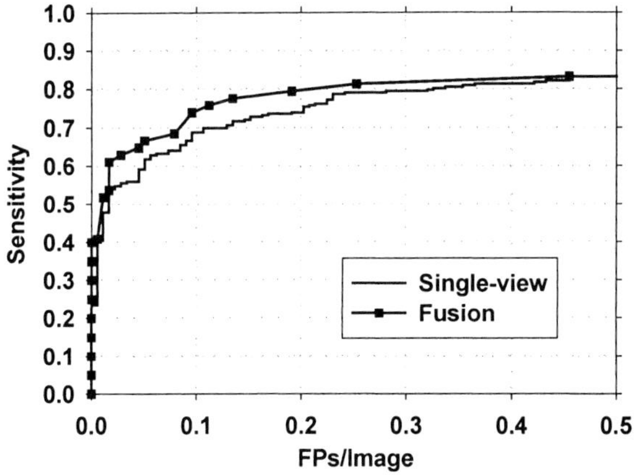

Fig. 2. The comparison of the FROC curves for the single-view detection and fusion methods.

Table 1. The comparison of the FP rates generated by the fusion method and the single-view detection method at selected sensitivity levels.

Sensitivity	False-Positives per Image	
	Fusion	Single-view
70%	0.09	0.13
75%	0.11	0.20
80%	0.22	0.33

4. Conclusion

The fusion of the single-view and two-view scores resulted in a reduced number of FPs at comparable sensitivities to single-view detection. Alternatively, it could improve the detection sensitivity at the same FP rate. Future work includes the optimization of the similarity measures, improvement of the fusion technique, and the application of two-view detection techniques to improve the overall detection sensitivity.

Acknowledgments

This work is supported by USPHS Grant CA 48129, USAMRMC grant DAMD17-01-1-0823, and a Career Development Award (L.H.) from the USAMRMC (DAMD 17-98-1-8211). The content of this publication does not necessarily reflect the position of the government and no official endorsement of any equipment and product of any companies mentioned in the publication should be inferred.

References

1. Warren, R., Duffy, S., and Bashir, S.: The value of the second view in screening mammography. British Journal of radiology, 1996, 69: 105-108.
2. Paquerault, S., Petrick, N., Chan, H.P., Sahiner, B., and Dolney, A.Y.: Improvement of mammographic lesion detection by fusion of information from different views. Proc. SPIE, 2001, 4322: 1883-1889.
3. Paquerault, S., Petrick, N., Chan, H.P., Sahiner, B., and Helvie, M.A.: Improvement of computerized mass detection on mammograms: Fusion of two-view information. Medical Physics, 2002, 29: 238-247.
4. Sahiner, B., Petrick, N., Chan, H.P., Paquerault, S., Helvie, M.A., and Hadjiiski, L.M.: Recognition of lesion correspondence on two mammographic views - A new method of false-positive reduction for computerized mass detection. Proc. SPIE, 2001, 4322: 649-655.
5. Chan, H.P., Lo, S.C.B., Sahiner, B., Lam, K.L., and Helvie, M.A.: Computer-aided detection of mammographic microcalcifications: Pattern recognition with an artificial neural network. Medical Physics, 1995, 22: 1555-1567.
6. Chan, H.P., Doi, K., Vyborny, C.J., Schmidt, R.A., Metz, C.E., Lam, K.L., Ogura, T., Wu, Y., and MacMahon, H.: Improvement in radiologists' detection of clustered microcalcifications on mammograms. The potential of computer-aided diagnosis. Investigative Radiology, 1990, 25: 1102-1110.
7. Heath, M., Bowyer, K., Kopans, D., Moore, R., and Kegelmeyer, P.: The digital database for screening mammography, in Digital Mammography; IWDM 2000, Yaffe, M.J., Editor. 2001, Medical Physics Publishing: Toronto, Canada. p. 457-460.

A Normal Mammogram Classifier using Binary Decision Trees with Multiresolution Features

Yajie Sun†,Charles Babbs‡, Edward J. Delp†·

†Video and Image Processing Laboratory
School of Electrical and Computer Engineering
Purdue University
West Lafayette, IN 47906-1285

‡Department of Basic Medical Sciences
School of Veterinary Medicine
Purdue University
West Lafayette, IN 47907-1246

Abstract. The majority of screening mammograms are normal, and it may be beneficial if a normal mammogram detection system were designed to help radiologists identify normal regions, allowing them to focus on suspicious areas. In this paper, we present a binary decision classifier based on global features extracted from different levels of 2-D Quincunx Wavelet Decomposition of pre-processed regional mammograms. This is fundamentally different than other approaches, which identify normal mammograms by detecting the type of lesion. Our approach presented here is independent of the types of abnormalities present. The experiment clearly shows that one can classify most normal mammogram regions, keeping the clinically critical misclassification rate of abnormal regions small.

1. Introduction

Early detection is the most effective way to prevent breast cancer death. Screening mammography is still the gold standard. Research reveals that the mortality rate could decrease by 30% if all women age 50 and older routinely have mammograms [1].

There have been many proposals for using computer-aided systems as a second opinion to improve radiologists' mammographic screening performance [2]. Since most screening mammograms are normal, another potential way to design a computer-aided system is to identify normal mammograms or regions with very high specificity and allow radiologists to focus more on suspicious areas. This strategy could improve detection efficiency and true positive rate in screening. Little has been done on computer-aided normal mammogram detection, though many individual cancer detection systems have been developed in the last decade. In [3], a statistical method was developed for identifying normal areas from abnormal regions, using a microcalcification detector. In [4, 5], a method was presented for the analysis of normal mammograms, but without an automatic normal mammogram classifier. In this paper, we present a normal detection scheme to distinguish normal mammogram

·Address all correspondence to E.J. Delp, ace@ecn.purdue.edu. This work was supported by a grant from Qualia Computing.

regions from suspicious regions. Our focus is on the classification of normal regional images, and not on the detection of particular abnormalities.

2. Normal Regional Classification

In this section we describe our approach to normal detection. We assume that we are examining regions of the mammogram and not the entire image.

2.1 Linear Structure Removal and Wavelet Decomposition

As a pre-processing step, a line detection scheme is used to remove the linear markings characteristic of clinically normal tissues [5]. After linear structure removal, the "residual" image of a normal mammogram appears relatively featureless. For abnormal mammograms, the "residual" images consist of enhanced abnormalities on a relatively featureless background. This step is used to suppress normal features, enhance abnormal features, and increase the "difference" between them.

The linear-phase 2-D Quincunx wavelet transform described in [6] is used to obtain a multiresolution decomposition of the "residual" images. This 2-D nonseparable transform does not introduce phase distortion in the decomposed image. We only select first four even-level decomposition images for feature extraction and further processing.

2.2 Feature Extraction

For every decomposition image, five features, *mean*, *variance*, *skewness*, *kurtosis* and *entropy*, are obtained from the histogram of the regional image. Therefore, there are twenty features, which form a feature vector for the four decomposition images. These features are labeled as *mean2, mean4, mean8, mean16, variance2, variance4, variance8, variance16, skewness2, skewness4, skewness8, skewness16, kurtosis2, kurtosis4, kurtosis8, kurtosis16, entropy2, entropy4, entropy8,* and *entropy16*. Since we are classifying normal regions and not the type or locations of a lesion, global features are appropriate for this purpose.

2.3 Decision Tree Classifier

We selected a decision tree as our normal classifier because a binary decision tree is easy to interpret and it has an automatic feature selection property. The decision tree is constructed using the method described in [7, 8]. Each leaf node of the decision tree is labeled as one of two classes: S represents the class of suspicious mammograms, and N represents the class of normal mammograms.

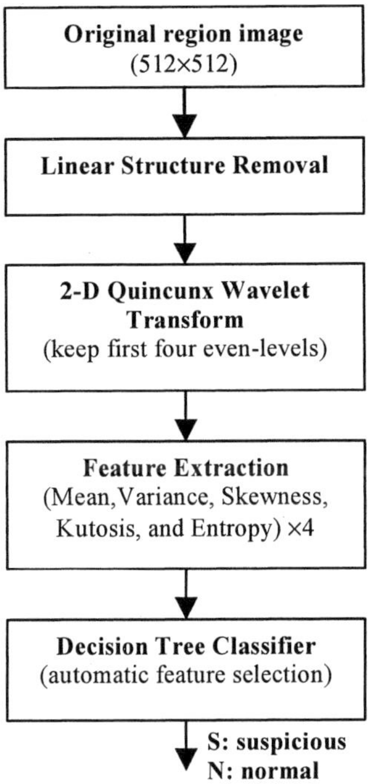

Figure 1. The normal classifier.

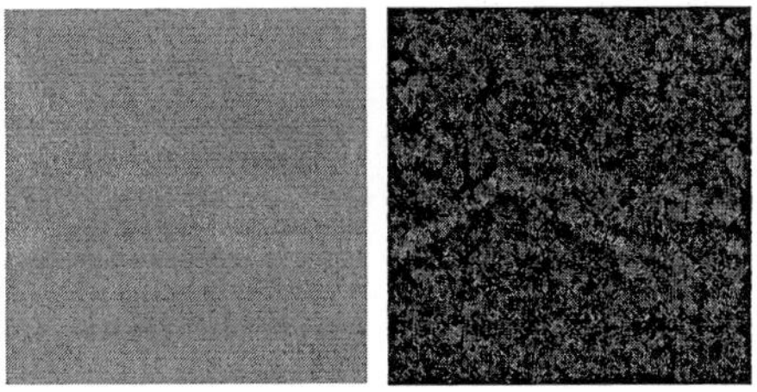

(a) (b)

Figure 2. (a) original normal region image (512×512); (b) the "residual" image after linear structure removal.

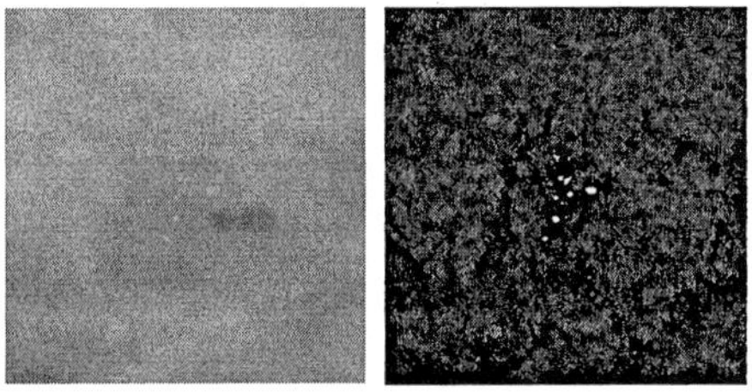

(a) (b)

Figure 3. (a) original abnormal (calcification) region image; (b) the "residual" image after linear structure removal

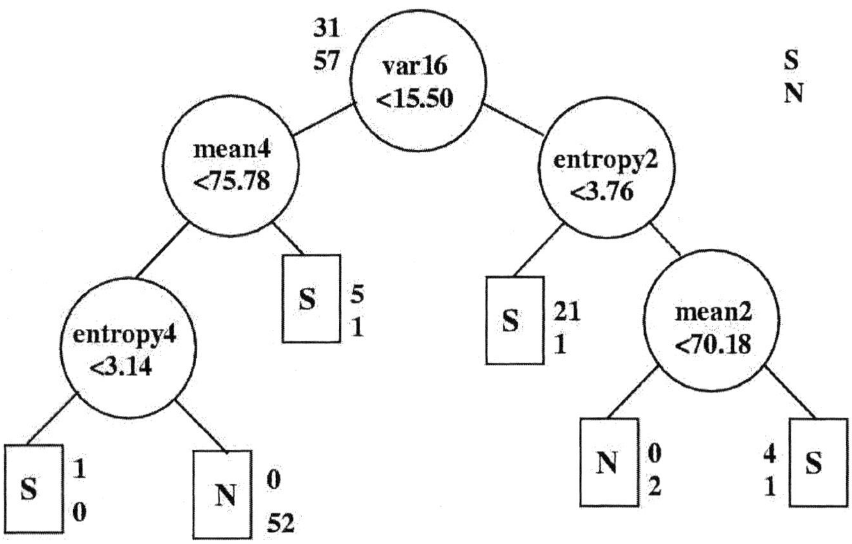

Figure 4. The Decision Tree with classified test sample numbers at each leaf node.

Figure 1 shows the schematic diagram of our normal mammogram classifier. Though this is a normal classifier, one should keep in mind that the misclassification rate of abnormal regions detected as normal regions should be as near zero as possible. It would be costly and dangerous in mammographic screening if an abnormal is misclassified as normal, or an abnormal lesion fails to be detected. Therefore, we set the cost of the misclassification of an abnormal mammogram as a normal one much larger than the cost of the misclassification of a normal case as a suspicious one.

3. Results

All mammograms used in our study were obtained from the Digital Database for Screening Mammography (DDSM) distributed by the University of South Florida [9]. Since we are interested in the regions of mammograms, normal region images (512×512 pixels) were extracted from normal cases. According to the "ground truth," abnormal region images (512×512 pixels) were extracted from cancer cases with the known cancer in the center of the region. A total of 239 region images were obtained from the DDSM. These region images were randomly separated into two sets. The first set is used to train the binary decision tree and consisted of 70 normal sample images and 81 abnormal/suspicious region images (27 circumscribed masses, 22 spiculated masses and 32 microcalcifications). A second set is used to test the constructed decision tree, which consisted of 57 normal region images and 31 abnormal region images (13 circumscribed masses, 11 speculated lesions and 7 microcalcifications).

Figure 2 (a) shows a typical normal region image, Figure 2 (b) is the "residual" image after linear structure removal. Figure 3 (a) and (b) show a typical abnormal (microcalcification) region image and its "residual" image.

In the training set, 3 of 81 of abnormal images were misclassified as normal and 7 out of 70 normal cases were misclassified as suspicious or abnormal. Figure 4 shows the classified regions using the trained decision tree, where S is the class label for the abnormal regions, and N is the class label for the normal regions. It shows that 3 of 57 normal regions were misclassified as suspicious mammograms, and none of the abnormal mammograms was misclassified as normal.

4. Discussion and Conclusions

From the trained decision tree, we observe that *entropy2* and *entropy4* are two prominent features for classifying normal and abnormal mammograms. It was observed that the histogram of the normal residual image is flat or unimodal, so the entropy is large. The histograms of abnormal lesions have peaks near the highest gray-level (multi-modal) since a cancer is a bright area, therefore the entropy is smaller. The decision tree also selected *variance16* as an important feature. This is a bit surprising, however, after examining the decomposition images, it is evident that the darkness due to filtering of the cancers causes a high global variance in the abnormal cases. We also observe that *skewness* and *kurtosis* are not very sensitive to normal and abnormal regions.

The three abnormal regions that were misclassified as normal cases are cases of very low-contrast and small masses. The normal regions that were misclassified as abnormal are mass-like very high dense regions.

This approach is able to classify most normal regions correctly. Moreover, it has a very low misclassification rate of abnormal regions detected as normal regions, which is critical in the clinical situation.

References

1. Cancer facts and figures. Technical Report, American Cancer Society, 1991.

2. C.J. Vyborny and M.L. Giger, "Computer vision and artificial intelligence in mammography", American J. of Roentgenology, 162(3), 699-708, 1994.

3. J.J. Heine, S. R.Deans, D.K. Cullers, R. Stauduhar, and L.P. Clarke, "Multiresolution Statistical Analysis of High-Resolution Digital Mammograms", *IEEE Trans. Med. Imag.* 16(5), 503-515, 1997.

4. S. Liu, C. F. Babbs, Z. Pizlo, E. J. Delp, "Characterization of Normal Mammograms," *Proceedings of the 5th International Workshop on Digital Mammography,* June 11-14, 2000.

5. S. Liu, C.F. Babbs, and E.J. Delp, "Normal Mammogram Analysis and Recognition," *Proceedings of the IEEE International Conference on Image Processing,* Chicago, Illinois, 727-731, October 4-7,1998.

6. J. Kovačević and M. Vetterli, "Nonseparable multidimensional perfect reconstruction filter banks and wavelet bases for R^n," *IEEE Trans. Inform. Theory,* 38(2), 533-555, March 1992.

7. S.B. Gelfand, C.S. Ravishankar, E.J. Delp, "An iterative growing and pruning algorithm for classification tree design," *IEEE Trans. Pattern Anal. Machine Intell.*, 13, 163-174, 1991.

8. S. Liu, C.F. Babbs, and E.J. Delp, "Multiresolution Detection of Spiculated Lesions in Digital Mammograms," IEEE Trans. Image Processing, vol. 10, no. 6, 874-884, June 2001.

9. M. Heath, K.W. Bowyer, D. Kopans et al., "Current status of the Digital Database for Screening Mammography", *Digital Mammography*, 457-460, Kluwer Academic Publishers, 1998.

Development of CAD system for 3D breast ultrasound images

Takeshi Hara [a], Daisuke Fukuoka [b], Hiroshi Fujita [a]

Tokiko Endo [c], and Woo Kyung Moon [d]

Department of Information Science, Gifu University
Yanagido 1-1, Gifu, Gifu 501-1193, Japan.
[b] Department of Electrical Information, Gifu National College, Japan.
[c] Department of Radiology, National Hospital of Nagoya, Japan.
[d] Department of Radiology, College of Medicine, Seoul National University Hospital, Seoul, South Korea.

Abstract. We have developed a CAD system for masses on 3D breast ultrasound images and estimated the preliminary performance with about 200 cases. The detection and classification methods were based on edge detection and active balloon models to segment the mass regions. Volume rendering technique was also applied to prepare the 3D images to readers. It showed a good classification performance as an initial result. Especially, the classification performance showed a good rate because the cases employed in classifications scheme were difficult ones to discriminate by the ultrasound images in a physician's opinion, however the number of the case we used was not so large at this time. keywords: ultrasound, mass, classification, CAD

1. Introduction

The technology of ultrasound devices for breast imaging significantly improved the resolutions of lesions of breast diseases. The usefulness is widely recognized not only for the detection of small masses but also for the classification of the lesions. We have developed a 3D breast imaging computer-aided diagnostic system by using 3D ultrasound breast images, although we have been developing a mammogram CAD system for detecting clustered microcalcifications and masses, because the diagnosis by using ultrasound images is strongly recommended for some younger people whose breasts tend to be dense one. Recently, mass screening with ultrasound devices for young women has proposed and has already started in some region in Japan. One of those examination employed Octson mechanism device, not handy-probe, to store stable regions of whole breast. By using the mechanism, patients have to lie prone on the examination equipment, because large four ultrasound probes move mechanically between adequate length below the breast. The device can archive over 50 scans with 3mm intervals per breast and can stores the image data on optical video disc. The reproducibility and ease-of-store of the breast image data is very useful to read them after the examination, because physicians can read the images of whole breast by slice-by-slice as 3D imaging data, although the device is too large to visualize lesions like magnification radiography.

The new technology for the 3D imaging devices for breast diagnosis has been introduced by Medison Co. South Korea. The device bases on hand-probe mechanism that store the three-dimensional images corresponding to almost 5cm x 5cm area. The 3D images are created by moving a tiny probe set in the handy case.

The purpose of this work is to develop a computer-aided diagnosis system to detect and classify mass signals on the 3D breast ultrasound images, and to estimate the classification performance with over hundred images with biopsy proven. This paper mainly describes the classification scheme of masses indicated within 3D images from the equipment by Medison Co.

2. Materials and methods

2.1. Image Dataset

The 3D images we employed were archived by the equipment by Medison Co.. There was a single prove that could scan within approximately 5cm x 5cm area on surface of a breast. This Medison device was mainly applied to classify the breast masses previously detected by other modality such as mammography or palpable examinations because of the narrow area of the scanning. The pixel size of images was within 256x256x256, and the scanning was examined in a few seconds moving the probe mechanically.

2.2. Segmentation of mass areas

The segmentation of masses region on ultrasound image was generally difficult tasks because the signal was week and noisy. Moreover, the posterior echo was eliminated by the nature of masses. Some approximation techniques were required to compensate the boundary to extract the feature values from the shape and/or the regions of masses. We applied the active balloon models (ABM), a kind of active contour models [1] in three dimensional spaces, to determine the boundaries around masses.

2.3. Feature extractions

The features to classify masses were consisted of eight components as follows: (1) Depth-width ratio in 3D. This feature was calculated by dividing the mass area [pixels] on x-z plain by on y-z plain. (2) Ratio between Min-max length. Each of the length was determined by measuring the maximum and minimum distance within the mass region. (3) Volume of mass. The volume was defined by the regions indicated by the ABM. (4) Variance of density within anterior echo area. The anterior area was automatically determined based on the expanded region by the ABM. The mass and the surrounding regions were divided into three areas. The regions were determined automatically by expanding the mass region in 20 pixels by using three dimensional morphological processing. The anterior echo area was indicated the bottom region. (5) Variance of density in internal area. The internal area also determined by the ABM. (6) Variance of length from center of gravity to boundary. All of the length was calculated by measuring from the center of gravity to the nodes of the ABM. (7) Circularity of the region. This feature was determined by the ratio of the volume and surface area. (8) Density ratio between anterior and posterior echo area. The posterior and anterior regions were determined by the ABM such as the region of feature (4). The intensity of anterior echo tends to be attenuated when the mass was malignant one.

2.4. Classification by artificial neural networks

The artificial neural network (ANN) technique was employed to classify the masses by using those eight features. The ANN we applied consisted of three layers with eight input units, twelve hidden units, and an output unit to express the malignancy of the input feature. The ANN structure was determined experimentally and was trained based on back-propagate algorithm by using some typical cases. The features were standardized between 0.0 and 1.0 to enter into the ANN.

2.5. Image Display

The display of the 3D images is very important to recognize the mass shape and distribution of echo signals. We have tried to visualize the mass regions by using volume rendering and surface rendering approaches.

Fig. 1 shows the example of three dimensional display by using volume rendering technique clipping at the mass region. The scan images in any directions were shown by moving mouse to indicate the angle of view.

Fig. 2 and Fig. 3 show an example of surface rendering of benign and malignant masses, respectively. Rough surface of mass was well recognized as compared with the benign one. Emphasizing the shadows created by artificial lights in the space was very effective to tell the shape of the mass.

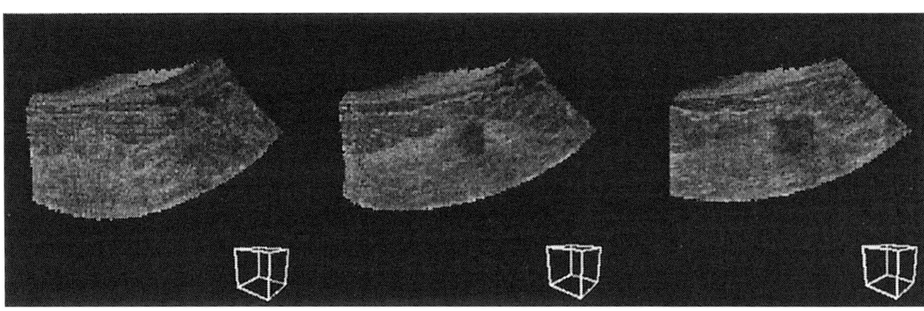

Fig.1 Examples of volume rendering images around a mass region.

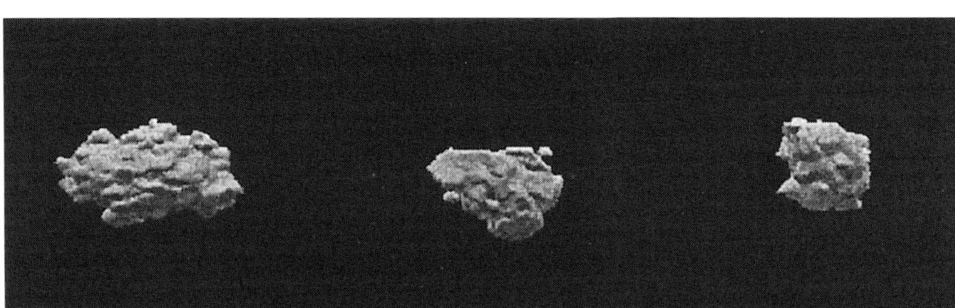

Fig.2 Examples of surface rendering images of a typical malignant mass

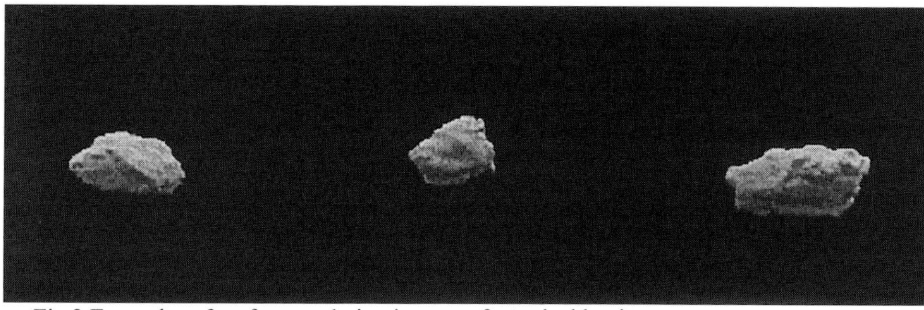

Fig.3 Examples of surface rendering images of a typical benign mass

3. Results and discussions

By employing 227 cases (147 benign, 80 malignant) with biopsy proven, the classification performance was 76%(61/80) sensitivity at 71% (104/147) specificity, although the consistency test approach was applied. The cases we tested were difficult to classify by well-experienced physicians by using only ultrasound images, so that this result may be adequate performance as an initial experiment.

Volume rendering images and patients list were shown on the same window. The volume images were rotated by moving mouse at the desired degree of view, and the position of clipping plain was determined by the same procedure of mouse movements. It was concluded that this scheme would be effective for the diagnostic aid of ultrasound images for breast diseases.

Acknowledgements

This work was partly supported by a Grant-In-Aid for Cancer Research from the Ministry of Health, Labour, and Welfare, and by a Grant-In-Aid for Scientific Research, from the Ministry of Education, Culture, Sports, Science and Technology.

References

1. M. Kass, A. Witkin, and D. Terzopoulos: "Snakes: Active contour models", Int. J. Comput. Vision, 1, 1, 321-331, 1988.
2. D. Fukuoka, T. Hara, H. Fujita, et al.: "Dynamic Region-contour-extraction method with automated initial-contour production and unification of contours", the transactions of the institute of electronics, infomartion and communication engineering, J81-D-II, 6, 1448-1451, 1998.

Incorporating Explanations into a CAD tool for the classification of calcifications

Paul Taylor, Richard Lee and Eugenio Alberdi

Centre for Health Informatics and Multiprofessional Education, University College London, Archway Campus, Highgate Hill, London, N19 3UA, United Kingdom
p.taylor@chime.ucl.ac.uk

Abstract. We argue that CAD systems should be designed as aids to decision-making. We have developed a prototype aid for the classification of calcifications that can present an explanation of the reasoning behind the classification.

A study was carried out to identify a set of terms commonly used by radiologists to describe calcifications. A second study assessed the capacity of the these terms to discriminate between benign and malignant calcifications. A set of discriminating terms was identified. Image-processing measures were then implemented to identify calcifications for which the descriptors applied. Linear discriminant functions were derived for the classification of a set of 40 groups of calcifications.

Two experiments were performed to test a prototype CAD system using the terms to advise on the differential diagnosis of calcfications. Image regions identifed by a commercial prompting tool were classified according to the descriptors assigned by the linear discriminant functions. A panel of expert radiologists reviewed the system and assessed its value as an aid to decision-making.

1. Introduction

A clinician requesting an imaging investigation does so in order to obtain information that will help in making a clinical decision. The motivation for our work is the conviction that we can improve the effectiveness of this decision-making by bringing together research on medical image processing with that on clinical decision support. This 'bringing together' however raises a number of questions, chief among them being that of how to map between the results of the numerical analysis of signal data on the one hand and the symbolic terms used in decision support systems on the other.

The algorithms used in CAD systems can be understood as functions that transform an input image into an output image representing local probability assessments of the image contents. The output is displayed to the user following a thresholding operation that places prompts on a small number of image locations where there is a particularly high risk of finding an abnormality. The detection of an abnormality is only part of the process. The radiologist must then come to a view about its likely significance, based on his or her experience, education and awareness of the relevant research as well as other information about the patient. Our aim has been to design a computer aid in which a knowledge base reflecting the experience of practicing radiologists could be used to help in the assessment of ambiguous clinical signs. The innovative aspect of the system is the attempt to drive the symbolic reasoning from a description of the salient features of the case, a description derived automatically from processing the image.

This approach remains distinctive and, we believe, may become increasingly important as other research shows that the current generation of prompting systems are failing to have an effect on radiologists' decision-making (see, for example, [1]). We believe that systems based on symbolic reasoning, which are able to provide explanations for why particular regions are prompted may prove more acceptable to radiologists. Access to this kind of reasoning may prove particularly important when radiologists are learning to use such systems, and this may be a more complex task than had been thought.

2. Implementation

2.1 Representing Radiological Expertise

Two studies were carried out to establish, validate and assess descriptors for use in the differential diagnosis of mammographic calcifications. In Study 1, eleven radiologists were asked to 'think out loud' as they interpreted 20 sets of calcifications. We recorded, transcribed and analysed what they said. We used this data to design a standard terminology for describing calcifications. The second study, in which ten radiologists used this scheme to describe 40 sets of calcifications, served to validate the terminology.

In the second of the studies we also assessed the capacity of the terms to discriminate between benign and malignant calcifications, testing them against the radiologists' assessments of malignancy as well as follow-up data. We used the correlation data and the sensitivity and specificity measures to identify four sets of descriptors: weak and strong arguments for benign and malignant interpretations. These arguments provide the basis for the decision support used in our prototype decision aid. This work is described in more detail in [2].

2.2 Implementing Image Processing Algorithms

Although algorithms for the detection of calcifications have been published since the 1970s, data comparing the performance of the different approaches are relatively scarce. We selected four quite different approaches to the detection of calcifications and reimplemented them according to a common scheme. The details of this work and of the subsequent comparison were published as [3]. Disappointingly, we found, with all four algorithms, that the performance on the test set we used fell far short of that obtained by the authors responsible for the original development of the algorithms. Nevertheless our results were sufficient to identify one algorithm as the most appropriate for use in our system. We were able to improve performance by adjusting the parameters of the algorithm to optimise it for two separate tasks; calcification detection and accurate segmentation of calcification boundaries.

The measures used in the characterisation of calcifications were, in part, taken from the literature on the classification of calcifications and in part devised to meet the particular needs of this project. We devised a number of new measures intended to capture the characteristics mentioned in the terminology, as described in [4].

2.3 Integration of Image Processing and Symbolic Inference

We used linear discriminant analysis to derive rules for classifying clusters of calcifications according to our terminology. The measures were applied to the groups of calcifications used in Study 2 above. We derived a rule for the classification of calcifications based on the measurements of individual calcifications. We then settled on a threshold for the application of a term to the cluster based on the classification of the calcifications in the cluster. In certain cases the discrimination functions were applied in stages, so that – for example – calcifications had first to be classified as linear and only then as branching or not branching or as straight or curvilinear, essentially building up a classification tree. This work is described in [4].

2.4 Design and Evaluation of a Prototype Workstation

We implemented a prototype tool using Visual C++ within Windows NT running on a PC. The interface is shown in Figures 1 and 2.

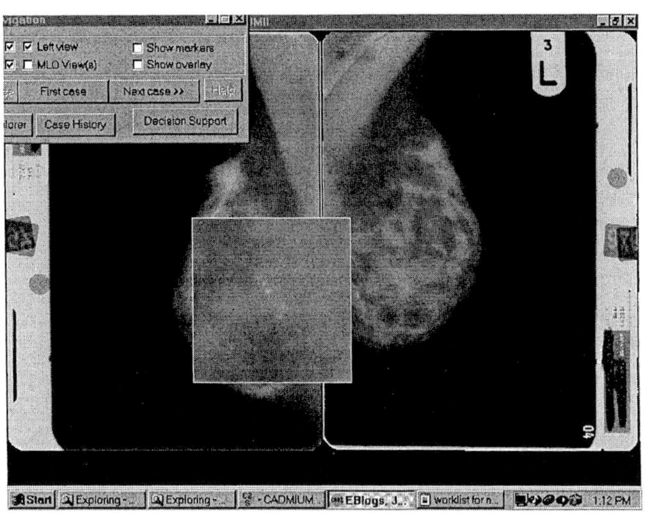

Fig. 1. The user interface of the decision support client. Higher resolution images are stored in memory and viewed by section in a small window that provides a magnifying-glass.

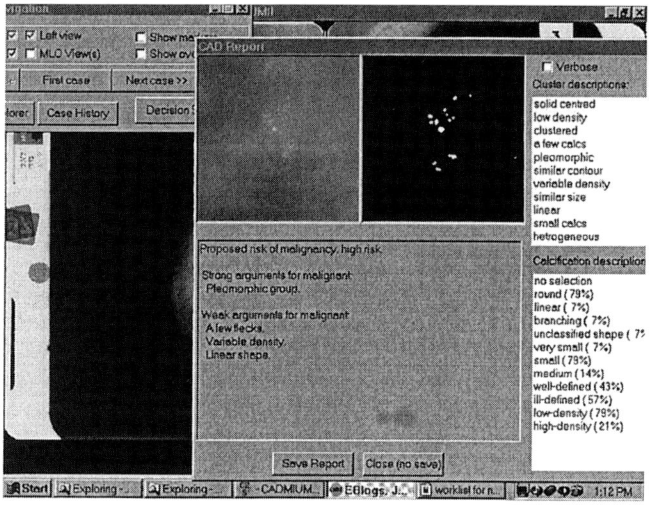

Fig. 2. The position of the magnifying glass defines a region of interest for the decision support analysis. The decision support window displays the region of interest, the results of segmenting the image using the output of the calcification detector, the supported arguments and a list of all the descriptors that apply to the identified calcifications or to the cluster of calcifications contained in the region.

3. Evaluation

We performed a number of evaluations to assess the prototype. One particularly promising result came from a study comparing the performance of our prototype with the R2 ImageChecker 2000 (a commercially available CAD tool). We were granted access to a set of films being used in an evaluation of R2, but which only included a limited number of calcifications. The ImageChecker produced 27 prompts for calcification on these films. We looked at the arguments generated by CADMIUM II for these regions. For six of the prompts, CADMIUM II generated equal numbers of benign and malignant explanations. The data for the remaining 21 regions are presented in Table 1.

Table 1. The balance of arguments generated by CADMIUM, compared to the actual diagnosis for a set of image regions prompted by R2.

		Actual diagnosis	
		Malignant	Benign
CADMIUM II	Malignant	5	8
	Benign	1	7

In eight cases CADMIUM II correctly identifies a benign explanation in a region where the R2 ImageChecker places a false positive prompt. In one region containing clear benign and subtle malignant calcification, CADMIUM II failed to detect the malignant calcification leading to the single false negative in the table. R2 missed three further cases of calcification, for two of these CADMIUM II correctly identifies a malignant cause. This simple study shows the potential of our tool to improve on the performance of the current market leader in this field.

In a second study a panel of three expert radiologists was convened to assess the value of the tool. They were given a short presentation on the research behind the prototype and then given a demonstration and a chance to use the prototype on a set of test cases. They were asked a series of questions to elicit assessments of the interface, the advice and the approach. It was clear from this that the approach generates more advice than radiologists find helpful and that a different mode of use would have to be considered if the tool is to be developed further. One potential application is in computer-assisted learning.

4. Conclusions

We have developed a prototype decision aid that incorporates reasoning based on the characteristics of calcifications. Preliminary experiments suggest that this kind of tool could have a role in assisting in the differential diagnosis of calcification prompts. Further work is required if the information that can be generated by such a tool is to made available radiologists without imposing an additional cognitive load.

Acknowledgements

This work is funded by the Engineering and Physical Sciences Research Council. The co-operation of Drs R. Given-Wilson, J. Davies, A. Schneidau, J. Cooke, S. Rankin, I. Nockler and their colleagues is gratefully acknowledged.

References

1. Warren Burhenne LJ, Wood SA, D'Orsi CJ et al. Potential contribution of computer-aided detection to the sensitivity of screening mammography. Radiology 215 (2000) 554-62
2. Alberdi E, Taylor P, R. Lee, J. Fox and A. Todd-Pokropek. Eliciting a terminology for mammography. Clinical Radiology *(in press)*
3. Lee R, Alberdi E, Taylor P et al. A Comparative study of four techniques for calcification detection. In: Yaffe (ed.) Proc. Fifth International Workshop on Digital Mammography Medical Physics Publishing, Madison, Wisconsin. (2000) 264-271
4. Taylor P, Lee R and Alberdi E. Combining image processing and rule-based decision making in computer-aided diagnosis in mammography (*submitted to Medical Image Analysis)*

Using Information from Two Mammographic Views to Improve Computer-Aided Detection of Mass Lesions

Saskia van Engeland, Nico Karssemeijer and Jan Hendriks

Department of Radiology, University Medical Center Nijmegen,
Geert Grooteplein 18, 6525 GA Nijmegen, The Netherlands
saskiave@radiology.azn.nl

Abstract. A new approach to combine information from two mammographic views for CAD of mass lesions is presented. Suspect regions in corresponding views are linked using feature probability distributions, and feature vectors are combined. Two k-Nearest Neighbor classifiers, one for single regions and one for regions with a corresponding region in the other view, are compared. Preliminary results show that this two view information improves the classifier performance.

1 Introduction

Most development of computer-aided detection (CAD) has been based on the analysis of single views. By combining information from multiple mammographic views (temporal, mediolateral oblique (MLO) and cranio-caudal (CC), or bilateral) it should be possible to improve the accuracy of CAD methods.

In literature some approaches have been described to establish correspondence between multiple views. However, few studies have been conducted to use the multiple view information to improve classification. Hadjiiski et al. [1] developed interval change analysis of masses and found that their classification accuracy improved significantly. Recently, Paquerault et al. [2] developed a two view matching method which results in a correspondence score for each possible mass pair. By combining this correspondence score with their single view detection score, their classification results also improved significantly.

This paper describes a new approach to combine information from two mammographic views (MLO and CC) to improve the accuracy of our CAD of mass lesions using fully automated detection, region matching and classification methods.

2 Methods

An initial detection stage [3] produced a limited number of suspect regions for each mammographic view in 172 MLO/CC image pairs (resolution 200 μm) from the DDSM database [4]. The detection software was used with a very low threshold, giving an average of 15 marked regions in the MLO view and 13 in the CC view. The number of regions used for matching was reduced to a maximum of 10 per view, using only the 10 most suspect regions.

It is generally believed that the distance between a lesion and the nipple remains fairly constant for different views. Radiologists use this distance to correlate a lesion in MLO and CC views. Therefore, this is the most important feature in our matching algorithm. The nipple location was determined automatically [5].

2.1 Matching

To describe the location of a lesion in each mammographic view, a polar coordinate system, centered at the nipple, and with a reference orientation perpendicular to the chest wall (CC view) or pectoral line (MLO view) (Figure 1), is used.

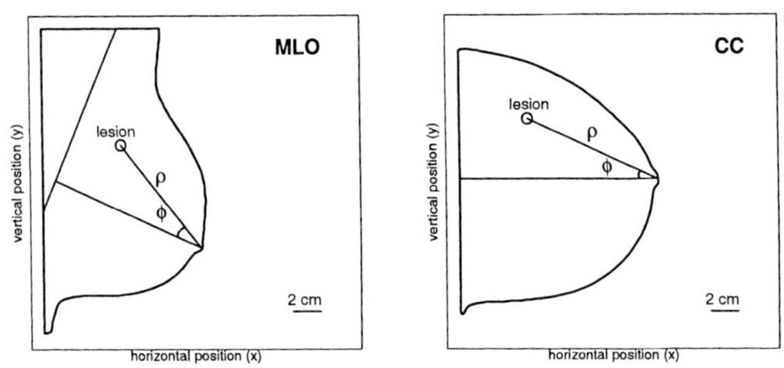

Fig. 1. Schematic representation of both mammographic views, indicating also the polar coordinate system used to define the location of a lesion.

Features from the first detection stage, the angle, and the distance between a region and the nipple were used to find matching regions in corresponding views. The used features (Figure 2) represent: distance between a region and the nipple, the angle between the region and the pectoral or chest (as shown in Figure 1), the likelihood of malignancy, a feature used for the detection of stellate patterns using second order line-orientation estimates [3] (stellate feature), a feature based on a multiscale statistical analysis of gradient orientation patterns for mass detection [6] (gradient feature), an estimate of the region size, and the relative y location of the region. Feature probability distributions of feature values for corresponding regions were created with Gaussian kernel density estimation [7] using an image set containing 275 MLO/CC annotated image pairs from the Dutch breast cancer screening program.

The distributions for the distance and the angle features are different from those found by Paquerault et al. [2]. They found a slightly higher correlation for the radial distance, correlation coefficient 0.94 against 0.88 for our dataset. On the other hand, their angle correlation is significantly lower, correlation coefficient 0.42 against 0.56 for our dataset. This deviation can be due to differences in positioning techniques. Since for our dataset the angular coordinates are not completely uncorrelated, including the angle feature may help to improve matching.

The used features are assumed to be independent. Therefore, by multiplying several feature probabilities, the likelihood that a region in one view belongs to a certain region in the other view could be obtained. After these likelihood measures had been determined for all possible region combinations, the most likely combination of regions was selected until all regions in one view were matched.

The performance of the matching algorithm could be evaluated using lesion annotations. Using these annotations, it was only possible to check whether the regions pointing to the true lesions were correctly matched. Since there does not have to be a corresponding region for a false positive, this is the most important indication for the performance of the matching algorithm. It is expected that for linked false positive regions the likelihood of malignancy will decrease by combining features.

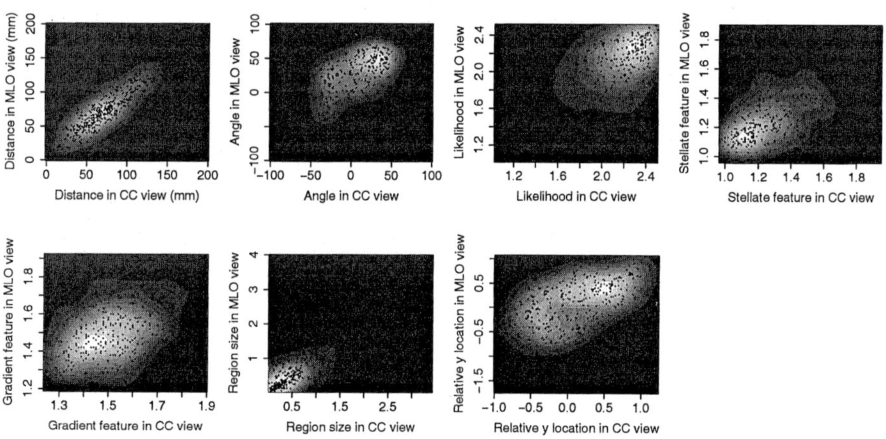

Fig. 2. Feature distributions of the features used for matching (for feature descriptions see text).

2.2 Classification, Combining Feature Vectors

After the initial detection stage and region matching, a final classification stage is used to classify the regions into true abnormalities and false positives.

The features used for the classification stage are region based and describe the position of a region in the breast (for instance the distance to pectoral and skin), region size, contrast, texture, compactness and acutance measures.

Two different k-Nearest Neighbor classifiers [8] were compared; one for regions without a corresponding region and one for regions with a corresponding region in the other view, using forward feature selection. The two view classifier used single view features, average features and absolute difference features.

Since we are still working on the matching algorithm, in this preliminary study we only combined features for regions in image pairs for which the true lesion in the MLO view was correctly linked with the true lesion in the CC view.

Classifier performance was measured by FROC analysis.

3 Results

In 87 % of the cases the lesions were detected in both views by the initial detection stage. Because our method does not yet handle the situation where there are multiple regions on the lesion in one or both views, an additional 2 cases, where the lesion diameter was larger than 3 cm, had to be removed from the image set. The remaining set thus consisted of 147 MLO/CC image pairs. Our matching algorithm could establish a correct link between the lesion in the MLO view and the CC view in 105 out of the 147 cases (71 %) (see Figure 3(a)). An example of the results of the matching algorithm can be found in Figure 3(b).

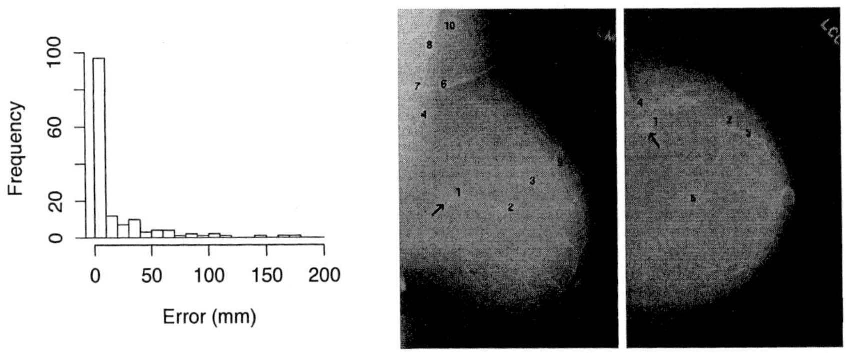

(a) (b)

Fig. 3. (a) Matching results for the 147 corresponding image pairs (using the distance feature, the likelihood feature, the stellate feature, and the gradient feature). (b) Example image pair showing matching results; equal numbers indicate matching regions. The lesion is indicated by an arrow on both views.

When using only the cases for which correct correspondence was found, the performance improved when using the two view classifier (Figure 4).

4 Discussion

Using a number of features, including the distance between a region and the nipple, regions could be matched in mammographic views taken at different angles. Using this correspondence, feature vectors of both views were combined, resulting in an improvement of the classifier performance.

When comparing our results with the results of Paquerault et al., it can be noted that both their image and case based performance increase significantly, while ours improve only slightly.

For comparison: their image based performance improves from a sensitivity of 62 % to 73 % (for 1 false positive per image), while ours increases from 93 %

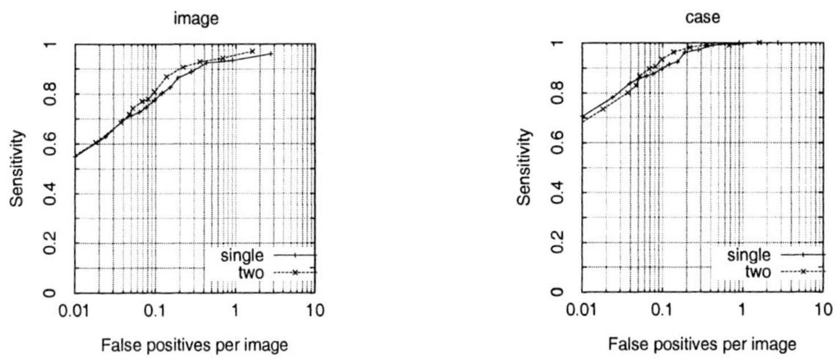

Fig. 4. Image and case based FROC curves for the single and the two view classifier. Note that the first part of the curve is not reliable because of the relative small dataset.

to 96 %. Their case based performance improves from a sensitivity of 77 % to 91 %, while ours is 99 % for both single and two view.

The smaller increase in performance for our set could be due to the fact that our starting performance for the single view classifier is already significantly higher, making it harder to improve. This difference in single view performance might be the result of the difference in used datasets. Moreover, we only used cases for which correct correspondence was found, which could result in simplification of the dataset.

References

1. Hadjiiski, L., Sahiner, B., Chan, H., Petrick, N., Helvie, M., Gurcan, M.: Analysis of Temporal Changes of Mammographic Features: Computer-Aided Classification of Malignant and Benign Breast Masses. Med Phys **28(11)** (2001) 2309–2317
2. Paquerault, S., Petrick, N., Chan, H., Sahiner, B., Helvie, M.: Improvement of Computerized Mass Detection on Mammograms: Fusion of Two-View Information. Med Phys **29(2)** (2002) 238–247
3. Karssemeijer, N., te Brake, G.: Detection of Stellate Distortions in Mammograms. IEEE Trans Med Imag **15(5)** (1996) 611–619
4. Heath, M., Bowyer, K., Kopans, D., Kegelmeyer, Jr. P.: The Digital Database for Screening Mammography. In Digital Mammography, Medical Physics Publishing, Madison, (2000) 212–218
5. van Engeland, S., Karssemeijer, N.: Matching Breast Lesions in Multiple Mammographic Views. In Medical Image Computing and Computer-Assisted Intervention, LNCS 2208, Springer (2001) 1172–1173
6. te Brake, G., Karssemeijer, N.: Single and Multiscale Detection of Masses in Digital Mammograms. IEEE Trans Med Imag **18(7)** (1999) 628–639
7. Terrell, G., Scott, D.: Variable Kernel Density Estimation. Annals of Statistics **20(3)** (1992) 1236–1265
8. Mount, D., Arya, S.: ANN: Approximate Nearest Neighbor software. University of Maryland (1998)

Classification of Breast Tumors in Digitized Mammograms

C. Varela, N. Karssemeijer, J.M. Muller, P.G. Tahoces

Department of Radiology, University Medical Center Nijmegen,
Geert Grooteplein 18, 6525 GA Nijmegen, The Netherlands
celiav@radiology.azn.nl

Abstract. An automatic computer-aided diagnosis algorithm to classify malignant and benign tumors in digitized mammograms was developed. Images selected from the publicly available data set "Digital Database for Screening Mammography" were used for evaluation of this algorithm. A new segmentation algorithm was used to segment the lesion. To represent spiculation we used features previously developed for mass detection. Features based on margin sharpness, location and contrast were also extracted. A k-nearest neighbor algorithm was used for feature selection. The average test results corresponded to A_z value of 0.84 and 0.79 in a case and in an image based classification scheme respectively.

1 Introduction

The positive predictive value of mammographic screening is not as high as desirable. In some countries, only 15-30% of detected lesions which are biopsied are subsequently determined malignant. Computer-Aided Diagnosis (CAD) has the potential to assist the radiologists in characterization of mammographic masses and reduce the benign biopsy rate.

In this study we present a digital image processing algorithm to classify breast lesions in digitized mammograms. This classification method is mainly based on quantitative measures of spiculation and margin sharpness. The spiculation of the margin of a lesion was characterized with spiculated measures previously developed for detection of masses and stellate lesions [1,2]. The margin sharpness of a mass was estimated based on gradient distributions at the contour of a lesion. In order to obtain an accurate contour a new mass segmentation algorithm was used to extract the lesions from the mammograms [3].

It is known that the use of different data sets, mostly with a small number of images, makes comparison among different CAD methods very difficult and hence it is hard to be certain that a proposed new CAD algorithm makes a practical advance in the state-of-the-art. To allow comparison of results, our method to characterize mammographic masses has been developed and tested using images contained in the publicly available data set Digital Database for Screening Mammography (DDSM)[4]. An accurate identification of the cases used is presented. Therefore, results may be easily reproduced or compared with future methods evaluated on the same data set.

2 Material and Methods

Our study consisted of three main steps: 1) Mass segmentation and transformation of its border, 2) Feature extraction and 3) Feature selection and classification between malignant and benign masses by means of a k-nearest neighbor algorithm.

2.1 Database

The images used in this study were obtained from the DDSM [4]. In this work we only used cancer and benign volumes of cases digitized with a Lumisys scanner. From the cancer volumes we used: cancer_01, cancer_05, cancer_09, and cancer_15. From the benign ones we used: benign_04, benign_06, benign_13, and benign_14. From these volumes we selected only those images that contained at least one mass lesion. Images containing only microcalcifications were rejected. We only included proven cases. Lesions with pathology indicated as unknown or benign_without_call_back were not used. DDSM cases are provided with a truth file containing the annotation of the tumor. The center of mass of this annotation was used as a reference point for our segmentation method. In some cases a single annotation provided by the DDSM included several lesions resulting in a center of mass that was outside of the lesion. For this reason 2 cases were not used in this study (cancer_01/case0019 and cancer_05/case0182). Some cases were further removed from the data set due to different reasons. Two cases were removed from the data set due to the presence of metal clips in the tumors (cancer_15/case3511 and cancer_15/case3513). Images contained in case cancer_15/case3043 were unreadable.

Excluding the 5 cases mentioned above, we used a total data set of 788 images containing 882 masses. Some images contained more than one lesion. The number of malignant and benign lesions were 481 and 401, respectively. Original digitized images were sub-sampled to a resolution of 200 microns maintaining the original gray value resolution of 12 bits.

2.2 Segmentation algorithm

In the literature, most methods developed to discriminate between malignant and benign lesions use regions of interest (ROI) containing the mass. In our study, the entire mammogram is used. Hereby, the size of our region of study is not limited. Our mass segmentation algorithm was based on the idea of finding optimal path in a cost function [3]. This cost function was built using as reference the center of mass of the annotation provided by the DDSM database. Once this cost function was calculated the contour was obtained by means of a dynamic programming algorithm [3](Fig. 1(c)). Next, a border region outside and inside the contour of the segmented mass were transformed into a rectangular band [5]. In this way, the radially oriented pattern of a mass was transformed into a vertical one. Different features were extracted from either the mass or the transformed image depending on the algorithm being applied.

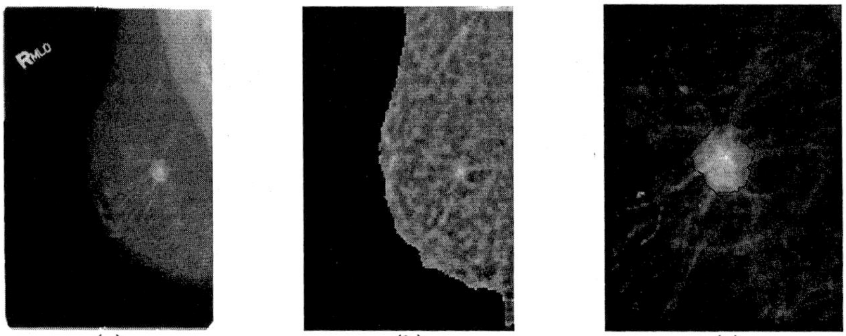

(a) (b) (c)

Fig. 1. a) Mammogram with a spiculated mass, b) Spiculation likelihood image, and c) Contour of the spiculated mass

2.3 Feature extraction

The margin and the shape of a mass are two of the major characteristics used by radiologists in classifying masses. Malignant masses have generally spiculated or ill-defined margins. However, benign masses usually have circumscribed sharply defined margins. The spiculation of the margin of a lesion was characterized by means of an operator previously developed for mass detection [1,2]. It was applied to the entire breast region of the mammogram obtaining an orientation concentration image (Fig. 1(b)) where orientations were computed with second order Gaussian derivatives. From this image two different features were calculated: i) The value in the center of mass of the annotation and ii) The average value of this image in the segmented lesion.

A sharp margin usually implies an abrupt change in the pixel value from the margin to the surrounding tissue. To estimate this variation, the first and the second directional derivatives in the normal direction to the contour were calculated. These were obtained applying Gaussian derivative filters at a low scale (σ=1.5 mm). Both distributions were smoothed with an averaging window that corresponded approximately to a sector of 60 degrees on the contour. Different measures were calculated from these smoothed gradient distributions: maximum, minimum, and the average value.

To introduce information about location in our feature space, the distance to the chest of the segmented region was also considered as a feature. Contrast of the mass was calculated as the difference in gray level between the mass and a border region surrounding it. The size of the segmented region was also included as a feature.

Features were also extracted from the transformed border image. A moving average window was used to calculated the distribution of the pixel values at every point of the contour. The maximum and the average of this distribution were calculated.

Finally the feature space included a total of 13 features.

2.4 Classification

Our classification method consisted of two independent steps, feature selection and classification between malignant and benign tumors. In order to validate the prediction abilities of the classifier, the data set was partitioned randomly into training and test subsets on a 1:1 ratio, under the constraint that the images from the same patient were grouped into the same subset. The training set in each partition was used for feature selection and the test set was used for the classifier validation. The data set was repartitioned randomly ten times and the experiment was repeated for each partition.

A k-Nearest Neighbor (KNN) algorithm was used on a leave-one-out basis to select the most useful features from the entire feature space. Features were selected from each training set in a sequential forward procedure. New features were included if they increased the performance of the classifier. For each step the performance was evaluated by means of the area under the Receiver Operating Characteristic Curve (ROC) [6].

Once features were selected, the classifier was evaluated with the corresponding test set. For every lesion in each view a probability of malignancy was calculated with KNN. Evaluation was performed in two ways, film-based and case-based. In the film-based method, the likelihood of malignancy provided by the classifier was used as a discrimination score. In the case-based method, the purpose was to classify each case as malignant and benign using the information from all available images. The discrimination score for each case was the maximum of the discrimination scores of the lesions belonging to it. This discrimination score was defined as the average of the classifier output for all different views of a lesion. The discrimination scores were analyzed using ROC methodology [6]. For each test partition, the classification accuracy was evaluated as the area A_z under the ROC curve. An A_z test value was obtained by averaging the A_z obtained for the ten different partitions.

3 Results

The average number of selected features in the training sets was 6. Spiculation measures turned out to be the most important features. The average value of the spiculation image in the mass region was selected for every partition. Features extracted from the distribution of the second directional derivative, mainly the maximum and the mean value, were selected in nine out of ten partitions. Fig. 2 shows scatter plots of the two most relevant features. The average test results for film-based performance corresponded to A_z value of 0.79. The average A_z for a case-based evaluation was 0.84. The average number of cases in the test partitions was 192.

4 Discussion and Conclusions

A computer-aided diagnosis scheme to automatically classify masses was developed. The new segmentation algorithm [3] turned to be robust and accurate

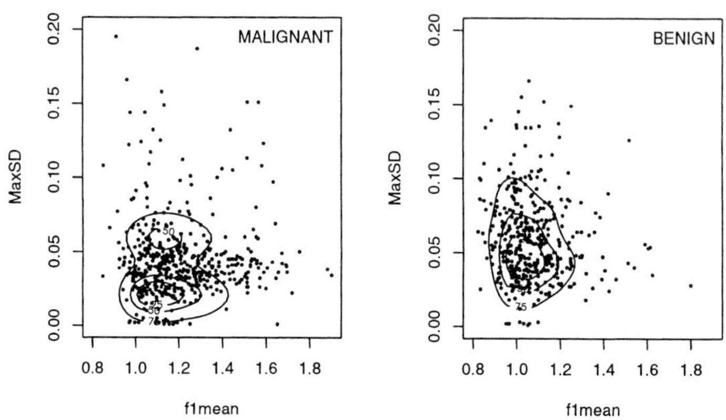

Fig. 2. Density distribution of the average value of the spiculation image in the mass region (f1mean) and the maximum of second directional derivative (MaxSD).

since features extracted from the contour of the mass were useful for our classification goal. Spiculation measures previously developed for detection of stellate patterns proved to be important also for benign/malignant classification. New features were developed to measure the sharpness of the margin and they turned out to be relevant for the classification task. As in the case of clinical practice, the combination of information of different views improved the performance of the classifier. Our study has been developed using a publicly available database so results should be easily reproducible. The large number of cases used in this study allowed the implementation of training and testing procedures in a completely independent way.

References

1. Karssemeijer, N., te Brake, G.M.: Detection of stellate distortions in mammograms. IEEE Trans. Med. Imaging 15 (1996) 611-619
2. Karssemeijer, N.: Recognition of stellate lesions in digital mammograms. In: Gale, A.G., Astley, S.M., Dance, D.R., Cairns, A.Y., (eds.) 2nd International Workshop on Digital Mammography. Elsevier, Amsterdam (1994) 211–220
3. Timp, S., Karssemeijer, N.:Comparison of three different segmentation methods. In press. 6th International Workshop in Digital Mammography, Bremen (2002)
4. Heath, M., Bowyer, K., Kopans, D., Kegelmeyer, Jr.P.: The Digital Database for Screening Mammography. In: Yaffe, M.J., (eds.) 5th International Workshop on Digital Mammography. Medical Physics Publishing, Madison (2000) 212–218
5. Sahiner, B., Chan, H.-P., Petrick, N., Helvie, M.A., Goodsitt, M.M.: Computerized characterization of masses on mammograms: the rubber band straightening transform and texture analysis. Med. Phys. 25 (1998) 516–526
6. Metz, C.E.: ROC methodology in radiographic imaging. Invest. Radiol. 21 (1986) 720–733

Experience with Computer-Aided Detection in a Low-Volume Mammography Clinic

Carl J. Vyborny[a,b], Catherine Kukec[b], Yulei Jiang[a] and Kunio Doi[a]

a) Department of Radiology, The University of Chicago, Chicago, Illinois
b) Department of Radiology, LaGrannge Memorial Hospital, LaGrange, Illinois
cvyborny@chi-rad-soc.org

Abstract. The effect of the R2 ImageChecker computer-aided detection system was evaluated in a low-volume mammography clinic in the suburbs of Chicago. Prompts from the ImageChecker resulted in an additional 1.0% of patients being recalled for additional imaging while increasing the yield for early detection of impalpable breast cancer by 5.2% over a 24 month period. Cancer detection rates before and after installation of the computer-aided detection system were not statistically different.

1. Introduction

It is well documented that present generation computer-aided detection (CAD) devices in mammography can detect breast cancers that are visible retrospectively on mammograms but that were not reported by the original interpreting radiologist [1,2]. The utility of CAD devices has now also been evaluated prospectively in screening centers [3,4]. We report our experience with the R2 ImageChecker at a small imaging clinic doing approximately 10 to 12 mammograms a day.

2. Materials and Methods

The study described here was performed after approval by, and under supervision of, the applicable Institutional Review Board. The R2 ImageChecker was installed at Grant Square Imaging in the suburbs of Chicago on April 1, 1998. A number of conventional mammography practice parameters were monitored between January 1, 1997 and March 31, 2000 in order to assess the effect and utility of the ImageChecker. Additionally, commencing on August 1, 1998, radiologists were asked to record cases in which patients were recalled to the department for additional imaging as the result of CAD prompts.

The volume of mammography at the clinic averaged between 10 and 12 cases per day throughout the course of the study. A single radiologist staffed the site and, in addition to mammograms, also interpreted plain film studies, as well as computed tomography, nuclear medicine and ultrasound examinations with the total case volume being approximately 40 studies per day. The volume and mix of the examinations was such that radiologists at the clinic were about "half as busy" as at other sites staffed by the radiology professional group. Four radiologists read more than 95% of the mammograms at the clinic during the 39 month study period.

It was the policy of the clinic that no added charges be assessed for additional mammography views. The technologists therefore routinely reviewed the cases before patient discharge and brought potential abnormalities to the radiologist's attention who then decided whether additional views might be needed before the examination was considered complete. This practice style did not change after installation of the ImageChecker, with technologist review coming before the films were digitized for CAD analysis. The approach described tended to reduce significantly the percentage of patients "called back" to the department on a separate date for additional views. It also reduced the potential for observational oversights due to a single reading by one radiologist.

3. Results

Between August 1, 1998 and March 31, 2000, 51 of 5359 (1.0%) patients were called back to the department based on prompts by the ImageChecker. An independent assessment of the average recall rate for the three radiologists who interpreted examinations throughout the entire study period showed an increase from 3.1% between January 1, 1997 and March 31, 1998 (before installation) to 4.2% between the August 1, 1998 and March 31, 2000 ($p=0.037$; Pearson Chi-square test with Yates correction). As described above, the practice style at the clinic tended to reduce recall rates appreciably.

The 51 additional patient recalls resulted in 6 biopsies, one of which yielded a malignant diagnosis. This represented an increase of 5.2% (1/19) in the yield of impalpable cancers at the clinic during the monitored period.

No statistically significant difference in the detection rate for impalpable breast cancer was noted before and after ImageChecker installation. Between January 1, 1997 and March 31, 1998 the detection rate was 4.5/1000 (13/2866). Between April 1, 1998 and March 31, 2000 the detection rate was 3.8/1000 (24/6345), ($p=0.73$). The positive predictive values for biopsy before and after installation were 38% and 30% respectively ($p=0.55$). In cases for which T staging was available, the minimal cancer detection rate (percentage Tis, T1a and T1b lesions) was 50% (4/8) before installation and 75% (9/12) after installation ($p=0.36$; 2-tailed Fisher exact test).

4. Discussion

The practice setting in this study is one that could be reasonably expected to minimize the benefits of computer-aided detection. The radiologists reviewed a relatively small number of cases every day and did so in a rather relaxed environment. Additionally, the technologists prescreened examinations for potential abnormalities in order to reduce recall rates. In so doing, they often served effectively as second readers, an approach taken at some institutions to improve the sensitivity of screening mammography [5]. It is therefore of interest that the ImageChecker alerted radiologists to abnormalities, overlooked on original film review, but warranting patient recall in nearly 1.0% of the cases. Further, biopsy recommendations resulted in more than 10% of the recalled patients (6/51). These results suggest that even in a favorable practice environment, radiologists do not perceive all findings that, retrospectively, can be considered worthy of concern.

The question does arise whether CAD information is as beneficial in a low-volume reading situation. In particular, one could postulate that CAD prompts might make the unhurried radiologist hyperattentive to borderline findings that ultimately prove to be benign. It has been shown that such borderline findings, at least when identified by experts, almost never are the result of malignant lesions [6]. The percentage of patients additionally recalled due to CAD prompts in this study was approximately 1.0%, a value similar to that reported by Freer and Ulissey. At the same time, the incremental increase in yield for breast cancer detection was much less in this study, i.e., 5%, than the nearly 20% reported by Freer and Ulissey in a study carried out in a much busier mammography center. Given the relatively small number of cancer cases involved, however, the difference is not statistically significant ($p=0.27$; 2-tailed Fisher exact test). Radiologists using CAD information in any setting should nevertheless be aware of the very low yield in the recall of borderline findings.

There are obvious difficulties in arriving at statistically meaningful observations in low-case-volume practice. We were fortunate to have a very stable practice environment for the 39 month study period during which slightly more than 9000 examinations were performed. Given the very low incidence of breast cancer, however, our results fail to prove or disprove the benefit of CAD in terms of the most reliable indicator, i.e. absolute detection rates at screening. Such a benefit, if any, may be difficult to prove satisfactorily at centers that perform a low volume of the examination.

5. Conclusions

The utilization of the R2 ImageChecker at a low volume mammography center resulted in an apparent small (5.0%) increase in the detection of impalpable breast cancer while an additional 1.0% of patients were recalled for additional imaging as a result of CAD prompts. The benefits of CAD at clinics doing a low volume of mammography may be less than those obtained at high-volume centers.

Acknowledgements

This work was supported in part by U.S. Army DAMD 17-96-1-6228. The authors thank Timothy Merrill, M.D., Joseph Chessare, M.D. and Allan Haggar, M.D. for their participation in this study. Melissa Tischman, R.T.(R)(M) and Geraldine Calzaretta, R.T.(R)(M) performed the mammograms during the period described in this paper. C. Vyborny and K. Doi are shareholders in R2 Technology Inc.

References

1. Nishikawa, R.M., Giger, M.L., Schmidt, R.A., Wolverton, D.E., Doi K.: Prospective Testing of a Clinical CAD Workstation for the Detection of Breast Lesions on Mammograms. In: Doi, K., MacMahon, H., Giger, M.L., Hoffmann K.R. (eds.) Computer- Aided Diagnosis in Medical Imaging: Proceedings of the 1st International Workshop on Computer-Aided Diagnosis, Elsevier, Amsterdam (1997) 209-214
2. Burhenne, L.J.W., D'Orsi, C.J., Feig, S.A., Kopans, D.B., Sickles, E.A., Tabar, L., Vyborny, C.J., Castellino, R.A.: The Potential Contribution of Computer-aided Detection to the Sensitivity of Screening Mammography. Radiology 215 (2000) 554-562
3. Freer, T.W., Ulissey, M.J.: Screening Mammography with Computer-aided Detection: Prospective Study of 12,860 Patients in a Community Breast Center. Radiology 220 (2001) 781-786
4. Cupples, T.E.: Impact of Computer-aided Detection in a Regional Screening Mammography Program. Radiology 221(P) (2001) 520
5. Tonita, J.M., Hillis, J.P., Lim, C.H.: Medical Radiologic Technologist Review: Effects on a Population-based Breast Cancer Screening Program. Radiology 211 (1999) 529-533
6. Wolverton, D.E., Sickles, E.A.: Clinical Outcome of Doubtful Mammographic Findings Identified Prospectively on Screening Mammograms. AJR 167 (1996) 1041-1045

Artificial Neural Network Method for Detecting Clustered Microcalcifications in Masses on Mammograms

Xuejun Zhang, Takeshi Hara, Hiroshi Fujita, Norimitsu Shinohara, Yoshitaka Ooe, Takuji Iwase and Tokiko Endo

(XZ, Graduate School of Engineering, Gifu University, Gifu City, Japan, 501-1193) (TH and HF, Division of Intelligent Image Information, Regeneration and Advanced Medical Science, Gifu University Graduate School of Medicine, Gifu City, Japan, 501-1193) (TI, Department of Breast Surgery, Aichi Cancer Center Hospital, Aichi, Japan, 464-8681) (TE, Department of Radiology, National Hospital of Nagoya, Nagoya, Japan, 460-0001)
zhang@fjt.info.gifu-u.ac.jp

Abstract. To get a higher performance of detecting the clustered microcalcifications in mass area, we combined the shift-invariant artificial neural network (SIANN) with triple-ring filter (TRF) method in our computer-aided diagnosis (CAD) system. After eliminating the false-positive (FP) detections by variable-ring filter and a conventional three-layer artificial neural network, the sensitivity of detecting clusters was improved from 90% by our previous method to 95%, while the number of FP clusters was decreased from 0.85 to 0.40 clusters per image.

1. Introduction

The existence of a cluster of microcalcifications in mass on mammograms is one of important features for distinguishing the breast cancer between benign and malignant. However, it often fails to be detected because of its low subject contrast in denser background and small quantity of microcalcifications. To aid radiologists in detecting the clustered microcalcifications in mass area efficiently with least number of false positives (FPs), we combined the shift-invariant artificial neural network (SIANN), which had been shown to be a powerful tool to eliminate over half of FP clusters without any loss of the true-positive (TP) clusters [1], with our previous TRF method [2] to our CAD system. Finally a conventional ANN was applied to reducing FPs.

2. Materials and Method

40 cases with clusters in mass were selected from the database at Aichi Cancer Center Hospital in Japan. Our overall scheme proposed for detecting microcalcifications in masses includes the following steps: 1. Extraction of Breast Region; 2. Detection and Extraction of Mass Area; 3. Contrast Correction; 4. Density

Gradient Calculation; 5. Triple-ring Filter (TRF) and SIANN Analysis; 6. Variable-ring Filter Analysis; 7. ANN Analysis for Eliminating FP Microcalcifications; 8. Feature Analysis; 9. Classification of Cluster and Display.

2.1 Detecting the candidates of microcalcification by TRF

In order to find out the suspected cone-shaped microcalcifications, we used a feature-extracting filter called triple-ring filter (TRF) based on analyzing the calculated density gradient vectors on direction and magnitude images. Calculated vector patterns, direction and magnitude values in each 3 subfilter were compared with the basic vector pattern represented by a particular cone shape. In this procedure, two features called the "directional feature" and the "magnitude feature" were employed in differentiation of microcalcification from normal tissues [2].

2.2 Detecting by shift-invariant neural network

The TRF performed well in the shape-based detection of microcalcifications, however, it failed to detect some irregular candidates, which were hard to model into a predetermined mathematical algorithm. A shift-invariant artificial neural network, which was a layered feed-forward neural network with local interconnections, was proposed by W. Zhang et al. [1]. As illustrated in Figure 1, units in the input layer and output layer corresponding to pixels of the input and output were divided into groups. Every unit in a subsequent layer was connected with the units of a small region called the receptive field in every group in the preceding. This structure was of benefit to the detection of clusters with highly independent of the quantity and position of the microcalcifications. Meanwhile, the learning procedure became more effective compared with the conventional full-connected neural network.

In our experiment we selected 100 region-of-interests (ROIs) around mass containing both of positive and negative microcalcifications for training the network with an improved error back-propagation algorithm [1] with a 21x21-17x17-13x13 structure. Another 30 cases were selected for testing the trained ANN.

2.3 Elimination of FPs

To eliminate the FPs like blood vessels or glandular tissue, we employed a variable-ring filter based on a region growing technique [3] to the detected candidates by the TRF and SIANN. The remained FPs were applied to a conventional full connected three-layer (121-60-1) neural network. Since the coordinate of microcalcification candidates were given by detecting filters, the ANN can be trained without learning any information on location, as they were all centralized in every ROIs. The training was undertaken by BP algorithm including datasets of 80 ROIs extracted from the output of variable-ring filter on detecting 30 mammograms. Finally all the suspected microcalcifications were reconfirmed by contrast, circularity and size as well.

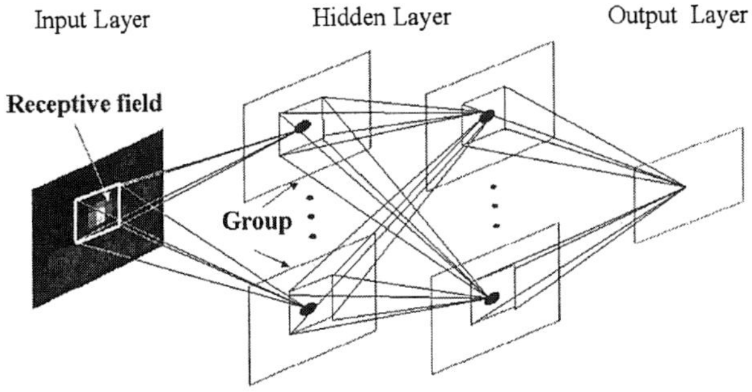

Fig. 1. The interconnections of a shift-invariant artificial neural network

3. RESULTS AND DISCUSSION

In a practical detection of 30 cases with 40 clusters in masses, 36 clusters were obtained from TRF and variable-ring filter while two other clusters could be found by adding SIANN. Therefore, the sensitivity of detecting clusters was improved from 90% by our previous method to 95% by using both SIANN and the TRF with the same number of FPs of 0.85 per image. Eliminating by both ANN and VRF method, FPs in the above experiment were reduced to 0.4 with keeping the same TP rate of 95%.

4. CONCLUSIONS

This study demonstrated that the SIANN method combined with our previous TRF method improved 5% additional true clusters compared with the TRF method only. Moreover, the conventional ANN was also an effective way in eliminating FPs in mass area.

References

1. W. Zhang, K. Doi, ML. Giger, et al., "An improved shift-invariant artificial neural network for computerized detection of clustered microcalcifications in digital mammograms," Med. Phys. 23, pp. 595-601, 1996.
2. K. Hirako, H. Fujita, T. Hara, et al., "Development of detection filter for microcalcifications on mammograms: A method based on density gradient and triple-ring filter analysis," Trans. Inst. Electron. Inform. Commun. Eng. J78-D-II, pp. 1334-1335, 1995.
3. K. Hirako, H. Fujita, T. Hara, et al., "Detection scheme for clustered microcalcifications with newly introduced contrast correction technique and variable-ring filter analysis, " Med. Imag. Tech. 14, pp. 665-679, 1996.

Removal of Curvilinear structure from Mammograms to improve Mass Detection

Keith Yates, Carolyn Evans and Michael Brady

Department of Computing and Mathematics, Manchester Metropolitan University, Chester Street Manchester M1 5GD - K.Yates@mmu.ac.uk Medical Vision Laboratory, Department of Engineering Science, University of Oxford, OX1 3PJ, UK. - {cje,jmb}@robots.ox.ac.uk

Abstract. We propose a method for improving te Brake and Karssemeijer's mass-detection algorithm [1, 2]. The method involves a pre-processing step, in which narrow, locally linear, ridge structure is removed from the image whilst retaining the larger underlying mass structure. We contrast two removal techniques for the fine structure: the first is based on wavelets and a feature detection measure known as phase congruency [3], and the second is based on a 'ridge' finding and connection algorithm developed by the authors. We display a ROC curve showing how the removal of the locally linear structure significantly improves the performance of te Brake and Karssemeijer's algorithm.

1 Introduction

Often a malignant mass appears in the mammogram to be surrounded by spicules: thin strands of tissue acting as anchors holding the mass in position. In [1] Te Brake and Karssemeijer compare the performance of three algorithms,including their own gradient orientation algorithm, designed to detect candidate mass regions in general (whether they be malignant or benign). The work reported here began with a re-implementation of their widely-cited algorithm, which pools local gradient orientation information to hypothesize the existence of masses. As suspected in [1], we found that the linear breast texture, corresponding to curvilinear structures CLS - composed of milk ducts, blood vessels, and connective stroma - degraded the performance of the algorithm. Such structures are locally linear but may curve on larger length scales. This paper reports on a novel technique for estimating the CLS, then applies the te Brake algorithm to the CLS-removed image. We demonstrate using ROC analysis the improvement that our CLS removal pre-processing step entails.

2 Method

Our method uses te Brake and Karssemeijer's gradient orientated mass detection algorithm, [1], and feature detection methods based on phase congruency, [3], and ridge finding. We review the main ideas in these methods.

2.1 Mass detection by Gradient Orientation Analysis

Te Brake and Karssemeijer's algorithm assigns to each pixel a value, which is a measure of the level of suspicion of that pixel. Te Brake's algorithm visits each pixel, α, in turn counting the number of surrounding pixels that satisfy the following two criteria,

1. They are within a distance R_{size} of the α pixel. This bounds the size of the sought for mass structure to be less than R_{size}.
2. The extrapolated gradient vector at each of the surrounding pixels passes with a distance R_{teBrake} of the central pixel.

If the resultant value is higher than that obtained from vectors oriented randomly, then this is indicative of an underlying structure. A fuller description of the method can be found in [1].

2.2 Detection of CLS using Kovesi's feature detection

Our first approach to CLS detection is based on the ideas of phase congruency and local energy, first applied to feature detection by Kovesi [3]. The local energy/PC theory is attractive because the vast majority of feature detection in image analysis is based upon differential operators that are optimized for detecting step edges, which CLS are avowedly not. The great strength of the local energy/PC model is that it is capable of detecting features of many diverse types, even those that involve complex combinations of steps, roofs, and delta-function-like spikes. The local energy model of feature detection postulates that features are perceived at points where the local Fourier components of a signal are maximally in phase, *i.e.* where phase congruency is a maximum [3].

2.3 Detection of CLS using local ridges

We now present an alternative CLS detection method which is simpler, than Kovesi's method. The algorithm begins by constructing a list of image pixels, $S = x_1, x_2, ..x_n$, whose image intensity is greater than some fixed threshold value. Each x_i is taken in turn and the algorithm searchs its neighbours for a local intensity ridge. If the search is succesful the pixel is added to list i and this added pixel is taken as the new growth point. When it is impossible to add any more CLS structure to any pixel in list i than the strand is deemed complete and the algorithm restart with x_{i+1} *etc.* A pixel can only belong to a single strand of CLS, once part of a CLS structure it is flagged and unavailable to the algorithm. The above algorithm assumes, incorrectly, that any CLS strand is only one pixel thick. We adapt it to work at multiple spatial scales by down-sampling the image: The CLS algorithm is then applied and the results rescaled to the original image scale. The union of all the images over the different spatial scales forms the final CLS image. A comparison of the two techniques is shown in figure 1

3 Removal of CLS from images

The binary image of the CLS obtained by either of the methods discussed above is now used as a template for removing CLS from the original mammogram. We first dilate the binary image using a 3×3 structuring element so that all the boundary pixels in the dilated image are positioned just outside CLS in the original mammogram. Finally, the CLS are removed from the original mammogram by replacing the original values of pixels located in the interior of detected CLS, with values smoothly interpolated from just outside the boundaries of detected CLS.

4 Results

We explain how we interpreted our results using ROC analysis. Te Brake's method assigns a value to each pixel, the higher the value the more suspicious the pixel.

The resultant image is thresholded, values less than (greater than) the threshold value are deemed to be normal (mass) tissue. Every image in the database [4] as an accompanying truth file - an image file with the mass structures marked by a radiologist. We threshold the image and then using its truth file we calculate the tru positive, TP, and the, FP, fractions. Each point on the graph is, for a fixed threshold α, the mean (TP, FP) evaluated over our database of images. By altering the threshold parameter the curves in fig 2 are plotted. Four lines are displayed: raw image data, CLS removed using ridge-finding, CLS removed using Kovesi and the result on smoothed image data.

From figure 2 we see that CLS removal using phase congruency improves te Brake's algorithm, for any value of FP its TP value is always greater than the results for the initial image. The results for the CLS removed using ridge finding and averaging are not so clear. Remembering the standard deviation of the points is approximately 0.02, the improvement in performance is only marginal. We believe the reason for the superiority of the phase congruency method over ridge finding was the wider range of scales it used to detect CLS.

5 Conclusion

We have shown quantitatively that the performance of teBrake and Karssemeijer's gradient orientation algorithm is improved by removing curvilinear structures from mammograms first. By removing CLS in a pre-processing step, we remove the structure that obscures masses in real mammograms, structure which is not taken into account in the gradient orientation algorithm's model of mass. After CLS are removed, a higher proportion of points about a bright mammographic region have local gradient vectors that point towards the centre of the region and contribute to the hypothesis of the existance of a mass.

References

1. G.M. te-Brake and N. Karssemeijer Single and multiscale detection of masses in digital mammograms. IEEE Trans. Medical Imaging vol 18 p 628-639 (1999)
2. G. te-Brake Computer Aided Detection of Masses in Digital Mammograms (Phd) University of Nijmegen (2000)
3. P. Kovesi Image Features from Phase Congruency Journal of Computer Vision Research 1999
4. USF Digital Mammography Home Page

   `http://marathon.csee.usf.edu/Mammography/Database.html`

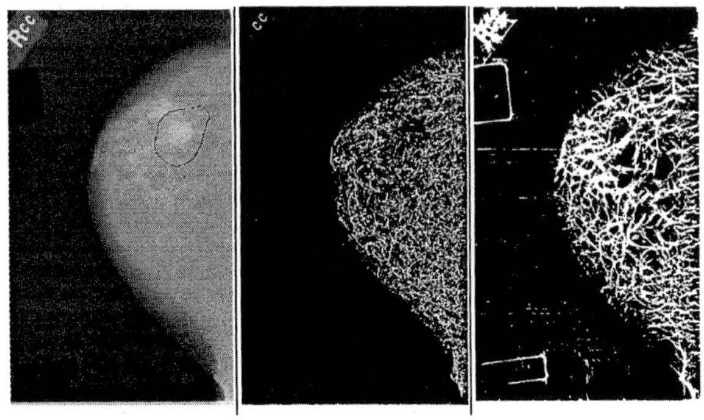

Fig. 1. (a) The original image, mass circled. (b) CLS binary using ridge method. (c) CLS binary using Kovesi.

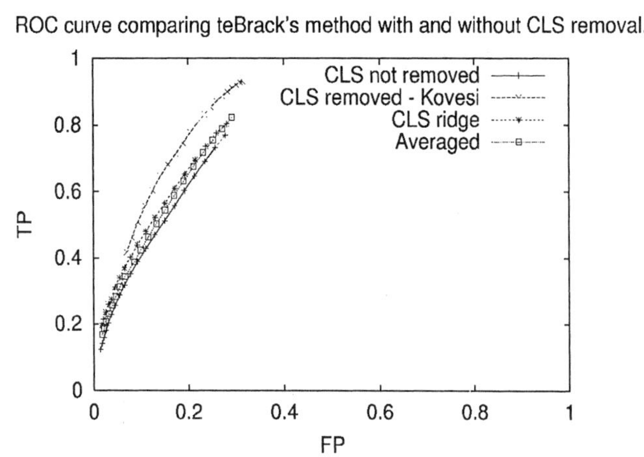

Fig. 2. Results of Mass Detection using the gradient orientation algorithm on digitized mammograms containing CLS, the same mammograms smoothed by a local averaging filter, the same mammograms without CLS detected using phase-congruency and the same mammograms without CLS detected by ridge-following.

A novel approach to mass detection in digital mammography based on Support Vector Machines (SVM).

Renato Campanini[1], Armando Bazzani[1], Alessandro Bevilacqua[2], Dante Bollini[1], Danilo Dongiovanni[1], Emiro Iampieri[1], Nico Lanconelli[1], Alessandro Riccardi[1], Matteo Roffilli[3] and Roberto Tazzoli[1]

[1] Physics Dpt., University of Bologna, Viale Berti-Pichat 6/2, 40127 Bologna, Italy
[2] DEIS, University of Bologna, Viale Risorgimento 2, 40136 Bologna, Italy
[3] Computer Science, University of Bologna, Via Sacchi 3, 47023 Cesena, Italy
nico.lanconelli@bo.infn.it

Abstract. In this paper we present a novel approach to mass detection in digital mammograms. The great variability of the masses appearance is the main obstacle of building a mass detection method. It is indeed demanding to characterize all the varieties of masses with a reduced set of features. Hence, in our approach we decide not to extract any feature, for the detection of the region of interest; on the contrary we exploit all the information available on the image. No a priori knowledge and no appearance model are used. A multiresolution overcomplete wavelet representation is achieved, in order to codify the image with redundancy of information. The vectors of the very-large space obtained are classified by means of an SVM classifier. Training, validation and test are accomplished on images coming from USF DDSM database. The sensitivity of the presented system is 84% with a false-positive rate of 3.1 marks per image.

1. Introduction

The incidence of breast cancer among women has been increasing during last years and this cancer is one of the leading cause of death in civilized countries. Mammographic screening programs result in earlier detection of breast lesions, thus permitting earlier treatment. Masses and clustered microcalcifications are the most common lesions associated with the presence of breast carcinomas. The automatic detection of masses can be hampered by the wide diversity of their shape, size and subtlety. It is indeed very difficult for a CAD system to discover all types of lesion; the reason is that detection methods often rely on a feature extraction step: here the masses are isolated by means of a set of characteristics which describe the opacities. Due to the great variety of the masses, it is extremely difficult to get a common set of features helpful for every kind of masses.

In this paper we present a mass detection system which does not rely on any feature extraction task; on the contrary, the algorithm automatically learns to detect the masses by the examples presented to it. In this way there is no *a priori* knowledge needed by the trainer: the only thing the system wants is a set of positive examples (masses) and a set of negative examples (non-masses). The detection scheme codifies the image with a wavelet overcomplete representation; the great amount of information handled by the algorithm is classified by means of a Support Vector Machine (SVM) classifier, a learning machine based on a well-founded statistical theory [1]. SVMs have already been applied to microcalcifications detection methods [2], giving rise to very good results. The advantages of SVM over other classifiers are that its setting is easier, it usually performs better on novel data and it is able to extract useful information in high-dimensional spaces. To improve SVM performance a bootstrap learning technique is performed. We validated the detection scheme with images coming from the USF DDSM database: images have a spatial resolution ranging from 43 to 50 ∝m and 12 bit gray-level resolution.

2. Methods

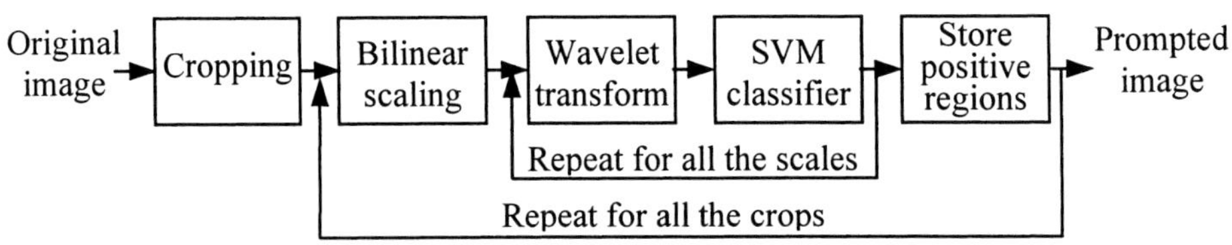

Fig. 1. Scheme of the detection method.

Figure 1 shows an overview of the CAD system presented in this paper. Since the system needs a fixed size crop (in our case 64×64 pixels), in order to detect masses of different size we first chose a window from the original image and then scale this window to a 64×64 crop, by means of a bilinear interpolation. The number of analyzed scales is strictly related to the range size of the masses we are interested in. A multiresolution analysis is then performed on the scaled crop, by transforming it with the Haar wavelet basis function. To exploit all the information available in the image, a redundant representation is obtained, by means of an overcomplete dictionary [3]. In the traditional wavelet transform, the wavelets do not overlap; they are shifted by the size of the wavelet support. An overcomplete transform allows the achievement of a richer set of features, with a shift equal to ½ (or ¼) of the size of the support of each wavelet. Unfortunately the number of coefficients obtained is extremely high: in our case more than 14000. These data represent the horizontal, vertical and diagonal coefficients of the considered levels in the multiresolution analysis. For each crop, we have a 14000 dimensional vector, which is used as input for the SVM classifier. SVMs are capable of learning in sparse, high-dimensional spaces, by using very few training examples. Once trained, the SVM classifies each crop and positive (suspect) regions are then stored and prompted. The system is able to detect lesions of different size; this is achieved by the shifting of a 64×64 window over the entire image combined with the scaling of the image, to get a multi-scale detection.

The training of the system is obtained by presenting a set of 64×64 pixels windows containing masses (positive examples) and a set of crops without lesions (negative examples): this combined set forms the initial training database. While the positive examples are well defined, there are no typical negative examples. To overcome the problem of defining this extremely large negative class, a bootstrap technique is used: after the initial training, the system is retrained with false-positive examples added to the negative set. Those examples are obtained from the detection of images not present in the initial training set. This procedure is iterated until an acceptable performance is achieved. In this way the system is forced to learn by its own errors.

3. Results and conclusion

The CAD system has been tested on images coming from USF database; about 600 images have been used: 300 for training, 150 for validation and 150 for test. In figure 2 there is shown the performance of the detection algorithm on the test images. Results are promising, especially if we consider that those images contain masses of different types: oval, circumscribed, spiculated. It is also worth remarking that our procedure automatically extracts the useful information directly from the images, without needing an external set of features for classifying the suspect regions.

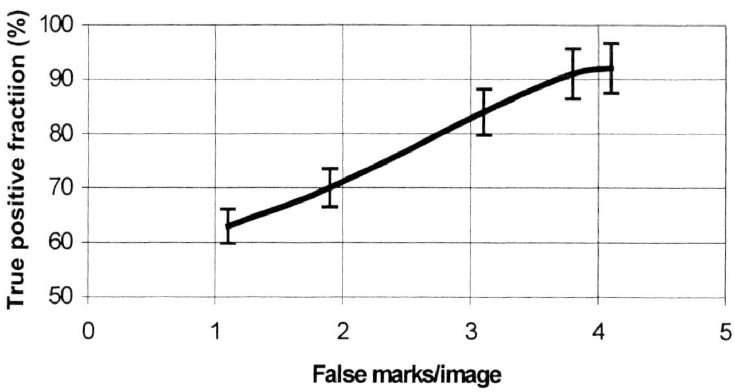

Fig. 2. FROC of the CAD system.

This work is partially supported by “Fondazione del Monte di Bologna e Ravenna”.

References

1. Vapnik, V.: The nature of Statistical Learning Theory. Springer-Verlag, 1995
2. Bazzani, A., Bevilacqua, A., Bollini, D., Brancaccio, R., Campanini, R., Lanconelli, N., Riccardi, A., Romani, D.: An SVM classifier to separate false signals from microcalcifications in digital mammograms. Physics in Medicine and Biology, 46 (6), (2001) 1651-1663
3. Oren, M., Papageorgiou, C., Sinha, P., Osuna, E., Poggio, T.: Pedestrian detection using wavelet templates. Computer Vision and Pattern Recognition, 1999, 193-199

Optimal texture feature extraction in digital mammograms

Thor Ole Gulsrud

Stavanger University College, Department of Electrical and Computer Engineering
Stavanger, Norway
thor.gulsrud@tn.his.no
http://ied.ux.his.no/

Abstract. In the present work we propose novel techniques for preprocessing and texture feature extraction in digital mammograms: The preprocessing scheme is based on dividing the input mammograms into blocks and compute an estimate of the normal background tissue contained in each block. Texture feature extraction is performed using an single filter optimized with respect to the relative distance between the average feature values. The methods are applied to a database of 43 mammograms - 23 containing one cluster of microcalcifications, and 20 containing no clusters. The results show that our CAD system performs very well in the detection of clustered microcalcifications. In particular, at a rate of about 1.5 false positive clusters per image the method reaches a true positive rate of 100%.

1 Introduction

In [1] we proposed a computer-aided diagnosis (CAD) system designed for the detection of clustered microcalcifications in digital mammograms. In short, the system consists of four parts: Preprocessing, texture feature extraction based on an optimal filter, postprocessing, and segmentation. In this paper we suggest new techniques for texture feature extraction and preprocessing which further optimize the performance of our CAD system.

2 Filter design

The obvious aim of our optimal finite impulse response filter is extraction of local frequencies in the mammogram where one of the textures (normal tissue) has low signal energy and the other texture (clustered microcalcifications) has high. If this is achieved, a mammogram can be segmented and the regions classified by analysis of their energies. Generally, the energy of a signal, y, is defined as $E\{y^2\}$ and a local measure is obtained by *smoothing* y^2. That is, the features are computed by a nonlinearity and smoothing.

In order to achieve good feature separation we try to optimize our filter, $\mathbf{h}$, with respect to the relative distance between the average features

$$J(\mathbf{h}) = \frac{(\mu_{v_1} - \mu_{v_2})^2}{\mu_{v_1} \cdot \mu_{v_2}} \tag{1}$$

where μ_{v_i} is the feature mean. Filters designed with respect to this object function have previously not been used in the detection of microcalcifications in digital mammograms. In [1] we optimized our filter with respect to the Fisher criterion [2], which are based on both the feature mean and the feature variance. A drawback with the Fisher criterion is that in order to obtain a closed form solution we have to assume that the filter outputs can be modeled as separable first order autoregressive (AR(1)) processes. For some cases this assumption may be a crude approximation.

3 Block-processing of input mammograms

In [1] we applied a difference-image technique for the preprocessing of our mammograms. A drawback with this technique is that in addition to enhance signals from microcalcifications, small signals caused by random noise in the image will also be enhanced.

Normal breast tissue has been modeled by using a stochastic model consisting of a nonstationary mean plus a stationary "residual" component [3]. If we are able to remove the nonstationary mean we may obtain a better estimate of the normal breast tissue. With this in mind we introduce block-processing as a possible preprocessing technique:

1. Divide the original mammogram into blocks of size $M \times N$. If the original mammogram is of size $M_{org} \times N_{org}$ the number of blocks will be $M_{org}/M \times N_{org}/N$.
2. For each block, compute a suitable feature for the normal tissue.
3. Interpolate the feature (background) image such as its size becomes $M_{org} \times N_{org}$. The interpolated background image represents an estimate of the normal tissue.
4. Subtract the interpolated background image from the original mammogram.

Individual microcalcifications appear as small impulslike spots on the mammogram, implying that they are represented by pixels having relatively high gray level values. Intuitively, the average of a certain number of the *smallest* gray level values in each block could be a useful feature for the normal tissue. In the following we refer to this preprocessing technique as the MIN method.

4 Results and conclusion

In our experiments we use 43 subimages from the Mammographic Image Analysis Society (MIAS) [4]. All subimages are of size 1024 $\times$ 1024 pixels - 23 containing one cluster of microcalcifications, and 20 containing no clusters (i.e. normal tissue only). The optimal filters have been designed based on preprocessed 40×40 subimages of the mammogram *mdb227lm*. Thus, we have excluded this mammogram from the test set (i.e. we are left with 22 clusters).

In Figure 1 we show the best *free-response receiver operating characteristic (FROC)* curve obtained for our detection scheme. As feature for the MIN method we have used the average of the 3 smallest gray level values in each block of size 8×8. The curve has been generated using a 8×8 optimal filter in combination with a 2×2 smoothing filter. Note that the number of false detections has been reduced by postprocessing the feature images using a smoothing filter of size 11×11. For a *True Positive* (TP) rate of 100% the corresponding *False Positive* (FP) rate is only about 1.5 detections per image. In [1] the tradeoff for achieving a TP rate of 100% was about 2.8 false detections per image. Thus, we have demonstrated that our new system configuration has improved the overall system performance.

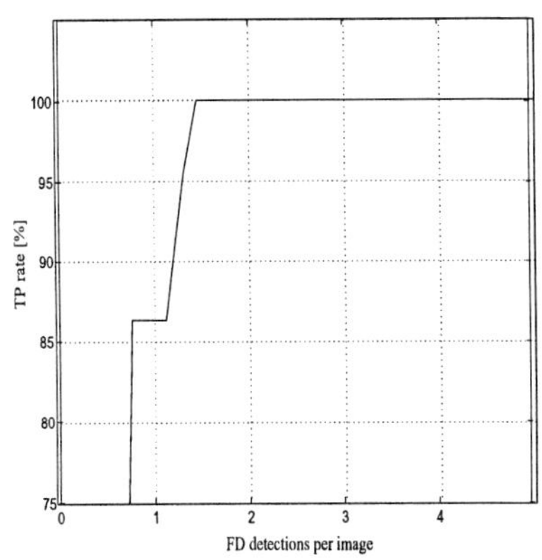

Fig. 1. FROC curve for the optimal filter based detection system.

References

1. T. O. Gulsrud and J. H. Husøy, "Optimal filter based detection of microcalcifications," *IEEE Transactions on Biomedical Engineering*, vol. 48, no. 11, pp. 1272–1280, 2001.
2. K. Fukunaga, *Statistical Pattern Recognition*. San Diego: Academic Press, 2nd ed., 1990.
3. R. N. Strickland and H. I. Hahn, "Wavelet transform for detecting microcalcifications in mammograms," *IEEE Trans. Med. Imag.*, vol. 15, no. 2, pp. 218–229, 1996.
4. J. Suckling, J. Parker, D. R. Dance, S. Astley, I. Hutt, C. R. M. Boggis, I. Ricketts, E. Stamatakis, N. Cerneaz, S.-L. Kok, P. Taylor, D. Betal, and J. Savage, "The Mammographic Image Analysis Society digital mammogram database," in *Proceedings of the 2nd International Workshop on Digital Mammography*, (York, England), pp. 375–378, Jul 1994.

Classifying masses: Significance of Az scores after feature space selection

Gobert N. Lee and Murk J. Bottema

School of Informatics and Engineering, IST Building, Flinders University of South Australia, PO Box 2100, Adelaide SA 5001, Australia
glee@infoeng.flinders.edu.au

Abstract. In order to develop a method for classifying masses in digitized screening mammograms as benign or malignant, 260 image texture features were measured on 43 images of known malignant masses and 28 images of known benign masses. A genetic algorithm was used to select the optimal subset of 4 features based on Az scores. The Az score for the optimal 4 features was 0.8879. Since feature space reduction can result in optimistic estimates of classifier performance, the significance of this score was estimated by computing the empirical distribution of Az scores in the context of the experimental parameters. Results indicate that probability of obtaining the observed performance by chance alone is 0.0080.

1. Introduction

Many authors have demonstrated that the texture of image intensity surfaces of screening mammograms provides information regarding the disease state of tissue [1],[2],[3]. Generally, these texture features are ones that are not seen by radiologists during visual inspection of the mammogram and are not based on models of the appearance of cancer in mammograms. Accordingly, the nature of texture features that are likely to provide positive predictive power is not well constrained. The result is that researchers are obliged to search far afield in order to discover optimal combinations of features. In addition, obtaining large numbers of training images on which to base the development of algorithms is not trivial and so a natural consequence is that studies comprise relatively small numbers of training images compared to the dimension of the feature space [1],[4].

Classification based on high dimensional feature spaces and small numbers of training images can be misleading. For example, if the dimension of the feature space is greater than, or equal to, one less than the number of training images, then for *any* assignment of the training images into two groups, there exists a hyperplane which separates the two groups perfectly. Moreover, the hyperplane can be chosen so that the distance between an image in the feature space and the hyperplane (magnitude of the linear discriminant score) is the same for each training image.

One way to overcome this problem is to extract from the original feature space, a low-dimensional subspace that is realistic with respect to the size of the training data set. Selecting an arbitrary low-dimensional subspace defeats the purpose of considering many features, so the natural choice is a subspace that is optimal in some sense with respect to distinguishing between benign and malignant cases. However, the performance of the selected subspace in terms of classification is bound to be high. For example, if an artificial feature space is constructed for two groups of training data by choosing feature values from the same distribution for the two groups, then a certain classification performance score will be observed. If this experiment is repeated several times, a distribution of performance scores will result. The performance score of the true experiment cannot be compared to this distribution of performance scores since the score in the true experiment represents the best performance score among several performance scores encountered directly or indirectly during the feature selection step.

Here we consider an experiment in which 260 texture features are measured on 71 training images. A genetic algorithm is used to select the four-dimensional feature subspace that is optimal with respect to Az score. The significance of the Az score is measured by constructing an empirical distribution of Az scores based on the full feature selection process.

2. Methods and materials

Images for training data were obtained from the archives of BreastScreenSA and digitized at 20 pixels per mm and 12 bit depth. From these images, 43 regions of interest (ROI) with malignant masses and 28 ROI with benign masses were extracted. A total of 260 texture features were measured. These included 12 features based on image energy, 8 based on gradients, and 240 based on cooccurrence matrices [4]. A genetic algorithm was used to search for the best four features. The fitness measure used in the genetic algorithm was the Az score computed by passing a hyperplane through the feature space in the direction determined by the Fisher transform.

The reliability of the genetic algorithm was verified by applying the algorithm to a smaller experiment comprising 50 original features and comparing the results with the true optimal set of four features determined by exhaustive search.

To test the significance of the Az score for the resulting optimal set of four features, an empirical distribution of Az scores was computed. This was done by using a bootstrap method to generate 500 different 260 dimensional feature spaces with 71 data points and randomly assigning the data points to one group of 28 and one group of 43. For each of the 500 feature spaces, the genetic algorithm was used to search for the optimal four-dimensional subspace.

3. Results

The 500 simulated optimal Az scores were used to determine an empirical distribution (Fig. 1). The optimal Az score found in the true experiment based on measured feature values was 0.8879. Based on the empirical distribution of Az scores, the probability of obtaining this Az score by chance under the assumption that there is no difference between the two groups of images is 0.0080.

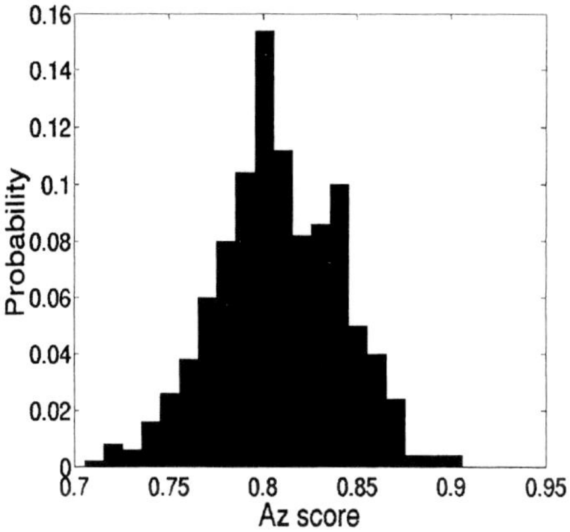

Fig. 1. Empirical distribution of Az scores

4. Discussion and conclusion

Drawing conclusion regarding classification experiments comprising data sets that are small in size relative to the dimension of the feature space is always tenuous. Merely reporting the classification scores without incorporating the bias originating from the optimization steps used to arrive at these scores does not provide sufficient information to judge the classification. Reporting confidence intervals for the classification performance score still does not acknowledge the bias of the method used to arrive at the score. By generating an empirical distribution of classifier performance values, it is possible to address the question of the significance of the classification performance measured experimentally.

References

1. Sahiner, S., Chan, H.-P., Petrick, N., Helvie, M. And Goodsitt M.: Computerized Characterization of Masses on Mammograms: The Rubber Band Straightening Transform and Texture Analysis. Med. Phys. 25(4) (1998) 516-526
2. Magnin, I., Bremond, A., Cluzeau, F., and Odet C.: Mammographic texture analysis-An Evaluation of Risk for Developing Breast Cancer. Opt. Eng. 25 (1986) 780-784
3. Thiele, D., Johnson, T., McCombs, M. And Bassett, L.: Using Tissue Texture Surrounding Calcification Clusters to Predict Benign vs Malignant Outcomes. Med. Phys. 23(4) (1996) 549-555
4. Lee, G. and Bottema, M.: Classification of Masses in Screening Mammograms as Benign or Malignant. Proceedings of the 5th International Workshop on Digital Mammography, June 11-14, 2000, Toronto, Canada. 259-263

Classifying DCIS and Lobular Clustered Microcalcification Using Different Schemes

Shijia Lu and Murk J. Bottema

School of Informatics and Engineering, IST Building, Flinders University of South Australia, PO Box 2100, Adelaide SA 5001, Australia
Lu@infoeng.flinders.edu.au

Abstract. Three sets of structural texture features were compared for classifying clusters of microcalcifications. Each set was based on a different method for defining image regions associated with local intensity maxima: (1) a circular patch of fixed radius, (2) Voronoi tessellation, and (3) watershed algorithm. Best classification was obtained using the simple circular patches.

1. Introduction

The presence of clustered microcalcifications in a screening mammogram is a significant indicator of breast cancer [1]. Clustered microcalcifications can be seen on mammograms in 30%-50% of breast cancers. As a result number of research groups have been developing CAD programs for the detection of microcalcifications. Calcification can also be seen in many normal mammograms, so it is important to find automatic ways for distinguishing between clusters associate with cancer and clusters associated with benign processes.

In this paper, a comparative study is performed on three methods for defining stuctural texture features for classifying clusters of micrcalcifications.

2. Methods and materials

2.1 Data

Film mammograms were obtained from the archives of BreastScreen SA, the organization responsible for breast cancer screening in South Australia. They were digitized at 50μ spatial resolution (20 pixel/mm) and 12-bit depth using a Lumisys Luminscan 150 digitizer. All cases of cancer were included only if verified by histopathology, and normal mammograms were included only if no cancer was diagnosed in three-year period following acquisition. A total of 45 mammograms were used in the study, of which 23 contained clusters associated with small DCIS, 22 contained clusters of lobular calcifications.

2.2 Structural texture

We have developed a fully computerized scheme for the automated detection of clustered microcalcifications. Microcalcifications are detected by analyzing all local image intensity maxima. Classification is based on statistical analysis of the local maxima. Here we use these structural texture measures to distinguish between one type of malignant clusters (DCIS) and one type of benign clusters (lobular). Structural texture features depend on the segmentation used to define the local maxima structures. We compared three methods of segmentation and three associated sets of structural texture features. (A) A circular region of a fixed radius of 7 pixels for every local maximum. (B) Voronoi tessellation using local maxima as Voronoi generators. (C) Watershed model. In the case of circular regions, 9 structural texture features were measured, and 14 features were measured for the Voronoi and watershed regions. Different numbers of features were used because some features are not defined or inappropriate for some methods. For example, the area of the region provides information when methods B and C are used, but not if A is used.

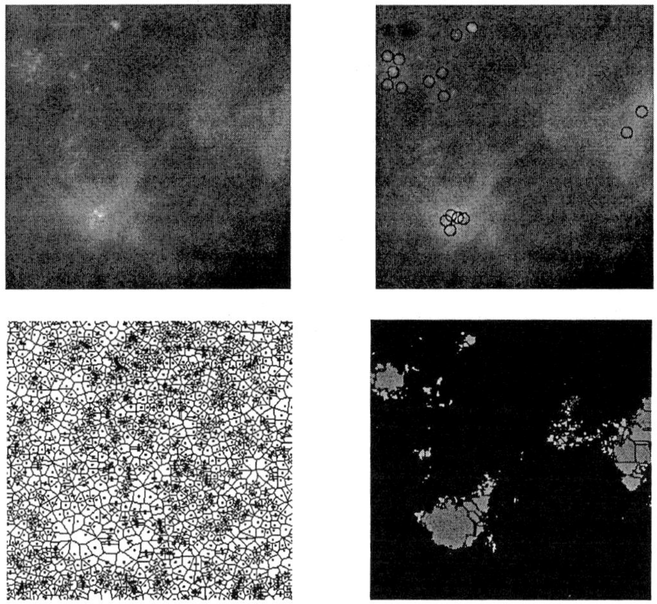

Fig. 1. Upper left is a portion of a mammogram. Upper right shows uniform circles centered at microcalcifications. Lower left shows the Voronoi tessellation and lower right shows the segmentation using the watershed algorithm.

The experiments were repeated using wavelets to compute detail images before extracting texture features.

3. Results

ROC analysis was used to measure classification performance. For each of the three segmentation methods, the Az score was computes using all features. The Az score was also compute for the best subset of features in each case.

Table 1. Az scores for the three segmentation methods. For each methdod, the Az score was computed using all features and the optimal subset of features. The top two rows show results without preprocessing using wavelets and the last two rows show results with preprocessing.

		Circles	Voronoi	Watershed
Full image	All features	0.8408	0.8027	0.7735
	Subset	0.8560	0.8195	0.7759
Wavelet details only	All features	0.8001	0.8269	0.8037
	Subset	0.8191	0.8369	0.8165

4. Discussion and Conclusion

One problem with using the watershed and Voronoi methods is that if a microcalcification appears near the top of a local background maximum, then the an unrealistically large region can be assigned to the microcalcification. Thus it is not surprising that background subtraction improved classification for these two methods. Since neighborhood sizes and shapes are fixed in the first method, background subtraction was not expected to improve classification. The drop in performance might be the result of distortion of the microcalcification shape during background subtraction. From an implementation point of view, it is convenient that the simplest method provided the best classification performance.

References

1. Holland, R, J.H. Hendricks (1994) 'Microcalcification associated with ductal carcinoma in situ: Mammographic-pathologic correlation'. Seminars in Diagnostic Pathology, 11(3), pp 181-192.
2. Boots, B. and O. Atsuyuki (1995), Spatial Tessellation: Concepts and Applications of Voronoi Diagrams, John Wiley.
3 Betal, D, N. Roberts, and G.H. Whitehouse, (1997) 'Segmentation and numerical analysis of microcalcifications on mammograms using mathematical morphology', The British of Radiology, 70(1997), 903-917.

Improved computerized detection of individual microcalcifications to integrate cluster detection and classification schemes

Maria F. Salfity[a], Robert M. Nishikawa[b], Yulei Jiang[b] and John Papaioannou[b]

[a]Instituto de Física Rosario, CONICET, Bv. 27 de Febrero 210 bis, 2000 Rosario, Argentina
salfity@ifir.edu.ar
[b]Kurt Rossmann Laboratories for Radiologic Image Research, Department of Radiology, MC2026, The University of Chicago, 5841 South Maryland Avenue, Chicago, IL 60637

Abstract. Computer-aided diagnosis (CAD) schemes for the detection and classification of microcalcification clusters have been developed at our laboratory. The classification scheme takes as input the location of each microcalcification present in the cluster. The cluster detection scheme is optimised for the detection of clusters and identifies in average half of the actual microcalcifications present in each cluster. Therefore, the input of the classification scheme was generated by manually identifying the individual microcalcifications. In this work we present a microcalcification detection scheme that acts as an interface between the cluster detection and classification schemes. This eliminates the need for manually identifying the location of each microcalcification. The new scheme analyses the region that contains a cluster previously identified by a radiologist or by an initial computer scheme, and requires as input the cluster location and size and the approximate number of microcalcifications in the cluster. This a priori information is used to identify the individual microcalcifications more accurately.

1. Mammogram Databases

We used two independent mammogram databases. Database I contained 107 microcalcification clusters (40 malignant, 67 benign) and Database II contained 246 microcalcification clusters (123 malignant, 123 benign). All films were digitized with a grey-scale resolution of 10 bits and a pixel size of 0.1 mm/pixel. A researcher manually identified the microcalcifications present in each film and regions of interest were extracted for each cluster. We used Database I to determine the appropriate parameters of the calcification-detection scheme, and Database II for evaluation.

2. Microcalcification Detection Scheme

The scheme takes as input a region of interest that contains a cluster of microcalcifications and a category to which the cluster belongs according to its number of microcalcifications, N. Three categories were used [1]: class 1 if $N < 6$, class 2 if $6 \leq N \leq 10$, and class 3 if $N > 10$.

The microcalcifications were enhanced with a Difference of Gaussians (DoG) filter. The Gaussian kernels of the DoG filter had standard deviation values of 1.1 and 1.4 and kernel sizes of 7x7 and 9x9 pixels respectively [2].

2.1 Segmentation Using *a priori* Information

First, a global threshold based on the histogram of the image segmented an initially large number of candidate microcalcifications. The value of the global threshold was iteratively changed until a certain number of potential microcalcifications, which was previously defined as a function of the cluster class [2], were segmented. Second, a local thresholding reduced false-positive detections and maintained a minimum number of potential microcalcifications, which also depended on the cluster class [2]. The local threshold value was calculated in regions of 100x100 pixels, centred on each previously identified potential microcalcification, and its value was set as $\mu + k*\sigma$, where μ and σ are the mean and standard deviation values of the region, and k is a variable parameter. If necessary, the value of k was iteratively decreased 0.01 until the number of segmented signals was above the predetermined minimum value. The output of the microcalcification detection scheme consists of the locations of the detected signals and can be used as input to the classification scheme.

3. Results and Conclusions

The performance of the microcalcification detection scheme was substantially higher than the performance of the cluster detection scheme in the task of identifying individual microcalcifications (Fig. 1). For $k = 3.2$, 85% of the actual microcalcifications were identified in Database I (Fig. 1). In the independent Database II, 77 % of the microcalcifications were detected at the same operating point. When these computer-detected microcalcifications were input to the cluster classifier [3], the classification performance was comparable to that obtained by using manually-identified microcalcifications (Table 1). In this way, with a minimal human intervention the cluster detection and classification schemes can be linked by the microcalcification detection scheme.

In a completely automated system, i.e. when the output of the cluster detection scheme constitutes the input of the microcalcification detection scheme, 61% of the actual calcifications are identified. This lower performance can be explained by the underestimation of the number of microcalcifications by the cluster detection scheme. As expected, the performance of the cluster classifier is also lower when compared to the results shown in Table 1. The area under the ROC curves (A_z) were 0.67 on a per patient basis and 0.75 on a per cluster basis. To completely automate the detection and classification CAD schemes, while maintaining high classification performance, it will be necessary to compensate for the underestimation of the number of microcalcifications by the current cluster detection scheme.

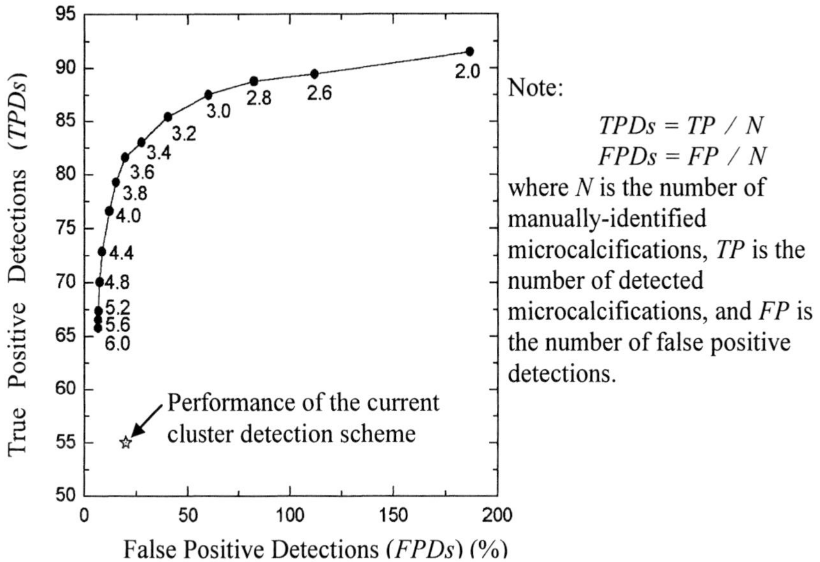

Fig. 1. FROC curve of the microcalcification detection scheme for Database I. The different numbers correspond to the value of the local threshold variable parameter *k*. For comparison, the performance of the cluster detection scheme for the detection of individual microcalcifications is also indicated on the plot.

Table 1. Area index A_z values obtained by using as input of the cluster classifier manually-identified and computer-identified microcalcifications (with the proposed detection scheme).

Database I			Database II		
Manual	Computer		Manual	Computer	
Per patient A_z			Per patient A_z		
0.92	0.92	$p = 0.91$	0.91	0.85	$p = 0.02$
Per cluster A_z			Per cluster A_z		
0.82	0.83	$p = 0.98$	0.93	0.89	$p = 0.08$

References

1. American College of Radiology: Breast Imaging Reporting and Data System. American College of Radiology, Reston VA (1998)
2. Nishikawa, R.M., Salfity, M.F., Jiang, Y., Papaioannou, J.: Improving the automated classification of clustered calcifications on mammograms through the improved detection of individual calcifications. Proc. SPIE 2002 Medical Imaging (2002) In press
3. Jiang, Y., Nishikawa, R.M., Wolverton, D.E., Metz, C.E., Giger, M.L., Schmidt, R.A., Vyborny, C.J., Doi, K.: Malignant and benign clustered microcalcifications: automated feature analysis and classification. Radiology 198 (1996) 671-678

Rapid Segmentation of Calcification Clusters using Multi-resolution Guided Fuzzy C-Means and Wavelet Processing

Christopher Sentelle, Sheri Sentelle, and Melanie Sutton

University of West Florida
Computer Science
11000 University Parkway
Pensacola, Florida, 32514 USA
msutton@uwf.edu

Work presented here focuses on employing wavelets, multi-resolution guided fuzzy c-means (FCM), and coarse-to-fine feature analysis for rapid detection of microcalcification clusters in uncropped images. FCM segmentation is guided through a multi-resolution approach to rapidly distinguish medically relevant tissue from background. Sets of overlapping sub images, containing only relevant tissue, are extracted from the image for further high-resolution analysis. A minimum number of features are used in a simple fuzzy system to detect candidate microcalcifications. This coarse detection is shown to provide high detection rates while minimizing the data points requiring further feature analysis. Feature extraction and classification is performed with a radial basis function (RBF) neural network. Cluster analysis provides final detection.

1. Introduction and Methodology

The goal of this research is to explore methodologies for improving execution times while maintaining good detection and specificity for calcifications in an uncropped, full-resolution mammogram image. This is done by applying fuzzy c-means algorithm (FCM) in a multi-resolution fashion and combining wavelet processing to rapidly segment candidate calcifications [1]. The overall design of the algorithm employed in this research is detailed in Figure 1. FCM is used to initially extract medically relevant tissue from background. FCM is applied to a low-resolution, down-sampled image (1:4096 pixels) to develop a set of prototypes, which are applied to another down-sampled version of the image (1:16 pixels). The classified (1:16) down-sampled image is dissected into a set of overlapping sub images and each sub image is analyzed to determine if it contains tissue or background. Those containing relevant tissue guide extraction of a high-resolution sample from the original image for calcification analysis.

A 4 level biorthogonal wavelet analysis is performed for each high-resolution (~500 x ~500 pixels) sub image. The level 1 detail and level 4 approximation coefficients are removed, and level 4 detail coefficients are rescaled to reconstruct a "contrast" image.

FCM with 3 clusters is performed on the 4th level approximation coefficients, directly, and then prototypes are applied to the wavelet reconstruction of the 4th level approximation coefficients only. Noise equalization, as a function of intensity, is performed by estimating the standard deviation of the contrast image corresponding to the 3 segmented areas in the "smoothed" 4th level approximation image.

Next, fuzzy images are created for each of the intensity and contrast images using a trapezoidal membership function. The intensity membership function scales intensity values between the 2nd and 3rd FCM prototypes to 0 and 1, and the contrast membership function scales contrast values between 0.9σ and 6.5σ to 0 and 1. A minimum function is then employed for a fuzzy "AND" to combine intensity and contrast. This final step appears to have additional equalizing properties adjusting for the fact that average contrast is higher in the areas of darker intensities [1].

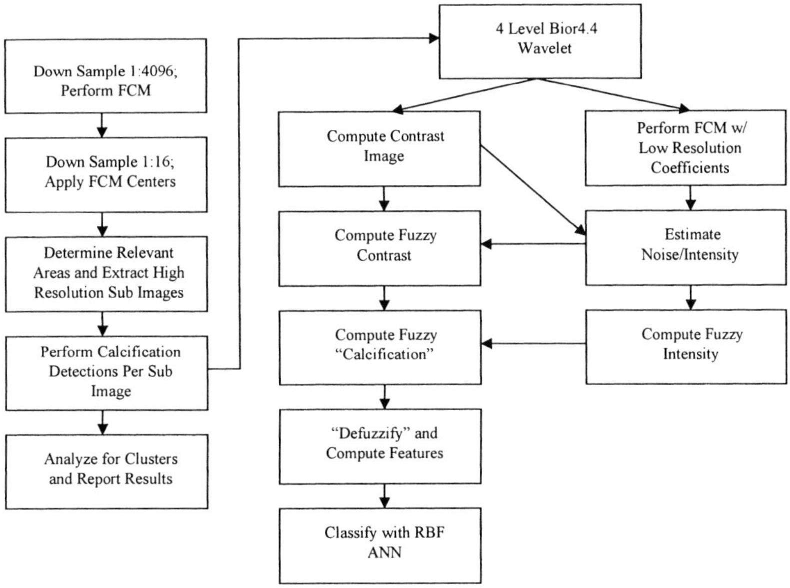

Fig. 1. Overflow of calcification detection algorithm.

Several features are extracted from candidate calcifications using 20 x 20 pixel regions to include (1) area, (2) contrast, (3) maximum wavelet contrast value, and (4) four different Law's texture measures (R5R5, L5S5, L5E5, S5S5). The Law's energy measures is computed for both background and foreground pixels. Due to the size of the analysis regions, it is possible for neighboring calcifications to appear as foreground pixels. The Law's energy features and contrast are measured with the extraneous detections as both foreground pixels and background pixels. A radial basis function (RBF) network is then used to classify the candidates. Cluster analysis determines cluster locations and density with thresholds set at 3 calcifications/cm^2.

2. Results and Conclusion

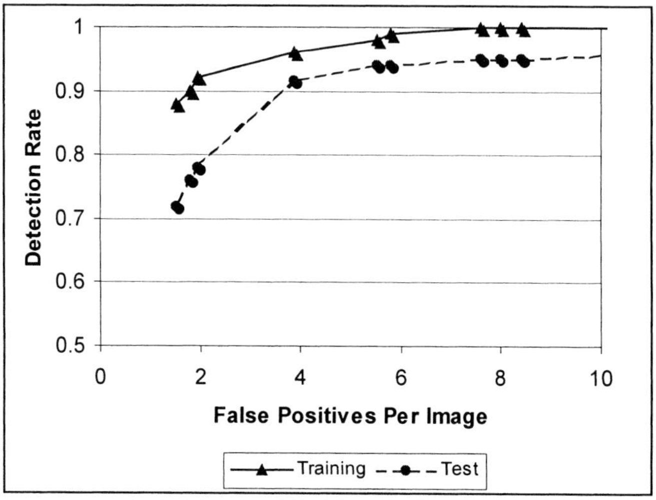

Fig. 2. ROC detection performance.

Results for four training images and twenty testing images with malignant microcalcifications from the Digital Database for Screening Mammography (DDSM) [2] are shown in figure 2. While Karssemeijer reports a processing time of 3 minutes, our average processing time per image was 4.5 minutes running in MATLAB on a Sun Ultra60 with 1GB of RAM. However, our times are based upon processing of higher resolution data, automatic extraction of relevant tissue from background, and running within an interpretive language environment. This algorithm also does not outperform results reported by Karssemeijer [3] for the long-range interaction model in terms of specificity. False positives from our algorithm appear to be attributed to linear structures and vascular calcification detections. Future work includes porting to a non-interpretive language where a multi-fold increase in image throughput is expected. We are also seeking input from clinicians who have access to the R2 ImageChecker® system.

References

1. Sentelle, S., Sentelle, C., & Sutton, M. A.: Multiresolution-based segmentation of calcifications for the early detection of breast cancer. Real-Time Imaging 8 (2002) In press
2. Heath, M., Bowyer, K., Kopans, D., Moore, R., & Kegelmeyer, P. The digital database for screening mammography. IWDM 2000 5th International Workshop on Digital Mammography. Medical Physics Publishing, Madison WI (2001) 212-218
3. Karssemeijer, N.: Adaptive noise equalization and recognition of microcalcification clusters in mammograms. State of the Art in Digital Mammographic Image Analysis. World Scientific Singapore (1994) 148-166

Soft Copy Reading

Soft Copy Mammography Reading: Influence of Monitor Luminance & Tone Scale

Elizabeth Krupinski & Hans Roehrig

Department of Radiology University of Arizona Tucson, AZ USA
Krupinski@radiology.arizona.edu

Abstract. The goal of this study was to evaluate reader performance viewing softcopy mammograms as display luminance and display tone scale are changed. The luminance study compared 80 ftL with 140 ftL, and the tone scale study compared a perceptually linearized tone scale with a non-perceptually linearized tone scale. Eye-position was recorded in both studies. Performance was better with the higher luminance display and with the perceptually linearized display, but in terms of diagnostic performance and visual search efficiency. The results suggest that it is very important to consider luminance and tone scale settings on a display monitor when viewing softcopy mammographic images.

1. Introduction

One of the most exciting advances in mammography in the past ten years has been the development and finally the clinical implementation of full-field digital mammography (FFDM) systems for the acquisition of mammographic images. The FDA has approved FFDM acquisition devices and they are currently being used in a large number of hospitals. Although the FDA has also approved softcopy viewing of FFDM images, there are still a number of issues that need to be addressed. Although issues such as how does one read an image that is approximately 5000 x 6000 on a monitor that is only 2000 x 2500 will eventually be solved by the development of better or alternative (e.g., flat-panel displays) displays, image quality will always be a crucial issue for any softcopy display system.

Two aspects of image quality and display that are important in film viewing are luminance and tone scale (basically the H & D curve). Several studies have shown that changes in viewbox luminance for film images can affect lesion detection in mammographic images. [1-4] Studies have also shown that using a perceptually linearized tone scale to display images also has an effect on diagnostic performance. [5-7] There are few studies, however, that have investigated these issues for softcopy display of mammograms, and none that have also looked at the issue of visual search behaviors and how these might be affected by luminance and tone scale differences. Thus, the goal of the present investigations was to examine whether display (monitor) luminance and choice of tone scale affects either diagnostic or visual search performance of radiologists as they search softcopy display of mammographic images for lesions.

2. Methods & Materials

For both studies a set of 50 pairs (right or left breast, craniocaudal and mediolateral views) of mammograms were selected for use in the study. 18 cases had a single, subtle mass, 18 had a single subtle microcalcification cluster and 14 were lesion free. The images were digitized with a spot size of 80 microns and a contrast resolution of 12 bits. For both studies, the images were displayed on DataRay DR110 monitors (DataRay Corp., Westminster, CO). For the luminance study, two monitors were used. One had a maximum luminance of 140 ftL and the other had a maximum of 80 ftL. The monitors were the same in every respect. The resolution of the monitors was 1728 x 2304, they used a P45 phosphor and had a refresh rate of 70 Hz. The brightness and contrast controls were set using the SMPTE pattern, so the 95% versus 100% and 0% versus 5% contrast objects could be seen equally well. For the tone scale study we used only the 140 ftL monitor. In one phase of the study the monitor was calibrated as before with the SMPTE pattern (a non-perceptually linearized tone scale). IN the other phase it was calibrated using the perceptually linearized Barten curve as incorporated into the DICOM-14 grayscale display standard.

In both studies, six radiologists participated as observers. Three observers were experienced in reading mammograms and three were senior residents who had read mammograms previously but were not considered experienced. Both studies used a counterbalanced design in which they saw half of the images first in one viewing condition and half in the other. They returned about 2 months later and saw them in the reverse conditions, so that all images were viewed twice – once in each condition. Eye-position was recorded as the readers searched the images for lesions using an Applied Science Labs (Bedford, MA) ASL 4000SU eye-tracker with head-tracker system. It is an infrared-based system that samples the eye every 1/60 of a second and records eye-position to within one degree of accuracy.

For each case, the readers were asked to first determine if a lesion was present or absent and then report their confidence in that decision using a 6-point scale. They then reported whether it was a mass or microcalcification and noted its location. Readers were not allowed to adjust window or level in either study. The room lights were turned off in both studies and readers had unlimited viewing time.

3. Results

The confidence data from both studies were analyzed using Alternative Free Response Receiver Operating Characteristic Analysis (AFROC) techniques since the readers could indicate more than one lesion location per case if they wanted to. All cases were malignant and the readers were informed of this prior to the study so it was a detection task only without classification. The average area under the curve A_1 values in the luminance study were 0.9695 and 0.9594 for the 140 ftL and 80 ftL monitors respectively. The difference was not statistically different ($t = 1.685$, $df = 5$, $p = 0.1528$). However, there were significant differences observed in the visual search patterns of the observers. Total viewing time lasted 3.71 seconds longer per case with the 80 ftL monitor compared to the 140 ftL monitor ($t = 1.994$, $df = 299$, $p = 0.046$), with the difference being greatest for the images without any lesions. Median dwell times for true and false, positive and negative decisions were also calculated from the eye-position recordings. The median dwells for the 140 ftL versus 80 ftL monitors for true-positive decisions were 1684 msec and 1737 msec, for false negatives 1329 msec and 1647 msec, for false positives 1527 msec and 1741 msec, and for true negatives 604 msec and 627 msec. The median dwell times were consistently lower for every decision with the 140 ftL monitor and were significantly lower for the true-negative decisions ($X^2 = 4.08$, df = 1, $p < 0.05$). In terms of the number of fixation clusters generated during search, there were no differences in the number of fixation clusters generated with the lesion-containing images, but there were significantly more clusters generated on the lesion-free images with the lower luminance monitor than with the higher luminance monitor.

The tone scale study also showed some interesting results in terms of diagnostic and visual search behaviors. The average A_1 for viewing with the Barten/DICOM curve was 0.9720 and was 0.9511 with the non-perceptually linearized SMPTE calibration curve. The difference was statistically significant ($t = 5.423$, df = 5, $p = 0.003$), with the true-positive rates being higher and false-positive rates lower for the Barten/DICOM perceptually linearized display. The visual search data also revealed some interesting differences. Total viewing time were only slightly different on average with the DICOM than with the SMPTE displays (49.53 sec versus 47.85 seconds), but again the median decision dwell times were consistently shorter with the perceptually linearized display. True-positive dwells were 1636 msec vs 1748 msec respectively, false negatives were 1299 msec vs 1411 msec, false positives were 1853 msec vs 1945 nsec, and true negatives were 586 msecd vs 613 msec respectively for DICOM vs SMPTE calibrated monitors. As with the luminance study, only the difference for the true-negative decisions was statistically significant ($z = 1.9$, $p = 0.05$). In terms of the number of fixation clusters generated during search, the results again paralleled those of the luminance study. Overall, significantly more clusters were generated on the lesion-free cases with the SMPTE calibration than with the DICOM perceptually linearized calibration.

4. Conclusions

The major conclusions to be drawn from the two studies presented here are that monitor luminance and tone scale can affect diagnostic and visual search behavior and thus should be taken into account when selecting a monitor for use in the clinical environment and when tracking image quality. Although diagnostic performance was not affected as much as visual search performance, diagnostic accuracy was better with the higher luminance monitor and with the perceptually linearized monitor. Whether there is an upper limit on monitor luminance has yet to be determined, but it is clear that a monitor of at least 140 ftL is appropriate for viewing softcopy mammographic images. As noted previously, a number of studies have demonstrated that perceptual linearization improves performance, and in fact it has become a part of the DICOM gray scale display standard. This study has demonstrated that it does indeed have an affect on observer performance.

The results of the eye-position recordings in both studies also revealed some important information. It seems as if providing a better or more perceptually optimized display improves the efficiency of visual search. Total search times tend to lower, decision dwell times are shorter, and fewer fixation clusters are generated with the higher luminance and perceptually linearized displays. The effect is even more pronounced with images that are lesion-free. What these results suggest is that the readers were quite capable of detecting the presence of the lesions under a variety of viewing conditions, but that when conditions were degraded (lower luminance and non-perceptually linearized) it became more difficult to determine that the images were indeed lesion free. More fixation clusters were generated and decision dwell times became significantly longer. The readers were still able to correctly identify the areas/images as lesion free as indicated by the lack of significant differences in the false-positive rates, but it took them significantly longer to do so. Longer viewing times and more fixation clusters suggest more intense processing or search of these lesion-free areas/images, perhaps because the lower luminance and non-perceptually linearized displays made it more difficult to discriminate normal image characteristics.

Although the differences may not appear important at first glance, they do have some important implications for clinical use of softcopy displays. In mammography, the majority of cases examined are normal or lesion free. If viewing times are longer and the allocation of visual resources are more intense with these images, it could very well take longer to get through the same stack of images using a non-optimized display compared to a perceptually optimized display. The use of a non-optimized display could also lead to greater and earlier fatigue than with optimized displays, affecting reader content. Overall, the results of the present studies suggest that care should be taken when selecting display monitors for viewing softcopy mammography images.

5. References

1. Robson, K.J., Kotre, C.J., Faulkner, K.: An experimental investigation of the effect of light-box luminance on the detection of low contrast objects in mammography. Br J Radiol. (1996) 153-159.
2. Wang, J., Gray, J.E.: Detection of small low-contrast objects in mammography: effect of viewbox masking and luminance. AJR (1998) 105-108.
3. Wayant R.W., Chakrabarti K., Kaczmerak, R., Suleiman, O., Rowberg, A.: Improved sensitivity and specificity of mammograms by producing uniform luminance from viewboxes. J Digit Imag (1998) 189-191.
4. Kimme-Smith, C., Haus, A.G., DeBruhl, N., Bassett L.W.: Effects of ambient light and view box luminance on he detection of calcifications in mammography. AJR (1997) 775-7778.
5. Hangiandreou, N.J., Fetterly, K.A., Bernatz, S.N., Cesar, L.J., Groth, D.S., felmlee, J.P.: Quantitative evaluation of overall electronic display quality. J Digit Imag (1998) 180-186.
6. Wang J., Langer, S.: A brief review of human perception factors in digital displays for picture archiving and communication systems. J Digit Imag (1997) 158-168.
7. Hemminger, B.M., Johnston, R.E., Rolland, J.P., Muller, K.E.: Introduction to perceptual linearization of video display systems for medical presentation. J Digit Imag (1995) 21-34.

SCREEN-TRIAL: Softcopy Reading in European Screening Mammography

Carl J.G. Evertsz(1), Nico Karssemeijer(2), Anke Bödicker(1), Ton Roelofs(2), Christian Beck(1), Sander van Woudenberg(2), Jan H.C.L. Hendriks(2), Guido Prause(3), Sascha Bohnenkamp(1), Dietmar Dechow(1), Dominik Böhm(3), Nora Wedekind(3), Barbara Lazzari, Patrice Heid, Nils Bjurstam, David Beijerinck, Hans Junkermann, Marco Rosselli Del Turco, Brigitte Séradour, Magnus Kokk, Julian Marshall, Heinz-Otto Peitgen (3)

(1) MeVis BreastCare, Universitätsallee 29, 28359 Bremen, Germany
(2) University Medical Center Nijmegen, Nijmegen, The Netherlands
(3) MeVis at the University of Bremen, Bremen, Germany
evertsz@mevisbreastcare.de

Abstract. Reading digital or digitized mammograms from computer monitors is called softcopy reading. Softcopy reading is the only way to fully exploit the diagnostic, logistic and financial benefits of the direct digital acquisition of mammographic images. We focus here on high-volume reading in breast care centers and in population-based screening mammography as it is practiced in the nationwide screening mammography programs in some European countries. Development, evaluation and demonstration of high-volume softcopy reading, is the objective of the SCREEN and SCREEN-TRIAL projects, funded by the European Commission.

1. High-volume Screening Mammography: Current Practice

Population-based mammography screening programs have been implemented nationwide in Finland, Sweden, the Netherlands, UK, Iceland, Norway and Luxemburg. France and Germany are in the process of implementation. In screening mammography it is important to achieve highest sensitivity at a very low false-positive rate. Double reading and elaborate quality control is widely practiced. Mammography images are taken by skilled technicians in (mobile) "screening units". Typically, the films resulting from a day's work are collectively sent to "reading centers", where medical experts - mostly radiologists - read them. Alternatively, the first-reading is done by general radiologists at the mammography site, while the second reading is done by expert radiologist elsewhere. Usually both current and prior images are available at reading. On the bases of the results of double reading, it is then decided whether or not to recall the women for further assessment.

For example, in the Netherlands, with a population of 16 million, there are about 1.9 million women in the age bracket 70-75. Technicians make screening mammograms in about 62 screening units. Reading is done in about 25 reading centers by specially trained and certified radiologists who take between 1 to 2 hours per day to read the films on motorized light boxes (alternators). Each case consists of current and prior two-view (CC and MLO) bilateral screening mammograms. Experts read between 50 to 200 cases in an hour.

Worldwide, mammography lags behind in its use of modern information technology, and the complete organization of European screening mammography is based on X-ray film. There are two main reasons for this situation. First, digital mammography (DM) systems only became commercially available recently. Second, suitable softcopy reading (SCR) systems designed for use in screening have been lacking [1]. Since 2000, the special challenges arising in the context of high-volume reading in European population-based screening mammography are being addressed in two projects (SCREEN and SCREEN-TRIAL) funded by the European Commission in the Information Society Technologies (IST) program in the fifth Framework.

Advantages Unique to Digital Mammography & Softcopy Reading

The reasons for pursuing digital mammography include better DQE, potential for significant dose reduction, superior dynamic range, and linear dose vs. optical density response. In addition, softcopy reading is the key to a more efficient integration and exploitation of various technologies, processes, as well as quality assurance and control procedures in the reviewing process. Amongst these are computer-aided detection (CAD); use of CAD for second opinion; immediate access to image enhancement; prevention of image retakes caused by film over-exposure or deficient film processing; electronic patient records; efficient and flexible organization of double reading; tele-mammography and tele-consultation on a regional and international level; electronic image archiving and retrieval (PACS); integration of other modalities such as US and MRI; integration of RIS; automated radiologist's performance monitoring; supplying quality healthcare in remote areas through tele-mammography; continuous computer-assisted education and training. Softcopy reading presents very promising new opportunities to increase both the sensitivity and specificity of screening radiologists via CAD, computer-aided interpretation, computer-assisted training, and automated reader in-service monitoring.

Challenges for Softcopy Reading

The major problems faced in the development of a softcopy reading environment for screening mammography are: **Spatial resolution.** The most widely used commercial high-resolution CRT displays have a 2,048 x 2,560 pixel matrix. This is sufficient to display one image at 100μm, but not to display, e.g., the 50μm CR images (3600x4800). High-resolution image display is particularly important for the detection and characterization of subtle microcalcifications. **Grayscale resolution.** Currently only BarcoView manufactures a graphics card capable of displaying 10bit grayscale on these high-resolution monitors. Digital acquisition devices, however, provide up to 16bits of grayscale information. This grayscale resolution is particularly important to diagnose subtle lesions especially in the regions of the breast with the highest density (parenchyma) and lowest density (skin-line). **Luminance and contrast.** The luminance of current high resolutions CRT monitors (± 300 cd/m^2) is about a factor of 10 less than that of a conventional light box. Moreover, also their contrast is less. **Insufficient diagnostic throughput**. In screening mammography each case consists of up to 8 mammograms. At 50μm and 12-bits this adds up to 450MB per case. This information has to be presented on 2 or more high-resolution monitors allowing an experienced screening radiologist to read 100 to 200 cases in one hour. **Workflow.** To compensate for the technical limitations of current display technologies, a new digital workflow is needed to access the relevant spatial and grayscale information in the data. **Algorithms.** Because of the number of large images involved, all image processing algorithms used in a high-volume softcopy reading system need to be sufficiently fast for either real-time application or for batch processing, and need to be extremely robust, i.e. the need for manual adjustments need to be exceptionally rare. **Validation.** The effectiveness of *film-based* breast cancer screening mammography to reduce mortality has been analyzed, discussed, and confirmed. However, conclusive studies on *digitally-based* breast cancer screening are still lacking [4]. **Training**. Until now, mammography training has been film-based. Adequate teaching and training systems for softcopy reading in high-volume screening mammography are a prerequisite for the success of digital screening mammography. It is essential that the training system itself be integrated in a high-volume softcopy reading system.

2. The SCREEN Project

The 2-year European SCREEN project (www.mevis.de/projects/screen) started in January 2000 and addressed the above-mentioned challenges. The objective was to develop a prototype high-volume softcopy reading system that can replace film-based reading in European screening mammography. This research and development project was executed by MeVis at the University of Bremen (Bremen, Germany), University Medical Center in Nijmegen (the Netherlands), Chancellor Masters and Scholars of the University of Oxford (UK), MeVis Technology (Bremen, Germany), and BarcoView (Kortrijk, Belgium). R2 Technology (Los Altos, CA, USA) provided CAD to the project.

The prototype SCR system that resulted from the SCREEN project consists of 2 high-resolution (2,048 x 2,560) CRT monitors with 10bit grayscale resolution, and a high-end PC. The high demands on image throughput from the computer hard disk onto the monitors were solved by optimizing the interplay between user demand, software, and hardware. The resulting combination of pre-processing, exploitation of hardware features including the graphics boards, and anticipation of user workflow demands through pre-fetching shows that it is possible to achieve system display responses of about 0.2 sec for all user demands, including change from one case to the next [29]. The complete display of 8 images, four on each monitor, takes about 1 sec.

The SCR-system provides the reviewer single key access to individual functions and features, eliminating functional hierarchy. Thus, the user does not have to struggle through pull down/up menus. This ViewByKey™ concept ensures that the user always has an overview of the available functions, making the system easy to use and learn. The newly developed digital workflow is reader-driven via a dedicated workflow keypad that concentrates most of the action in 6 keys. In addition, a feature has been developed enabling the reader to navigate through an individually predefined workflow with just one-key (FlowNext™ and FlowBack™) on the keypad. The cases can be annotated digitally. Predefined templates allow very efficient and detailed annotation for each lesion individually. Reports for each case are then automatically generated, and the results of double reading matched. To compensate for the limited grayscale resolution of the monitors and the human visual system, dedicated pre-processing, and special look-up-tables were developed to ensure that typically no changes to window-level are needed during reading. Pre-defined display sequences for the mammograms provide the reader with various levels of spatial resolution, including a digital magnifying glass.

With a dedicated key the reader can instantaneously access CAD results on micro-calcifications or masses, which are integrated into the screening mammograms on the display in various levels of details. Via CAD [2], computer aided interpretation, computer assisted training, and automated reader in-service monitoring softcopy reading presents new opportunities to increase both the sensitivity and specificity of screening radiologists. It is known that between 15% and 30% of screening and interval cancers in screening programs could have been detected on the previous mammograms[3]. Earlier detection in these cases could have a considerable impact on the effectiveness of screening mammography in reducing mortality. Over 700 fully annotated digitized film-screen cases from the Dutch screening program have been integrated into the system, to support in Continuous Medical Education (CME) and training of mammography reading skills and softcopy reading. The system is able to fully automatically compare the digital annotation by the radiologist with ground-truth in the database. This is also the basis for radiologist's in-service monitoring. The SCR system is able to randomly include known cases in real reading sessions. In this way, the in-service performance of readers can be monitored and suitable measures can be taken.

In addition to pre-defined hanging protocols, the reviewer needs additional control on the presentation of the image material on the monitors. This is particularly important when dealing with non-standard views, such as mosaic, magnifications, preparation radiographies, US, MRI, etc. To the end a dedicated viewing module - MammoNavigator™ - has been developed that contains thumbnails of all diagnostic images of a patient that are currently available on the system. The reviewer can control the display of mammograms on the monitors, simply by drag-and-drop. The system is capable of handling images with full-field digital images with pixel sizes ranging from 40 micron to 100 micron. This covers image-sizes from manufacturers such as Hologic-Lorad, Siemens, GE, Fuji and Fischer. Radiologist's performance evaluation on the system is discussed in T. Roelofs et al. in this volume.

The SCR system is further developed by MeVis BreastCare, and is the basis for softcopy reading systems by Siemens (MammoReport^{Plus}) and Hologic-Lorad (Selenia).

3. SCREEN-TRIAL Project

Now that the fundamental technological obstacles of softcopy reading have been removed, European screening organizations are faced with a major challenge of incorporating the digital technologies, so as to benefit from the diagnostic, logistic and financial advantages. These challenges include, validation, archiving, communication, workflow, training, and the transition from analog to digital and financing. To develop solutions to these challenges, and thus expedite the use of digital mammography, softcopy-reading and CAD in the European screening programs, a new project, called the SCREEN-TRIAL project, started in April 2002. The basis for the softcopy reading part in this new project is the system developed in the SCREEN project. The project's strategy is to bundle and manage existing technological, scientific, and clinical expertise to install softcopy reading and digital mammography at User Demonstration Sites at the University of Northern Norway (Tromsø, N), Preventicon (Utrecht, NL), Bremen Breast Cancer Screening Program (Bremen,D), University Medical Center Nijmegen (Nijmegen, NL), Danderyd Hospital (Danderyd, S), Centre for Oncological Study and Prevention, Tuscany (Florence, I), and ARCADES - Association pour la Recherche du Dépistage des Cancers du Sein (Marseille, F). These sites promise to serve as role models and nucleation points for the further uptake of digital mammography in the various screening programs. Clinical studies in the project will compare softcopy and film-based reading, and the impact of CAD and training. The project also addresses the management of the transition from film-based to digital screening mammography.

SCREEN-TRIAL is a take-up action in the Information Society Technologies (IST) program with the fifth Framework coordinated by MeVis BreastCare (Bremen, D). The scientific and clinical coordination in the project are done by MeVis at the University of Bremen (Bremen, D) and the University Medical Center in Nijmegen (Nijmegen, NL). The industrial partners are MeVis BreastCare (Bremen, D) and Siemens-Elema (Solna, S). R2 Technology (Los Altos, CA, USA) is supplier of CAD to the project.

References

1 Shtern F et al.: Report of the Working Group on Digital Mammography: Digital Displays and Workstation Design. Washington DC, USA. March 19-10, 1998. Acad. Radiol. 1999 Apr; 6 Suppl 4: S195-219.

2 Burhenne LJW, et al.: Potential contribution of computer-aided detection to the sensitivity of screening mammography. Radiology, 2000. 215(2): p. 554-562.

3 van Woudenberg S, et al: Interpretation skills of Radiologist in a nation-wide screening program, in IWDM 2000, 5th International Workshop on Digital Mammography. Medical Physics Publication, Madison Wisconsin, 2000, p.537-543.

4 Skaane P, Skjennald L, Gangeskar L, Pedersen K: Population-based full field direct digital mammography (FFDDM) screening: The Oslo Project, in IWDM 2000, 5th International Workshop on Digital Mammography. Medical Physics Publication, Madison Wisconsin, 2000, p.566-572.

On the Problem of Bilateral Comparison of Mammograms

Fredrik Georgsson

Department of Computing Science, Umeå University, SE-901 87 Umeå, Sweden
fredrikg@cs.umu.se

Abstract. Since radiologists use anatomical symmetry quite extensively in their judgement of mammogram, we should try to include this knowledge into automatic systems. There are several different approaches to this problem, in this paper a general framework is presented, and some of the difficulties are pointed out.

1. Motivation

One of the most important instructions to radiologists when learning to judge mammograms is: compare left and right images and look for asymmetrical developments. When constructing automatic system for judging mammograms we should aim at implementing bilateral comparison of mammograms. In this paper, a general framework for bilateral comparison is described and some of the difficulties are pointed out.

2. Definitions

With reference to Figure 1; given a breast, say the right one, and a mammogram of this breast, say a MLO-projection, the intensity in a point *p*, on the mammogram is the accumulated attenuation along a ray *r* from the point to the x-ray foci through the compressed breast. By modeling the projection geometry, *P*, and the breast compression, C_{MLO}, we are able to draw the curve of *r* in the 3D-dimensional breast. We can call this curve r_{3D}. An approximation of the three dimensional breast is possible to construct by interpolating between the skin-air interfaces in the MLO and CC projections (given that we know the angle in which the MLO was acquired). By applying CC-compression to the 3D model of the breast and projecting r_{3D} down to a new image plane, it is possible to obtain an epipolar line in CC corresponding to the possible projections of *p*. If we instead map r_{3D} from the right breast to the left breast with the mapping *A*, compress the right breast with a MLO compression and then project compressed breast we obtained the transferred epipolar line in the left breast. This means that we have a way of finding the bilateral correspondence of *p*.

More formally, we say that r_{3D} are the points that are projected onto *p* and the intensity in *p* is the accumulated attenuation along r_{3D}. r_{3D} can be calculated according to $r_{3D} = C_{MLO}^{-1}(P^{-1}(p))$.

3. Problems

In the previous section, a method for finding possible bilateral points to a given point p was described. It was shown that given knowledge of the projection of points P, knowledge of how tissue moves while under compression C and knowledge of how to map anatomical points from left to right breast A, it is easy to calculate to corresponding points.

3.1 Modelling the projection

It is possible to model an x-ray projection of a body to a very high degree [1], so it could be argued that we actually know P.

3.2 Modelling the compression

The female breasts are very heterogeneous objects and mechanical properties such as the movements of tissue are thus rather hard to model accurately. By making assumptions and hence simplifying the problem we are, however, able to, at least, gain a rough understanding of the movements of tissue. Compression modelling have been studied in [2, 3, 4, 5] but there still remain quite a substantial amount of work to be carried out before we have a full understanding of the problem of compression modelling.

3.3 Modelling the anatomical symmetry

Little or no work is believed to have been carried out in the field of modelling anatomical symmetry. It seems hard to model anatomical symmetry in mathematical models, but on the other hand it could be argued that since radiologists carry out a comparison based on anatomical features on a daily basis, there must be something that is possible to model. The simplest approach is to mirror and scale all points from one breast to map them to its bilateral counterpart. More sophisticated models would have to take into consideration that the distribution of tissue types varies between breasts.

3.4 Direct methods of bilateral comparison

As indicated above there are several difficulties in building good models required for solving the mapping of bilateral points. One way of avoiding this is to rely on direct methods of bilateral comparison. In these methods no attempt to directly model the steps are carried out, but bilateral points are compared more or less directly. It could be argued that these methods rely on three-dimensional models, but they may not be directly visible. Examples of direct models can be found in [6,7,8].

4. Conclusion

The area of bilateral comparison of mammogram is an important one and there still remains work to be done. Trying to find bilateral points directly, without three-dimensional modelling, has rendered some success. However, it is still believed that even though we have to make assumptions when building the models, it is the most feasible way to go.

References

1. R. Highnam, M. Brady, *Mammographic Image Analysis*, Kluwer Academic Publishers, 1999.
2. R. Novak, *Transformation of the female breast during compression at mammography with special reference to the importance for localization of a lesion*, Ph.D.-thesis, Stockholm, 1988
3. F.S. Azar, D.N. Metaxa and M.D. Schnall, "Methods for Modelling and Predicting Mechanical Deformations of the Breast under External Perturbations", *Medical Image Analysis*, 6, 1-27, 2002
4. M. Yam, M. Brady, R. Highnam, C. Behrenbruch, R. English, and Y. Kita, "Three-Dimensional Reconstruction of Microcalcification Clusters from Two Mammographic Views", *IEEE Transactions on Medical Imaging*, 20, 479-489, 2001
5. F. Georgsson, N. Björnestål, "On the Problem of Breast Compression Modelling" in H.U. Lemke, M.W. Vannier; K. Inamura, A.G. Farman, K. Doi & J.H.C. Reiber (Editors), *proceedings of CARS 2002,* Springer Verlag, to Appear.
6. N. Karssemaijer, and G. Brake, Combining single view features and asymmetry for detection of mass lesions, In N. Karssemeijer, M. Thijsen, J. Hendriks, L. van Erning (Editors), Digital Mammography, Kluwer Academic Publishers, pp. 95-102, 1998.
7. P. Miller and S. Astley, Automated detection of mammographic asymmetry using anatomical features. International Journal of Pattern Recognition and Artificial Intelligence, 7 (6), pp 1461-1476, 1993.
8. F. Georgsson, Differential analysis of bilateral mammograms, In I. Austvoll (Editor), proceedings of SCIA 2001, pp. 70-77, 2001.

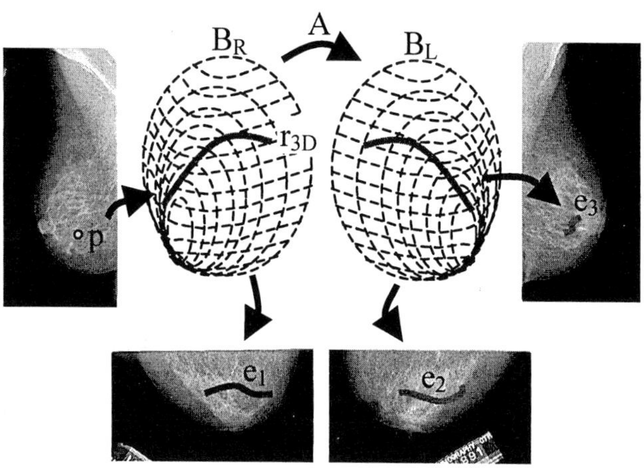

Fig. 1. Given a point p in a mammogram, in this case right MLO, and knowledge of the projection parameters P and compression parameters C_{MLO} we are able to calculate what points in the breast that are depicted on p, we call these points r_{3D}. These points can be projected down to the other projection, in this case CC and we obtain the epipole e_1. With a mapping A between points in the left and right breast, we are able to find the bilateral corresponding points of r_{3D}. By projecting these points down to the bilateral CC and MLO images we obtain the transferred epipoles e_2 and e_3. Images from case A-0041-1 from the Digital Database for Screening Mammography, University of South Florida.

Stereoscopic digital mammography: perceptual and display factors leading to improved early detection of breast cancer

David J. Getty

BBN Technologies, 10 Moulton Street, Cambridge, Massachusetts, 02138, U.S.A.
getty@bbn.com

Abstract. Stereoscopic digital mammography holds the promise of improving the early detection and diagnosis of breast cancer compared to standard planar views. A stereo mammogram provides the radiologist with an in depth view of the breast, in which a subtle lesion is directly seen volumetrically. The increased detection sensitivity from stereo seems to arise from the separation of overlying and underlying normal tissue from the lesion, and also from capabilities provided to the reader to manipulate characteristics of the displayed stereo image. In a recently completed project, stereo mammography was shown to significantly improve diagnostic accuracy and led to detection of a significant number of new lesions in the stereo mammograms *that were not detected in the films.*

1. Stereoscopic versus Planar Digital Mammography

Standard planar mammography is widely regarded as one of the most difficult radiographic exams to interpret. It is often difficult to detect a very subtle lesion because of superimposed overlying and underlying normal tissue that masks its presence. To confirm a lesion as real, a radiologist has to find it in each of two orthogonal views. And constructing a mental image of the three-dimensional structure of a lesion from two orthogonal projections is a difficult task, at best.

Stereoscopic digital mammography holds the promise of significantly reducing these problems. In a stereo mammogram, a radiologist is able to directly view tissue and the internal structure within the breast in depth. With stereo, detection of subtle lesions is improved because overlying and underlying normal tissue, superimposed on the lesion in 2D projections, is separated away from the lesion in depth. With stereo, false alarms are reduced because normal tissue lying at different depths, aligned by chance in a 2D projection, does not superimpose to resemble a focal abnormality.

With stereo, classification accuracy is improved because the stereo mammogram enables a direct perception of a lesion's volumetric shape. Also, by separating the lesion from superimposed tissue, the stereo mammogram can present the critical diagnostic features in a clearer and sharper form. For a cluster of microcalcifications, the volumetric distribution of the elements can be directly appreciated. This is novel information since finding a one-to-one correspondence of many elements in orthogonal 2D projections is essentially impossible.

2. Stereoscopic Image Acquisition and Display

We have been acquiring stereoscopic digital mammograms, illustrated in Fig. 1, on a GE Senographe 2000D with the x-ray source rotated by 6 degrees between exposures while the position of the breast and the digital detector remains fixed, as shown in Fig. 2. The stereo pair of mammographic images is viewed by the radiologist on a stereo display workstation, shown in Fig. 3, while wearing special stereo-viewing glasses made by StereoGraphics,. The two images are presented alternately in rapid succession (at a 120 Hz. refresh rate) on a high-resolution (2300 x 1900 pixel) MegaScan monochrome monitor. The stereo-viewing glasses contain LCD lenses that function as optical shutters. They are synchronized to the display and alternately block each eye's view of the display—effectively routing each image to the appropriate eye. The radiologist's visual system fuses the two images into a single in-depth perceived image of the internal structure of the breast.

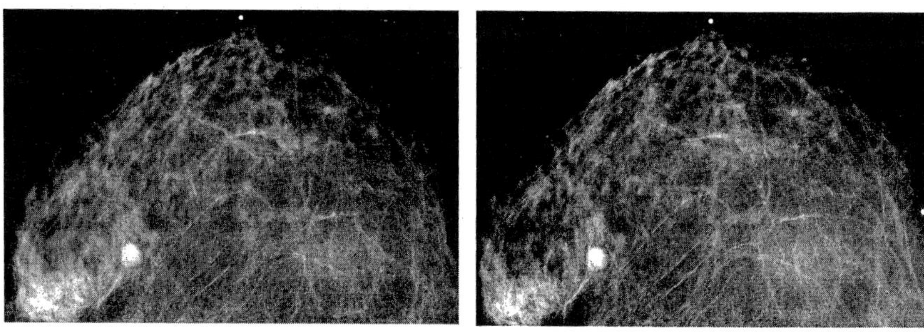

Fig. 1. Stereoscopic pair of digital mammograms, with a benign mass at 8 o'clock. It is possible to fuse these two images into a single image seen in depth by crossing one's eyes.

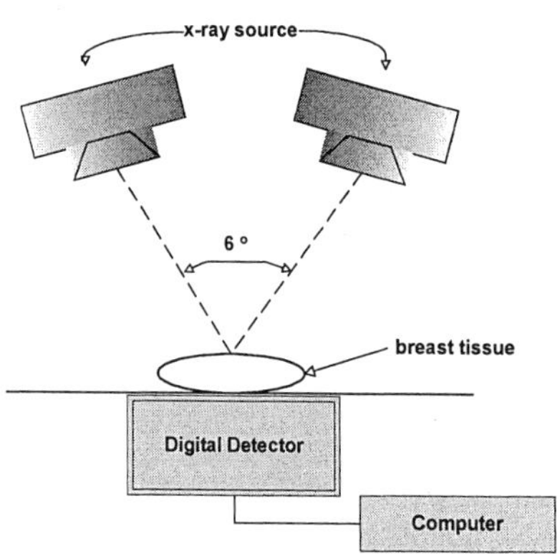

Fig. 2. Stereo mammogram acquisition.

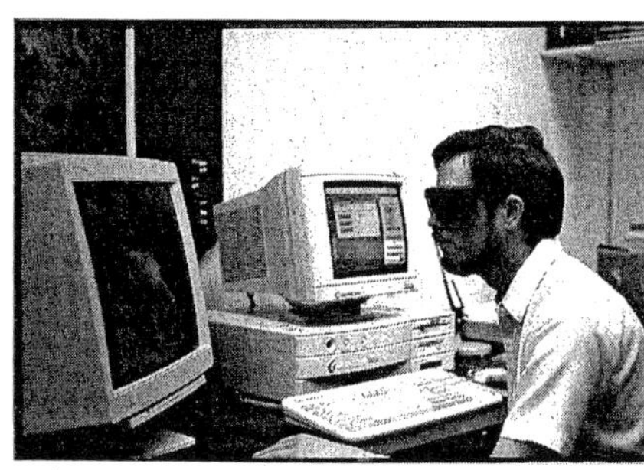

Fig. 3. Stereo display workstation.

Because of their separation, our two eyes have slightly different views of the world. There is sufficient information in these two differing views for the visual system to determine the relative depth of different objects in the visual scene. The perceptual result is a single fused image with objects seen as distributed in depth.

This visual process is called "stereopsis." The basis of stereopsis is the angular horizontal disparity between corresponding points of an object in the two retinal images. When you fixate an object, your eyes rotate, or "converge," to bring the point of fixation onto the fovea of each retina. There is zero retinal disparity in the depth "plane" defined by the point of fixation. A point on an object that lies farther away from you than the fixation point creates images on the two retinas that have "positive" retinal disparity, determined by the angular difference of the corresponding points from the fovea on the two retinas. Similarly, a point that lies closer to you than the fixation point creates retinal images that have "negative" retinal disparity. The magnitude and sign of the retinal disparity are sufficient to determine an object's depth relative to the point of fixation.

In a stereo display, retinal disparity is created by horizontal parallax—the separation of corresponding points in the left- and right-eye images on the display screen. There are three types of parallax, illustrated below in Fig. 4. If a point belonging to an object is displayed at exactly the same position in the left- and right-eye images, then it is said to have "zero parallax." The perceptual effect is that the object is seen to lie at the surface of the display screen.

In the other two cases, a point belonging to an object is displayed at different locations in the left- and right-eye image. If the right-eye point is displaced to the right of the left-eye point, then the object will be perceived to lie behind the screen surface. The larger the separation, the farther the object will be from the screen surface. This case is called "uncrossed" or "positive" parallax.

In the third case, if the right-eye point is displaced to the left of the left-eye point, called "crossed" or "negative" parallax, then the object will be perceived to lie in front of the display surface. Again, the larger the separation, the farther the object will be from the screen surface.

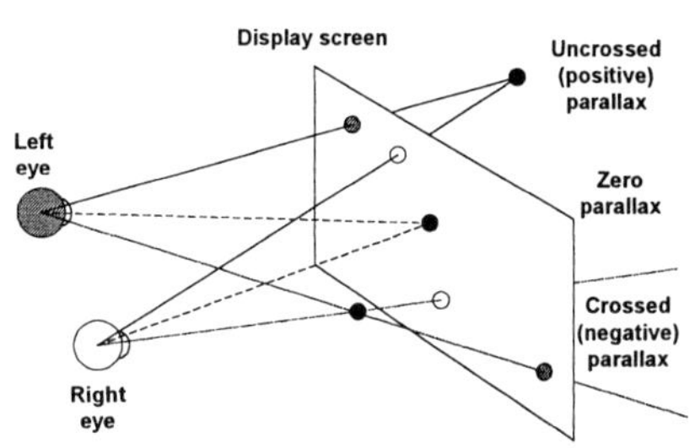

Fig. 4. Three cases of horizontal parallax. Images for the left eye (filled dots) and right eye (open dots) are shown superimposed on the display screen.

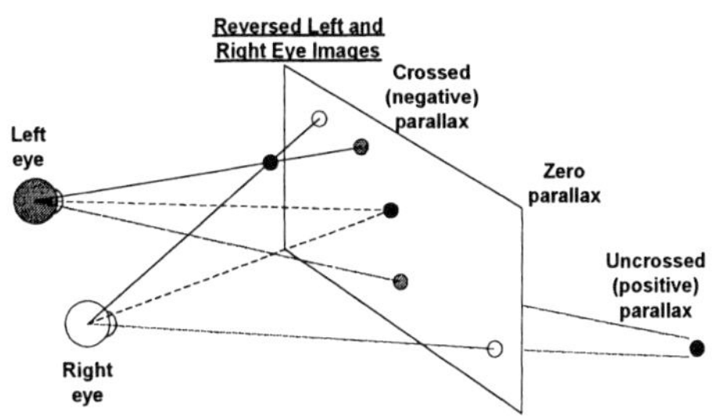

Fig. 5. Inversion of depth resulting from swapping left- and right-eye images. Compare to Fig. 4.

While the stereo point-of-view of the displayed breast tissue is determined by the point-of-view at image acquisition, there are two other aspects of the viewed volume that the user can manipulate. First, one can invert depth by swapping the two images—presenting the left-eye image to the right eye and the right-eye image to the left eye. Consider the two points corresponding to uncrossed parallax in Fig. 4. When we swap the images, as shown in Fig. 5, the filled dot becomes the open dot and vice versa. So now we have crossed parallax and the object will be seen not behind the screen, but in front of it. Similarly, dots originally displaying crossed parallax will now have uncrossed parallax. Thus, objects originally seen in front of the screen will now be seen behind it, and vice versa. Dots with zero parallax will still have zero parallax, and remain seen at the screen surface. Thus, the effect of swapping images is to invert depth—much like reaching into a glove in a pressurized bio-isolation chamber and pulling it inside out. If, in addition to swapping the two images, one also spins each image 180 degrees about a vertical axis, then the inverted depth image is seen as if one had walked around the object to view it from the backside.

Inverting depth can be important in stereo viewing, especially of stereo mammograms. The visual system is set up to attend much more strongly to objects seen in the foreground, as opposed to the background. By allowing a radiologist to invert depth, tissue originally at the back of the displayed breast volume can be moved to the front of the volume, making it easier to perceive structure there.

A second aspect of the viewed volume that can be manipulated is the location of the displayed volume in depth with respect to the screen surface. If one shifts the right-eye image slightly to the left while holding the left-eye image fixed, as shown in Fig. 6, then the horizontal parallax of all points will be changed in the direction of uncrossed parallax. Points originally with uncrossed parallax will have larger uncrossed parallax, and points with crossed parallax will have decreased crossed parallax. The perceived effect is to shift the entire viewed volume forward in depth, with the amount of shift in depth proportional to the amount of left lateral shift of the right-eye image. Shifting the right-eye image in the other direction, to the right, will shift the viewed volume away from the viewer relative to the screen surface. It is only the amount of relative shift of the two images that matters, so one could just as well make shifts to the left-eye image, or to both.

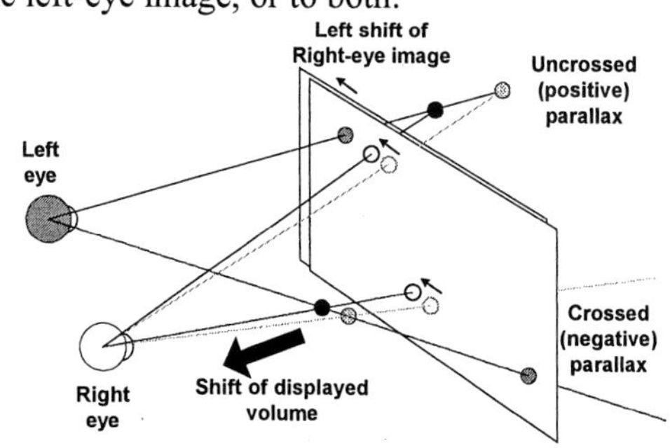

Fig. 6. Shift of the displayed volume towards the viewer with a left shift of the right-eye image.

Control of volume location is useful in that many people initially find it difficult to perceive a displayed volume that begins at the screen surface and comes towards one in space. Usually, they are more comfortable with a displayed volume that starts at the screen surface and goes back into the monitor. It's always possible to achieve this condition by using relative shifts of the two images. On the other hand, with increasing experience, people often come to prefer a displayed volume that comes out into space. As an interesting note, when the stereo image is occupying accessible physical space in front of the screen, one can actually use a pencil to point to an object of interest within the volume that other viewers can see.

3. Evaluation of Stereoscopic Digital Mammography

A project has recently been completed to evaluate the improvement in diagnosis of breast cancer achieved by stereo mammography. Over several years we acquired both standard film and stereo digital mammographic images on a number of women scheduled for biopsy of a suspicious focal breast lesion. We conducted a reading study to determine the diagnostic accuracy achieved by standard film alone compared to standard film read together with the stereo mammogram. A second goal, added as the project progressed, was to obtain preliminary data on the capability of stereo mammography to detect subtle lesions that are not visible in the corresponding film studies.

The reading study was conducted with 5 experienced mammographers individually reading 129 path-proven cases with 137 malignant and benign lesions. The reading of each case was conducted in two successive stages. The reader first examined the full set of film mammograms from the diagnostic study that led to biopsy, rating the probability that the lesion was malignant on a scale of 0 to 100. The reader was then shown the stereo view of the lesion and asked to again rate the probability of malignancy. The stereo image was always a CC view acquired just prior to biopsy. For each case, the reader was also asked to report on any additional lesions seen in either the films or the stereo mammogram, in addition to the known, biopsied lesion.

We conducted an ROC-based analysis of the accuracy of the readers' predictions of malignancy for the two viewing conditions. Diagnostic accuracy, measured by Az (the area under the ROC curve), was .83 when the readers viewed the film study alone, rising to .86 when readers also viewed the stereo mammogram. This is a statistically significant improvement.

Perhaps a more important finding was that readers detected a very significant number of likely new lesions in the stereo mammogram—ones that were not detected in the films. In all, 39 new lesions were reported in the 129 cases, corresponding to 30% of the cases. Of these 39 lesions, 30 were reported as masses, 6 as new calcification clusters, and 3 as architectural distortions. We are still awaiting confirmation of some of these lesions from later mammograms. However, we do have truth now on one subset: masses detected only in the stereo mammogram in association with prior film-detected calcifications. Of 12 such cases, the path report for 11 of the 12 cases reported that the calcifications were located *within a mass*.

4. Conclusions

Stereo mammography, as an adjunct to film, significantly improves classification accuracy of detected lesions. Perhaps of more importance is the finding that stereo mammography appears to be more sensitive than standard film mammography in detecting subtle masses and architectural distortion, enabling mammographers to detect possible lesions that are not visible on standard films. The increased detection sensitivity from stereo seems to arise from the separation of overlying and underlying normal tissue from the lesion, and also from the reader's ability to manipulate characteristics of the displayed image, including inversion of depth and grayscale windowing. Significantly, stereo mammography would be relatively easy to implement on the new digital mammography systems now being developed.

Modeling the time course of the detection of lesions on digitized mammograms

Harold L. Kundel and Calvin F. Nodine

Department of Radiology, University of Pennsylvania Health System,
Philadelphia, PA 19104 USA
kundel@rad.upenn.edu

Abstract. The elapsed time for the detection of suspected abnormalities on digitized mammograms has fast and slow components for both mammographers and trainees. Nonlinear regression of the positive predictive value using a biexponential model shows that the half time of the fast component is about 9 seconds for mammographers and 5 seconds for trainees. The slow component is almost constant. Since most of the true cancers are detected early in viewing using global perception, the initial appearance of the displayed digital mammogram is very important.

1. Introduction

We have proposed that searching for objects such as breast tumors embedded in a structured background starts with a global analysis of the entire visual field followed by scanning the image with the central vision [1,2]. Both perceptual processes are augmented by clusters of checking fixation on image regions that attract visual attention (see Fig. 1).

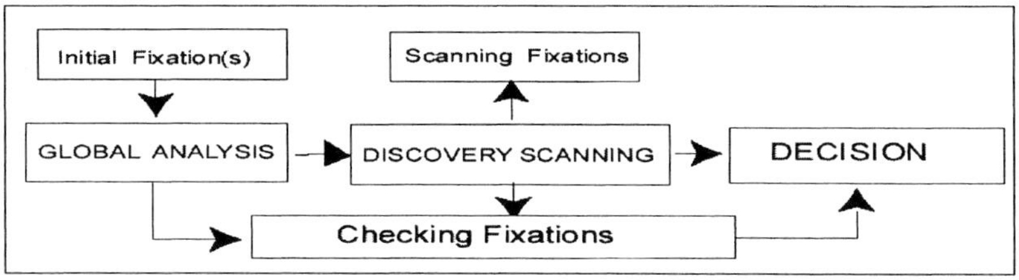

Fig. 1. A flow chart of the perceptual processes involved in searching images.

The interspersed scanning and checking fixations that occur as decisions are made about possible lesions can produce very complex visual scanpaths that can be parsed according to the model in Figure 1 (see Fig. 2.). Lesion detection on chest images proceeds very rapidly [3,4,5]. Radiologists can detect abnormalities with only a brief (250-300) ms glance look at chest images [4,6]. Christensen et al. [3] made decision time measurements during the reading of chest radiographs and concluded that perception has a fast and a slow component. We have made similar observations for mammograms [7,8] and present here a two-component regression model that corresponds with observations on decision time and visual scanning.

2. Materials and Methods

Three full-time mammographers and six trainees (3 residents and 3 fellows) viewed 20 normal and 20 abnormal mammograms consisting of craniocaudal (CC) and mediolateral oblique (MLO) views. There were 20 subtle biopsy proved cancers of which 12 appeared as masses, 6 as calcifications and 2 were mixed. The mammograms were digitized to 50 υm with a digitizer (Lumisys 100 ,Lumisys, Sunnyvale, CA) and displayed at natural size, side by side on a 21-inch high-resolution (2560 X 2048) landscape monitor (DS5000L: Clinton Electronics, Rockford IL). The display used a perceptually tempered grayscale tailored to the density range of the mammogram and the contrast sensitivity of the reader [9]. Eye-position was monitored using an ASL Model 4000SU (Applied Science Laboratory, Bedford, MA). Decision time and lesion location were recorded by having the reader put a cursor over the center of the lesion and click on the computer mouse. A drop down menu opened and the reader selected one or more diagnoses (mass, calcification and architectural distortion) and a confidence level. Viewing and event timing continued after each response [7,8].

The elapsed time was calculated from the onset of viewing until each mouse click. The responses on each view were grouped into 5-second intervals and true and false positive categories. A false positive response was scored on a tumor-containing case if the location of the cursor was more than 2.5 cm from the center of the true lesion. Means and standard deviations were calculated for each interval and category. The averaged standard deviation was used in the Chi square goodness-of-fit calculation.

The ideal method for characterizing the positive responses uses either the likelihood ratio or one of the indices of detectability (d') defined in signal detection theory [10]. However, both require the calculation of the false positive fraction, which cannot be done in a free response experiment without applying simplifying methods such as selecting images with only one lesion, restricting the readers to one response per case or only using the response with the highest confidence rating. We were interested in all false positive responses and, therefore, the positive predictive value (PPV) was used as a measure of performance because it only requires the frequency of true positive (TPn) and false positive (FPn) responses.

$$PPV = \frac{TPn}{TPn + FPn} \quad (1)$$

The main disadvantage of the PPV is that it cannot be generalized because it is highly dependent on the prevalence of positive cases. However, it is useful for comparing performance within readers viewing the same cases.

In keeping with the notion that perception is a two-stage process (global analysis and discovery search), we modeled the change in the PPV with viewing time as a bi-exponential process using the following equation with four free parameters:

$$y = ae^{-bt} + ce^{-dt} . \quad (2)$$

The equation was fit using nonlinear regression [11] and minimizing Chi square to test the goodness-of-fit.

3. Results

Figure 2. shows the scanpath of a mammographer viewing side-by-side CC and MLO views containing a mass.

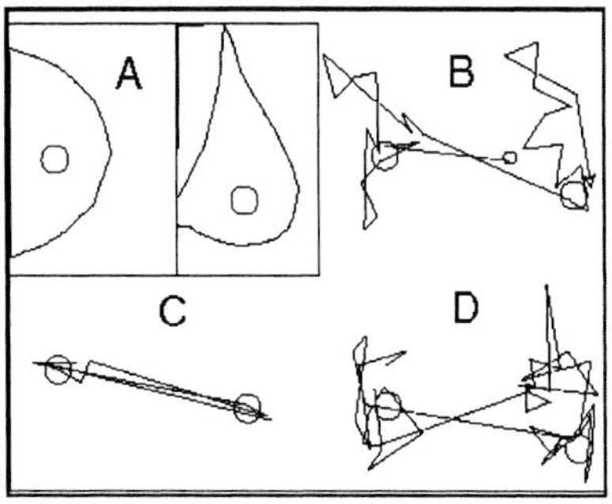

Fig. 2. A: Outline of the CC and MLO views with circles showing the location of a mass lesion. The circles are repeated in B, C and D as reference marks. B: The scanpath during the first 15 seconds of viewing. The small circle marks the start of the scanpath and the fixation point when the image appeared. The first movement is directly to the lesion in the CC view as a result of the global analysis. C: Seconds 16 to 20 are checking fixations comparing the appearance of the tumor in the CC and the MLO views. D: Seconds 21 to 40 show discovery scanning.

The average time required by the mammographers and the trainees to make an overt decision by pointing to a lesion and click the mouse button is shown in Figure 3.

The trainees make fewer true positive decisions and more false positive decisions than the mammographers. This is reflected in the plots of the PPV shown in Figure 4. The mammographers start and equilibrate at a higher value (PPV = 1.0 and .67 v .65 and .42). The solid line in the figure is a plot of Equation 2 using the parameters shown in Table 1.

Table 1. The parameters resulting from the nonlinear fit of Equation 1 to the PPV data. The coeficients are a and c. The exponents are b and d. The T ½ is the time in seconds required for the PPV to decrease by half.

	Fast Component			Slow Component		
	Coef	Exp	T ½	Coef	Exp	T ½
Mammographers	. 59	.078	8.9	.71	.0003	1925
Trainees	.65	.13	5.3	.42	.0013	5331

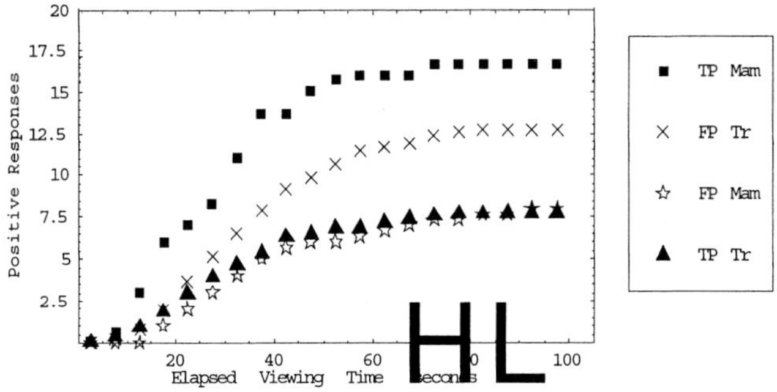

Fig. 3. The cumulative true positive and false positive responses made during the viewing time by mammographers and trainees. The true positive responses are shown by squares for mammographers and crosses for trainees. The false positive responses are shown by triangles for mammographers and stars for trainees.

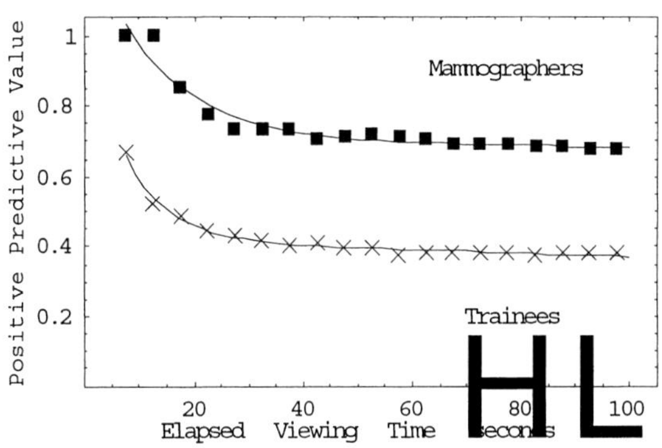

Fig. 4. The symbols are the observed positive predictive value of the responses of the mammographers (squares) and trainees (crosses) during the course of viewing the mammograms. The lines are the curves fit by Equation 2. using the parameters in Table 1.

4. Discussion

The time course of perception for mammographers and trainees as represented by the positive predictive value (PPV) can be modeled by a fast and slow component. The fast component is attributed to the global perceptual analysis of the image that occurs at the onset of viewing, which identifies and checks the most suspicious regions.
The PPV is greatest at the beginning of viewing because true abnormalities are most likely to be conspicuous and are, therefore, inspected first.

The least conspicuous candidates for abnormality are inspected during the discovery phase when the image is being scanned in a quasi-systematic manner. During this phase the PPV is almost constant (the second exponent is not statistically different from zero). The mammographers and trainees both show the two-phase time course but the performance of the trainees is worse. During discovery search the mammographers report more true than false lesions (PPV > .5) while the trainees report more false than true lesions (PPV<.5). The main difference between the trainees and mammographers is not in the ability to detect candidates for abnormality but to separate true and false lesions.

The early, rapid identification of abnormalities suggests that the initial appearance of the image is very important to perception. We have focused our efforts in workstation design for digital mammograms on presenting an initial display that automatically matches the range of intensities in the mammogram to the perceptual system of the observer rather than have the observer set the initial parameters [8].

References

1. Kundel, H., Nodine, C. , Thickman, D. , et al.: Searching for lung nodules: A comparison of human performance with random and systematic scanning models. Invest. Radiol. 22 (1987) 417-422
2. Nodine, C., and Kundel, H.: Using eye movements to study visual search and to improve tumor detection. RadioGraphics 7 (1987) 1241-1250
3. Christensen, E., Murry, R., Holland, K., et al.: The effect of search time on perception. Radiology. 138 (1981) 361-365
4. Oestmann, J., Greene, R., Kushner, D., et al.: Lung lesions: Correlation between viewing time and detection. Radiology. 166 (1988) 451-453
5. Berbaum, K., Franken, E., Jr., Dorfman, D., et al.: Time course of satisfaction of search. Invest. Radiol. 26 (1991) 640-648
6. Kundel, H., and Nodine, C.: Interpreting chest radiographs without visual search. Radiology 116 (1975) 527-532
7. Nodine, C., Mello-Thoms, C., Weinstein, S., et al.: Blinded review of retrospectively visible unreported breast cancers: an eye-position analysis. Radiology 221 (2001) 122-129
8. Nodine, C., Mello-Thoms, C. Kundel, H. Weinstein, S.: The time course of perception and decision making during mammographic interpretation. AJR (2002) in press.
9. Kundel, H., Weinstein, S., Conant, E., et al.: A perceptually tempered display for digital mammograms. RadioGraphics 19 (1999) 1313-1318
10. Macmillan, N., and Creelman, C.: Detection Theory: A user's guide. Cambridge University Press,Cambridge, UK (1991)
11. Wolfram Research, Mathematica 4.0 Standard Add-on Packages, Wolfram Media, (1999)

MammoTrainer – Computer-based Training for Soft-Copy Reading of Mammograms on PC

Guido Prause, Jan H.C.L. Hendriks*, Roland Holland*, Henny Rijken*, Heike Seyffarth, Olaf Klinghammer and Heinz-Otto Peitgen

*National Expert and Training Centre for Breast Cancer Screening, University Hospital Nijmegen, Geert Grooteplein 18, 6500 HB Nijmegen, The Netherlands

MeVis – Center for Medical Diagnostic Systems and Visualization, Universitätsallee 29, 28359 Bremen, Germany
prause@mevis.de

Abstract. The introduction of digital mammography into the clinical practice will considerably change the radiologists' reviewing process. The MammoTrainer is a self-training software for PC that allows physicians, technicians, and medical students to improve and test their skills in soft-copy reading of screening mammograms. It is built on a database of 350 screening cases (300 non-suspicious cases and 50 histologically proven cancers) with more than 2.000 mammograms from the Dutch national breast cancer screening program. A training session is divided into three phases: (1) specification of an individual training set, (2) reading and classification into suspicious (recall for further diagnosis) or non-suspicious (no further diagnosis required) cases, and finally (3) results and solution based on the ground truth obtained from follow-up mammograms (normals) and pathology (cancers). The MammoTrainer is designed to run on standard PCs under Windows.

1. Introduction

We are currently in the transition phase from film-based to digital mammography (Full-Field Digital Mammography, Computed Radiography). While the image acquisition process will experience only little changes, the introduction of digital mammography into the clinical practice will have a considerable impact on the radiologists' reviewing process both for diagnostic and screening mammography.

Compared to the reading of film-based mammograms on a conventional lightbox, digital mammography allows for direct soft-copy reading, automatic and interactive image manipulation, as well as easy image transfer and computer-aided diagnosis [1,2]. These new capabilities of digital mammography are changing the workflow of mammography reading and create a strong need for training of radiologists.

It is known from literature that the reading performance in diagnostic and screening mammography depends on the experience of the radiologist and may be improved by training [3,4]. Since the availability of professional soft-copy reading workstations with high-resolution monitors is currently still very limited, we developed a self-training software (MammoTrainer) that allows physicians, technicians, and medical students to improve and test their skills in soft-copy reading of digital mammograms on a common personal computer.

2. Material and Methods

The MammoTrainer software was developed at MeVis in Bremen in close cooperation with the expert and training center for breast cancer screening in Nijmegen. The self-training software is a result of the research project MammaVision which was funded between 1997 and 2000 in part by the German Ministry of Education and Research (BMBF), the Springer-Verlag in Heidelberg, and MeVis Technology in Bremen.

2.1 Cases

The training software is built on a database of 350 actual screening cases (300 non-suspicious cases and 50 cancers) with more than 2.000 film-based mammograms from the Dutch national breast cancer screening program. All cancer cases are histologically proven. All non-suspicious cases showed no signs of cancer in the screening mammograms taken at least 2 years after the current round.

Each screening case has up to eight mammograms: four images of the previous screening round (priors, usually taken 2 years before) in the upper row and four images of the current screening round in the lower row. The four mammograms of each round may comprise medio-lateral oblique (MLO) and cranio-caudal (CC) views of the left and the right breast.

2.2 Digitization and Compression

The mammograms (180x240 mm^2) were digitized with a laser scanner (Lumiscan 85 by Lumisys) with a resolution of 50 micron/pixel and 4096 gray levels. The digitized mammograms were downsampled to three levels of magnification with 256 gray values:

- low resolution with 650 micron/pixel or 39 dpi, respectively (for overview mode with all eight mammograms of a case)
- medium resolution with 325 micron/pixel or 78 dpi, respectively (for pairwise magnification of two mammograms)
- high resolution with 100 micron/pixel or 254 dpi, respectively (for magnifying glass).

The medium and high resolution mammograms are JPEG images compressed with an average compression factor of about 15. The overview images are losslessly compressed TIFF images.

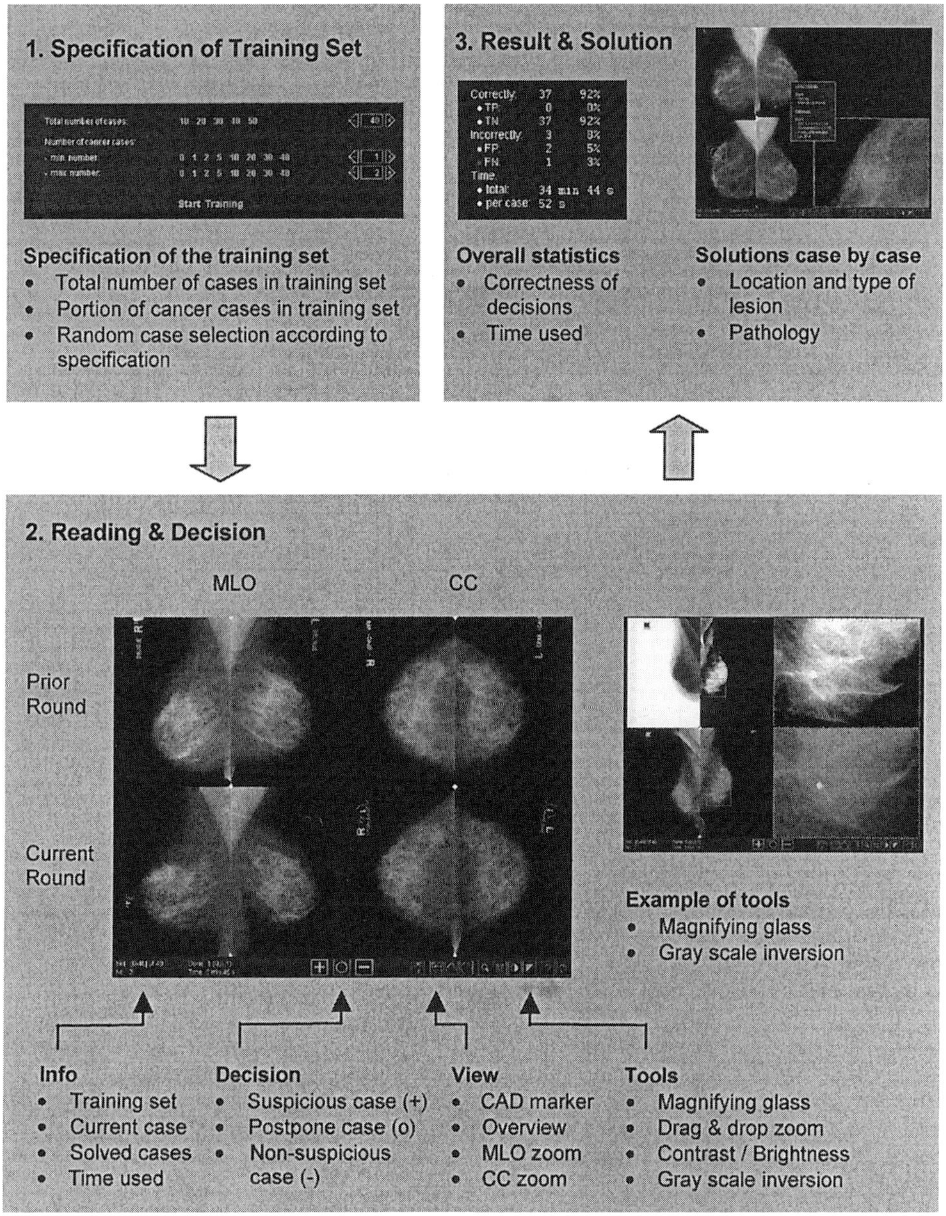

Fig. 1. Overview of the three phases of a training session with the MammoTrainer: (1) specification of training set, (2) reading and decision, (3) results and solution.

2.3 Training

A self-training session with the MammoTrainer software is divided into three phases: (1) specification of the training set, (2) reading and decision, and (3) results and solution. An overview of a training session is given by the flowchart in Fig.1.

2.3.1 Specification of Training Set

A new training set may be specified either by amount or in a case-by-case fashion. Alternatively, an existing training set, either pre-defined by an expert or previously self-defined by the user, may by loaded. The most common way is the specification by amount. Here a total number of cases is chosen for training plus a number or range of cancer cases to be included.

2.3.2 Reading and Decision

The cases of a specified training set are randomly selected from the case database and are presented in an randomized order. For soft-copy reading of the cases, the user may choose between various standard views in different resolutions and among tools for interactive image manipulation (magnifying glass, drag & drop zoom, contrast/brightness, and gray scale inversion). In addition, CAD markers may be superimposed to prompt for microcalcifications. Each case has to be classified by the user as "suspicious" (refer for further diagnosis) or "non-suspicious" (no further diagnosis required). In suspicious cases, the findings are localized in the mammograms by drag-and-drop markers representing one of three lesion types (density, calcification, architectural distortion).

2.3.3 Result and Solution

Finally, the results of the training session are presented. An overall statistics summarizes the time used as well as the correctly (true positives, true negatives) and incorrectly (false positives, false negatives) classified cases in absolute and relative values. For each case the user's decision is opposed to the correct decision using a traffic light color coding scheme. In the solution mode, the user can compare his/her own findings with the correct positions and types of the mammographic lesions. Finally, the pathologies of the cancer cases are presented including lesion type and lymph node status.

3. Conclusions

The MammoTrainer software is successfully employed in a pilot project for mentor-guided training and self-training of radiologists and gynecologists in an electronic classroom. The system enables the user to make first steps into soft-copy reading of digital mammograms and to experience the workflow and the capabilities of computer-based reading. The self-training on PC might be a useful preparation for the work on a professional soft-copy reading station for digital mammography.

Limitations of the display quality of the mammograms on a PC may be overcome by selection of appropriate cases and the use of CAD markers.

The minimum system requirements to run the MammoTrainer are a PC with Windows 98, Pentium II 366 MHz, 128 MB RAM and CD-ROM drive. For improved image quality the use of a CRT monitor is recommended.

References

1. Pisano, E.D., Cole, E.B., Major, S., Zong, S., Hemminger, B.M., Muller, K.E., Johnston, R.E., Walsh, R., Conant, E., Fajardo, L.L., Feig, S.A., Nishikawa, R.M., Yaffe, M.J., Williams, M.B., Aylward, S.R.: Radiologists' Preferences for Digital Mammographic Display. The International Digital Mammography Development Group. Radiology 216(3) (2000) 820–830
2. Giger, M.L., Karssemeijer, N., Armato, S.G.: Computer-Aided Diagnosis in Medical Imaging. IEEE Trans Med Imaging 20(12) (2001) 1205-1208
3. Nodine, C.F., Kundel, H.L., Mello-Thoms, C. Weinstein, S.P., Orel, S.G., Sullivan, D.C., Conant, E.F.: How Experience and Training Influence Mammography Expertise. Academic Radiology 6(10) (1999) 575-585
4. Sickles, E.A., Wolverton, D.E., Dee, K.E.: Performance Parameters for Screening and Diagnostic Mammography: Specialist and General Radiologist. Radiology 224(3) (2002) 861–869

Effect of Default Display and Presentation Protocol on Softcopy Mammography

Maria Kallergi,[1] Claudia G. Berman,[1] John J. Heine,[1] Marla R. Hersh,[1] Lisa D. Hooper,[1] Jihai J. Kim,[1] Marcia M. Miller,[1] Jerry A. Thomas,[2] and Robert A. Clark[1]

[1] H. Lee Moffitt Cancer Center & Research Institute, University of South Florida, Tampa FL
kallergi@moffitt.usf.edu
[2] Uniformed Services University of the Health Sciences, Bethesda, MD

Abstract. The purpose of this study was to determine the impact of default image display, presentation protocol, and workstation configuration on the softcopy interpretation of mammograms. Results from ROC studies that compared film to softcopy mammography were analyzed for this purpose. On average, no difference in performance was observed between the two modalities. However, differences were identified in individual observer performance and the qualitative evaluation of the two platforms that were related to the system's speed, the default grayscale display of the images, and possibly the CRT phosphor. Speed and default display were ranked as the top two impact factors on softcopy reading.

1. Introduction

The advent of FDA approved full field digital mammography systems with dedicated computer workstations for softcopy reading of digital mammograms have made the transition from film to softcopy (computer monitor) display an irrevocable process.[1] Digital mammography has also cleared the path for softcopy digitized mammography and supported findings of earlier studies that have shown equivalency between standard film and softcopy digitized mammogram interpretation. Current studies investigate the type and numbers of monitors to use, the characteristics of the display hardware and software, the display protocol and greyscale settings, and the image processing tools that should be available to the reader.[2],[3] These investigators have developed, independently and in collaborative efforts, several generations of mammographic workstation-user interfaces based on clinical models and observer preference studies.[4],[5] In this paper we will report findings from the evaluation of our most recent systems through observer studies.

2. Materials and Methods

The results from two ROC studies that compared film to softcopy digitized mammography and a 2 AFC study that compared different initial display approaches were analyzed in terms of user preferences and performance to determine the impact of the hardware and software configuration on the interpretation of softcopy mammograms. The studies were performed at USF and USUHS and involved 200 cases each of cancer, benign, and negative mammograms and 7 mammographers.

The Display Softcopy Protocol (DSP) system, developed at USF, attempted to follow as closely as possible the protocol followed in film mammography without consideration to speed and optimization of display space. The MammoCAD system, developed at USUHS, focused on speed optimization and workspace usage as well as default display. Both interfaces offered similar processing and manipulation tools including greyscale adjustment (linear and nonlinear), zoom and pan, measuring options, and computer-aided diagnosis (CAD) output overlay, although different approaches were followed in the implementation of these tools. Table 1 summarizes the characteristics of the two systems in terms of hardware and software design.

Table 1. Characteristics of the DSP and MammoCAD workstations and interfaces used to compare film to softcopy digitized mammography. The systems were designed to display four-view cases, namely the RCC, LCC, RMLO (or RML), and LMLO (or LML) views and CAD. LM corresponds to the Left Monitor display and RM corresponds to the right monitor display.

Features	DSP	MammoCAD
Speed	60-90 secs per case	Less than 5 secs per case
Display scenarios	(1) LM: 2 reduced CC views; RM: 2 reduced MLO views (2) LM: High resolution regions of the CC views; RM: High resolution regions of 2 MLO views	LM: 4 reduced views RM: Selected view to fit the window
Hardware	Single Sun UltraSparc2200	Double Intel PC 480 MHz
Monitors	Two DataRay DR110 5Mpixel CRTs with P104 phosphor driven by DOME Md5 video boards	Two Barco MGD521 5Mpixel CRTs with P104 phosphor driven by BarcoMed 5MP1H boards
Software	Sun (XIL), Motif, SPARCworks Visual C++/C, and Java	Visual C++/C
CAD option	Available as overlay to both views	Single image overlay

3. Results and Discussion

Both ROC studies showed no differences between film and softcopy interpretation of breast lesions. Individual differences and preference differences were more likely due to system design and performance, type of initial display, type of phosphor used, and setup of the observer studies and less to inter-observer variability. Specifically, ROC and 2AFC results suggested that: (a) Speed is a critical feature of a clinical interface and a key element in the design process. The MammoCAD with the significantly higher speeds than the DSP was better received and had overall more positive evaluations than the DSP. (b) The high quality of the initial display that requires minimum reader intervention and adjustment is the second critical feature of a mammography workstation. Initial image quality introduces a strong preference bias and impacts the readers' acceptance of the system as well as his/her performance. High quality initial display cannot be achieved with conventional methodologies.

Multiresolution wavelet processing seems to offer significantly better alternatives. (c) The hanging protocol of the digital images is not of extreme importance and it is not critical to maintain the protocol followed in film mammography. The ability to modify protocols and match them to the user's preference is desirable but not critical. (d) Superposition of CAD output to the original image in a toggle-on/off mode was favoured over a side-by-side display as was the simultaneous display of CAD for the two views of the same breast. (e) Senior mammographers with expertise in computer monitor reading performed better in softcopy mammography than junior mammographers with less experience. Junior readers, however, improved with time as shown by a temporal analysis of the data. (f) Five readers performed worse on softcopy than film mammography. Although this difference was statistically significant for only one of the readers, this trend may be attributed to the phosphor used and the type of default greyscale display selected for the studies. The latter was further confirmed with the 2AFC experiment.

4. Conclusions

High speed and high quality of initial image display were determined as the most critical features of a workstation/user interface for primary reading of softcopy, digitized or digital mammograms. Readers prefer certain hanging protocol features and image manipulation tools but these are of secondary importance in performance.

Acknowledgments

This study was sponsored by The Naval Medical Research and Development Command, contract nb. # 42952, funds managed by The Henry M. Jackson Foundation for the Advancement of Military Medicine.

References

1. Lewin, J.M., Hendrick, R.E., D'Orsi, C.J., et al: Comparison of full-field digital mammography with screen-film mammography for cancer detection: Results of 4,945 paired examinations. Radiology 218 (2001) 873-880.
2. Krupinski,E.A., Roehrig,H., Furukawa,T., and Tang, C.: Influence of film and monitor display luminance on observer performance and visual search. Acad. Rad. 6 (1999) 411.
3. Shtern, F., and Winfield, D. (Eds.): Report of the working group on digital mammography: Digital displays and workstation design. Acad. Rad. 6 (1999) S193-S220.
4. Gohel, H.J., Kallergi, M., Vossberg, M., et al: A workstation interface for ROC studies in digital mammography. *SPIE* 3031 (1997) 440-447.
5. Loscocco, M.F., Thomas, J.A., Chakrabarti, K., and Kaczmarek, R.V.: Preference studies of workstation monitor performance. Proc. 5th International Workshop on Digital Mammography, June 11-14, Toronto, Canada, 2000, pp. 612-616.

Computer-Based Reading of Full-Field Digital Mammograms

Silvia Obenauer, Susanne Luftner-Nagel, Klaus-Peter Hermann and Eckhardt Grabbe

Department of Diagnostic Radiology, Georg-August-University Göttingen, Robert-Koch-Str. 40, 37 075 Göttingen, Germany
soben@med.uni-goettingen.de

Abstract. Mammograms of 50 patients performed on a full-field digital mammography system were evaluated. The images were judged as hardcopy prints and on 2k x 2.5k high resolution monitors. 19 of the 50 patients had histologically proven carcinomas, the remainder showed no malignancies after a follow-up of 2 years. The mammograms were evaluated with respect to image quality, presence of masses and microcalcifications. All detected lesions were categorized according to the BI-RADS™ classification. Time was recorded. Postprocessing in softcopy evaluation (windowing and levelling, zooming, inversion) and additional views like spot views in both methods were also timed. Possible changes in the BI-RADS™ classification were included in the evaluation protocol. Diagnostic accuracy of the classification of the malignant lesions according to the BI-RADS™ categories showed no significant differences between soft- and hardcopy. More time was needed for the evaluation of the softcopies than for the hardcopies. Additional views were recommended in hardcopy more often than in softcopy evaluation (26 versus 21 for reader 1, 20 versus 18 for reader 2). Postprocessing was used in 9 cases by reader 1 and in all cases by reader 2 resulting in an further increase of the evaluation time. Furthermore softcopy reading enables radiographers to use the advantages of a digital system (e.g. CAD, teleradiology, PACS).

1. Introduction

The major potential advantages of digital mammography systems are improved handling, processing, computer assisted diagnosis (CAD), communication (teleradiology) and archiving of image information (Cowen et al. 1997, Feig et al. 1995, Pisano 2000, Shtern 1992). However, these benefits can be fully used only with softcopy reading. But softcopy reading is not yet the standard in mammography. The goal of this study was to evaluate the feasibility of using a mammography review workstation of a commercially full-field digital mammography system for the interpretation of mammograms (Muller 1999).

2. Material and Methods

The review workstation of the FFDM system (Senographe 2000D, GE Medical Systems, Buc, France) consists of 2 prozessors with 512 MB RAM. In the softcopy situation the images were evaluated on two high-resolution monitors (2kx2.5k) (Fig. 1). The images could also be printed on a high-resolution imager (Scopix LR 5200, Agfa, Leverkusen, Germany). Pixel size of the printer is 40 μm with 8.820 x 10.710 pixels at the format 14x17 inch in 11 seconds (Hermann et al. 2000, Muller 1999, Obenauer et al. 2000)

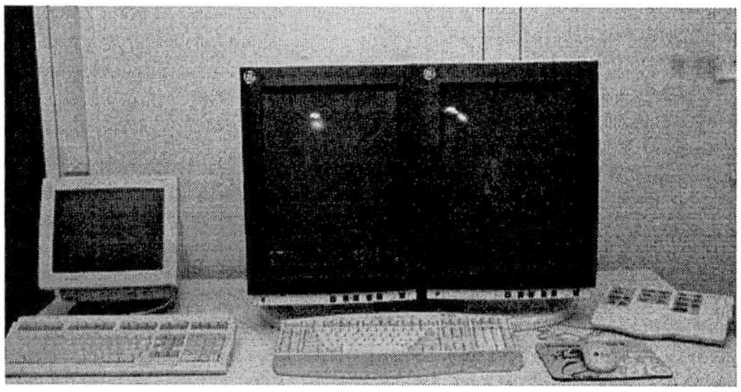

Fig. 1: Softcopy reading situation. Two 2k x 2.5k monitors.

Digital images of 50 patients were evaluated by 2 readers either in softcopy or hardcopy reading. The radiologists had full freedom to adjust window and level and to magnify each image at the monitor (windowing and levelling, zooming and inversion). The interpretation of the mammograms was done in a darkened room. 19 of 50 patients had histologically proven carcinomas, the remainder showed no malignancies after a follow-up of 2 years. The mammograms were evaluated with respect to image quality, presence of masses and microcalcifications. All detected lesions were categorized according to the BI-RADS^{TM} classification (ACR 1998). Time was recorded. Postprocessing in softcopy evaluation (windowing and levelling, zooming, inversion) and additional views like spot views in both methods were also measured. Changes in the allocation to the BI-RADS^{TM} classification were included in the evaluation protocol.

3. Results

There was no differences in diagnostic accuracy in the BI-RADS^{TM} classification of malignant lesions. More time was necessary for the evaluation in softcopy than in hardcopy reading. Observer 1 needed 26 sec versus 16 sec and the second observer 25 sec versus 17 sec in the softcopy versus the hardcopy interpretation, respectively. Less additional views were recommended in softcopy than in hardcopy reading (observer 1: 21 versus 26 and observer 2: 18 versus 20 views, respectively) (Fig. 2). Postprocessing was used in 9 cases by observer 1 and in all cases by observer 2.

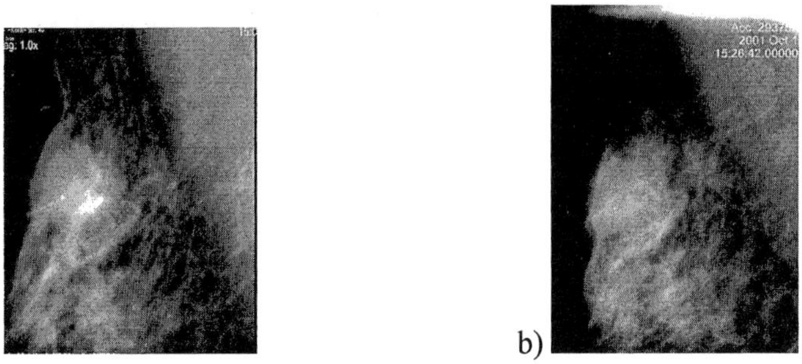

a) b)

Fig. 2a+b: Spiculated mass with microcalcifications in projection of the mass. Zoomed view of the contact mammogram (a) and magnified view (b).

4. Discussion

With the available high resolution monitors softcopy reading is possible. Longer evaluation time is needed in softcopy than in hardcopy reading, especially when postprocessing is used. However, the procedure to develop the mammograms is faster and the images have more information. Fewer additional views are recommended in softcopy reading without any change in diagnostic accuracy. This reduces the dose to the patient and improves the workflow. The main benefits of a digital system are postprocessing, the possibility to integrate computer-assisted diagnosis, digital and cost-effective image archiving (telemammography, e.g. double reading and second opinion) (Feig et al. 1995, Pisano 2000). In the softcopy situation these advantages of a digital system will improve reading of mammograms. However, habit and experience influence the preference of radiologists for hard- and softcopy reading.

5. References

1. American College of Radiology (ACR). Breast imaging reporting and data system (BI-RADS), Ed 3. Reston, VA: American College of Radiology, 1998
2. Cowen A.R., Parkin G.J.S., Hawkridge P. Direct digital mammography image acquisition. Eur. Radiol. (1997) 7 : 918-930
3. Feig S.A., Yaffe M.J. Digital mammography, computer-aided diagnosis, and telemammography. Breast Imaging (1995) 33: 1205-1230
4. Hermann K.-P., Obenauer S., Grabbe E. Comparison of radiation exposure between a digital amorphous silicon and a screen-film based mammography system. Fortschr. Röntgenstr. (2000) 172: 940-945
5. Muller S. Full-field digital mammography designed as a complete system. Eur. Radiol. (1999) 31: 25-34
6. Obenauer S., Hermann K.-P., Schorn C., Funke M., Fischer U., Grabbe E. Full-field digital mammography: A phantom study for the detectability of microcalcifications. Fortschr. Röntgenstr. (2000) 172: 646-650
7. Obenauer S., Hermann K.-P., Schorn C., Fischer U., Grabbe E.. Full-field digital mammography: dose–dependant detectability of simulated breast lesions. Fortschr. Röntgenstr. (2000) 172: 1052 - 1056
8. Pisano E.D. Current status of full-field digital mammography. Radiol. (2000) 214: 26-28
9. Shtern F. Digital mammography and related technologies: a perspective from the national cancer institute. Radiology (1992) 183: 629-630

Display of mammograms on a CRT

Hans Roehrig, William J. Dallas, Elizabeth Krupinski, Jiahua Fan, Amarpreet Chawla and Kunal Gandhi

University of Arizona, Department of Radiology,
1609 N. Warren Ave, Building 211, Tucson, AZ, 85724, USA
hans@radiology.arizona.edu

In most radiological imaging workstations the monochrome cathode ray tube (CRT) is the electronic display of choice. The CRT offers the best performance; it is the most highly developed, mature and reliable display in common use. Unfortunately, because of limited spatial resolution and because of limited dynamic range, the efficacy of soft-copy versus hard-copy diagnosis has been challenged.

It has been shown for chest radiography that, when the images are display-specifically processed before the display to compensate for the reduced MTF of the CRT and its reduced dynamic range, current high-resolution monochrome CRT display systems will present all information in mammograms without interaction by the reader [1], [2]. The basic idea is then to perform an operation on the image before it is displayed that will counteract the degradation that will come from the action of the display system's MTF. This paper indicates in a preliminary experiment that this may be true also for the area of mammography even though processing was restricted to compensation for the display system's MTF .

MTFs were derived from the square wave response and with the aid of a CCD camera. Here small-amplitude square waves of different spatial frequencies are displayed on the CRT on a uniform background in horizontal and vertical direction, and the CCD camera records the displayed patterns. Elements of linear system theory were applied to the evaluation of the inherently non-linear CRT display system by using the small-signal approximation. The Fourier Transforms of the data recorded by the CCD camera and representing the square wave response of the display, provide the output modulations of the fundamental sine wave and their harmonics.

The method we use to prepare the image for display is Wiener (sometimes called Wiener-Helstrom) filtering. For the following explanation, we use continuous mathematics. If we call the original image $u(x,y)$ then its Fourier transform is $U(\xi,\eta)$. Modeling the display as an approximately linear shift-invariant system, we would expect the output to be degraded on display by the optical transfer function $OTF(\xi,\eta)$ according to the equation

$$V(\xi,\eta) = U(\xi,\eta)[OTF(\xi,\eta) + N(\xi,\eta)] \tag{1}$$

where N represents the Fourier spectral density of the noise. The mathematical justification for the use of the Wiener filter in this situation comes from the fact that the actual restoration we are attempting is variations in the point spread function, not in the image.

Because the *OTF* is positive over the entire region of frequency space that we are considering, we may replace it by its absolute value, the modulation transfer function.

$$MTF(\xi,\eta) = \left|OTF(\xi,\eta)\right| \tag{2}$$

The filtered signal version is then

$$U_f(\xi,\eta) = \frac{V(\xi,\eta)OTF^*(\xi,\eta)}{\left|OTF\right|^2(\xi,\eta)+\left|N(\xi,\eta)\right|^2} = \frac{V(\xi,\eta)MTF(\xi,\eta)}{MTF^2(\xi,\eta)+\left|N(\xi,\eta)\right|^2} \tag{3}$$

In actual practice, we replace the noise power spectral density by a constant that we adjust as a parameter in the filter. The filter we use is

$$F(\xi,\eta) = \frac{MTF(\xi,\eta)}{MTF^2(\xi,\eta)+N_0^{\ 2}} \tag{4}$$

We make an additional simplification, we assume the *MTF* to be separable so that we can actually perform the measurements and the filtering as 1-D operations.

$$F(\xi,\eta) = \frac{MTF_\xi(\xi)}{MTF_\xi^{\ 2}(\xi)+N_\xi^{\ 2}} \cdot \frac{MTF_\eta(\eta)}{MTF_\eta^{\ 2}(\eta)+N_\eta^{\ 2}} \tag{5}$$

As a practical matter, because we do the filtering in real time for a window that is moved across the image, we have optimized the filter operation for speed. One of the chief components in this optimization is the use of the Intel Signal Processing library. The library is obtainable from the Intel WEB site URL: http://developer.intel.com/software/products/perflib/index.htm. The routines contained in this library are highly efficient for Intel processors.

Fig. 1 presents the MTFs of a high performance 5 M-pixel CRT in the horizontal and vertical direction and the MTFs in the horizontal direction, arising from the filtering as calculated for various estimates of noise N. N = 1 represents low noise, while n = 8 represents high noise. Notice that the original horizontal MTF of the display is inferior to its original MTF in the vertical direction. Notice also that the maximum spatial frequency included in the processing becomes lower as the estimates of the noise increase. At N = 1, the new (compensated) MTF in the horizontal direction is almost equal to the vertical MTF before processing.

In order to test the effectiveness of the MTF-correction method, a preliminary observer performance study was conducted. 2 observers viewed two sets of 250

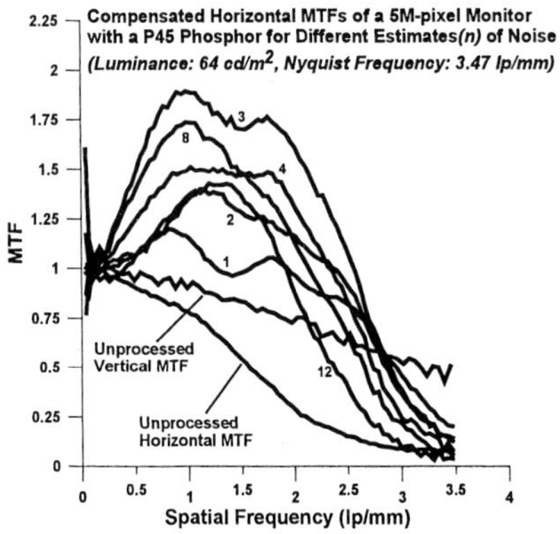

Fig. 1. Original MTFs and MTFs after processing

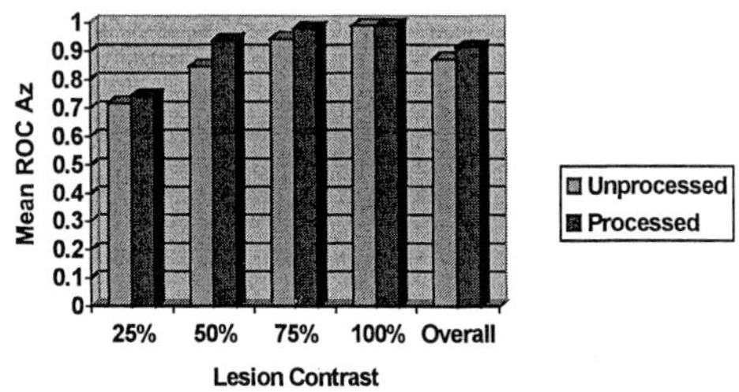

Fig. 2. Results of the Pilot-ROC Study

images each with micro-calcifications of different size and each at 4 degrees of contrast: 100%, 75%, 50% and 25%. One set of the images was frequency processed in the horizontal direction using N = 1, the other set was not processed. Performance was measured by ROC Az (Receiver Operating Characteristic Area Under the Curve). The result is shown in Fig 2. Performance was higher at all contrast levels for the MTF-correction processed images compared to the unprocessed versions, but the difference was not statistically significant. However this result is encouraging. Future work will include compensation for the limited dynamic range of the CRT display

Acknowledgement

This work is funded by two grants from NIH.

References

1. Reiker GG, Blume H, Slone RM, Woodard PM, Gierada DS, Sagel SS, Jost RG, Blaine GJ: Filmless Digital Chest Radiography within the Radiology Department; SPIE Vol 3035, 355-368, 1997
2. Roehrig H, "The Monochrome Cathode Ray Tube Display and its Performance"; Volume 3, Chapter 4 of Yongmin Kim and Steven C. Horii, eds, "Display and PACS"; in Jacob Beutel, Harold L. Kundel and Richard L. Van Metter, eds, "Handbook of Medical Imaging", SPIE Press, Bellingham,WA, June 2000.

Performance Evaluation of a Digital Reading Station for Screening Mammography

Ton Roelofs, Sander van Woudenberg, Jan Hendriks, Anke Bödicker, Carl Evertsz, and Nico Karssemeijer

University Medical Center St. Radboud, Department of Radiology, P.O. Box 9101, 430 Radiology, 6500 HB Nijmegen, The Netherlands
T.Roelofs@rad.umcn.nl

Abstract. In this paper the use of a soft-copy reading station for screening mammography is investigated and results are compared with analog reading. In the analog part of the study prior mammograms of 183 normal and 88 cancer cases selected from the Dutch breast cancer screening program were used. Only positive cases where the abnormality was visible on the prior screening mammogram were included. The prior mammograms were digitized and reread about 1.5 years after their first reading, on a dedicated screening workstation. All mammograms were processed by a CAD system. Unsharp masking was applied to the images to compensate for image degradation during digitization and display. Five experienced screening radiologists participated in the study. Performance was evaluated by ROC analysis and determination of reading speed. Soft-copy screening performance was found to be as good as conventional reading, both in terms of detection and reading speed.

1. Introduction

In the context of the SCREEN project (IST-1999-10246) a digital reading station for screening mammography was developed in a consortium of Mevis and Mevis Technology (Bremen, Germany), Nijmegen University Medical Center (Nijmegen, The Netherlands), and Oxford University (Oxford, UK). The dedicated reading station offers many advantages over a conventional alternator. Mammograms can be magnified, inverted, and presented in various combinations. Also, window-and-level and contrast can easily be adjusted, Computer-Aided Detection (CAD) can be incorporated, and the performance of radiologists can be monitored by mixing known cases in the screening (in-service monitoring). However, a digital reading station will only be accepted in daily screening practice if radiologists can perform their task equally well or better using the reading station instead of a conventional alternator.

This paper describes a study in which the utility of the digital reading station is investigated by making a performance comparison with analog reading. An experiment was set up in which radiologists read a number of cases both on a conventional alternator and on the SCREEN reading station. Since mammograms from two screening rounds are presented simultaneously, the experiment resembles a normal screening. Also the workflow in the experiment is close to the usual screening practice. Since in the current screening only analog acquisition is applied, the experiment was performed with digitized mammograms.

2. Materials and Methods

2.1 Image Database

The Dutch breast cancer screening program is a population based program that has been implemented in the Netherlands since 1989. All women in the age group 50-75 are invited every two years to participate in this program. The attendance rate is almost 80 percent. In this program, at the initial screening two view mammograms (MLO and CC) are taken, while subsequent screenings are limited to MLO views only, unless there is indication that additional CC views would be beneficial.

A large database was created from cancer and normal cases, all taken from the Dutch breast cancer screening program. For all cancer cases in the database the mammogram at time of detection was available, as well as the mammograms taken in the two screening rounds prior to detection, separated by time intervals of two years. We will refer to these mammograms, respectively, as the diagnostic mammogram, the prior mammogram, and the former prior mammogram. The diagnostic mammograms were either clinical mammograms (of the interval cancers) or screening mammograms. They originated from screening between 1997 and 1999. For the normal cases two screening mammograms were collected, the ones corresponding to the two prior screening rounds of the positive cases. However, only normals were taken for which a next screening mammogram was made in the same period as the diagnostic mammogram from the cancer cases. In this new screening round the mammogram again was found to be normal. By selecting in this way, biases due to variation in image quality can be assumed to be minimal.

2.2 Reader Study

A number of experienced screening radiologists from the Netherlands were invited for a "blinded" review of 500 cases from the database (250 negatives, 250 positives). The readers read all cases during five sessions spread out over two days. All cases were presented on alternators in a randomized order. As is common practice in screening mammography, mammograms of two screening rounds are presented to allow radiologists to judge mammographic changes over time. In this study we mounted the priors and former priors on the alternators. Only original films were used. An expert radiologist reviewed all positive cases, using the diagnostic mammograms and pathology reports to draw the location of the cancers on paper prints of the diagnostic and prior mammograms.

The radiologists were instructed to use a very low threshold in reporting their findings, so that all regions that they interpreted as possible locations of cancers can be analyzed. For every case they were provided with a scoring form, which included a printed copy of the prior mammogram. For each finding they were asked to draw its contours in the MLO and CC views on paper. To assess the likelihood of malignancy of each finding a rating scale was used, with fourteen levels ranging from 0 to 100 percent. Percentages were only used to guide the radiologists in using the scale. It was explained to them before the reading sessions started that their subjective interpretation of the scale would not influence performance measurement; they should try to be consistent in their interpretation and spread their scores over the full range of the scale. Time for reading was limited. The radiologists could use a maximum of 1.5 hours for 50 cases. In practice they read 50 cases in about an hour.

A subset of the mammograms was reread on the dedicated SCREEN reading station for screening mammography by a subset of five radiologists, about 1.5 years after their first reading. From all women where breast cancer was detected 45 positive screen detected cases and 43 interval cancers were chosen, in which the lesion was visible on the prior mammogram. Furthermore, 183 normal cases were selected. Cases with insufficient image quality or poor positioning were excluded. The total number of used films was exactly 1800. An additional CC view for the prior mammograms was available in 21 percent of the cases, for the former prior mammograms in 49 percent. All films were digitized using a R2 Imagechecker (Los Altos, CA) equipped with a Lumisys 85 film scanner. The images were archived after scaling the resolution down to 100 micron per pixel. All cases were processed by the R2 Imagechecker CAD-software. The algorithms use a classification of lesions into two categories: masses and microcalcifications. However, in this experiment only the CAD-markers for the microcalcifications were made available to the radiologists. All five radiologists received training on the SCREEN workstation before the experiment was started. A separate set of 150 cases was used for this training.

The workstation is equipped with two high-resolution monitors (BARCO, 21-inch, 2048x2560 pixels) using a 10 bits gray level. Unsharp masking was applied to the images to compensate for image degradation during digitization and display (see, for example [1]). Microcalcifications lend themselves well to enhancement by digital unsharp masking. This processing technique enhances the high spatial-frequency components of the image, thereby improving the contrast of small structures [2].

2.3 Data Analysis

Performance was evaluated by ROC analysis, calculation of A_z scores and determination of reading speed. Results obtained using the dedicated workstation were compared to the results obtained with analog reading.

The SCREEN system contains an action recorder, which logs all actions of the radiologist. Timestamps in the action recorder files were analyzed for four out of five radiologists in order to determine the reading speeds. In the analysis reading times shorter than five seconds were ignored, assuming that these cases were just passed by repeated use of the "Next" or "Previous" button. When a radiologist took a break or was interrupted from the experiment, the time registration in the action recorder was not stopped. Therefore, an upper limit was set to four minutes. When a case was revisited, reading times were added up. This resulted in one reading time per case for each of the four radiologists.

3. Results

For the experiment with the digital reading station three radiologists needed three sessions while two radiologists needed only two sessions. During the analog reading the radiologists made on average 353 (σ=44) annotations for the 271 cases, which is about 1.3 (σ=0.16) annotations per case. Using the digital reading station they made 209 (σ=133) annotations, which is about 0.8 (σ=0.5) annotations per case.

The results for the radiologists, expressed in A_z values for both analog and digital reading, are given in Table 1.

Table 1. Radiologists' A_z values

Radiologist	A_z value analog	A_z value digital
1	0.70±0.07	0.77±0.04
2	0.80±0.04	0.80±0.06
3	0.81±0.03	0.78±0.04
4	0.66±0.08	0.71±0.04
5	0.75±0.04	0.80±0.04
Mean	0.74	0.77

For the digital reading, discarding reading durations because they were either too short or too long, resulted in three and 48 eliminations respectively. The average reading time per case for positive cases and negatives (controls) is shown in Table 2.

Table 2. Time used in digital reading

	Negatives	Positives
Number:	183	88
Average (s):	72	98
Stdev (s):	27	28

The average reading time per case was 85 seconds (non-weighted average; based on equal numbers of negative and positive cases, as is the case in the study with the analog mammograms), which is about 42 cases per hour. On the conventional alternator, 1.5 years earlier, the radiologists read about 50 cases per hour.

4. Discussion and Conclusions

We conclude that a dedicated reading station allows soft-copy reading of digitized mammograms without loss of quality, provided that CAD is available for microcalcification detection.

The results suggest that screening on the SCREEN reading station is somewhat slower than conventional reading. However, we believe this is due to the fact that the annotation process is more laborious on the prototype version of the SCREEN reading station. This is not a significant factor in normal screening practice, in which only few positives occur. Other factors reducing the reading speed may have been the use of CAD and a possible residual learning effect, in spite of extensive training. Taking these factors into account, the two ways of screening are probably about equal in terms of reading speed.

As part of a recently started project (SCREEN-TRIAL; IST-2001-33439) a trial with the digital reading station will be carried out during the next two years. During this trial the reading station will be used in daily screening practice at a number of European sites. Additional experiments related to performance (both quality of diagnosis and speed) will be carried out on a larger scale during this project, as well as experiments to test the effects of Computer-Aided Detection, to optimize image quality, and to evaluate the in-service monitoring capabilities of the system.

Acknowledgements

The authors wish to thank the radiologists who participated in the observer study: Dr. D. Beijerinck and Dr. J.J.M. Deurenberg from Preventicon, Utrecht, The Netherlands, Dr. P.A.M. Bun from SKPW and the LUMC, Leiden, The Netherlands, Dr. A.C.W. Borstlap from the Department of Radiology, St. Maartensgasthuis, Venlo, and Dr. F.H. Janssen from the Catharina Hospital in Eindhoven, The Netherlands. They also would like to thank Dr. J.M. Muller and Ir. S. van Engeland for their helpful suggestions.

References

1. Loo, L-N., Doi, K., Metz, C.E.: Investigation of Basic Imaging Properties in Digital Radiography. 4. Effect of Unsharp Masking on the Detectability of Simple Patterns. Med. Phys. 12 (1985) 209-214
2. Chan, H-P., Vyborny, C.J., MacMahon, H., Metz, C.E., Doi, K., Sickles, E.A.: Digital Mammography ROC Studies of the Effects of Pixel Size and Unsharp-Mask Filtering on the Detection of Subtle Microcalcifications. Investigative Radiology 7 (1987) 581-589

Clinical Presentation of Breast Tissue Composition Metrics

J. Kaufhold, Ph.D.*, J.W. Eberhard, Ph.D.*, C.E. Galbo, M.D.**, and J.A. Thomas, M.Sc.**

*GE Global Research Center, X-ray systems and applications laboratory, 1 Research Circle, Niskayuna, NY, 12309, USA; **Uniformed Services University of the Health Sciences, Department of Radiology, 4301 Jones Bridge Road, Bethesda, MD, 20814, USA
kaufhold@crd.ge.com

Abstract. Breast tissue composition is linked to both risk of developing breast cancer as well as the sensitivity of mammography. Thus, breast tissue composition assessment is important for patient management. However, it is not clear from published work if the visualization of breast tissue composition is relevant for clinical screening or diagnosis. We investigated the usefulness of different approaches to presenting quantitative tissue composition metrics to radiologists on a review workstation to address this question. Five different display methods were used to present the tissue composition metrics, 1) a word label, 2) a number, 3) superimposed contours, 4) a histogram, and 5) all together. For the specific presentation methods, we found that the radiologists polled preferred the first two methods to methods 3) and 4). All radiologists believed that it would be useful to present accurate, quantitative tissue composition information for establishing a consistent breast tissue composition score for each patient/mammogram.

1. Introduction and Background

It is widely recognized that mammography sensitivity decreases with increasing breast density. Further, the breast tissue composition is an indicator for breast cancer risk [1], [2]. For these reasons, understanding breast tissue composition is important for patient management reasons. To date, however, the question of whether quantitative assessment of patient tissue composition is relevant to radiologists for the purposes of screening, diagnosing and/or reporting has not been addressed. Recently, a number of investigators have proposed new methods for measuring the breast tissue composition quantitatively [3], [4], [5]. These developments make it possible to study whether the radiologist would find that information useful as a review workstation feature. In this paper, using recently proposed methods for measuring breast tissue composition [5], we experiment with different tissue composition presentation methods to assess whether any or all of these presentation methods on a review workstation may be useful to a radiologist in a screening, diagnostic, or reporting role.

2. Methods

The percent glandular-like tissue composition image is calculated (as in [5]) for 10 randomly selected patients from a screening study at the National Naval Medical Center in Bethesda, MD. From these percent glandular-like images, we compute four different metrics which can each be presented independently or in combination. 1) The average percent glandular tissue composition for each mammogram, $\%G_i$ (between 0 and 100), is computed. 2) By thresholding $\%G_i$, we associate a density *label* to each mammogram. 3) *Contours* of specific percentages of glandular-like tissue are computed for each mammogram. These contours can be displayed on the mammogram using different colors (black or white) and different line weights. 4) A *histogram* of the glandular-like composition greater than 0% is computed. A screen shot from the workstation (Mammocad of Image-Smiths, Bethesda, MD) used to perform the preference study is shown in Figure 1.

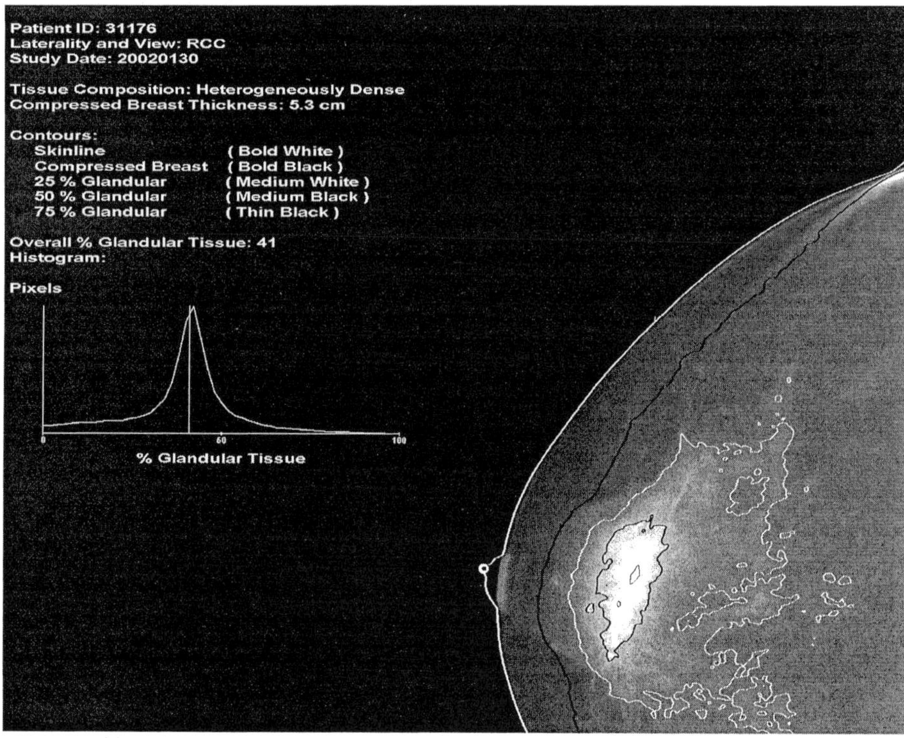

Fig. 1. All 4 tissue composition metrics displayed in combination on one mammogram. The label metric is 5.3 cm Heterogeneously Dense, the numerical metric is 41%, the contours are superimposed on the mammogram, and the histogram is shown with a line indicating the mean percent glandular composition.

Each radiologist is first shown a standard mammogram with no breast tissue composition metric displayed, and then is shown the same mammogram with one breast tissue composition metric displayed using 5 different presentation methods 1),

2). 3), 4), and the combination of 1)-4). After viewing at least 5 mammograms with these different presentation methods, the radiologist is asked two questions. They are asked to rate the usefulness numerically from 0 to 5 (0 is not useful, 5 is most useful). They are also asked to judge if the presentation method is distracting.

3. Results and Discussion

Table 1. Radiologist usefulness rankings for each presentation method (1-4) and all (5)

	1) Label	2) Number	3) Contours	4) Histogram	5) All
Radiologist A	3	3	0	0	1
Radiologist B	5	5	4	0	3
Radiologist C	3.5	3.5	1.5	1	3

In addition to the usefulness rankings, the radiologists also called presentation methods 3), 4) and 5) distracting. The early evidence from this preference study indicates that the categorical label and numerical value associated with the tissue composition was most useful to the radiologists, and that contours and histograms distract the radiologist while contributing little, if any, value in tissue composition assessment. All radiologists believed that it would be useful to present accurate, quantitative tissue composition information for establishing a consistent breast tissue composition score for each patient/mammogram. All radiologists indicated the importance of consistent tissue composition scores between CC and MLO views for the same breast. The presented information could ultimately be used to aid in writing reports using a standard metric for breast tissue composition. From this preference study, we believe there may be potential utility to tissue composition metric presentation on workstations for review by radiologists.

Acknowledgements: This work was supported by the Office of Naval Research under Grant Number MDA905-00-1-0041.

References

1. J.N. Wolfe. "Breast Patterns as an Index of Risk for Developing Breast Cancer" *American Journal of Roentgenology* 126:1130-1139, 1976.
2. J.J. Heine, P. Malhotra, "Mammographic Tissue, Breast Cancer Risk, Serial Image Analysis, and Digital Mammography, Part 2. Serial Breast Tissue Change and Related Temporal Influences", *Academic Radiology* , Vol. 9(3), 317-335, March 2002.
3. R.P. Highnam, M. Brady, "Mammographic Image Analysis", Kluwer Academic Publishers, 1999.
4. A. Bloomquist, B. Augustine, O. Pawluczyk, G.E. Mawdsley, M.J. Yaffe, "Estimating Breast Density Using a Volumetric Technique and Full-Field Digital Mammograms—Preliminary Results," *Proceedings of the 5th International Workshop on Digital Mammography*, pp705-712, Toronto, Canada, April 2000.
5. J. Kaufhold, J.A. Thomas, J.W. Eberhard, C.E. Galbo, D.E. Gonzalez Trotter, "A Calibration Approach to Glandular Tissue Composition Estimation in Digital Mammography," *Accepted to Med. Phys.*, (in revision) April, 2002.

Using Observer Models to Predict Softcopy Performance With Digital Mammography

Elizabeth Krupinski, Jeff Johnson, Hans Roehrig & Jeff Lubin

Department of Radiology University of Arizona Tucson, AZ USA
Sarnoff Corporation Princeton, NJ USA
Krupinski@radiology.arizona.edu

Abstract. The goal of this study was to evaluate reader performance viewing softcopy mammograms as the type of phosphor in the monitor faceplate changes from P104 to P45. The human observer results were then compared to the output from a human visual system model that was developed by the Sarnoff Corporation for assessing the discriminability of targets embedded in complex scenes. The results indicate that performance for the human observer is better (for the detection of microcalcifications in mammograms) using the P45 monitor compared to the P104 monitor. Physical evaluation of the monitors indicates that the signal-to-noise ratio for the P45 is higher than for the P104, which likely explains the difference in performance. The human visual stem model was effective in predicting the performance of the human observers.

1. Introduction

Full Field Digital Mammography (FFDM) is one of the newest and most exciting advances in radiology in recent years. It offers the potential to acquire and view mammograms using softcopy displays, allowing the viewer to adjust window and level settings to better visualize lesions, and to use a variety of other image processing and computer-aided diagnosis (CAD) tools during the interpretation process. Softcopy viewing of these very large (~ 5000 x 6000) images is, however, still not completely optimized. The traditional CRT monitor does not have the spatial resolution needed to display the entire image at full resolution, and other questions regarding image quality still exist in terms of what is the optimal display. Although LCD flat-panel displays are becoming more common, the CRT monitor is still the most widely used and accepted device for displaying digital radiographic images. There are a number of parameters that differ from monitor to monitor, however, requiring a wide variety of studies to be done in order to determine what the optimal display parameters are. The ideal is to conduct Receiver Operating Characteristic (ROC) studies with large numbers of images and observers for each parameter studied, but this is for the most part quite impractical. For example, ROC studies [1-2] have been conducted (along with eye-position recording) that showed that monitor luminance and tone scale (perceptually optimized or not) can affect diagnostic performance as well as visual search behaviors, but these studies utilized a lot of resources to complete. Another approach that has been used to assess observer performance has been the use of models that simulate the human visual system. [3-6] The eventual goal is to be able to model human visual system performance accurately enough to avoid conducting time-consuming and expensive human observer studies. In order to do this, one component is to validate the human visual system model against human observers doing the same task. The goal of this project was to further develop and refine an existing human visual system model and validate it against human observer performance for the task of searching for lesion in mammograms displayed in a CRT monitor. The specific parameter studied was the influence of monitor phosphor on detection performance.

The model (JNDMetrix) used in the following study was developed by the Sarnoff Corporation [7,8] for predicting human performance in a variety of detection, discrimination and image quality tasks. Basically, the model is based on the concept of just-noticeable differences (JNDs) and frequency-channel vision-modeling principles. If the model is provided with two images or image sequences, it will return accurate estimates of their visual discriminability. The model starts with the pair of images and ends with a JND map defining the magnitude and location of visible differences between the two images. The first step of the model convolves the images with a function that approximates the point-spread function of the optics of the eye. In the second step the image is sampled by a Gaussian convolution and point sampling sequence of operations to simulate the retinal cone mosaic. The raw luminance image is then converted to units of local contrast and decomposed into a Laplacian pyramid that yields seven frequency bandpass levels. These levels are then convolved with 8 pairs of spatially oriented filters with bandwidths derived from psychophysical data. The pairs of filter output images are then squared and summed, giving a phase-independent energy response. The next level of the model is a transducer phase in which the energy measures for each pyramid level are normalized and then transferred by a sigmoid non-linearity to reproduce the dipper shape of visual contrast discrimination functions. Non-linear masking effects that make features less detectable on a non-uniform background are taken into account. The model also accounts for characteristics of human foveal sensitivity by using a pooling step that averages transducer outputs over a small neighborhood by convolving with a disc-shaped kernel. At this point the outputs for each spatial position can be regarded as m-dimensional vectors where m is the number of pyramid levels x the number of orientations. The distance metric stage computes the distance between these vectors and the final result is the spatial map of JND values showing the discriminability between the two input images.

2. Methods & Materials

The first phase of the study involved the assembly of a set of test images for use in the observer and model phases. A set of 25 cases was selected from the Database for Screening Mammography [9], 13 with malignant (biopsy proven) microcalcification clusters and 12 with benign microcalcification clusters. A variety of breast densities and calcification types were selected. Pixel resolution of the raw images was 42 to 50 microns with 12-bit grayscale resolution. Regions of interest around the clusters were extracted from the images to create 512 x 512 sub-images. Digital processing techniques were used to remove the microcalcification clusters to create lesion-free versions of the images. The clusters were superimposed on a second set of 25 image regions (lesion-free) to create another set of lesion images. More images were created by weighted superposition of the signal-absent and signal-present pairs to create calcifications at intermediate contrast levels (25%, 50% and 75%). The final set of images was decimated by a factor of 2 to produce a set of 256 x 256 images, and some of the images were reflected horizontally and/or vertically to prevent recognition during the human observer trials. The final set contained a total of 250 images.

A study was then conducted to insure that the readers would not be able to distinguish between the original images and those created for the study. The sets of 512 and 256 images were shown to three radiologists. 200 pairs of images were used in side-by-side presentations. The radiologists had to indicate which of the pair of images (2AFC design) was the simulated version.

Prior to the actual observer performance studies, the monitors used in the study were characterized physically. Two high performance monochrome Siemens monitors (2048 x 2560) were used. The only difference between them was that one had a P45 phosphor in the faceplate and the other had a P104 phosphor in the faceplate. Since the main way that phosphor can affect the display is via noise, the main parameter evaluated was the noise power spectrum (NPS). Photographs were also taken (with a CCD camera) of all of the images displayed on both of the monitors. The reason was that these images (how the raw images appear once they have been transmitted through the display) were then fed into the human visual system model.

For the human observer performance study, 6 radiologists were recruited to participate, 3 experienced in reading mammograms and 3 less experienced. The 256 x 256 set of images was used. The 250 images were randomized and displayed once on the P45 and once on the P104 monitor. A counterbalanced randomized design was used for image presentation with at least one month between sessions to promote forgetting. The radiologists were shown each image and were asked to decide if a microcalcification cluster was present or not, then report their confidence in that decision using a 6-level scale (1 = absent, definite; 6 = present, definite). Viewing distance was set at 20 $\pm$ 2 cm from the monitor and all room lights were turned off. They were not allowed to adjust the window/level settings. Prior to each session the monitor was calibrated using the DICOM-14 grayscale display function standard.

3. Results

The physical evaluation of the two monitors showed that the NPS was different for the P45 versus the P104 phosphor. Pixel ratios of 53:1, 8:1 and 4:1 were used in the measurements. The NPS for the P104 monitor was higher at all spatial frequency levels than for the P45 monitor. This indicates that the P104 monitor is noisier than the P45 monitor, possibly affecting detection performance, especially for small, subtle microcalcifications.

The image quality study to determine whether the radiologists were able to tell the difference between the original "real" images with microcalcifications and the "simulated" images revealed that they were not able to tell the difference. For the 512 x 512 set of images the readers had 47.5%, 57% and 39% correct detections of simulated images (mean = 47.83%, sd = 7.35). For the 256 x 256 set of images the readers had 46%, 47.5% and 49.5% correct detections of simulated images (mean = 47.67, sd = 1.08). The readers were barely operating at chance in their discrimination of the real versus simulated images, indicating that the use of these images in the ROC and model trials was acceptable.

The confidence data were analyzed using the Multi-Reader Multi-Case Receiver Operating Characteristic (MRMC ROC) analysis technique. The average area under the curve Az for the P45 phosphor was 0.8044 and the average for the P104 phosphor was 0.7267. The Analysis of Variance (ANOVA) that MRMC performs on the Az values revealed a significant main effect for type of phosphor ($F = 9.19$, $df = 1{,}1245$, $p = 0.0027$). All 6 of the readers had higher Az performance with the P45 than with the P104 monitor. The vision model predicted the same results. Future analyses will examine the data for each of the contrast levels of the lesions (i.e., 25%, 50%, 75% and 100%).

4. Conclusions

The results of the physical evaluation of the P104 and P45 monitor indicate that there are indeed physical differences between them, at least in terms of NPS. The P104 monitor has a higher NPS than the P45. With higher noise levels it is likely that the signal-to-noise ratio (SNR) of images displayed on these monitors would likely be better for the P45 monitor since the NPS is lower. The result in terms of human observer performance should be reflected as better detection performance with the P45 than with the P104. Indeed, that is precisely what was found in both the human and model observers. The Az values overall were higher for the P45 than P104 monitor indicating better performance in terms of higher true-positive and lower false-positive rates for the detection of microcalcification clusters in mammograms. These results are similar to those found for a similar study comparing P45 with P104 monitors (mid-resolution) using a series of chest images with subtle pulmonary nodules. [10] The chest study also recorded eye-position during search and found that search was more effective with the P45 than with the P104 monitor. This was true in the studies noted earlier that compared luminance and tone scales for monitor displays [1,2] as well. Overall, it seems as if deficiencies in the display on a number of parameters results in both a decrease in observer performance and a decrease in the efficiency of visual search. The ideal display, therefore, should take these differences into account and be a combination of those parameters shown to promote better performance (i.e., higher luminance, perceptually linearized tone scale, and a P45 phosphor). There are certainly other display parameters that are likely to affect performance (e.g., veiling glare) and future studies will be aimed at investigating these issues.

5. References

1. Krupinski, E.A., Roehrig, H., Furukawa, T.: Influence of film and monitor display luminance on observer performance and visual search. Acad Radiol (1999) 411-418.
2. Krupinski, E.A., Roehrig, H,: The influence of a perceptually linearized display on observer performance and visual search. Acad Radiol (2000) 8-13.
3. Abbey, C.K., Eckstein, M.P., Shimozaki, S.S.: Comparison of human and model-observer templates for detection of simulated lesions in mammographic images. Proc SPIE Medical Imaging (2002) In Press.
4. Kupinski, M.A., Clarkson, E., Barrett, H.H.: Matching statistical object models to real images. Proc SPIE Medical Imaging (2002) In Press.
5. Eckstein, M.P., Abbey, C.K.: Effect of image compression on human and model performance in signal known statistically tasks. Proc SPIE Medical Imaging (2002) In Press.
6. Johnson, J.P., Lubin, J., Chakraborty, D.P.: Visual discrimination modeling of lesion detectability. Proc SPIE Medical Imaging (2002) In Press.
7. Johnson, J.P., Lubin, J., Krupinski, E.A., Peterson, H.A., Roehrig, H., Baysinger, A.: Visual discrimination model for digital mammography. SPIE Medical Imaging Proc 3663 (1999) 253-263.
8. Jackson, W.B., Said, M.R., Jared, D.A., Larimer, J.O., Gille, J.L., Lubin, J.: Evaluation of human visual models for predicting human-observer performance. Proc SPIE Medical Imaging 3036 (1997) 64-73.
9. Heath, M., Bowyer, K.W., Kopans, D., et al.: Current status of the digital database for screening mammography. In: Digital Mammography. Karssemeijer, N., Thijssen, M., Hendriks, Van Erning, J.L. (eds), Kluwer Academic Publishers, Boston, MA (1998).
10. Krupinski, E.A., Roehrig, H.: Pulmonary nodule detection performance and visual search: differences with P45 and P104 monochrome versus color monitor displays. Acad Radiol (2002) In Press.

Clinical Studies of Digital Mammography or Related Modalities

An Evaluation of a Commercial Prompting System in a Busy Screening Centre

Astley SM, Boggis CRM, Walker K, Wallace S, Tomkinson S, Hillier V, Morris J

Imaging Science and Biomedical Engineering, University of Manchester, Stopford Building, Oxford Road, Manchester, M13 9PT, and Nightingale Breast Centre, South Manchester University Hospitals NHS Trust, Nell Lane, Withington, Manchester, M20 OPT
Sue.Astley@man.ac.uk

We have investigated the feasibility of using a commercial prompting system in our screening centre. Its sensitivity was 92% for two-view screening mammograms and 66% for one-view, with three times as many false prompts as true ones. We attempted to integrate the system into clinical practice, assessing the impact on four readers who each reviewed 800 cases. Prompted reading did not significantly change their assessment of the films. Finally we took 90 incident round screening cases in which cancer was detected, and a similar control group of non-cancer cases. The previous screening mammograms were reviewed by an expert radiologist, then analysed by the system. The radiologist detected very early signs of cancer in 10% of the cancer cases, rising to 14.4% with the benefit of the subsequent diagnostic films. The system recorded a sensitivity of 27.8%, with an average of 1.32 false prompts per film in a one-view case and 1.56 per film in two-view cases.

1. Introduction

Breast screening generates a large number of mammograms, all of which need careful scrutiny to detect signs of abnormality. In the Nightingale Breast Screening Centre in Manchester, some 200 women's screening mammograms require interpretation each day, in addition to those of symptomatic women, and those of women attending because they have a family history of breast cancer. This workload is demanding both for the radiographers who acquire the images and for the radiologists who do the bulk of the film reading. One approach which has been widely promoted is the use of computer aided detection (CAD) technology to detect potential abnormalities and to draw them to the attention of the human film readers. Under suitable conditions, this approach, which is also known as prompting, can improve the performance of the reader. If CAD could improve the standard of an expert reader so that double reading was no longer necessary, or could improve the performance of a less well qualified reader to a level in which he or she could participate in double reading, this would enable the existing workforce to be used more efficiently. Furthermore, it could alleviate some of the problems caused by shortages of suitably trained staff.

In this paper, we describe three different aspects of our evaluation of a Second Look CAD system, from CADx Medical Systems, which was sited in the reading room at the Nightingale Breast Centre for a twelve month period during 2000/2001. Firstly, we measured the performance of the system, by processing a test set of films and comparing the positions of prompts with the known locations of abnormalities. Secondly, we attempted to simulate the clinical use of the system, and looked at the effect of prompting on four film readers. Thirdly, we looked at the potential of the system to detect very early breast cancers, by processing the previous screening films of women that had screen-detected cancers.

2. System Performance

In the first place, our aim was to establish the performance of the Second Look system in detecting cancers from the National Health Service Breast Screening Programme. In order to do this, we examined the prompts produced by the system when it had analysed a set of normal and abnormal screening films.

2.1 Method

One hundred and six unequivocally normal mammograms were obtained from the Nightingale Breast Centre. These were the previous screening films from all the women who had a normal screening examination on 17th May 2000. A second group of films comprised 116 biopsy-proven cancer cases, selected at random from those screened in a one year period ending in May 2000. About two thirds of the cases were one-view mammograms, and the rest had two views. All the cases were analysed by the Second Look system, which produces a paper printout showing the locations of prompts superimposed on the mammogram. A radiologist then annotated the malignant areas on the mammograms, drawing the boundary around each lesion and cluster of microcalcifications. The annotated films were run through the system to produce an annotated printout corresponding to each abnormal case.

2.2 Results

Second Look generated on average 1.43 prompts per film for the normal mammograms. Of these, 1.07 were mass prompts and 0.37 microcalcification prompts. Overall, the system prompted 73.8% of the abnormalities. However, it performed better where two views were available, with abnormalities prompted in at least one view in 83.3% of those cases. On average, the system generated 1.22 false prompts (i.e. prompts placed in normal locations) per film in the cancer cases.

2.3 Discussion

Previous studies have shown that, for prompting to be successful in improving detection performance, the prompt generator must not only be sensitive, but must also be specific [1]. False prompts have the potential to distract the observer from genuine regions of interest. If there are many false prompts, the importance attached by the observer to any prompt is reduced, since the likelihood of it corresponding to a genuine target is low. In mammographic screening, the vast majority of cases are unequivocally normal [2], so that, if one extrapolates the figures above to a situation in which about 0.75% of women screened had cancer, for each true prompt, there would be about 380 false prompts. This is an unacceptably high ratio.

3. Simulation of Clinical Use of the System

Having looked at the baseline performance of the system, we wanted to attempt to integrate it into clinical practice, to see how practical it would be to use it for screening on a daily basis, and to determine its effect on film readers.

3.1 Current Screening Practice

At the Nightingale Centre, films are reviewed from women attending screening at five mobile vans. All films exposed on the same day are reviewed together two working days later. They are displayed, where possible, with the previous screening films.

The readers take between one and a half and two hours to review 200 cases, depending on experience. In addition to the radiologists based at the Centre, films may also be read by trainee breast radiologists and by trained radiographers. Films deemed technically adequate are graded from one to five. A grade of one is normal and is not recorded, although each reader marks the edge of the film to show that they have read it. Those graded two to five are noted on a form. At the end of each day, the film readers meet to discuss these cases; any woman whose films are rated three or more by an experienced reader is recalled. Those with a rating of two may be recalled after discussion.

3.2 Method

The Second Look system was sited in the main reading room at the Nightingale Centre. The films used in this study were taken directly from eight days of routine screening, and may be regarded as typical screening cases. All had been reviewed by at least one consultant radiologist. Three hundred and seventy one (23.5%) of cases had two views, 76.3% had one view and the remainder had previously undergone a mastectomy, and had two views of one breast. Nearly nine percent of the women had had previous breast surgery. Ten women had breast cancer, detected as a result of the mammograms in the trial, and three women had abnormalities which were probably benign, but of sufficient concern for an early recall for screening in 6-12 months. Eight of the cancers were graded four or five by the consultant, one had grade three and the other grade two. Three radiologists and a trained radiographer each read approximately half of the 1581 cases after training and practice in prompted reading. For each reader, half of their reading sessions were prompted. All cases were independently reviewed by two readers, who graded each case and indicated whether they would recall the patient. Prompted cases were graded both before and after prompting.

3.3 Results

There was no significant difference between recall rates with and without prompting. Since the number of malignancies was small, the study provided little information about any effect on readers' sensitivity. There were only two cases for which the Second Look prompts changed a reader's grading. Both cases had been graded one by the expert; the reader changed her assessment from one to two after seeing the prompts. The effect of prompting on reading time was neither consistent nor significant. The least experienced reader, who had 12 months experience reading symptomatic mammograms, and had read approximately 1800 screening mammograms before the study, actually took less time when prompted, but the other three took between 22% and 33% longer with prompts.

Second Look processes 15 one-view or 9 two-view cases per hour, loaded into a 50-film hopper. This should have enabled a throughput of about 90 cases per day at the Nightingale Centre, but in practice we were not able to achieve this due to digitizer picking problems caused by our use of stick-on film labels, and system problems caused by static in the reading room. We would need two such systems to cope with our normal screening workload, and we would need to employ an extra clerk to deal with the systems and associated activities. In addition, there would be an extra day's delay before films were available for reading.

3.4 Discussion

At the time of the study, the majority of cases were one-view mammograms. This is no longer the case, which has implications both for throughput and for reading, since the sensitivity of second Look is much higher where two views are available. We knew from the outset that we would have insufficient data to study reader sensitivity. We were, however, able to assess the impact on readers' degree of suspicion for cases, and we found that the prompts had little effect, possibly because of the high false prompt rate. The most revealing information from this study was the throughput problem, which, in association with the running costs, severely limits the cost-effectiveness of using such systems unless a significant improvement in reader performance can be achieved.

4. Potential to Detect Early Cancer

One of our aims was to assess the potential of a CAD system to detect early cancer, whether or not the system is currently able to make a difference to the way in which human film readers interpret the films. To do this, we looked at the prompt positions in prior screening films, that is, the previous screening mammograms of women who subsequently had screen-detected cancers.

4.1 Method

A random sample of 90 women who had incident round, screen-detected, biopsy-proven cancers discovered between April 1999 and April 2000 was taken. The previous screening films (priors), the majority of which were taken about three years before cancer was detected, were obtained, and formed the study group. This contained 59 one-view and 31 two-view mammograms. Our control group comprised the prior screening films from 71 consecutive normal screening cases. All the prior mammograms were analysed by the SecondLook CAD system. The study and control group mammograms were randomized and reviewed by an expert breast radiologist who knew the approximate proportion of women who subsequently went on to develop cancer. The radiologist was not provided with any indication of which films corresponded to patients in the study group, and was required to mark the locations of any signs of early cancer. The radiologist was then provided with the subsequent diagnostic screening films, and reviewed the study group films again.

4.2 Results

Twenty five (27.8%) of the locations which subsequently developed cancers were prompted in at least one view. The average number of prompts in other locations in films in the study group was 2.64 per one-view case, and 6.26 per two-view case. The average number of these prompts per film was 1.45. In the study group, 7.8% of the cases had no prompts at all, and 18.9% had the maximum number of prompts allowed by the system. In the control group, there was an average of 1.25 prompts per film, 8.5% of the cases had no prompts, and 8.5% had the maximum number of prompts. Out of the 577 prompts in total, 29 (5%) marked developing cancers.

On first review of the mammograms, the radiologist identified nine cases (10%) in which signs of early cancer were visible; for another 18 cases, the radiologist had some degree of suspicion, but not enough to merit recalling the patient. When reviewing the mammograms with the aid of the diagnostic films, the radiologist identified visible cancers in 13 (14.4%) of the cases. In a further 15 (16.7%) of the cases, there were some equivocal signs.

4.3 Discussion

The Secondlook system demonstrated both its strength and its weakness in this study. The proportion of films in which some signs of cancer were visible – and prompted – was higher than we expected. It is likely that some of the on-target prompts appeared in the right locations because those locations shared properties with the kind of cancerous appearances that the system is designed to detect. These properties are also responsible for the many prompts which did not correspond to locations subsequently developing cancer. In summary, this study demonstrated the potential of CAD systems to detect very early signs of cancer, but for such a system to make a difference to readers' assessments, specificity must be improved.

References

1. Hutt I. The Computer-Aided Detection of Abnormalities in Screening Mammograms. PhD Thesis, University of Manchester, 1996.
2. J.Patnick (Ed) Breast Screening Programme Annual Review 2001. NHS Breast Screening Programme Publications.

Should we use humans or a machine to pre-screen mammograms?

Astley SM, Mistry TC, Boggis CRM, Hillier VF

Imaging Science and Biomedical Engineering, University of Manchester, Stopford Building, Oxford Road, Manchester, M13 9PT, UK, and Nightingale Breast Centre, South Manchester University Hospitals NHS Trust, Nell Lane, Withington, Manchester, M20 0PT, UK.
Sue.Astley@man.ac.uk

With an acute shortage of breast radiologists to cope with increasing demands, we are seeking ways of reducing the radiologists' workload. In this study, we consider whether either a commercial prompting system or trained non-medical readers could be used to identify unequivocally normal mammograms. Nine hundred screening mammograms, of which 10% showed cancer, were processed by an R2 ImageChecker. Six non-medical readers who had been trained to identify signs of abnormality read the same 900 mammograms, randomized into test sets. The cases in which the computer system did not place any markers and those believed by the non-medical readers to be normal were compared with the ground truth. The ImageChecker failed to mark only three of the cancer cases; however, fewer than 30% of cases were unprompted. The non-medical readers' performance varied widely; they missed between four and twenty-one of the cancers, but they were better able than the computer to label normal cases correctly.

1. Introduction

There is an acute shortage of radiologists in the United Kingdom National Health Service Breast Screening Programme. This is partly due to the already heavy workload; nationally, the programme generates approximately 1.5 million mammograms per year [1]. The eligible population is expected to increase by about 25% over the next twenty years, as a result of the 'baby boom'. Recent changes to the programme, including increasing the number of radiographic views and extending the age range of women invited for regular screening, will also add to the radiologists' workload. At the Nightingale Breast Centre in Manchester, radiologists interpret screening mammograms from women screened both at the Centre and on five mobile vans, along with those of women who are symptomatic or at higher than average risk of suffering from breast cancer. The screening workload is approximately 1,000 mammograms per week. There are the equivalent of two full-time radiologists working at the Centre.

The National Health Service (NHS) imposes very high standards of interpretation. One important measure is the Standardised Detection Ratio [2], which should be greater than one. In addition, the recall rate should be less than 7% [1], and the preoperative diagnosis should be known for over 90% of patients [3]. These standards are clearly met at the Nightingale Centre. For the most part, mammograms are 'double read', that is, two radiologists (or one radiologist and one trained radiographer) independently interpret each film, and a decision to recall is made following discussion between the two. It has, however, been shown that double reading with independent arbitration provides the most accurate interpretation [4], but this is not widely used because of the staffing implications.

One way of overcoming a shortage of readers is radiographer reading [5], which has been successfully implemented in a number of centres. There is, however, a national shortage of radiographers in the screening programme. This has led us to consider other options, such as using non-medical readers or a CAD system, to find a cost-effective way of reducing the radiologists' workload. Non-medical readers are used for other visual tasks within the NHS. For example, in the national cervical screening programme, readers paid at laboratory technician rates are trained to look for a range of abnormal patterns. Sperm counting is also done by lay readers, although this task requires the identification of fewer types of entity, and is not of the same level of visual complexity as mammography. Another potential solution to the shortage of readers is the use of computer-based aids. Computer-aided detection (CAD) systems for mammographic screening are generally designed to improve the performance of radiologists. If a single reader using a CAD system could perform as well as two radiologists double reading, this would clearly be a good solution to the manpower problem. Similarly, we might investigate whether a less experienced (or less highly qualified) reader with a CAD system could bring their performance up to an acceptable standard for double reading.

In this study, we investigate an alternative model of the screening process. Pre-screening involves sorting mammograms into two groups: those which are possibly abnormal, and those which are almost certainly normal. The sorting process is carried out prior to interpretation by the radiologist. The radiologist will view only the 'possibly abnormal' group and a small subset of the others for quality control purposes. Thus the expert radiologist will be spared from viewing a large number of unequivocally normal mammograms, and will be able to focus his or her attentions on the more difficult or suspicious examples. This would make much more efficient use of the time of highly trained experts, but its success depends critically on the ability of the pre-screener to separate the films appropriately. Here, we compare a commercially available CAD system (the R2 ImageChecker) with six non-medical readers, to determine their performance as pre-screeners.

2. Method

We have obtained from the Nightingale Breast Centre 265 randomly selected, four film screening mammograms in which cancer was detected (all biopsy-proven) and 855 normal screening mammograms. We consider these cases typical of those encountered in the screening programme. The normal mammograms were the previous screening films of women who have subsequently had a second normal screening examination, to avoid the possibility of small or subtle developing cancers being present. The majority of the mammograms were on standard (18 by 24cm) film, but about 10% of the women had bigger breasts and required large format films (24 by 30cm). Eight hundred and ten normal and 90 abnormal mammograms were allocated randomly to six test sets, each comprising approximately 150 mammograms of which about 10% were abnormal. The remaining mammograms were formed into training and practice sets.

All the mammograms in the test sets were put through an R2 ImageChecker Computer-Aided Detection system. The system places markers in locations where the probability of malignant abnormality is high. There are two types of markers, one for microcalcifications and one for masses. Each location may be additionally labeled as having a particularly high degree of suspicion ('SuperCheck' markers). The locations of the markers were compared with the known locations of the cancers.

Six non-medical readers were recruited. They ranged in age from 17 to 57, and in occupation from student to housewife. None had any previous medically-related training. These readers were split into two groups of three, each group attending for two working weeks. On days one and two, they underwent intensive training in mammographic interpretation under the supervision of an experienced breast radiologist who is also a trainer of breast radiologists. The training used 120 cases, of which 100 showed cancer. On day three, the non-medical readers had practice sessions in which 75% of the mammograms were normal, with detailed feedback from the radiologist. On day four, they independently read one of the six test sets. This was split randomly into three subsets of 50 mammograms, and the three readers rotated around the subsets. The readers were informed of the approximate percentage of abnormal films, and were instructed to rate each film according to their degree of suspicion that cancer was present. They indicated their judgement by making a mark on a 5cm line; they were instructed to circle the appropriate end of the line if they were completely confident that a mammogram was definitely normal or definitely showed a cancer. At the end of the day, feedback was given to each individual, so that they could learn from their own mistakes and from those of the other readers. They also filled in evaluation forms. The pattern of day four was repeated until the readers had read each of the six test sets, and on day ten, they were presented with test set one again. This had been re-randomized, and the readers were not made aware that they were reviewing films they had already seen. The results were collated and analysed.

3. Results

The R2 ImageChecker placed markers in 556 of the 810 normal mammograms, and 87 of the 90 cancer mammograms in the test set. The distribution of markers in normal mammograms is shown in Table 1, and that in cancer-containing mammograms in Table 2. Should the system be used for pre-screening, and any mammogram with one or more markers was considered to be potentially abnormal, it would be necessary for the radiologist to view at least 71% of the mammograms and approximately 3% of cancers would definitely be missed. Of the 1242 markers on normal cases, 234 (18.8%) were labeled as highly suspicious. Of the 331 markers on the cancer cases, 122 (36.9%) were labeled as highly suspicious. The average number of markers per film for normal mammograms was 0.38, and for abnormal mammograms was 0.92. In the cancer cases, 65 (72.2%) had at least one prompt labeled highly suspicious.

Table 1. Distribution of CAD system markers in 810 normal 4-film mammograms. The upper row shows the number of markers, and the lower row the number of normal mammograms with that number of markers.

no. markers	0	1	2	3	4	5	6	7	8	9	10	11
mammograms	254	239	144	85	47	19	7	7	5	2	0	3

Table 2. Distribution of CAD system markers in 90 4-film screening mammograms showing cancer.

no. markers	0	1	2	3	4	5	6	7	8	9	10
mammograms	3	6	20	15	20	11	8	2	3	1	1

On average it took 5.3 minutes for each standard format 4 film mammogram to be processed by the CAD system, and 6 minutes for each large format 4 film case.

The non-medical readers took an average of 40 seconds to read (and record) a 4-film mammogram, although there was a significant increase in reading speed as they progressed through the test sets. By the end of the trial, reading speed had settled to about 35 seconds. Detailed analysis of the performance of the non-medical readers revealed substantial differences in their performance. Two of the readers were clearly inconsistent in their use of the rating scale, whilst the other four performed well, with areas of between 0.82 and 0.89 under their Receiver Operating Characteristic curves. Statistically, there was no significant difference in performance when comparing results for test set one at the start and end of the trial period.

Two of the readers achieved a sensitivity of 94%, which corresponds to missing about 5 cancers from the test sets. One of these readers had a false positive rate of 44% and the other 33%. None of the others achieved a sensitivity over 90% with a false positive rate less than 50%.

4. Discussion

The R2 ImageChecker placed markers on a high proportion of the cancer cases. However, three cancer cases, which had been graded 3 (and hence recalled) by the screening radiologist who first reviewed the films, had no prompts. The first such case was a small cluster of calcification in the upper outer quadrant of the left breast. Three of the non-medical readers missed it completely, another thought it was probably normal, and the other two thought it might be cancer. The second case missed by the ImageChecker was a 4.5mm deformity in the outer half of the left breast. One non-medical reader labeled this as 'definitely cancer', and another marked the middle of the decision line. The remaining four readers missed it. The third case was a small mass with associated microcalcification in the upper outer quadrant of the left breast. This was detected by four of the non-medical readers, two of whom thought it was 'definitely cancer'. It is important to note that in this study we are considering the potential of using a CAD system for pre-screening, rather than prompting, and make no judgement about the locations of markers within a given case.

The performance of the non-medical readers varied widely, indicating the need for aptitude testing. Two of the readers performed particularly well, considering the very limited training that they were given. They missed only 5 cancers, and they also managed to correctly classify a high enough proportion of normal films to significantly reduce the workload of the radiologist in a pre-screening situation. However, it is debatable whether their sensitivity (or even that of the CAD system) would be acceptable, since there is no guarantee that the radiologist would detect all of the cancers in the more difficult, reduced set of mammograms. It may, however, be possible to pre-screen a more limited set of films, such as those which are predominantly fatty, with greater success.

5. References

1. Patnick J (Ed.). Breast Screening Programme Annual Review 2001. NHS Breast Screening Programme Publications.
2. Blanks R, Day N, Moss S. Monitoring the Performance of Breast screening Programmes: Use of Indirect Standardisation in Evaluating the Invasive Cancer Detection Rate. J Med Screening 3:79-81 1996
3. Wilson R, Asbury D, Cooke J, Michell M, Patnick J (Eds.) Clinical Guidelines for Breast cancer Screening Assessment. NHS Breast Screening Programme Publications 2001
4. Blanks RG, Wallis MG, Moss SM. A comparison of cancer detection rates achieved by breast cancer screening programmes by number of readers, for one and two view mammography: results from the UK National Health Service breast screening programme. J Med Screening 1998; 5(4) 195-201
5. Pauli R, Hommond S, Cooke J, Ansell J. Radiographers as film readers in screening mammography: an assessment of competence under test and screening conditions. British Journal of radiology 69: 10-14, 1996

Intraindividual Comparison of Full-Field-Digital-Mammography and Conventional Film-Screen Mammography for Early Detection of Breast Cancer

Arne Fischmann, Katja Siegmann, Annika Wersebe, Nicos Fersis *, Claus D. Claussen, Markus Müller-Schimpfle

Radiologische Universitätsklinik, Department of Diagnostic Radiology, Hoppe-Seyler-Str. 3, 72076 Tübingen, Germany
*Universitätsfrauenklinik, Schleichstr. 4, 72076 Tübingen, Germany
arne.fischmann@med.uni-tuebingen.de

Abstract. Full field digital mammography (FFDM; Senographe 2000D, GE Medical Systems) of one breast and conventional film screen mammography (FSM; Senographe DMR+, GE Medical systems) of the other breast were performed in 75 women with no symptoms or known breast lesions. Imaging parameters were set automatically. Hardcopies were used for analysis. Parameters were rated by three readers independently. In automatic mode no significant difference of skin dose was found. Rating of image quality showed a tendency in favour of FFDM. With FFDM more calcifications were detected than with FSM ($p = 0.02/0.13/0.06$). Contrast in parenchymal and fatty tissue and detection of opacities did not differ significantly. FFDM provided better visibility of skin and nipple ($p<0{,}05$). Also the visibility of the pectoral muscle was better with FFDM ($p<0.05$). In conclusion, FFDM does provide at least equal to better image quality compared to FSM using automatic mode and hard-copy reading.

1. Introduction

Digital technology is replacing conventional film screen systems in all aspects of clinical radiology. Due to higher requirements in contrast and spatial resolution, digital mammography was the major exception of this development up to recently. The spatial resolution of the FFDM for high contrast objects is 5 lp/mm and below the minimal requirements for FSM, that require a spatial resolution of at least 8 lp/mm. Still the system has a higher detective quantum efficiency (DQE) and contrast resolution.[5] This allows for better resolution of structures at a resolution of 3 to 5 lp/mm, where the human eye has its maximal performance. Since November 2000 the University of Tübingen has an FFDM unit (Senographe 2000 D, GEMS) with review workstation for monitor diagnosis. The technical parameters of this system are in many ways comparable to the conventional FSM Senographe DMR+ (GEMS) used in our department for routine diagnosis. The aim of this study was to compare image quality of FFDM and FSM in a prospective randomised study in the same woman without double radiation exposure of her breast.

2. Materials and Methods

We included 75 women in this study who were sent to our department for mammography. Women with obvious asymmetry of the breasts or with known breast lesions, previous breast infections or surgery were excluded, as were women below the age of 40. Due to the limited size of the detector of 19x23 cm, women with macromasty were excluded as well. Informed consent was obtained by all women. The study was approved by the ethical board committee of the University.

Table 1. Quality criteria used for the rating of digital and conventional mammography.

detection of the pectoral muscle	detectable/not detectable
visualisation of nipple	excellent/good/mediocre/not visible with and without bright light
visualisation of the skin	excellent/good/mediocre/not visible with and without bright light
sharpness	sharp/mostly sharp/not sharp
contrast in parenchymal tissue	excellent/good/mediocre/little
contrast in fatty tissue	excellent/good/mediocre/little
parenchymal density	complete involution/markedly involuted/little involution/no involution *(see table 2)*
detection of microcalcifications (MK)	no MK/probably no MK/ probably MK/MK
diagnostic classification of MK	excellent /good/poor/not possible
detection of opacities	no opacities/probably no opacities/ probable opacities/opacities
diagnostic classification of opacities	excellent /good/poor/not possible
general image quality	excellent/good/mediocre/acceptable/poor/ inadequate

All participants were randomised in two groups. Patients of the first group received a digital mammography of the left breast and a conventional mammography of the right. Patients in the second group received a digital mammography of the right breast and conventional of the left. With this proceeding we were able to perform an indirect intraindividual comparison without additional radiation exposure[7]. To enable a comparison on routine examinations, the imaging parameters were chosen automatically by the systems in standard mode. Imaging parameters of the conventional system were documented by the radiographer. FSM was performed on a Senographe DMR+, (GEMS) with a state-of -the -art film screen system (MinR, Kodak, Rochester, NY, USA), processed on a modern developing system (Xomat M35 with RP Xomat, Kodak). FFDM was performed on a Senographe 2000 D

(GEMS). Hardcopies were printed on a laser printer (DryView 8610, Kodak). Contrast and brightness of the hardcopies were set automatically in standard mode by both systems. Skin dose calculations were made based on reference measurements on a 4.5cm PMMA phantom. Modalities were rated separately according to different criteria *(See Table1)* by three independent observers experienced in mammography. Statistics were calculated with the software JMP 4.0 for Windows NT (SAS Institute Inc. Cary, NC, USA).

3. Results

In automatic mode, Rhodium/Rhodium (Rh/Rh) as anode-filter combination was used significantly more often by FFDM. Skin dose in cc-view averaged 10.28 mGy for FFDM and 11.14 mGy for FSM, in the mlo-view 10.75 mGy for FFDM and 12.04 for FSM. These differences were not significant but showed a tendency towards lower skin dose in FFDM. In cc-views, the pectoral muscle could be depicted by reader 1/2/3 more often with FFDM (n = 27/33/36) than with FSM (n = 18/22/27). The corresponding p-values of 0.11, 0.02 and 0.9 showed significance for reader 2.

The visibility of the nipple was excellent in 73/73/75 cases with FFDM and in 23/24/64 cases with FSM ($p < 0.001$). The visibility of the skin was rated excellent in 75/67/72 cases for FFDM compared to 21/5/58 cases with FSM ($p < 0.001$/$p < 0.001$/ $p = 0.04$). Image quality was rated to be excellent in 75/55/56 cases for FFDM and in 61/41/54 cases for FSM. These differences were significant for reader 1 ($p = 0.02$) and showed a tendency in favour of FFDM for reader 2 ($p = 0.055$). The rating of contrast in parenchymal and fatty tissue did not differ between the modalities. Still there was a tendency to rate the parenchymal tissue to be further involuted in FFDM compared with FSM, which was significant for reader 2 (p = 0.7/ 0.02/0.2).

Microcalcifications were detected with FFDM in 46/36/45 cases and with FSM in 28/29/32 cases. This difference was significant for reader 1 and showed a tendency in favour of FFDM for the other two readers (p = 0.02/0.13/0.06). There was also a tendency towards better diagnostic classification of microcalcifications for digital mammography (p = 0.36/0.003/0.85) No difference was found in detection and diagnostic classification of opacities. These were detected with FFDM in 13/11/13 cases and with FSM in 13/7/11 cases.

4. Discussion

As in the previously published phantom studies [2] we found a better detection of microcalcifications. This can be explained by the fact that the minimal size for detectable calcifications is 100-130 μm even with FSM and a high spatial resolution of 15 lp/mm [4]. Therefore the limiting factor for detection is not the maximal spatial resolution but the contrast to the surrounding tissue. As the latter is inversely related to the size of the calcifications, the higher contrast resolution of FFDM is of more clinical importance than the higher spatial resolution of FSM.

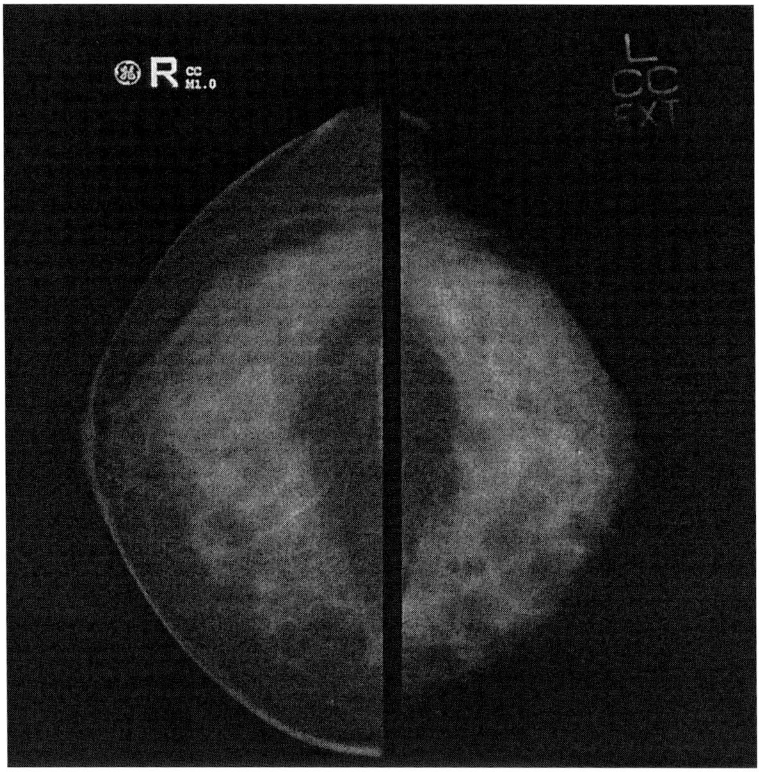

Fig. 1. Better depiction of skin, nipple and pectoral muscle in FFDM (left) than in FSM (right).

In contrast to phantom studies we found no increased detection of opacities with FFDM[6]. As in a clinical situation the detection of opacities is limited less by the contrast to the surrounding tissue but rather by the inhomogeneity of the background of the parenchymal tissue. Another interesting result is the better image quality of FFDM. Obvious differences were found in the visualisation of skin and nipple, which were better visible on digital mammographies. A less obvious advantage was the better depiction of the pectoral muscle in cc-view, which is an important parameter for quality control [3]. FFDM does not require a film-cassette or cassette holder, therefore the detector is a few mm closer to the thoracic wall of the patient. This small difference is enough to depict a small part of the muscle in many patients and allows a better detection of lesions close to the thoracic wall *(See Fig. 1)*.

To classify the degree of involution we use a classification system that is developed from the system described in the BI-RADS™-lexicon of the American College of Radiology [1]. The classification in 4 levels of parenchymal density is based on the size of lesions that cannot be excluded (see table 2). Our studies showed a good inter-reader correlation with this classification system with Kappa values of 0.517, 0.712, 0.590 in FFDM and 0.423, 0.591, 0.405 in FSM. With FFDM the breasts are classified to be less dense and further involuted than with FSM. This underlines once more the advantage of the better contrast resolution of FFDM.

Table 2. Classification of parenchymal density

Class	Size of a potential lesion that cannot be excluded
1	< 0,5 cm
2	0,5 to 1 cm
3	1 to 2 cm
4	> 2 cm

Due to its higher contrast resolution we expected that the digital unit would use a harder radiation spectrum, to achieve a dose reduction. Indeed, FFDM used more often the Rh/Rh combination. In contrast to phantom-studies, that showed a potential dose reduction with FFDM [6], the harder radiation did not cause a significant reduction in skin dose, although there was a tendency towards lower doses with FFDM.

5. Summary

Digital full field mammography proved to be at least equal to conventional film screen mammography. Higher image quality especially for dense breasts and better detection of microcalcifications were the main advantages. Future studies with histopathological correlation should be performed to assess the diagnostic characterisation of calcifications and opacities with FFDM compared to FSM.

References

1. (ACR) American College of Radiology: Breast Imaging Reporting and Data System (BI-RADS). Third Edition ed. Reston, Va (1998)
2. Diekmann, F., Diekmann, S., Bick, U., Rogalla, P., Blohmer, J.U., Winzer, K.J.,Hamm, B.: Comparing the visualization of microcalcifications with direct magnification in digital full-field mammography vs. film-screen mammography.
   Fortschr Geb Rontgenstr Neuen Bildgeb Verfahr **174** (2002) 297-300
3. Heywang-Köbrunner, S.H.: Plans of the German Roentgen Society and the Professional Association for Quality Assurance in Mammography. Radiologe **41** (2001) 352-358
4. Karssemeijer, N., Frieling, J.T.,Hendriks, J.H.: Spatial resolution in digital mammography. Invest Radiol **28** (2001) 413-419
5. Muller, S.: Full-field digital mammography designed as a complete system.
   Eur J Radiol **31** (1999) 25-34.
6. Obenauer, S., Hermann, K.P., Schorn, C., Fischer, U.,Grabbe, E.: Full-field digital mammography: dose-dependent detectability of breast lesions and microcalcinosis. Fortschr Geb Rontgenstr Neuen Bildgeb Verfahr **172** (2000) 1052-1056
7. Thilander-Klang, A.C., Ackerholm, P.H., Berlin, I.C., Bjurstam, N.G., Mattsson, S.L., Mansson, L.G., von Scheele, C.,Thunberg, S.J.: Influence of anode-filter combinations on image quality and radiation dose in 965 women undergoing mammography
   Radiology **203** (1997) 348-354.

Longitudinal retrospective study of breast tissue composition

J. Kaufhold, Ph.D.*, J. A. Thomas, M.Sc.** and J.W. Eberhard, Ph.D.*

*GE Global Research Center, X-ray systems and applications laboratory, 1 Research Circle, Niskayuna, NY, 12309; **Uniformed Services University of the Health Sciences, Department of Radiology, 4301 Jones Bridge Road, Bethesda, MD, 20814
kaufhold@crd.ge.com

Abstract. Links between subjective measurements of breast tissue composition and patient age have been demonstrated in the literature. Specifically, as women age, especially after menopause, radiologist-assigned breast tissue composition characterizations for a given patient regress from dense to less dense. Recently, a number of investigators have developed objective tools for quantitative breast tissue composition estimation. We evaluate the quantitative link between breast tissue composition and age, as well as other quantities, such as compressed breast height using the newer more quantitative methods for calculating breast tissue composition. We find that the compressed breast height is more strongly correlated with breast tissue composition than age. Further, we find that the quantitative tissue composition metric we calculate is correlated with the radiologist characterization of breast tissue composition.

1. Breast Tissue Composition Introduction and Background

The healthy breast is composed almost entirely of two distinct tissue types, fatty and glandular-like, each with characteristic x-ray attenuation properties. On a digital mammogram, the more fatty the volume projected onto the digital mammogram, the darker it appears; the more glandular-like the volume, the brighter it appears. Wolfe recognized that the tissue composition of patient breasts may be an indicator of patient risk for breast cancer—this hypothesis was borne out by subsequent studies. To test his hypothesis, Wolfe proposed a subjective 4-category ranking of breast compositions by radiologists [1]. There were 4 categories of breast tissue "patterns" which roughly indicated increasing glandular composition. In related studies, it was found that for typical patients, the radiologist characterization of breast category regressed over time from the dense, high-risk category, to a less dense, lower-risk category. This progression from high risk to lower risk categories was interpreted to be an indicator of post-menopausal involution of the endocrine function of the breast, in which the glandular compartments of the breast regress [2]. Recently, more objective quantitative volumetric methods [3,4,5,6,7] have become available to measure breast tissue composition. However, these new approaches have not yet been applied to measuring effects of involution quantitatively. Here we study the quantitative effects of involution in a patient population over 2 years.

2. Methods

2.1 Quantitative Analysis of Patient Mammograms

To quantitatively assess the tissue composition of the breast, we used the technique described in ([6][7]). Briefly, the steps required in the quantification are 1) Measure mean signal levels (converted to log domain) for raw digital mammograms of a range of phantom heights (2-7cm) for both glandular-equivalent and fatty-equivalent material (measurements are taken in an ROI where residual scatter through the grid is essentially spatially invariant). 2) Fit calibration curves to each tissue-equivalent material's x-ray technique and composition as a function of the phantom slab height. 3) Compute the –log of each raw digital mammogram. 4) Remove the pectoral from each MLO digital mammogram. 5) Estimate the compressed breast region (*CBR*) with an intensity threshold based on compressed breast height and calibration curves,

$$CBR = \{(i,j) \mid y(i,j) > y_{100\%\,fat}\} \tag{1}$$

6) The percent glandular image is formed by computing

$$\%G(i,j) = \frac{100\left(y(i,j) - y_{100\%\,fat}\right)}{y_{100\%\,glandular} - y_{100\%\,fat}} \tag{2}$$

$$P_G = \frac{1}{A_{CBR}} \sum_{(i,j)\in CBR} \%G(i,j), \text{ where } A_{CBR} = \sum_{(i,j)\in CBR} 1 \tag{3}$$

7) From the compressed breast height (*H*), the percent glandular-like tissue (P_G), and the *CBR* area (A_{CBR}), the glandular-like volume is computed as:

$$V_G = (P_G / 100)(A_{CBR})(H)(0.0001\,\text{cm}^2/\text{pixel}) \tag{4}$$

To test for temporal stability of calibration curves, we measured the calibration curve signal level and noise level 6 months apart.

2.2 Study Design

Sixty-five patients followed for 2 years on General Electric Senographe 2000D FFDM systems were selected at random from the digital mammogram screening population at the National Naval Medical Center in Bethesda, MD. Each patient had 4 views for each year. This study population excludes patients whose compressed breast thicknesses were > 7.5 cm.

3. Results

The calibration curves for each technique were measured 6 months apart to quantify machine drift. A representative set of calibration curves is shown with error bars indicating the standard deviation of the measurements in **Fig. 1**.

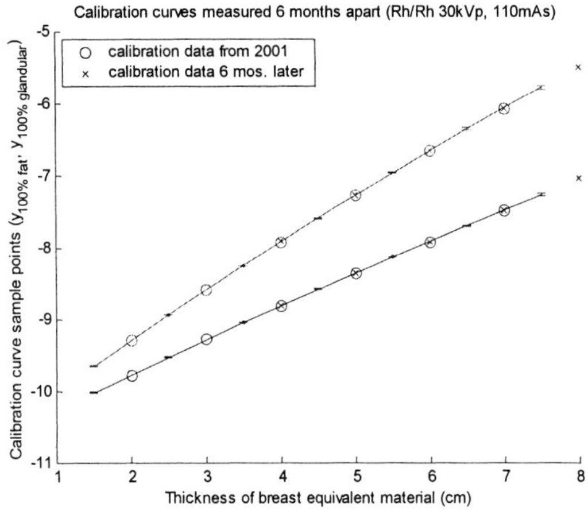

Fig. 1. Representative calibration curves acquired 6 months apart. Top curve is 100% glandular-equivalent material. Bottom curve is 100% fat-equivalent material.

The percent glandular for the population over all study years, P_G, as estimated by **equation (3)**, is plotted versus the compressed breast height as measured by the digital compression paddle height readout in **Fig. 2**.

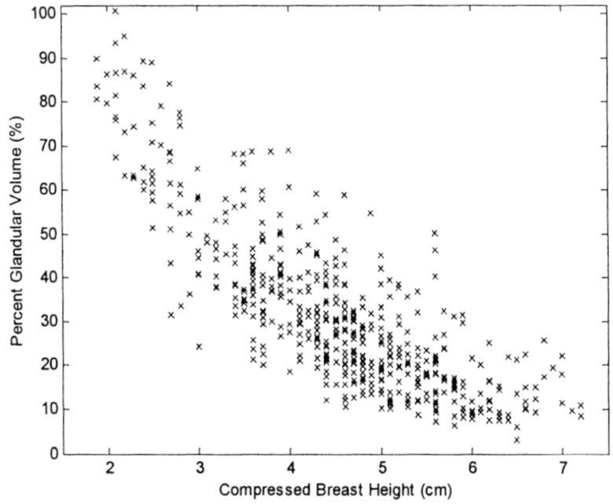

Fig. 2. Measured percent glandular tissue versus compressed breast height

The volume of glandular tissue for the population over all study years, V_G, as estimated by **equation (4)**, has a mean of 98.4 cc, a standard deviation of 48.9 cc, and does not appear to vary as strongly as a function of compressed breast thickness as does P_G (correlation coefficients –0.81 for P_G vs. H and –0.33 for V_G vs. H).

In **Fig. 3** the percent glandular tissue for the population over all study years, P_G, as estimated by **equation (3)**, is plotted versus the radiologist composition impression for each patient. The associated means and errorbars are displayed to the right of the data.

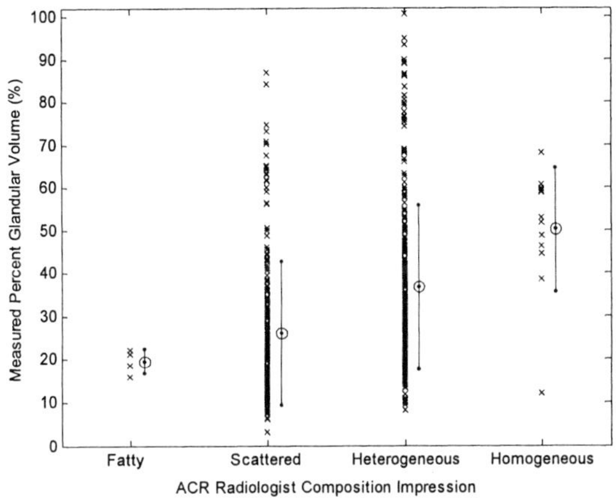

Fig. 3. Percent glandular volume versus radiologist composition impression

The volume of the glandular tissue for the population over all study years, V_G, as measured by **equation (4)**, is plotted versus the patient age in **Fig. 4**.

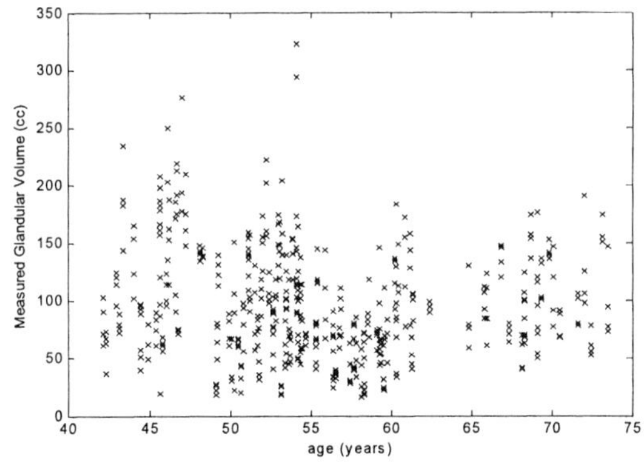

Fig. 4. Volume of glandular tissue versus patient age

4. Discussion

One striking result in the work presented is that the calibration curves for a given FFDM system are remarkably stable over time. The implication of such a result is that raw mammograms collected at virtually any site with such a system can be retrospectively analyzed using the method described. This is an advantage for FFDM systems compared to film-screen approaches for similar calibrated tissue measurement tasks. Similar measurements on film screen systems are best performed with a step wedge in each image to account for film speed differences from exposure to exposure.

Another new and interesting result is that we found the radiologist composition impressions of the mammograms in the study correlates with the percent glandular-like composition as measured by the volumetric tissue composition measurement technique described. This result suggests that there is also a link between the risk of breast cancer and the measured volumetric breast tissue composition.

We found that the glandular composition estimate versus age was not as strongly correlated as the composition estimate versus *H*. However, conclusions drawn from this study population can only be called preliminary due to, among other reasons, the paucity of data for pre-menopausal women. Further, because reported regression from high risk categories to lower risk categories is most noticeable pre- and post-menopause, it can be argued that the majority of women in this study have already experienced most of their glandular regression due to involution. Further, because the previously reported results for categorical regression from high to lower risk were for individual patients over time, and not for entire populations as a function of age, it may not generalize to the results presented here. A comparable analysis of breast tissue compositions measured using the approach described would follow individual patients over a number of years—this study is currently underway.

Acknowledgements: This work was supported by the Office of Naval Research under Grant Number MDA905-00-1-0041

References

1. J.N. Wolfe. "Breast Patterns as an Index of Risk for Developing Breast Cancer" *American Journal of Roentgenology* 126:1130-1139, 1976.
2. J.J. Heine, P. Malhotra, "Mammographic Tissue, Breast Cancer Risk, Serial Image Analysis, and Digital Mammography, Part 2. Serial Breast Tissue Change and Related Temporal Influences", *Academic Radiology* , Vol. 9(3), 317-335, March 2002.
3. L. Desponds, R. Klausz, "Automatic Estimation of Breast Composition with Mammographic X-ray Systems," *Proc. Of The RSNA*, Nov. 1994, Chicago, IL.
4. R.P. Highnam, M. Brady, "Mammographic Image Analysis", Kluwer Academic Publishers, 1999.
5. A. Bloomquist, B. Augustine, O. Pawluczyk, G.E. Mawdsley, M.J. Yaffe, "Estimating Breast Density Using a Volumetric Technique and Full-Field Digital Mammograms—Preliminary Results," *Proceedings of the 5th International Workshop on Digital Mammography*, pp705-712, Toronto, Canada, April 2000.
6. J. Kaufhold, J.A. Thomas, J.W. Eberhard, C.E. Galbo, D.E. Gonzalez Trotter, "A Calibration Approach to Glandular Tissue Composition Estimation in Digital Mammography," *Accepted to Med. Phys.*, (in revision) April, 2002.
7. J. Kaufhold, J.A. Thomas, J.W. Eberhard, C.E. Galbo, D.E. Gonzalez Trotter, "Tissue Composition Determination in Digital Mammography," *Proc. Of The RSNA*, p. 188, Nov. 2001.

Microcalcifications and Masses: Is high resolution digital luminescence mammography (without magnification) (CR) equal to concentional screen film mammography (SFM) ? A clinical, histologically proven study

R. Schulz-Wendtland, U. Aichinger, I. Kuchar, M. Tartsch, W. Bautz

Institute of Diagnostic Radiology, University of Erlangen-Nürnberg
91054 Erlangen, Germany
Ruediger.Schulz-Wendtland@idr.imed.uni-erlangen.de

Introduction

The mammography is the only method that reduces the mortality of breast cancer until 44 %, demonstrated in screening projects (Sweden, Netherlands, USA) [1]. Up to 20 % of the detected cancers are DCIS (ductal cancer in situ). The DCIS are differentiated into low grade and high grade DCIS and especially the high grade DCIS contains up to 80 % microcalcifications. In contrast to this, round lesions and masses are much more difficult to diagnose and the rate of detected small cancers with a diameter up to 1 cm is documentated with 70 % [2].

Screen film mammography (SFM) have a resolution up to 12-15 lp/mm. In Germany the regulations demand at least 8 lp/mm for a system used for mammography [3]. Therefore we use at our department of Gynaecological Radiology, Institute of Diagnostic Radiology, University of Erlangen-Nürnberg, a high resolution digital luminescence mammography system with storage phosphor plate technique (CR) and a resolution of 9 lp/mm. After a phantom study (Wisconsin RMI phantom) with the same results in the detection of details between conventional screen film mammography (SFM) and digital technique (CR) we received full permission to perform digital luminescence mammography in clinical routine [4].

Material and Method

From April 2001 and November 2001, we investigated 112 patients (mean age 55 years). All patients got a conventional SFM and after needle marking, before undergoing an open biopsy, a digital CR. The indications were suspect microcalcifications and masses.

The technical equipment:

1st Conventional screen film mammography (SFM) (Mammomat 3000 N (Siemens), resolution 12-15 lp/mm, for exposure we chose the screen film combination UM mammo Fine (screen) UM-MA (film) (Fuji), for development of the films the day light system MF FPM 2100 (Fuji)).

2nd High resolution digital luminescence mammography with phosphor storage plate technique (CR) (Mammomat 3000 N (Siemens), resolution 9 lp/mm, digital phosphor storage plate type IP HRV (Fuji), image reader FFDM-CR (Fuji / Siemens), printer dry view TM 8600 Laser Imaging System (Kodak)).

We compared the anonymous med.-lat. images (hardcopies) of the SFM and the CR (same exposure datas) by three observers without knowing the histological diagnosis. All observers were radiologists with at least one year of experience in mammography (observer 1, 12 years; observer 2, 5 years and observer 3, 1 year in a specialized department). Criteria were the diagnosis as either benigne or malignant for microcalcifications and masses.

Results

By the same image quality of the SFM and the CR we found the following results compared with the histological diagnosis: Screen film mammography (SFM): sensitivity 62,8 %; specificity 66,2 %; ppv 44,9 %; npv 80,3 %; accuracy 65,2 % respectively high resolution digital luminescence mammography with phosphor storage plate technique (CR): sensitivity 63,7; specificity 66,6 %; ppv 45,5 %; npv 80,8 %; accuracy 66,6 %.

Discussion

In conventional screen film mammography (SFM) the quality of the imaging system is determined by the limited resolution described in line pairs per mm (lp/mm). The German Quality Assurance Committee requires a higher resolution than 8 lp/mm corresponding to 63 µm pixel in mammographies [3]. Some investigators [5, 6, 7] could demonstrate that the recognition of details in phantom examinations was the same in SFM as in full field digital systems despite the lower resolution. These experimental results were already verified in clinical studies [8, 9, 10]. After our phantom study, proved that it is possible to replace equivalent the conventional screen film mammography (SFM) by high resolution digital mammography with storage phosphor plate without magnification technique (CR) [4], the now presented clinical study demonstrates the same results.

In summary we can say that the digital luminescence mammography (CR) is equal to screen film mammography (SFM) in the accuracy of diagnosis in view of microcalcifications and masses – with the advantages of the post-processing, digital archieving and teleradiology.

Literature

1. Schreer, I.: Auswertung der bisherigen Mammographie-Screening-Studien in Europa und in Nordamerika.Radiologe 41: 344-351 (2001)
2. Schulz-Wendtland, R., Krämer, S., Döinghaus, K., Säbel, M., Lang, N., Bautz, W.: Die Bedeutung der Röntgen-Mammographie für das Mammakarzinom-Screening. Röntgenpraxis 50: 103-109 (1997)
3. Säbel, M., Aichinger, U., Schulz-Wendtland, R., Bautz, W.: Digitale Vollfeld-Mammographie: Physikalische Grundlagen und klinische Aspekte.Röntgenpraxis 52: 171-177 (1999)
4. Schulz-Wendtland, R., Aichinger, U., Säbel, M., Böhner, C., Dobritz, M., Wenkel, E., Bautz, W.: Experimental investigations of image quality in X-ray mammography with conventional screen film system (SFS), digital phosphor storage plate in / without magnification technique (CR) and digital CCD-technique (CCD). Röntgenpraxis 54: 123-126 (2002)
5. Fiedler, E., Aichinger, U., Böhner, C., Säbel, M., Schulz-Wendtland, R., Bautz, W.: Bildgüte und Strahlenexposition bei der digitalen Mammographie mit Speicherfolien in Vergrößerungstechnik. RöFo 171: 60-64 (1999)
6. Funke, M., Hermann, K., Breiter, N., Hundertmark, C., Sachs, J., Gruhl, T., Spemer, W., Grabbe, W.: Digitale Speicherfolienmammographie in Vergrößerungstechnik: Experimentelle Untersuchungen zur Ortsauflösung und Erkennbarkeit von Mikrokalk. Fortschr Röntgenstr 167: 174-179 (1997)
7. Obenauer, S., Hermann, K., Schorn, C., Funke, M., Fischer, U., Grabbe, E.: Digitale Vollfeldmammographie: Phantomstudie zur Detektion von Mikrokalk. Fortschr Röntgenstr 172: 646-650 (2000)
8. Aichinger, U., Schulz-Wendtland, R., Dobritz, M., Mitze, M., Bautz, W.: Mikrokalkanalyse – welche Vorteile zeigt die Speicherfolientechnik gegenüber konventionellen Film-Folien-Systemen ? RöFo 170: 129 (1999)
9. Cowen, A., Launders, J., Jadav, M., Brettle, D.: Visibility of microcalcifications in computed and screen-mammography. Med Phys Biol 42: 1533-1548 (1997)
10. Schönhofen, H., Arnold, W., Hess, T., Allgayer, B.: Digitale Mammographie: Erfahrungen bei klinischer Anwendung.Fortschr Röntgenstr 169: 45-52 (1998)

Clinical Evaluation of CR Mammography in Comparison with Full-Field Digital Mammography

Uchiyama N[1], Kobayashi H[1], Tanikoshi M[1], Machida M[1], Tajima H[1], Kumazaki T[1], Moriyama N[2]

1: Department of Radiology, Nippon Medical School, 1-1-5 Sendagi, Bunkyo-ku Tokyo, Japan, nuc-7575@nms.ac.jp 2: Department of Radiology, National Cancer Center Hospital, 5-1-1 Tsukiji, Cyuo-Ku Tokyo, Japan

Abstract.. To prospectively evaluate the clinical diagnostic equivalence of a new CR mammography (CRM) system and a full-field digital mammography (FFDM) system using hard copy images. 103 patients were imaged with FFDM and 91 patients were imaged with CRM. Sensitivity, specificity, positive predictive value (PPV), and ROC analysis were used to compare the differences in observer performance between the two systems. The number of the readers was five. The overall sensitivity of the FFDM system was 76.8% versus 70.3% for the CRM system. The overall specificity for the FFDM system was 86.9% versus 91.5% for the CRM system. The overall PPV for the FFDM system was 67.2% versus 85.5% for the CRM system. The average area under the ROC-curve (A(z)) for the FFDM system was 0.905 versus 0.907 for the CRM system.

Introduction

A new CRM system utilizing dual-sided light collection during scanning and a 50µm pixel pitch has been recently introduced [1]. However, there has not been a clinical report on the diagnostic accuracy of this new CRM system. In this paper, we report intermediate results on a prospective clinical comparison study of CRM and FFDM.

Materials and Methods

Image Acquisition

CRM was performed with a film-screen mammography unit (Mammomat 3000; Siemens, Germany) with a new imaging plate system (FCR 5000MA, Fujifilm, Japan).The pixel pitch size was 50µm and Q algorism, MPF, and PEM processes were also acquired. CRM images were interpreted in hard copy (CR-AL, Fuji Film, Japan). FFDM was performed with a system that used an amorphous silicon area detector bonded to a cesium iodide phosphor (GE Medical Systems, Milwaukee). The pitch of the detector elements was 100 µm. FFDM images were interpreted in hard copy (CR-

AL, Fuji Film, Japan). The images were interpreted without post-processing other than an initial window and level setting derived from an image histogram. Quality control procedures were in accordance with the guidelines of the Mammography Quality Standards Act for both systems [2]. 103 women (average age; 48.4 years old) underwent FFDM during April 2001 and another 91 women (average age; 49.2 years old) underwent CRM during March 2001. Each case was verified by pathological examination or other radiographic modalities. In FFDM, 25 cases were diagnosed as breast cancer, 18 cases were diagnosed as benign diseases (fibrocystic disease, fibroadenoma, lipoma, and cyst) and 60 cases were diagnosed as normal In CRM, 33 cases were diagnosed as breast cancer, 18 cases were diagnosed as benign diseases (fibrocystic disease, fibroadenoma, lipoma, and cyst) and 40 cases were diagnosed as normal.

Image Interpretation and data analysis

Sensitivity, specificity, positive predictive value (PPV), and ROC analysis were used to compare the differences in observer performance between the two systems. The five readers independently interpreted all of the mammograms in the 194 patients, with attention to the findings compatible with breast malignancies. They were blinded to the clinical details of each patient. To compare the diagnostic accuracy of the two systems, the observers were required to report each finding with a corresponding confidence rating to indicate the clinical importance. Six confidence rating categories were predefined as the following: 1, definitely absent; 2, probably absent; 3, possibly absent; 4, possibly present; 5, probably present; 6, definitely present. The readers identified the lesion location for each finding. Confidence ratings 1-3 were defined as negative findings and confidence ratings 4-6 were defined as positive findings. Sensitivity, specificity and positive predictive value (PPV) were calculated for each reader and for all the readers combined. A receiver operating characteristic (ROC) analysis was also used to compare the differences in observer performance. ROC curves and the area under the curves (A(z) values) were obtained with the software ROCKIT program 0.9B Beta Version (Metz CE., Chicago University)[3] [4].

Results

Sensitivity, Specificity, and PPV

The overall sensitivity, specificity, and PPV averaged over the five readers of FFDM versus CRM were 76.8 % versus 66.6% ($P<0.05$), 86.9% versus 91.5%($P<0.05$), and 67.2% versus 85.5% ($P<0.05$), respectively. Sensitivity of FFDM was superior to CRM. On the other hand, specificity and PPV of FFDM were inferior to CRM.

ROC Analysis

A(z) values of FFDM and CRM were 0.937 versus 0.921(observer1), 0.916 versus 0.936 (observer 2), 0.859 versus 0.872 (observer 3), and 0.872 versus 0.866 (observer 4), and 0.943 versus 0938 (observer 5). An overall A(z) value was 0.905 with FFDM versus 0.907 with CRM. However, the result was not statistically significant (P>0.05).

Discussion

A new CRM system with the imaging plate reader utilizing dual light collection technology and a 50μm pixel size has been introduced. A FFDM system has been also introduced recently and studies have indicated this new system has a high Detective Quantum Efficiency and high contrast resolution. [6] In this study, we compared the two new digital mammography systems for cancer detection. The overall sensitivity of FFDM was superior to that of CRM. On the other hand, the specificity and PPV of FFDM were inferior to CRM. ROC analysis showed no statistical difference between the two systems. These results indicate that the observers could detect more malignant lesions with FFDM than with CRM. On the other hand, they tended to detect more false positive lesions with FFDM than with CRM. One possible explanation is that readers identified more suspicious structures with FFDM than with CRM, but they also tended to detect pseudo-lesions in normal breast tissues that readers using CRM did not detect. In conclusion, our intermediate results suggested that a new CRM system is at equivalent to a FFDM system in cancer detection, and thus, the new CRM system could also be used for digital mammography.

Acknowledgement

The authors acknowledge the reader-Tomoyuki Suzuki RT-for the analysis of observer performances. In addition, we appreciate gratefully Gen Iinuma MD, for his assistance with statistical analysis.

References

1. Arakawa S, Yasuda H, Kohda K et al: "Improvement of Image quality in CR Mammography by Detection of Emissions from Dual Sides on an Imaging Plate". SPIE Vol.3977, 590-600,2000
2. American College of Radiology. Breast imaging reporting and data system (BI-RADS). 2nd ed. Reston, Va: American college of Radiology, 1995.
3. CE Metz: ROC methodology in radiologic imaging. Invest Radiology 1986; 21: 720-733.
4. Swets JA.: Measuring the accuracy of diagnostic systems. Science 1988; 240: 1285-1293.
5. John M. Lewin MD, R. Edward Hendrick, PhD, Carl J. D'Orsi, MD et al.: Comparison of full-Field digital Mammography with Screen-Film Mammography for Cancer detection: results of 4,945 Paired Examinations. Radiology 2001; 218: 873-880.
6. Vedantham S.: Full breast digital mammography with an amorph. sillicon-based flat panel detector; physical characteristics of a Clinical prototype. Med. Phys 2000; 27: 558-567.

Comparison of Full Field Digital and Analog Mammograms

Sander van Woudenberg, Ton Roelofs, Jan Hendriks and Nico Karssemeijer

Department of Radiology, University Medical Center Nijmegen
Geert Grooteplein 18, 6525 GA Nijmegen, The Netherlands
sanderw@radiology.azn.nl

Abstract. We collected 34 pairs of digital and analog mammograms with visible lesions of 34 patients. All patients had a digital mammogram using a GE Senographe 2000D. These patients were either referred from the screening program (21) or by their GP's (13). Only the images of the suspect breast were used. The digital images were printed on laser image film. Eight trainee screening radiologists reviewed the cases using a conventional lightbox. Their analog and digital performance was measured by ROC technique. The readers' performance measured as an A_z value reveal an equal or better performance on the digital printed images. The improvement can be traced to improvement in characterization of benign masses.

1. Introduction

Film-screen combinations have been the primary breast imaging technique for many years. Over the years film-screen systems have provided an increasing image contrast, which enhances the detection of masses, provided they are exposed correctly. In order to detect small details like micro-calcifications image resolution is a critical factor. Digital mammography offers a new way to improve both contrast and spatial resolution.

Technical image quality is only one aspect affecting correct radiological interpretation. Even when images are perfect technically and double read, a significant fraction of lesions remain undetected. In a mammography screening setting the task is even more challenging; a repetitive task with a low number of positives is like searching for a needle in a haystack. Recommendations for improvement have suffered from a lack of practicality [1,2], but these may be overcome in future using the new information technology.

The advent of digital mammography calls for evaluation of this new technique. Apart from technical performance tests, the new technology must be prove its value when used by radiologists for detection of breast cancer.

In an American study [3], a group of about 5000 women was subjected to both techniques within a mammography screening framework. Imaging on both modalities was performed by the same radiographer on the same day using the same exposure settings. In this set-up about 30 malignancies were discovered. The study aimed to compare the detection of malignancies in analog and digital mammography in a screening setting using single read mammograms. No difference in cancer detection rate had been observed between digital and analog mammography.

Venta et al. [4] studied the causes of differences in interpretation of digital and analog mammograms, and concluded that inter-observer variability prevails over the differences in visibility of lesions.

The purpose of the present study is to investigate whether digital mammography can record mammographic lesions as least as good as film-screen mammography. To that purpose a set of patient images showing benign and malignant lesions was prepared in analog and digital hard-copy. The compatibility between soft-copy and hard-copy digital images needs to be established separately. A recent study by Pisano et al. [5] showed equivalency under low light levels, but that condition is not met under normal radiology room lighting conditions.

2. Materials and Methods

All digital mammograms were obtained with the General Electric Senographe 2000D in the so-called Standard Mode. This standard mode selects kilo-voltage, target, filtration and charge automatically based on compressed breast thickness and opacity for X-rays. The images were taken by one of six radiographers responsible for training of radiographers of the Dutch screening program.

Images were printed from the radiographers' acquisition station on a Kodak DryView 8600 laser imager, using Kodak DVB medical imaging film. The values for window and level were seldomly changed by the radiographers. In the clinical routine the printed images are evaluated on a viewbox, and therefore these default values for window and level are considered as leading to adequate image quality.

The analog mammograms from patients referred by their GP's were obtained using either a GE Senographe DMR 2 Plus or a Siemens Mammomat 3000. Both systems are used in combination with a Kodak M6B processor and both use Kodak Min-R 2000 film and Min-R cassettes. The GE DMR 2 Plus and the Siemens Mammomat 3000 are always used in Standard Mode and in full automatic mode, respectively. Mammograms of patients referred from the screening program were made in one of the five regional units, all using a Philips Mammodiagnost 4000 in combination with a Kodak M35-M processor, Min-R 2000 films and Min-R 2 cassettes.

All these units are subject to the quality control system of the Dutch screening program. Quality control procedures for the digital unit are under development.

Out of the flow of patients who had their mammograms taken in our center, attention focussed on two groups of patients. The group referred from the screening program and the group referred by their GP's. After the patients' consent was obtained, additional images were taken using the alternative technique. Data were collected during a period of nine months in the year 2000.

Screening referral leads to a clinical follow-up within typically 14 days. This group had a clinical digital mammogram while the analog screening images were available. The second group, referred by their GP's had a digital mammogram first, and with the patients' approval had an additional analog mammogram the same day. This approach reduces bias toward either imaging technique. All cases with alternative imaging in that period were included in the dataset

The total of 32 patients comprised 19 in the group referred from screening and 13 patients in the GP referred group. All the records of these patients were checked for results of pathology reports. In 17 patients a malignancy had been demonstrated. The remaining 15 patients had either a histologically proven benign lesion or no visible lesion at all. Details are summarized in Table 1. All of the benign and negative cases have been rechecked for further imaging and pathology, one year after the original image had been taken. None needed to be excluded from the study for that reason.

Table 1. Ccharacteristics of 32 abnormalities

Benign		Malignant	
Normal tissue	4	DCIS	6
Fribroadenoma	5	IDC	8
Cysts	4	ILC	3
Papilloma	1		
Mastopathy	1		
Total	15		17

DCIS Ductal Carcinoma In Situ
IDC Invasive Ductal Carcinoma
ILC Invasive Lobular Carcinoma

To investigate the possible differences between the two modalities we conducted an observer study. In this study only the images of the suspect breast were used in both MLO and CC-view. In three cases only the medio lateral oblique image was available. Eight junior radiologists finalizing the training course to become a screening radiologist, evaluated these mammograms. No earlier images were presented and no medical records were made available. None of these radiologists had ever read digital mammograms before. For each patient a score form for both techniques was supplied, used to *rate* the annotated area of the abnormality in the images, and to score lesion type, size, probability of malignancy and BI-RADS classification. Images were displayed using a RADX technology alternator of adequate brightness. Cases were displayed according to their date of entry in this study.

For practical purposes images from both modalities were read in one session. To avoid reading order effects the following precautions were taken. The digital images presented first in half of the cases. The analog images of the same case appeared beyond halfway of the belt, to separate the readings as much as possible. Each alternator frame held views of a given technique; the next frame held a views of the alternative technique. Half of the radiologists worked in reverse order. Within frames no specific image order was used, and varied between readers. The radiologists were beforehand introduced to the specifics of the test, but received no training.

3. Results

Receiver Operating Characteristic Analysis (ROC) is a widely used tool to evaluate performance measurements of radiological image evaluation. The characteristic is a curve of the true positive fraction against the false positive fraction. The A_z value equals the area under the curve, and is a measure of performance. For each of the 8 radiologists ROC-analysis was performed using the ROCFIT program [6]. In all analyses 10 categories of malignancy probabilities were used. The results are shown in Table 2.

Table 2. A_z scores by participant

Radiologist	Analog		Digital		Difference
1	0.82	±0.074	0.82	±0.087	0.00
2	0.82	±0.075	0.87	±0.070	0.05
3	0.74	±0.088	0.78	±0.083	0.04
4	0.72	±0.092	0.86	±0.068	0.14
5	0.88	±0.064	0.92	±0.053	0.04
6	0.72	±0.092	0.79	±0.081	0.07
7	0.57	±0.136	0.61	±0.140	0.04
8	0.69	±0.096	0.80	±0.079	0.11
Mean	0.75		0.81		0.06

The A_z scores for analog and digital scores were subjected to a one-sided paired Student T-test as implemented in Microsoft Excel 97 (Microsoft, Richmond) yielding that the digital Az scores are higher at a significance level of 0.0001.

Detailed analysis of the reader scores indicated that the improved performance was due to the enhanced characterization of benign masses, while the radiologist's microcalcification characterization did not suffer from the possible loss in image resolution.

4. Conclusions

The results of this study indicate that digital mammography utilizing the GE Senographe 2000D is comparable or better than film-screen mammography, while there may be an improvement in the characterization of benign masses. Caution must be taken to draw general conclusions because of the limited size of case samples, and the limited experience of the radiologists. A broader study -using experienced screening radiologists- needs to confirm these results, and investigate the validity of these results when images are read from the monitor.

References

1. Laming, D., Warren, R. : Improving the detection of cancer in the screening of mammograms. J Med Screen (2000) 7:24-30
2. Bird, R.E., Wallace, T.W., Yankaskas, B.C. : Analysis of cancers missed at screening mammography. Radiology (1992) 184:713-617
3. Lewin, M.L., Hendrick, R.E., et al.: Comparison of full-field digital mammography with screen-film mammography for cancer detection: results of 4945 paired examinations. Radiology (2001) 218:873-880
4. Venta, L.A., Hendrick, R.E., et al.: Rates and causes of disagreement in interpretation of full-field digital mammography and film-screen mammography in a diagnostic setting. AJR (2001) 176:1241-1248
5. Pisano, E.D., Cole, E.B., et al. : Interpretation of digital mammograms: comparison of speed and accuracy of soft-copy versus printed film display. Radiology (2002) 223:483-488
6. ROCFIT version june 1993, Dept. Of Radiology, University of Chicago, Il
7. Pepe, M.S., Urban, N., et al.: Design of a study to improve reading mammograms. J Clin Epidemiol (1997) 50/12:1327-1338
8. Blanks, R.G., Wallis, M.G. Moss, S.M. : A comparison of cancer detection rates achieved by breastc cancer screening programmes by number of readers, for one and two view mammography : results from the UK National Health Service breast cancer screening programme
9. Baker, S.G., Pinsky, P.F., A proposed design and analysis for comparing digital and analog mammography: special receiver operating characteristic methods for cancer screening. Journal of the American Statistical Association (2001) 96/454: 421-428

Average glandular dose with full-field digital mammography – Clinical results

Klaus-Peter Hermann, Sonja Kehbel, Silvia Obenauer, Uwe Fischer and Eckhardt Grabbe

Department of Diagnostic Radiology, Göttingen University Hospital, Robert-Koch-Str. 40, 37075 Göttingen, Germany
kherman@gwdg.de

Abstract. The goal of this study was to determine the average glandular dose with a full-field digital mammography (FFDM) system using a flat-panel X-ray detector based on amorphous silicon technology. The study was performed using the FFDM unit Senographe 2000D (GE Medical Systems). The number of women was 591 and the number of exposures was 1116. The mean average glandular dose was 1.51 mGy for a single view. In comparison with conventional screen-film mammography FFDM needs about 25% less dose.

1. Introduction

Statements about the patient dose with amorphous silicon full-field digital mammography are until now exclusively based on phantom surveys [1, 2]. However, the measurement of radiation dose delivered to an acrylic or other standard phantoms does not provide complete information about doses received by patients. Instead, a survey of actual patient dose is needed to assess the characteristics of the patient population and the risk to radiation-induced cancer. In addition, the distribution of exposure characteristics can provide guidance in selecting the relevant technique factors for equipment performance evaluation. Thus, in order to assess exposure factors and dose to the patient, a patient survey was undertaken at our department.

2. Methods and Materials

The survey consisted of a 4-month compilation of patient data collected from 1116 mammograms of 591 women and included contact, automatic exposure control (AEC) mammograms of cranio-caudal projections only from preventive examinations, screening and aftercare.

The study was performed using the full-field digital mammography unit Senographe 2000D (GE Medical Systems, Waukesha, USA). The 19 cm x 23 cm digital detector of this system consists of an amorphous silicon transistor/photodiode array deposited as a thin film over a large area glass substrate. A cesium iodide (CsI) phosphor layer above the silicon layer is used to convert X-ray photons to light photons that are then used to create a signal in the amorphous silicon. The pixel size is 100 μm.

The average glandular dose, AGD, cannot be measured directly, but was determined for each mammogram on the basis of the entrance surface air kerma free in air (i.e. without backscatter), ESAK, and the conversion factor g, which converts ESAK to AGD, by the relationship AGD = ESAK • g.

The ESAK for each exposure was calculated from the recorded mAs and tube output (measured in mGy/mAs for all relevant anode/filter combinations and settings of the tube voltage with an 1 cm^3 flat chamber type 77334 (PTW, Freiburg, Germany)), and corrected to the actual source-skin distance, according to the European Protocol on Dosimetry in Mammography [3]. The conversion factor g mainly depends on radiation quality and on thickness and tissue composition of the breast; g factors for standard breast composition was used.

3. Results

Table 1. Summary of survey results

	Mean ± Standard deviation	Minimum	Maximum
Age (a)	55.37 ± 10.01	34	81
Compression thickness (mm)	55.70 ± 13.21	17	94
AGD (mGy)	1.51 ± 0.34	0.66	4.05

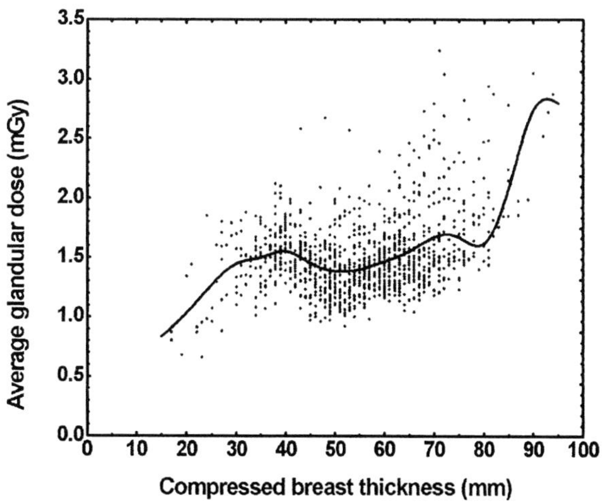

Fig. 1. AGD per exposure as a function of breast thickness.

4. Discussion

The results of the present study on an amorphous silicon full-field digital mammography system are compared with those of nine previous clinical surveys, performed between 1993 and 1998 with conventional screen-film systems by different working groups [4]. The mean value of the overall averaged AGD was 2.0 mGy (1.3 – 2.6 mGy) for a single view. The wide dose intervall is due to different optical density (1.15 – 1.7) used by the respective studies. The mean value of compressed breast thickness was 50 mm (45 –52 mm).

A more penetrating X-ray beam will usually reduce both patient dose and image contrast. Increasing the kVp in conventional mammography would inevitably lead to an unacceptable loss of image quality. In digital mammography it is possible to use higher energies, because image contrast can subsequently be increased by adjusting the window settings [5]. The dose at the detector is thus kept constant, while patient dose is decreasing simultaneously. This is our preferential way of acquiring dose-reduced digital mammograms. Whereas a tube voltage of 25 kVp in combination with the Mo/Mo anode/filter combination is the most common radiation quality in conventional mammography [4], our results identified the Rh/Rh anode/filter combination with 28 kVp, or higher, as the standard radiation quality used in digital mammography.

Various types of X-ray detectors are used for digital mammography systems. These detectors have different technical characteristics, in detail the detective quantum efficiency (DQE) is different, a measure which strongly influences the dose required for adequate image quality. Therefore we cannot generalize our results concerning the radiation exposure with amorphous silicon full-field digital mammography to mammography systems using other digital image receptors.

References

1. Hermann K-P, Obenauer S, Grabbe E. Radiation exposure in full-field digital mammography with a flat–panel x-ray detector based on amorphous silicon in comparison with conventional screen-film mammography. Fortschr Röntgenstr 2000, 172: 940-5
2. Hendrick R E, Berns E A. Optimization of technique factors for a silicon diode array full-field digital mammography system and comparison to screen-film mammography with matched mean glandular dose. Radiology 2001, 221(P): 338-9
3. European Protocol on Dosimetry in Mammography. Luxembourg: European Commission, 1996
4. Kruger R L, Schueler B A. A survey of clinical factors and patient dose in mammography. Med Phys 2001, 28: 1449-54
5. Diekmann F, Diekmann S, Bick U, Hamm B. Reduced-dose digital mammography of skin calcifications. AJR 2002, 178: 473-4

3D Techniques

3D Visualization of X-ray Tomosynthesis Digital Mammography Data: Preference Study

Abdalmajeid M. Alyassin, Jeffrey W. Eberhard, Bernhard E.H. Claus , John Kaufhold, Dinko E. González Trotter, Ajay Kapur, William P. Pakenas*, Cynthia E Landberg, Claudia Galbo**, Jerry A. Thomas**

GE Global Research Center , One Research Circle, Niskayuna, NY 12309, USA
*Imagesmiths Inc., Germantown, MD 20874, USA
**Uniformed Services University of the Health Sciences, Bethesda, MD 20814, USA
alyassin@crd.ge.com

Abstract. A 3D visualization preference study was conducted on digital mammography tomosynthesis datasets. Two volume rendering [VR] techniques were used in the preference study, the Maximum Intensity Projection [MIP] and the Composite Ray Casting [CRC]. These techniques were presented side by side to experts in the field of digital mammography on dual high resolution monitors. The two techniques were presented using each of three different modes, the thick slice VR, tumbling along the azimuth direction, and tumbling along the elevation direction. Several phantoms and mastectomy specimens were imaged and reconstructed for this study. The experts ranked MIP higher than CRC, and tumbling along the elevation direction was selected as the best mode. In addition, the experts indicated that the MIP technique is better in displaying microcalcifications, and the CRC technique is better in showing masses.

1. Introduction

One of the fundamental limitations of standard 2D mammography is that a 2D image does not separate overlying anatomical structures which can be confused with disease in screening or diagnosis. Visualization of tomosynthesis mammography data overcomes this fundamental limitation. Rendered tomosynthesis images suffer less overlap of 3D breast structures, contrast is enhanced and the morphological features of malignancies should be more evident than in 2D x-ray imaging.

There are numerous approaches to visualizing tomosynthesis data (e.g. slice by slice, cine of slices, or volume rendering). However, volume rendering helps visualize the tomosynthesis data in an efficient timely manner. This paper presents the results of a preference study designed to rate alternative volume rendering techniques.

2. Materials and Methods

Tomosynthesis images of several phantoms and several mastectomy specimens were used in this preference study. The phantoms used were 1) RMI-164A biopsy phantom, 2) CIRS-NS11A phantom, 3) a specially developed swirl phantom (inhomogeneously swirled fat & glandular-equivalent tissue slabs in a 50/50% aggregate mix) speckled with microcalcification-like objects inserted into the phantom, 4) RMI-164A sandwiched between two swirl slabs, 5) CIRS phantom sandwiched between two swirl slabs. The tomosynthesis datasets were reconstructed with 1624x2304xN voxels where N is the number of slices which ranged between 41-81 slices. The voxel size was .1x.1x1 mm^3.

Two volume rendering techniques were used in the 3D visualization preference study. These were the Maximum Intensity Projection (MIP) and the Composite Ray Casting [CRC] techniques. The visualization toolkit was used to prepare the MIP and the CRC images[1]. To facilitate the interactivity of rendering 3D Visualization images, we pre-processed the 3D views prior to the preference study. The VR images were generated with full resolution (1624x2304 image size). The sampling along the rays was set to half the slice thickness with nearest neighbour interpolation (0.5 mm). The dynamic range of the 3D rendered images was 8 bits. The transfer functions for the volume rendering techniques were generated automatically[2]. The 3D rendered images were displayed on dual high-resolution monitors (5 Mega Pixels each). The CRC data was presented on the right monitor and the MIP data was presented on the left monitor. For each technique, three different presentations were generated for the reviewers. The first presentation was generated from a set of thick slice volume rendered images where each slice was incremented by half the size of the slice thickness (slice thickness was set 1 cm). The second presentation was generated from rotating the tomosynthesis data +/- 10 degrees in increments of 1 degree along the azimuth direction, and the third presentation was generated from rotating the tomosynthesis data +/- 10 degrees in increments of 1 degree along the elevation direction. Figure 1 illustrates the latter presentation rendered with MIP and CRC techniques.

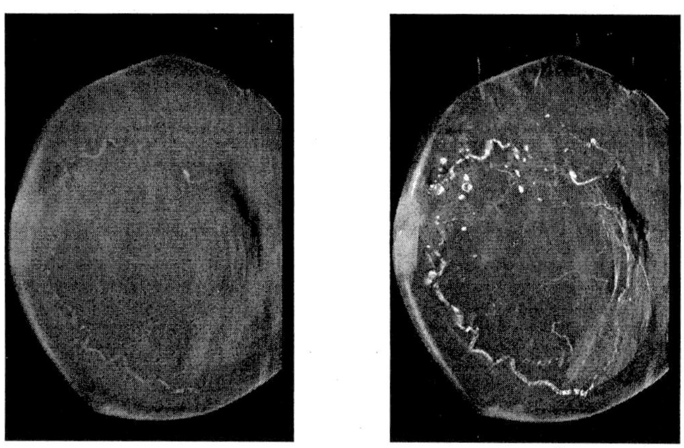

a b

Fig.1. Shows 3D volume rendering images of tomosynthesis mastectomy specimen data. Fig. 1.a displays a composite ray casting image and Fig. b shows a MIP image.

The 3D Visualization pre-processed images were presented to one radiologist and several imaging scientists who are experts in digital mammography. These experts were asked to compare MIP to CRC images for the three different presentations by scoring on a discrete, linear scale from –3 to +3 (-3 = much worse to 3 = much better). In addition, the experts were asked to rank separately the MIP presentations (2 = best, 1 = ok, 0 = worst) and were asked to also rank separately the composite presentations. Finally, the experts were asked to pick the best presentation among the 6 different presentations.

3. Results and Discussion

The outcome of this preference study showed that MIP was preferred over the composite ray casting technique on the azimuth as well as the elevation presentations. There was no major preference disparity in the thick slice presentation. The MIP elevation presentation was selected as the best MIP technique and composite thick slice was selected as the best composite technique. Overall, the MIP Elevation was ranked as the best 3D Visualization technique. The experts also indicated that the MIP technique renders micro-calcifications better and the composite ray casting renders spiculated masses better. These results were consistent for all of the phantoms and specimens.

4. Conclusions

A 3D visualization preference study was conducted on 3D digital mammography tomosynthesis data using the MIP and the CRC techniques. The two techniques were used to provide three different presentations; thick slice VR, tumbling along the azimuth, and tumbling along the elevation direction.

Experts ranked MIP higher than CRC technique and the elevation tumbling MIP was selected as the best presentation. In addition, the experts indicated that the MIP technique is better in displaying microcalcifications than CRC, and the CRC technique may be better in showing masses than MIP. In summary, 3D visualization techniques have the potential to effectively present important diagnostic information from the tomosynthesis data to the radiologist in a timely manner.

References

1- W. Schroeder, K. Martin, and W. Lorensen, "The Visualization Toolkit", 2nd Edition. Prentice-Hall, ISBN 0-13-954694-4, 1998.

2- A.M. Alyassin, "Automatic Transfer Function Generation for Volume Rendering of High Resolution X-ray 3D Digital Mammography Images," SPIE Medical Imaging – Visualization, Image-Guided Procedures, and Display, Vol. 4681, p338-p348, Feb, 2002.

Acknowledgements

This work was supported by the Office of Naval Research under Grant Number MDA905-00-1-0041.

Is Stereomammography Possible Without Increasing Dose?

Andrew D.A. Maidment, Predrag R. Bakic, and Michael Albert

Thomas Jefferson University, 111 S 11th St., Philadelphia, PA, 19107, USA
pbakic@esther.rad.tju.edu

Abstract. Stereoscopic viewing of mammograms is advantageous in reducing ambiguity due to background anatomic noise. This advantage is usually considered to be balanced by doubling the dose required for acquisition of a stereo image pair. In the case of a quantum-noise limited detector, detection theory suggests a possible decrease of the per-image dose by half. We tested this assumption by a series of contrast-detail observer experiments, using phantom images acquired over a range of exposures. Several performance measures were computed and compared for images under different display and viewing conditions. Experimental results support this hypothesis.

1. Introduction

Relevant findings in projection mammography are often either obscured or mimicked by the x-ray shadows of other anatomical structures. Stereomammography can reveal overlapped anatomic structures of different depth using parallax, at the price, as usually assumed, of doubling the dose. In the quantum-limited case, detection theory suggests that an ideal observer would be able to combine the information from two stereoscopic views and thereby suppress quantum mottle. Thus, two stereoscopic views each acquired with one half of the dose of a single-projection mammogram should provide the same level of resilience to quantum noise, but give the inherent benefits of stereoscopic viewing.

For many visual tasks, the use of two eyes is more efficacious than the use of one [1,2]. In particular, measurements of sinusoidal pattern visibility have shown a decrease in threshold (i.e., an increase in contrast sensitivity) of a factor of $\sqrt{2}$ when viewed binocularly as opposed to monocularly [3], precisely as expected for an ideal observer combining the signal from each eye. The noise in these experiments is different from the quantum mottle in mammograms, which is permanently recorded at the time of acquisition and presented to each eye as a fixed pattern. To address this difference and examine the role of dose in stereomammography, we performed an observer study. Our hypothesis was that in combining the left and right eye images by the human visual system, the dose needed for each of these two images is one half of the dose for a single x-ray image viewed monoscopically. This corresponds to an effective increase in SNR by a factor of $\sqrt{2}$.

2. Materials and Methods

2.1 Image Acquisition

The observer study consisted of a series of contrast-detail (C-d) experiments with images acquired over a range of exposures. We imaged an RMI-180 mammographic C-d phantom (Gammex RMI, Middleton, WI). The phantom has 90 objects aligned in nine columns. Objects within the same column decrease in diameter in steps of √2, in the range of 7.07-0.312 mm, with constant thickness. The thickness of the objects varies between columns in steps of √2, in the range of 1.0-0.062 mm. The images were acquired with a DirectRay detector (Hologic, Newark, DE) [4].

Imaging was performed at 60 kVp and six mAs stations in the range of 2-100 mAs, using a tungsten target tube (HVL=1.34 mm Al, at 60 kVp). To simulate tissue and appropriately harden the beam, 6 cm of lucite was positioned near the tube. The phantom was imaged in contact with the detector within a wide lucite frame of equal thickness, providing uniform scatter. Five images were acquired at each mAs station. To isolate the effects of quantum noise, each image was acquired with the same geometry, thus when viewed stereoscopically, all objects were in the imaging plane.

2.2 Image Processing

The raw phantom images were corrected to compensate for the effects of detector nonuniformity using a standard bright and dark field correction, followed by the detection and correction of malfunctioning detector elements [5]. In addition, the images were adjusted for the non-linearity of human contrast sensitivity based upon the DICOM grayscale standard display function (GSDF) [6].

The transformation from 12-bit pixel values to 8-bit monitor digital-driver values consisted of three parts. The monitor characteristic, relating luminance to digital driver levels was interpolated from photometric measurements. An appropriate GSDF transformation was applied. We then used two different strategies for displaying images. In the first display mode, the contrast of the largest detail in the phantom was held constant. In the second display mode, the background noise (variance) was held constant. In both modes, the transformation was image dependent.

2.3 Observer Study

Six medical physicists participated in the study. Each observer was presented with 60 images (30 monoscopic and 30 stereoscopic; 5 at each exposure level). The monoscopic images were displayed so that both the left and right eye saw the same image; for stereoscopy, the left and right eye images were different. The sequences of mono- and stereo images were permuted separately and then randomly interleaved into a single sequence.

The experiments were performed in a darkened room, with a black monitor background. The distance between the observer's eyes and the monitor was kept constant at approximately 1 m. Stereoscopic goggles (StereoGraphics, San Rafael, CA) were used for both mono- and stereo experiments. Several training sessions were held to establish a uniform decision criterion for scoring. The observers were trained to inspect the objects from largest to smallest and from greatest to least contrast. Each object was inspected as to whether or not more than 50% of the edge was visible, whether or not more than 50% of the object was present, and whether the object was in the expected position. The goal was to prevent misinterpretation of the clustered background noise as phantom details. A graphic user interface was developed allowing an observer to assign the smallest detail seen in a column by clicking over the detail position.

The stereoscopic acuity of the observers was tested using a standard clinical test, the RANDOT Stereotest (Stereo Optical Company, Chicago, IL). The test consists of random-dot image pairs with or without angular disparity over the range of 20-500 arc-sec. One of the observers could distinguish a minimum angular disparity of 200 arc-sec, significantly poorer than the others (average 35 arc-sec). Since this observer has also reported limited stereo vision, we have excluded his results from the analysis of the C-d experiments

3. Results

The observers took on average 39±2.8 min to score each set of 60 images. Fig. 1 shows the difference in the number of details per image, seen stereo- and monoscopically, as a function of the exposure. Plotted are the results for individual observers on images displayed with constant contrast and the average results for 5 observers in both display modes, excluding the observer with poor stereo vision. We have analyzed these data using three metrics.

3.1 C-d Analysis

For a low-contrast object with thickness, t, and diameter, d, contrast is proportional to t, and detectability is determined by the signal-to-noise ratio, SNR = $t\, d\, K \sqrt{X}$, where X is the exposure and K is a proportionality constant. C-d curves relate the diameter of the smallest objects visible to their thickness. Points in C-d experiments would ideally form a line with negative unit slope on a log-log plot, satisfying:

$$\log_{10} t + \log_{10} d = \log_{10} \mathrm{SNR}_\mathrm{T} - \log_{10} K - \log_{10} \sqrt{X} \qquad (1)$$

where SNR_T is the value of the SNR at the threshold of perception.

For each observer we calculated their C-d performance as the median diameter of the smallest visible detail in the same column over the set of images. We compared the difference in the intercept values between the linear fits of the stereo and mono results to determine the effective reduction of exposure for stereoscopy:

$$\log_{10} d_M - \log_{10} d_S = \log_{10} d_M / d_S = \log_{10} \sqrt{X_{Seff} / X_M}$$

where d_M and d_S are the diameters of the smallest visible details viewed mono- and stereoscopically, respectively; X_M is the exposure used for acquiring the mono images. X_{Seff} is the effective exposure of stereoscopic viewing, defined as the exposure needed to obtain an image which, when viewed monoscopically, would produce the same C-d performance. If our hypothesis is true and the dose in stereomammography is equal to half of the dose required for monoscopic viewing, then the corresponding linear fits would be separated by an intercept of $\sqrt{2}$.

Fig. 2 shows the relative reduction in exposure for stereo- rather than monoscopy, normalized with the hypothesized reduction by half. Plotted are the percent values of $[d_M/d_S]^2/2 = [X_{Seff}/X_M]/2$, averaged over the 5 observers, for both display modes. For clarity of presentation, the 2 datasets are displaced slightly. If our hypothesis is true, this measure would be equal to 100%. For both display modes, we observed better agreement with theory at lower exposures. At higher exposures, the images displayed with constant noise showed more benefit from stereoscopy than images with constant contrast.

Fig. 3 shows the effective stereoscopic exposure relative to the nominal monoscopic exposure of the next higher mAs station. Plotted are the percent values of $[d_{M,\,2\times(\mathrm{mAs})}/d_{S,(\mathrm{mAs})}]^2 = X_{Seff}/X_{nextM}$, averaged over the 5 observers for both display modes. In our study, the nominal exposures increase by a factor of 2 for all mAs stations except 2 mAs and 20 mAs (not plotted in Fig. 3). This measure is of interest since it directly compares the observer's performance at the mAs stations whose stereo- and monoscopic results should be equal. The values of this measure for images displayed with constant contrast showed little variation over the range of exposures used in the experiments.

3.2 Threshold SNR Analysis

Following the Rose model [7], the SNR of each object was computed from the subject contrast and the standard deviation in the pixel values. For each observer and each viewing condition, the threshold SNR is computed as the mean of the smallest SNR of the details detected and the largest SNR of the details not detected. The averages of these per-scoring values over the 5 mono images give the monoscopic threshold $(SNR_T)_M$ and similarly the 5 stereo images give $(SNR_T)_S$. A hypothetical observer, capable of reducing the quantum noise in the phantom images by using information from both stereo images, would then effectively find the SNR of each disk increased by a factor of $\sqrt{2}$, and $(SNR_T)_M/(SNR_T)_S=\sqrt{2}$. Fig. 4 shows the threshold SNR ratio averaged over the 5 observers, for both display modes. The ratio is near $\sqrt{2}$ at low exposures; at higher exposures, the ratio is less, but still greater than one. Higher values are seen for the constant noise mode.

4. Discussion

Stereoscopic goggles were worn for both mono and stereo images, to keep the brightness of both sets of images comparable and to prevent bias. The goggles reduce the brightness level of the scene. We have not analyzed the amount and uniformity of this reduction, and its effects on the appropriate compensation of the non-linear human contrast sensitivity. We repeated the C-d experiments, reading the images without the goggles. Displayed images in this case are equal to the average of the left eye and right eye images. Results were comparable for each display mode, whether or not the goggles were worn.

We tested two display modes (constant contrast and constant noise) in order to evaluate the effects of quantization, and window and level. Displaying high mAs images with constant contrast limits the background noise range to only a few digital driver levels, resulting in poor visualization of the quantum noise. This can potentially result in significant quantization distortion. Alternatively, keeping the noise constant in the images with different nominal exposure leads to possible saturation of the display (clipping).

Structured anatomic noise was not included in the test images, but its modeling is considered for future research. We are also evaluating other approaches for testing the hypothesized benefits of stereomammography.

5. Conclusions

A series of C-d experiments was performed testing the hypothesis that the radiation dose per image required for stereomammography is one half the dose for a single mammogram, due to combination of images by the human visual system. For images acquired at a fixed exposure, more objects were detected under stereoscopic than monoscopic viewing conditions. For images where the quantum fluctuations were easily visualized, the increase in the number of details observed was the same as expected for a theoretical observer combining the two projections to remove noise. The study results are influenced by the brightness reduction of the stereoscopic goggles, quantization effects, and the lack of anatomical noise. Future experiments may give a more accurate estimate of the advantages of stereomammography.

Acknowledgements

This work was funded by U.S. Department of Defense, Grant DAMD-17-98-1-8169.

References

1. Reading, R.W.: Binocular Vision: Foundations and Applications. Butterworths, Boston (1983)
2. Kundel, H.L., et al: Evaluation of Observer Performance Using Televised Stereofluoroscopy. Investigative Radiology. 2 (1967) 200-207
3. Campbell, F.W. and Green, D.G.: Monocular Versus Binocular Visual Acuity. Nature. 208 (1965) 191-192
4. Gingold, E.L.: Development of a Novel High-Resolution Direct Conversion X-ray Detector. In: Dobbins III, J.T. and Boone, J.M. (eds.): Physics of Medical Imaging. Proc. SPIE 3977 (2000) 185-193
5. Bakic.P.R., Albert, M., Maidment, A.D.A.: Dose Requirements in Stereoradiography. In: Antonuk, L. and Yaffe, M.J. (eds.): Physics of Medical Imaging. Proc SPIE 4682 (2002) in press
6. DICOM Standard PS-3.14-2000: Grey-scale Standard Display Function. NEMA, Rosslyn (2000)
7. Burgess, A.E.: The Rose Model, Revisited. J. Opt. Soc. Am. A. 16 (1999) 633-646

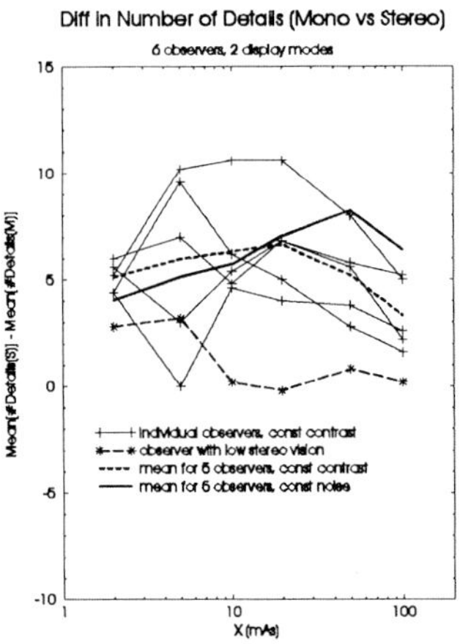

Fig. 1 Difference in the number of details seen stereo- vs. monoscopically, computed for 2 display modes. Individual results and the average over all the observers are shown.

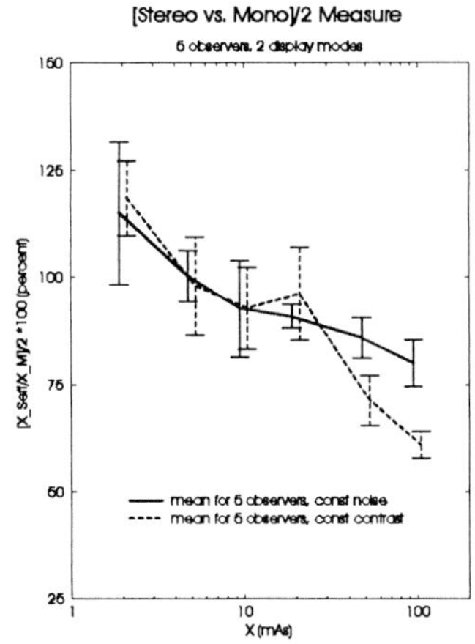

Fig. 2 Relative exposure reduction in stereoscopy, computed for 2 display modes. Average over all the observers, and the standard error are shown.

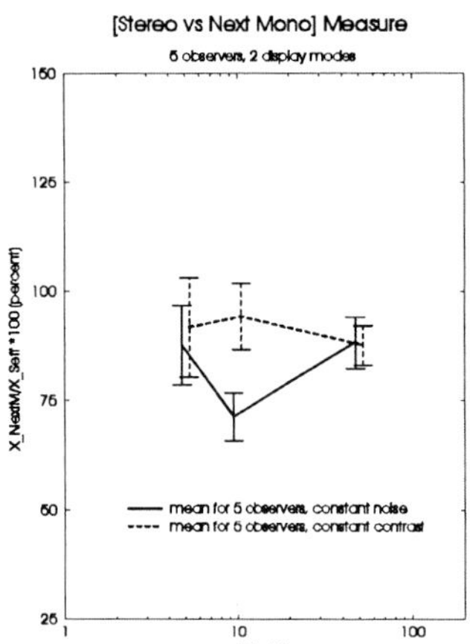

Fig. 3 Effective stereoscopic exposure, relative to the next (nominally double) monoscopic exposure, for 2 display modes. Average over all the observers and the standard error are shown.

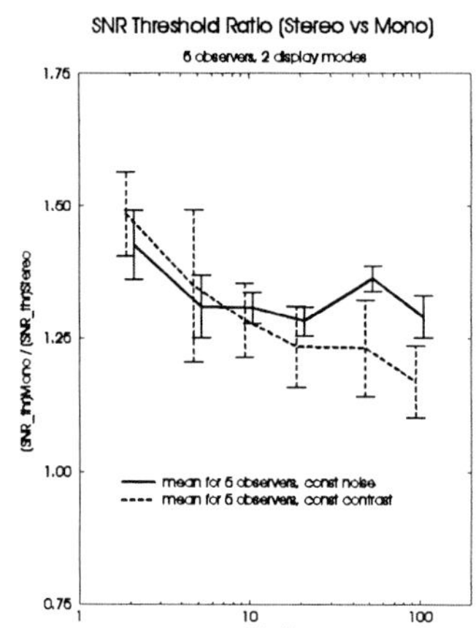

Fig. 4 Ratio of mono and stereo threshold SNR, computed for 2 display modes. Average over all the observers and the standard error are shown.

Preference Study of Reconstructed Image Quality in Mammographic Tomosynthesis

Bernhard E.H. Claus[1], Jeffrey W. Eberhard[1], Jerry A. Thomas[2], Claudia E. Galbo[2], William P. Pakenas[3], Serge L. Muller[4]

[1] GE Global Research Center, One Research Circle, Niskayuna, NY 12309
claus@crd.ge.com
[2] Uniformed Services University of the Health Sciences, Bethesda, MD 20814
[3] Image SMITHS, Inc., Germantown, MD 20874
[4] GE Medical Systems, Rue de la Miniere, Buc, France

Abstract. Digital tomosynthesis mammography is an advanced x-ray application that provides detailed 3D information about the imaged breast. The involved 3D reconstruction step is a difficult problem due to incomplete data and the limited projection angle. In this preference study we compared results obtained with advanced reconstruction techniques, in particular ART (Algebraic Reconstruction Technique), FBP (Filtered Backprojection), OSBP (order statistics based backprojection), and GFBP (generalized filtered backprojection) in terms of their image quality. The 3D datasets were displayed slice-by-slice in "cine loop" mode. As observers we included radiologists, physicists and image processing experts. Phantom and mastectomy specimen datasets were included in the study. The results obtained with our dataset indicate that ART was overall preferred for the phantom datasets while GFBP was preferred for mastectomy specimen reconstructions.

1. Introduction

One of the biggest problems in mammography today is the problem of superimposed tissue which may prevent the detection of cancers by masking the finding of interest, or may lead to false positives in situations where superimposed normal tissue in the mammogram resembles a lesion[1]. Digital tomosynthesis mammography addresses this problem by providing detailed three-dimensional (3D) information about the location and size of structures within the imaged breast. In particular, tomosynthesis aims at obtaining a representation of the 3D structure of the imaged object from a small number of projections acquired from different projection angles. Already with the simple backprojection reconstruction technique, which is the digital equivalent to the image formation process in motion tomography[2,3], the potential clinical impact of tomosynthesis as a 3D breast imaging technique becomes obvious[4]. However, simple backprojection reconstructions suffer from significant artifacts and low contrast for small structures. Obtaining high quality and high fidelity reconstructed 3D images is a difficult problem due to incomplete data and the limited angular range of the projections. In this study we focus on the evaluation of results obtained with four advanced reconstruction techniques, ART (Algebraic Reconstruction Technique)[5], FBP (Filtered Backprojection)[6], OSBP, an order statistics based backprojection technique[7], and GFBP, a generalized filtered backprojection technique. These reconstruction techniques are described in more detail in Section 2. Datasets obtained with these reconstruction techniques were displayed on a slice-by-slice basis (i.e., in "cine-loop" mode), evaluated by readers/radiologists, and rated in terms of their image quality as compared to ART, which was used as the "reference" reconstruction technique.

2. Materials and Methods

Tomosynthesis. A full field digital mammography tomosynthesis prototype system was used, based on a Senographe DMR (GE Medical Systems, Milwaukee, WI) film/screen mammography system retrofitted with an amorphous silicon flat panel x-ray detector and an x-ray tube motion drive. Each set of tomosynthesis projections consists of 11 images that were acquired with an effective angular range of ±17° with respect to the standard mammography projection angle. From these projections a three-dimensional dataset is reconstructed, which is represented as a set (or stack) of slices. Each slice represents a cross-sectional image through the object in a plane parallel to the detector, with the same pixelsize as the detector, 100 μm. Due to the limited angle of the projections, the resolution in "height" (i.e., in the direction perpendicular to the detector plane) is limited, and the slice separation in this study was chosen to be 1mm. See Figure 1 for an illustration of tomosynthesis reconstruction results.

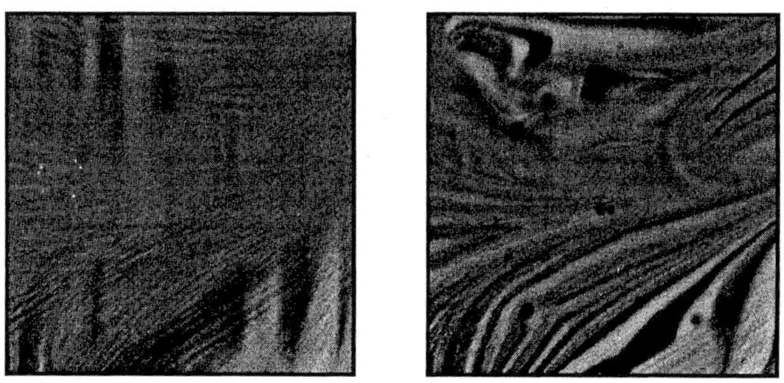

Figure 1: These two images regions of interest of slices at different heights through the same region of a phantom. The left image contains clearly visible calcifications, while the image on the right shows the reconstructed structured 50/50 fatty/glandular "swirl" background. The reconstruction technique shown is GFBP.

Tomosynthesis Reconstruction Methods. In simple backprojection reconstruction [3], the projection images are backprojected, i.e., "smeared back" across the imaged volume (in the corresponding direction of x-rays), and then averaged. This reconstruction method, however, exhibits significant drawbacks. First, relatively high-contrast structures in the projections generate so-called out-of-plane artifacts. At the correct height, where the corresponding structures is located, the backprojected structures line up, and form a high-contrast reconstruction of the structure. At other heights, however, the backprojected structures do not line up, and are visible as several low contrast copies of the structure. Second, there is low contrast for small structures (already in the projection images), that is not recovered in the reconstruction. For example, for a structure with a thickness of 1/N times the thickness of the imaged object, the contrast in the projection image is 1/N times its "true" 3D contrast. More advanced reconstruction algorithms address these fundamental problems (at least implicitly).

ART (Algebraic Reconstruction Technique)[5] represents an iterative improvement of the simple backprojection technique, which achieves (after convergence) consistency between the projection images and the reconstructed volume. This consistency constraint should theoretically translate into both fewer artifacts and improved contrast.

FBP (Filtered Backprojection)[6], is the standard reconstruction method used in most CT systems. The data is essentially high-pass filtered (1D filtering in scan-direction), and then backprojected and averaged. In CT, the high-pass filtering enhances the contrast of "small" structures, and in the process of backprojecting and averaging images from the full angular range, the artifacts cancel out. In our framework, while still achieving a significant contrast enhancement, this approach exhibits only incomplete cancellation of artifacts, due to the "missing data" problem.

OSBP, an order statistics based backprojection technique [7], is similar to the simple backprojection method, but aims at minimizing artifacts caused by high-contrast structures by replacing the averaging operator (which combines the backprojected images into a reconstructed slice) with an order-statistics operator. However, there is no contrast enhancement step included in this reconstruction.

GFBP, a generalized filtered backprojection technique, combines a two-dimensional filtering with an order statistics based backprojection step. The two-dimensional filter used in this study is a rotationally symmetric scale-enhancing filter, designed to counteract the low contrast that is inherent in the projection process, while the subsequent order statistics based backprojection step aims to minimize the occurrence of out-of-plane artifacts.

Comparison of reconstruction results. In this study we chose ART as the "reference" reconstruction technique, and the reconstruction results were displayed in a slice-by-slice "cine" mode. The ART reconstruction result was displayed first on the left monitor, and then the corresponding result for a different reconstruction technique was displayed on the right monitor. The reader was then asked to rank the image quality on the right monitor, as compared to the image quality on the left monitor, on a 7 step scale ranging from "much worse" to "much better". For every single case, the comparison against ART was performed for all three reconstruction techniques (FBP, OSBP, and GFBP), in random order. After going through the three comparisons, the next case was displayed.

The analyzed datasets included three mastectomy specimen, as well as a number of phantoms containing different structures. The phantoms included the CIRS NS11A[8], as well as combinations of custom-made phantom plates (CIRS[8]) containing micro-calcification or mass-like structures with other "complex background" plates consisting of an inhomogeneous "swirl-like" mix of material corresponding to 100% fatty and 100% glandular tissue, with an overall 50/50 composition. In Figure 2 we show reconstruction results for a region of a specific slice through a mastectomy specimen, for all four reconstruction algorithms.

3. Results

In the comparison the ranking of the reconstruction methods was different for the reconstructed phantom datasets, than it was for the mastectomy specimen.
For the phantoms, ART was overall slightly preferred over the other reconstruction methods. The order-statistics based backprojection (OSBP) was ranked on average "worse" than ART, while both filtered backprojection (FBP) and generalized filtered backprojection (GFBP) were ranked between "same", and "slightly worse", as compared to ART.
For the mastectomy specimen, generalized filtered backprojection (GFBP) was overall preferred, with an average ranking between "slightly better" and "better" as compared to ART. OSBP was ranked between "same" and "slightly better", while FBP was ranked between "same" and "slightly worse" than ART.

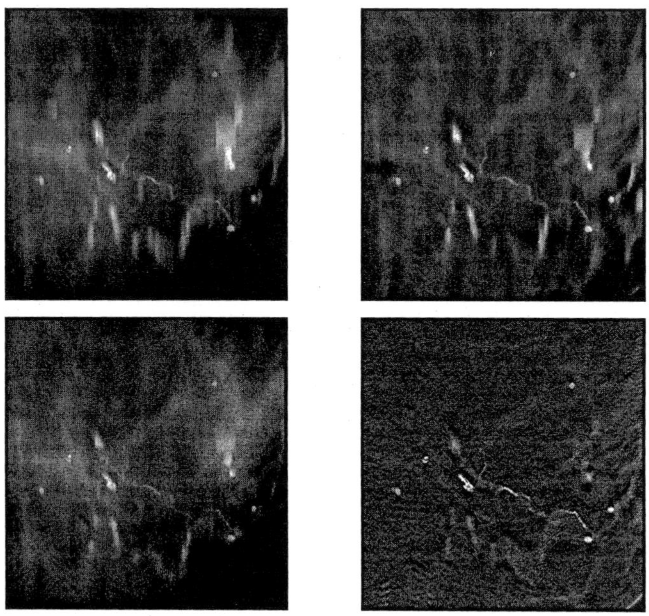

Figure 2: Reconstructions of corresponding regions of interest of a mastectomy specimen. Top-left: ART, top-right: GFBP, bottom-left: OSBP, bottom-right: FBP.

4. Conclusion

A preference study was performed comparing four different reconstruction algorithms for mammographic tomosynthesis. For phantom datasets, ART (Algebraic

Reconstruction Technique) was overall preferred, with FBP (filtered backprojection) and GFBP (generalized filtered backprojection) only slightly worse. For mastectomy specimen, GFBP was preferred overall, followed by OSBP (order statistics-based backprojection) and ART.
Due to the limited number of datasets in this study, the specific mammographic findings, or the specific objects of interest contained in the phantoms, were not taken into account in the analysis of the results. However, the different rankings obtained for phantom datasets, as compared to mastectomy specimen, do suggest that the preference for a specific reconstruction algorithm may depend on the specific "structures of interest" contained in the dataset. A future study including a significantly larger number of datasets, with various findings (calcifications, masses, spiculated lesions, etc.) will help to answer that question.

Acknowledgments

This work was supported by the Office of Naval Research under Grant Number MDA905-00-1-0041. Development of the tomosynthesis prototype was supported by the U.S. Army Medical Research and Materiel Command under grant DAMD17-98-8309.

References

1. L. Ma, E. Fishell, B. Wright, W. Hanna, S. Allan, N.F. Boyd: "Case-Control Study of Factors Associated with Failure to Detect Breast Cancer by Mammography", J. Natl. Cancer Inst., 1992; 84:81-785.
2. W.J. Meredith, J.B. Massey, *Fundamental Physics of Radiology*, John Wright & Sons, Bristol, England, 1977.
3. D.G. Grant, "Tomosynthesis: A Three-Dimensional Radiographic Imaging Technique", *IEEE Trans. on Biomed. Eng.*, **BME-19**, no.1, 20-28, 1972.
4. L.T. Niklason, B.T. Christian, L.E. Niklason, D.B. Kopans, D.E. Castleberry, B.H. Opsahl- Ong, C.E. Landberg, P.J. Slanetz, A.A. Giardino, R. Moore, D. Albagli, M.C. DeJule, P.F. Fitzgerald, D.F. Fobare, B.W. Giambattista, R.F. Kwasnick, J. Liu, S.J. Lubowski, G.E. Possin, J.F. Richotte, C.Y. Wei, and R.F. Wirth: "Digital tomosynthesis in breast imaging," Radiology 205:399– 406 (1997).
5. Andersen, A.H.: "Algebraic Reconstruction in CT from Limited Views", IEEE Trans. Med. Im., vol. 8, no. 1, March 1989.
6. Hiriyannaiah, H.P.: "X-ray Computed Tomography for Medical Imaging", IEEE Signal Processing Magazine, pp.42-58, March 1997.
7. B. Claus, J.W. Eberhard: A New Method for 3D Reconstruction in Digital Tomosynthesis, Proc. SPIE Vol. 4684, Medical Imaging 2002 – Image Processing, San Diego, CA, 2002.
8. CIRS-Breast Phantom – Computerized Imaging Reference Systems, Inc., 2428 Almeda Ave., Suite 212, Norfolk, VA 23513, USA.

Scatter Correction in Tomosynthesis Imaging for Mamography

Dinko E. González Trotter, John Kaufhold, Bernhard E.H. Claus and Jeffrey W. Eberhard

GE Global Research Center, Niskayuna, NY-12065, USA
trottedi@crd.ge.com

Abstract. Scatter is a significant source of bias and contrast-degradation in X-ray mammography. Accurately scatter-corrected projection images in tomosynthesis are expected to improve the performance of advanced 3D quantitative applications, such as tissue decomposition. In standard 2D mammography, scatter grids typically mitigate the scatter signal to an acceptable level. A scatter-rejection grid is not a practical option in X-ray tomosynthesis, where the X-ray source moves with respect to the detector. We have developed a scatter-correction algorithm based on inverse filtering, including *a priori* information about the tomosynthesis acquisition system. We investigated the performance of our scatter-correction method on a series of x-ray projection images of anthropomorphic breast phantoms, with thickness ranging from 3.0 cm to 6.0 cm, and acquired at angles ranging from 0 to 16 degrees with respect to the normal to the detector plane. A comparison of the scatter-corrected projection images with the scatter-free signal acquired using a slit collimator showed mean deviations of ~3% or less for all investigated phantom thicknesses and source angles. Because our scatter-correction method is almost entirely automated, we have readily incorporated it into the 3D breast tomosynthesis reconstruction procedure. We present the effect of scatter correction on breast phantom tomosynthesis projections.

1 Introduction

Tomosynthesis is a promising alternative to 2D x-ray mammography, where several low-dose 2D x-ray projection images are acquired for various orientations of the x-ray source with respect to a stationary breast/detector. Projection images are then employed in a 3D reconstruction image of the breast. In the reconstructed image there is less overlap of radiological 3D breast structures, contrast is enhanced and the morphological features of malignancies should be more evident than in 2D x-ray imaging.

The tissue density in the breast may be an important parameter in the assessment of cancer risk[i]. The accurate estimation of tissue density is hampered by the presence of the scatter signal in the images, which is strongly dependent on the geometry of the imaged breast[ii]. The use of a non-stationary x-ray source precludes the use of a traditional grid for scatter rejection. We present a scatter-correction algorithm (SCA) based on inverse filtering that explicitly takes into account the locally-varying thickness of the imaged object and the angular projection acquisition. The scatter-corrected projections are compared to the nearly scatter-free signal obtained using a slit collimator.

2 Materials and Methods

2.1 Scatter Correction Model

The measured image y in a 2D x-ray projection can be defined as

$$y = b + s = b + p * b, \tag{1}$$

where b are direct events detected and s is the scattered x-ray photons' signal. The term s is modeled as a convolution of a scatter kernel, p, and the direct image b[iii]. $b^{(0)} = y - p * y$ can be used as a rough initial estimate of the scatter signal. The scatter corrected image can then be calculated iteratively using the expression[iv]

$$b^{(n)} = \frac{y}{2^l} + \left(\frac{2^l - 1}{2^l}\delta - \frac{p}{2^l}\right) * b^{(n-1)}, \tag{2}$$

where l must satisfy $\overline{p} < 2^l$ (l is a positive integer) for convergence.

2.2 Scatter Kernel Asymmetry and Normalization

If the X-rays are parallel to the detector surface normal, then the probability of a photon from ray k to scatter and be detected in pixel j is assumed to be symmetric and dependent only on the distance between pixels k and j.

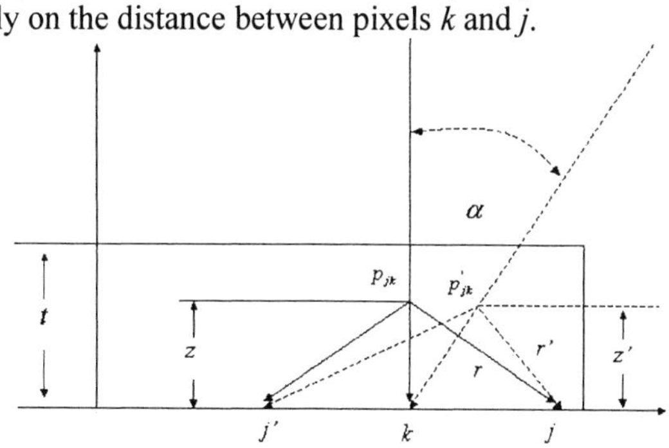

Fig. 1. Comparison of normal (unprimed) and angular(primed) scatter events.

If the angle of incidence of the radiation is $\alpha \neq 0$, then the length of the photon path from the point of scatter is different for pixels j and j' (which are equidistant to pixel k), and the probability of transmission of the X-ray photons scattered into pixels j and

j' will be $p'_{jk} \neq p'_{j'k}$ in general. We introduce correction factors that relate the scatter kernel at zero degrees with the angular scatter kernel so that

$$p'_{jk} = (\sum_{jk} \frac{e^{-\mu(r'-r)} rz}{r'z'})^{-1} f(t,\alpha) \frac{e^{-\mu(r'-r)} rz}{r'z'} p_{jk}, \quad (3)$$

where μ is the mean attenuation coefficient of X-ray photons in the breast tissue. Distance r is given by

$$r = \sqrt{z^2 + \rho^2}, \quad (4)$$

where ρ is the distance between pixels k and j.
The distance r' is given by

$$r' = \sqrt{(\rho - z' \tan\alpha)^2 + z'^2}. \quad (5)$$

The estimated height, z', (angular incidence) at which the scatter events take place is given by

$$z' = (\frac{t}{\cos(\alpha)} - (\frac{1}{\mu} - e^{-\mu\frac{t}{\cos(\alpha)}} (\frac{t}{\cos(\alpha)} + \frac{1}{\mu}))(1 - e^{-\mu\frac{t}{\cos(\alpha)}})^{-1}) \cos(\alpha). \quad (6)$$

The height $z = z'(\alpha = 0)$. The empirical normalization function $f(t,\alpha)$ was determined by measurements for object thicknesses t from 1 to 8 cm and radiation incidence angles α from 0° to 45°, where two images were taken for any given object thickness and incident X-ray angle:

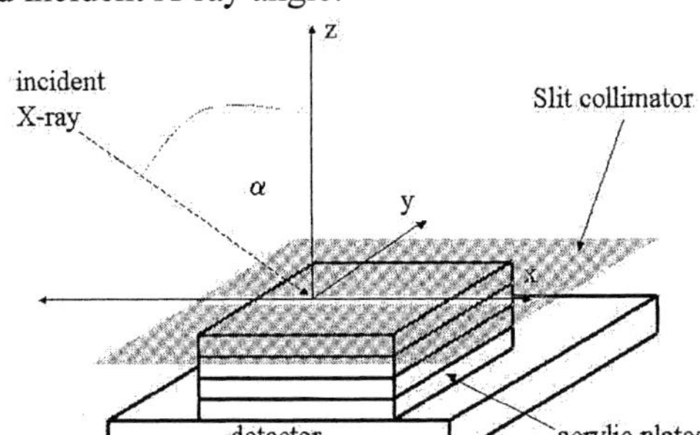

Fig. 2. Experimental setup for angular measurements of scattered radiation

1) Slit collimator image: Image was taken as shown in **Fig. 2**. The slit collimator was a sheet of Tungsten with a thickness of 20 mils (~0.5 mm). A 1 mm-wide slit allowed X-rays through. The signal directly beneath the slit is effectively scatter-free.
2) Open-geometry image: Same as 1) except that the collimator was removed, thus allowing for scatter in the image.

The reduced chi-squared between the scatter-free (b_k) and scatter-corrected ($b_k^{'}$) signals was calculated by

$$\chi^2 = \frac{1}{N-1}\sum_{k=1}^{N}(b_k - b_k^{'})^2 . \qquad (7)$$

An empirical kernel normalization factor was determined by minimizing χ^2 for a given t and α. An analytical surface function $f(t, \alpha)$ was then generated by regression.

3. Results: Validation Through Anthropomorphic Phantoms

Three breast phantoms[1] (nominal thickness of 3, 5 and 6 cm) were used for validation. Their glandular/fat percent composition was 50/50, 30/70 and 20/80, respectively. 11 projections were acquired for slit collimator and open geometry for each phantom with gantry angles ranging from +25° to –25° in 5° steps (+16° to -16° w/respect to the detector plane's normal) . The technique used was Rh/Rh, 32 kVp and 10 mAs per projection image.

		25 deg		15 deg		0 deg	
phantom thickness (cm)		with scatter correction	no scatter correction	with scatter correction	no scatter correction	with scatter correction	no scatter correction
3 cm	% mean deviation	0.15	-68.64	0.18	-67.26	-0.46	-65.40
	%standard deviation	4.10	16.90	3.92	14.06	3.79	14.26
5 cm	% mean deviation	0.20	-44.73	-0.72	-45.01	-0.73	-44.36
	%standard deviation	2.37	6.11	2.37	5.02	2.12	4.41
6 cm	% mean deviation	7.73	-87.29	2.66	-84.95	1.95	-83.16
	%standard deviation	4.99	12.67	5.67	10.63	5.30	10.60

Table 1. % mean deviation and % standard deviation of the open-geometry signal with and without scatter correction for all breast phantoms as a function of source pivot angle and phantom thickness.

The open-geometry projections were scatter-corrected using the scatter kernel $p_{jk}^{'}$, and compared to the scatter-free signal from the slit collimator measurement. The anthropomorphic phantoms were positioned in a similar manner as the acrylic plates in **Fig 2.**, with the chest-wall aligned with the x-axis. Comparison of the scatter-free and scatter-corrected images was accomplished by calculating their percent mean deviation

$$\Delta b = \frac{100}{N}\sum_{i=1}^{N}\frac{b_i - b_i^{'}}{b_i} . \qquad (8)$$

The resulting percent mean deviations and the standard deviation of their distributions are shown in **Table 1**.

[1] Computerized Imaging Reference Systems, 2428 Alameda Avenue, Suite 212, Norfolk, Va 23513, USA.

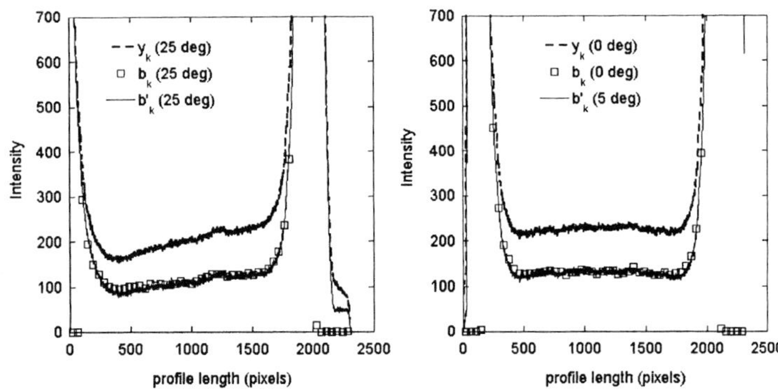

Fig. 3. Comparison between open-geometry (y_k), scatter-free (b_k) and scatter-corrected (b'_k) signals for a 25° and 0° angular acquisitions of a 5 cm-thick phantom.

Conclusions

Scatter suppression is not possible in tomosynthesis using commercially-available 2D anti-scatter grids. We introduce a scatter-correction algorithm (SCA) based on inverse filtering with asymmetry and re-normalization of the scatter kernel. Through phantom experiments we show that the percent mean deviation between the open-geometry and scatter-free signal is brought down from ~40-70% to ~3% after application of the SCA. The excellent agreement between scatter-corrected and slit-collimated projection images is encouraging and indicates that more advanced quantitative 3D analyses, such as 3D tissue composition on a voxel-by-voxel basis, may soon be possible.

Acknowledgements

This work was supported by the Office of Naval Research under Grant Number MDA905-00-1-0041.

---

[i] John J. Heine *et al., Mammographic Tissue, Breast Cancer Risk, Serial Image Analysis, and Digital Mammography* Acad Radiol 2002; 9:298–316

[ii] John M. Boone *et al. Scatter/primary in mammography: Comprehensive results* Med. Phys. 27(10), October 2000, p2408-2416

[iii] J.A. Seibert *et al., X-ray scatter removal by deconvolution*, Med. Phys. 15(4). Jul/Aug 1988, p567-575

[iv] D. E. González Trotter *et al. Thickness-dependent Scatter Correction Algorithm for Digital Mammography.* Medical Imaging 2002. Proc. SPIE vol. 4682.(2002) p 469-478

Mammographic X-Ray and MR Correspondence

Robert Martí[1], Caroline M.E. Rubin[2], Erika Denton[3], and Reyer Zwiggelaar[1]

[1] School of Information Systems, University of East Anglia, Norwich, UK
{marti,rz}@sys.uea.ac.uk
[2] Breast Screening Unit, Royal South Hants Hospital, Southampton, UK
[3] Department of Breast Imaging, Norfolk and Norwich University Hospital, Norwich,UK

Abstract. This paper presents a novel approach to tackle the problem of multi-modality correspondence in mammography. More precisely, this work focuses on finding a methodology to correspond areas in X-ray and MR images of the same breast. If correspondence between modalities is achieved, this information can be combined into a model providing a better understanding of the region of interest. Initial results show the validity of our approach although further evaluation is needed.

1 Introduction

We present a novel methodology for the correspondence of MR and X-ray mammographic images. MR is often used for diagnosis of unclear findings in mammographic images. Radiologists need to perform a correspondence between areas in those two modalities. Our aim is to provide a framework which will make this correspondence an automatic and therefore easier task. Correspondence will allow to match salient structures in X-ray images to the MR volume (2D to 3D). It should be mentioned that 3D to 2D correspondence can be achieved based on the same principles as described but will not be discussed here.

2 Methodology

We subdivide the correspondence into a 2D-2D (X-ray to a 2D MR projection) and 2D-3D (MR projection to 3D MR volume) correspondence. For both correspondence problems a similar approach is used which uses both mutual information to achieve a global linear correspondence and a local feature based non-linear model. Related work (see [3, 2]) describes the methodology for a 2D correspondence problem which forms the basis of the work described here.

The 2D-3D registration of X-ray and MR images is developed as follows: initially a projection of the MR volume is generated which simulates the same X-ray view. Subsequently, images are registered matching their most significant linear structures. Using this correspondence, matched points from the projection image can be tracked back to the MR volume, thus obtaining a correspondence between X-ray image and MR volume.

We aim to obtain an X-ray like image from the MR volume in order to match a particular X-ray view. To obtain a realistic projection we simulate the X-ray imaging process using MR data. This takes into account the thickness of the volume and the anatomical characteristics of the tissue. The projection image is generated using a simple X-ray energy attenuation model [1].

Correspondence points obtained in the 2D registration are used to find the MR slices that are most likely to have generated such points. Candidate points in each slice from the MR volume are obtained similarly to the 2D case. A 2D point will be likely to have been generated by a 3D point if it maximises a feature similarity measure.

3 Where is it? Evaluation and Results

We present evaluation of the proposed methodology and initial correspondence results. We measured the similarity between the MR projection and the real X-ray image using different transformations. A maximum similarity was obtained at the expected angle for a particular view (i.e. 30 degrees for an MLO view). The correlation between features from the projection image and the MR volume was also investigated. All features used showed a clear linear correlation (graphs not included).

The robustness of the proposed approach is assessed by observing the correspondence results between the X-ray image and projection images where a range of projection angles close to the most likely projection angle were used. The results of this evaluation can be found in Fig. 1, which shows an example of a good and a bad match. For each projection angle a point and its corresponding volumetric slices are plotted. For a robust correspondence point (see Fig. 1a) the resulting slices show little variation as a function of the projection angle. It should be noted that corresponding points have been found for all projection angles. We believe that the apparent oscillation is due to bi-linear interpolation but this will need further investigation. For a less robust correspondence point (see Fig. 1b) two changes occur. Firstly, the variation in the resulting slice increases which means that it becomes less certain to which slice the X-ray point should be matched. Secondly, it should be clear that for certain projection angles no matches have been found. It should be mentioned that the less robust correspondence as shown in Fig. 1b are outside the normal range that would be used in the matching process. Fig. 2 shows an example of matching a point in the X-ray image to a point in the MR volume.

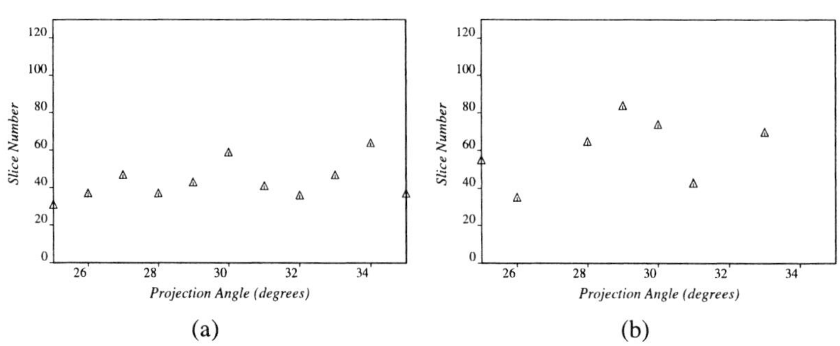

Fig. 1. Slice correspondence for various projection images (from 25 to 35 degrees).

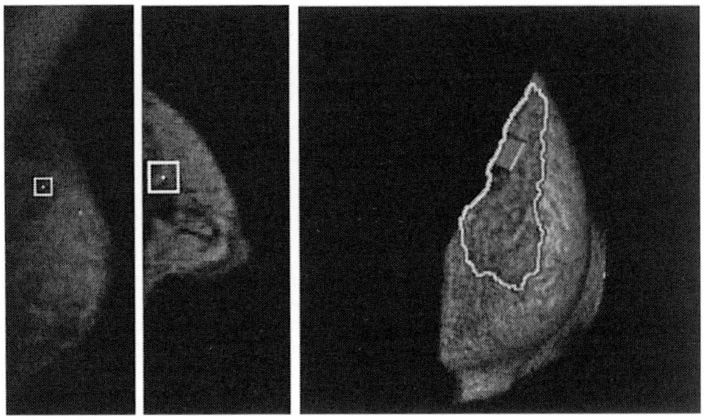

(a) (b) (c)

Fig. 2. Example of X-ray to MR correspondence: a point from (a) the X-ray image is matched to a point in the MR volume seen here as (b) a single slice and (c) a rendered volume. In all three cases the corresponding point is at the centre of the square.

4 Discussion and Conclusions

The novelty of this work is the development of a correspondence based on matching meaningful anatomical structures found in both images. Therefore in principle, differences (due to the presence of abnormalities or severe structural changes) are not used in the correspondence. This latter aspect can be seen as a drawback of methods based on similarity measures, which use the complete image (inclusive any abnormalities when present) to obtain correspondence. We believe that better results will be obtained when the quality of the data is improved and the size of the database is enlarged. One of the most difficult problems we encountered in the presented work was its evaluation. Quantitative and qualitative methods have been proposed which showed the validity of our approach.

Acknowledgements

This work was supported by EPSRC grant GR/M53387.

References

1. J. Hubbell and S. Seltzer. Tables of X-ray mass attenuation coefficients and mass energy-absorption coefficients. Technical report, National Institute of Standards ànd Technology, Gaithersburg, MD, 1997. http://physics.nist.gov/xaamdi.
2. R. Marti, R. Zwiggelaar, and C. Rubin. Tracking mammographic structures over time. In 12th *British Machine Vison Conference*, pages 143–152, 2001.
3. R. Marti, R. Zwiggelaar, and C. Rubin. Automatic point correspondence and registration based on linear structures. *International Journal of Pattern Recognition and Artificial Intelligence*, 16(3), 2002.

Assessment Tools for Breast Surgery Based on 3D Surface Anatomy Imaging

Beattie S, Siebert JP, Stevenson* JH & Yap* LH

The 3D-MATIC Laboratory – Department of Computing Science, University of Glasgow, Glasgow, Scotland G12 8NN
* Specialist Services Group, Ninewells Hospital, Dundee, Scotland DD1 9SY
psiebert@dcs.gla.ac.uk

Abstract. The authors present the results of a pilot investigation into the use of stereo-photogrammetry for capturing the 3D surface anatomy of the living breast to allow non-contact volumetric assessment for surgery planning purposes. Breast volume measurement is investigated in terms of chest wall-breast segmentation methods, inter and intra operator variability and pose.

1. Introduction

Techniques for 3D imaging the *surface anatomy* of the breast have become sufficiently mature to allow their investigation for assessment of key breast parameters prior to and following surgery. Clinically relevant parameters, such as breast surface area, volume and symmetry, can be computed in order to assist the selection of a particular surgery protocol and aid the assessment of the surgical outcome. This paper reports a pilot investigation[1] to gain an initial understanding of measurement errors and repeatability associated with this technique.

2. 3D Data Capture and Analysis

Subjects are imaged in 3D using the C3D [1] stereo-photogrammetry system originally developed by the Turing Institute, Glasgow. Software-based measurement tools [2] under development at 3D-MATIC, are then used to segment and analyse the breast region within the captured 3D surface anatomy data. Three different interactive breast segmentation methods have been evaluated: manual delineation, Coons patch [3] and cubic spline [4]. Each segmentation method estimates the chest wall underlying the breast based on the morphology of the chest area surrounding the breast region. The best approximation method will result in a surface patch which closely resembles the morphology of the physical chest wall and which can be reproduced accurately and reliably.

Additional facilities [5], originally developed for 3D facial measurement, have been adapted to allow longitudinally captured 3D images of breasts to be registered and their volume differences to be estimated. A similar procedure has been adopted to estimate the area and volume difference between breasts captured simultaneously based on the computation of a symmetry plane.

3. Phantom Breast Initial Results

In order to assess the volumetric accuracy of breast scans, three plasticine breast models of differing size were constructed and 3D imaged against a flat surface using the simplest approximation method, the centroid method. The volume of each plasticine model was then measured using water displacement, Table 1.

Table 1. Volumetric comparisons of phantom breasts

Volume (cm^3)				
Test Model	*Application*	*Water Displacement*	*Difference*	*% Error*
Model 1	540.30	535	5.3	0.99
Model 2	589.23	590	0.77	0.13
Model 3	812.11	800	12.11	1.51
			Average % Error	0.88

4. Real Breast Initial Results

Five breast reduction volunteers were recruited and imaged using C3D. Their breast volume was then evaluated in terms of intra-operator variability (Tables 2 & 3), inter-operator variability (Table 4), method of segmentation (Tables 2-4) and reliability of measurement with regard to posture (Table 5, Coons method).

Table 2. Volume variability over 5 segmentation trials, same subject & operator

Volume (cm^3)							
Patch method	*Trial 1*	*Trial 2*	*Trial 3*	*Trial 4*	*Trial 5*	***Mean***	***Std Dev***
Centroid	615.22	595.16	638.45	659.15	624.68	**626.53**	**24.1**
Coons	539.13	527.01	544.04	526.44	528.82	**533.08**	**8.00**
Spline	519.34	524.09	510.52	494.95	538.94	**517.56**	**16.31**

Table 3. Volume variability for three subjects, five trials each, same operator

Volume (cm^3)	**Subject 1**		**Subject 2**		**Subject 3**	
Subject	*Mean*	*Std Dev*	*Mean*	*Std Dev*	*Mean*	*Std Dev*
Centroid	626.532	24.09132	758.19	27.97834	637.738	17.70348
Coons	533.088	7.996966	630.062	10.15626	525.05	9.004921
Spline	517.568	16.30711	626.296	18.27934	526.382	14.38113

Table 4. Volume variability for three operators, five trials each, same subject

Volume (cm^3)	Operator 1		Operator 2		Operator 3	
Patch method	*Mean*	*Std Dev*	*Mean*	*Std Dev*	*Mean*	*Std Dev*
Centroid	624.7	24.1	632.46	19.6	571.79	20.11
Coons	533.09	8	520.9	10.37	520.292	8.79
Spline	517.56	16.3	501.67	17.1	499.03	16.89

Table 5. Volume variability with different postures, same subject & operator

Volume(cm^3) Coons Segmentation Method							
Posture	*Trial 1*	*Trial 2*	*Trial 3*	*Trial 4*	*Trial 5*	*Mean*	*Std Dev.*
Arms down	440.1	448.4	433.38	451.61	439.01	459.68	7.39
Arms out	498.9	498.1	492.25	505.21	507.3	496.41	6.01
Arms up	515.91	520.06	516.58	520.3	513.61	517.51	2.85

5. Conclusions

The principal findings are that the reported method is capable of estimating the volume of phantom targets to better than a few percent error. Based on the volunteer 3D data, both the intra and inter operator volume measurement standard deviations for the Coons patch segmentation method were approximately twice as low as those of the other methods investigated. The standard "arms raised" posture appeared to be significantly more repeatable compared to "arms lowered" and "arms out stretched" postures (segmented using the Coons method).

6. References

1. Siebert, J.P., Marshall, S.J.: Human Body 3D Imaging by Speckle Texture Projection Photogrammetry. Sensor Review, Vol. 20 No. 3, 218-226 (2000)
2. Moffat, A.M.: A Prototype Breast Surgery Planning and Assessment Tool. MSc Dissertation in Information Technology. Department of Computing Science, University of Glasgow, Glasgow (1999)
3. Fletcher, Y., McAllister, D.F.: A Tension Compatible Patch for Shape-Preserving Surface Interpolation. IEEE Computer Graphics, Vol. 9 No. 3, 45-55 (1989)
4. Knott, G.D.: Interpolating Cubic Splines. Birkhauser Boston, Cambridge MA (1999)
5. Mao, Z., Siebert, P. and Ayoub, A.: Development of 3D Measuring Techniques for the Analysis of Facial Soft Tissue Change. MICCAI 2000, 3rd International Conference on Medical Image Computing Computer Assisted Intervention. Pittsburgh USA 1051-1060 (2000)

---

[1] Funding support from NHS Tayside and EPSRC (Faraday Partnership scheme).

Volumetric Texture Analysis: Towards the Third Dimension

Lilian Blot and Reyer Zwiggelaar

School of Information Systems, University of East Anglia, UK

Abstract. In recent years, 3D volumetric imaging has been used increasingly for the detection and classification of mammographic abnormalities. This increase in usage has been accompanied by an increase, within the computer vision community, of the development of novel techniques. A review of volumetric texture synthesis and analysis is given. The first step towards realistic 3D texture modelling is the extension of existing 2D-texture model to the third dimension. Examples of these extensions are given in this paper as well as a discussion of the validity and limitations of the developed approaches.

1 Introduction

Texture analysis and synthesis are important fields in computer vision. In 2D images, the two fields of research have always been closely related and many techniques like Markov random fields, grey-level co-occurrence matrices and fractal modelling can be applied in both domains.

Unfortunately, in 3D the relation between the two domains is less exploited. This is partly due to the difficulty that exists in obtaining volumetric data from the real world. Synthesis of volumetric (also known as solid) texture has been driven mostly by empirical results and assessed by visual inspection of images rather than physical property.

Closely related to the synthesis of solid texture is the analysis of such data. In medical imaging, the most common techniques to deal with volumetric images is to slice the volume into 2D cross-sections and subsequently apply 2D texture analysis model on each slice. Then the volume is interpolated from the stack of analysed slices. However, such an approach is not satisfactory as most of the embodied information along the axial direction of the stack is not taken into account. Only a few techniques using full 3D information exist in the literature and those known to us are presented in this review.

2 Solid Texture Synthesis

Solid noise, the initialisation of most procedural synthesis approaches, is a function defined on $\mathbb{R}^3$ which attributes a random value at each point in the 3D-space. Lattice noise is one of the most popular implementations. At every point in the texture space one (or more) pseudo-random numbers are generated from a uniform distribution and subsequently interpolated. The characteristics of the resulting noise are determined by the interpolation method.

Gardner [3] described a model to texture volumes in images based on the use of selected mathematical functions T defined on the 3D-space. The texture is completely defined by the sets of parameters describing T. Another technique used is to perturb solid noise with a mathematical function. Among the disadvantages of such approaches are the difficulty to select the parameters and to predict the resulting texture. Nevertheless this approach has been widely developed and a large collection of procedural textures can be found in [2].

The principle of the physical simulation approach is to simulate natural phenomenon based on their physical properties. The use of such techniques results in realistic texture which closely resembles aspects of natural objects. The main drawback of this approach is the difficulty to obtain the theoretical model of the processes to be simulated. In most cases expert knowledge is needed and this is not always available (or even non-existing).

The analytical approach uses 2D texture information (such as spectral) from the volume (using slices) to generate a solid texture. The main difference of this technique compared to the procedural approach is that the parameters are automatically determined via spectral analysis of a 2D texture model. A more detailed overview of these three approaches can be found in [1].

3 Solid Texture Analysis

Lang *et al.* [6] analysed muscle fibre structures in 3D confocal fluorescence microscopic images by extending Laws' model to 3D. Laws' texture energy measure approach is based on two successive convolutions. The first convolution uses a micro-mask (constructed from seed vectors) and the result of this operation is a filtered image F. Subsequently the filtered image F is converted to a texture energy image E by convolving F with a window W (called a macro-mask). Several texture features are obtain by using micro-masks composed of different seed vectors. The extension of Laws' model to volumetric data is straightforward. Three seed vectors are used instead of two and a cube is used instead of a 2D window for the macro-mask.

Kovalev, Petrou and Bondar [5] presented two techniques to characterise texture anisotropy in 3D MRI images. The first model is the *gradient density measure* approach, where each voxel is convolved along the three axes with a 3D filter producing the three components of the gradient vector. The resulting gradient vector is assigned to the appropriate solid angle (ϕ, z) on the unit sphere and $H(\phi, z)$ is incremented by one. The second model is the *intensity variation measure* approach, where a grey-level co-occurence matrix ($GLCM$) with a translation $(d, (\phi, z))$ is calculated and the inertia $I(d, (\phi, z))$ of the image populates the histogram $H(\phi, z)$. A set of features is extracted from H in order to describe the texture properties.

Ip and Lam [4] have also used $GLCMs$ to segment volumes, but their model is not based on texture anisotropy properties. To construct the feature vector of a volume, they used nine *GLCMs* with different bi-directional orientations and a distances of one pixel. For each of these *GLCMs* three features are extracted to compose the feature vector V, the feature vector characterising the volume is the average of the nine vectors calculated from the nine *GLCMs*.

4 Discussion and Conclusions

To synthesise texture procedural approaches are powerful tools for computer graphics but their application to the medical domain is not recommended because the only validation is visual and this is not sufficient for the medical field. The two other approaches are more suited. The analytical approach enables the selection of texture features based on original medical image information and the physical simulation approach could create images based on a physical image acquisition model.

To analyse texture the model presented by Lang *et al.* [6] used axial information in the 3D space to separate directional texture but disordered texture was not discussed. In comparison, the model introduced by Ip and Lam [4] is able to describe such texture. Kovalev *et al.* [5] *intensity variation measure* is more robust than their *gradient density measure* but is less sensitive to micro-texture, it also incurs a much higher computational cost. However, these two techniques are suitable for segmenting anisotropic texture.

In this review we have presented an overview of the techniques related to the synthesis and analysis of solid texture. The choice to focus on solid texture was driven by the desire to open up the research area to include medical applications. The recent development of 3D medical imaging and its increased usage in diagnostic tools results in an increasing demand of image processing techniques dedicated to volumetric data. As illustrated in this paper, models based on the full 3D informations are rare. However, many 2D texture models can be extended to 3D but need to be validated on the appropriate medical data.

References

1. J.M. Dischler and D. Ghazanfarpour. A survey of 3d texturing. *Computer & Graphics*, 25:135–51, 2001.
2. D.S. Ebert, F.K. Musgrave, D. Peachey, K. Perlin, and S. Worley. *Texture & Modeling: A rocedural approach.* 2nd *edition.* Academic Press, 1998.
3. G.Y. Gardner. Simulation of natural scenes using textured quadric surfaces. *Computer Graphics (ACM Siggraph Annual Conference Series)*, 18(3):11–20, 1984.
4. H.H.S. IP and S.W.C. Lam. Using an octree-based rag in hyper-irregular pyramid segmentation of texture volume. *Proc. of the IAPR Workshop on Machine Vision Applications*, pages 259–62, 1994.
5. V.A. Kovalev, M. Petrou, and Y.S. Bondar. Texture anisotropy in 3-d images. *IEEE Transactions on Image Processing*, 8(3):346–60, 1999.
6. Z. Lang, R.E. Scarberry, Z. Zhang, w. Shao, and X. Sun. A texture-based direct 3d segmentation system for confocal scanning fluorescence microscopic images. *Proceeding of the* 23rd *Southeastern Symposium on System Theory. IEEE Comput. Soc. Press, Los Alamitos, CA, USA*, pages 472–6, 1991.

Tracking of 3D structures in MR Mammography

Robert Martí[1], Caroline M.E. Rubin[2], Erika Denton[3], and Reyer Zwiggelaar[1]

[1] School of Information Systems, University of East Anglia, Norwich, UK
{marti,rz}@sys.uea.ac.uk
[2] Breast Screening Unit, Royal South Hants Hospital, Southampton, UK
[3] Department of Breast Imaging, Norfolk and Norwich University Hospital, Norwich,UK

Abstract. This work presents a novel method to establish correspondence in MR images taken at different times which allows the tracking of regions of interest through time-series and dynamic MR studies. This is developed as an hybrid correspondence approach, where a correlation measure and a point based method are used. Evaluation results are obtained using simulated deformation of the breast volume. In addition, registration and tracking results using real data are shown.

1 Introduction

This paper describes a novel approach to the alignment (also referred to as registration) of MR images from the same patient. Registration could be applied to MR dynamic studies, where MR volumes are taken at different time intervals after a contrast agent is injected and tissue uptake is measured. In addition, various MR volumes could have been taken at different times and a comparison between them would help to assess changes in the breast such as the development of suspicious regions or the changes due to undergoing chemotherapy.

2 Materials and Methods

We address the correspondence problem proposing a methodology that aims to match meaningful internal structures such as linear structures (i.e. vessels, ducts) and tissue and breast boundaries [4, 3]. An overview of the methodology can be found in Fig. 1. Initially linear structures are detected using a three dimensional extension of the non-linear line operator [2]. This provides every voxel with line strength, scale and orientation information. Post processing is performed (using thresholding, non maxima suppression and thinning) to provide the backbone of the linear structures. Points of maximum local curvature are extracted by computing the tangent angle difference of neighbouring points on the linear structure.

Once points have been extracted, matches in MR volumes are found comparing their local features such as orientation, width, and position. Potential matches are assumed to lie in approximately the same area after a global alignment is carried out based on maximising a normalised mutual information measure using a rigid transformation. Volumes are aligned using a point based registration method such as volume, thin-plate, or elastic body spline. Here we use an elastic body spline (EBS) [1] mapping function based on a deformation model of an elastic material which can be regarded as a simple model of breast tissue.

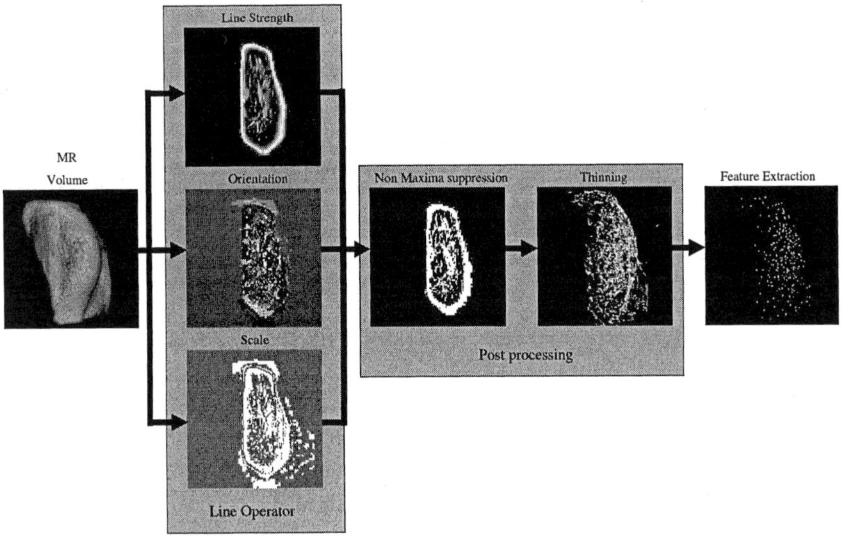

Fig. 1. Overview of the extraction of characteristic points.

3 Evaluation and Results

Evaluation is first performed using a synthetic registration case. A volume is matched to a deformed version of itself. The deformation is generated corresponding some points manually and applying an EBS transformation to the volume. The use of EBS for the generation of the deformed volume can be seen as a drawback of this evaluation, but it should be stressed that the experiment is to show that the points found by our method are reliable and not to evaluate the EBS method. A comparison of the results can be found in Fig. 2 which shows difference images (where darker means larger difference) between the registered and the original volumes for a particular slice. It should be noted that there is a large improvement compared to unregistered and even registration using a global rigid transformation.

The method has been applied to the registration of MR images. Fig. 3 shows the same slices from two MR volumes from a dynamic study. In this case the abnormal region is highlighted after the contrast agent has been injected. However, looking at the difference image, other dark areas are present due to misalignment. Applying registration reduces such areas resulting in a clearer image of the abnormal area.

4 Discussion and Conclusions

We have presented a novel method to register MR breast images based on correspondence between their internal linear structures. Initial results using synthetic and real data indicates the validity of our approach. However, the inclusion of other features (local intensity similarity) could improve robustness and will be investigated.

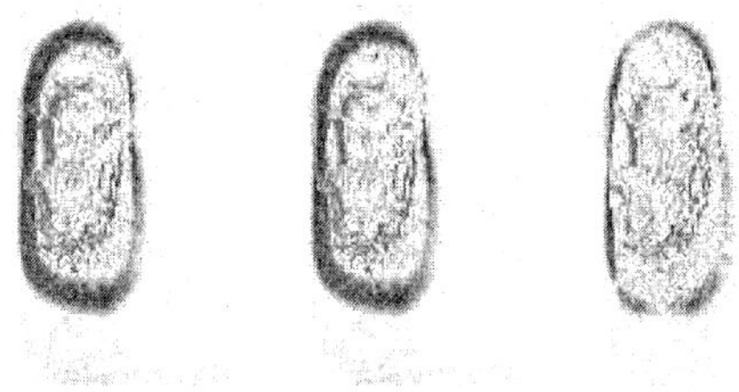

Fig. 2. Evaluation: difference image between registered and original volumes for a particular slice, using (a) no registration, (b) rigid registration (c) our approach

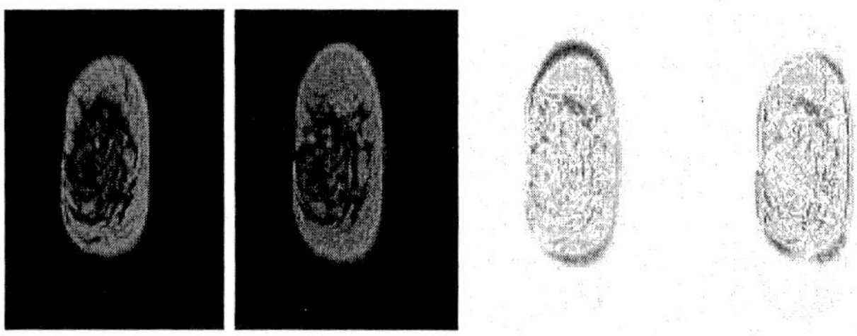

Fig. 3. Registration results: (a) slice from first volume, (b) same slice after a contrast agent has been injected, (c) difference image (d) difference image after registration.

Although the application field has been only breast images, it is our belief that the method can be applied to any three dimensional data which incorporated some sort of structural information as no data related assumptions have been introduced. This, along with further testing using a larger MR breast database will be the focus of future work.

Acknowledgements

This work was supported by EPSRC grant GR/M53387.

References

1. M. H. Davis, A. Khotanzad, D. P. Flaming, and S. E. Harms. A physics-based coordinate transformation for 3-D image matching. *IEEE Transactions on Medical Imaging*, 16(3):317–328, 1997.
2. R. Dixon and C. Taylor. Automated asbestos fibre counting. *Inst. Phys. Conf. Ser*, 44:178–185, 1979.
3. R. Marti, R. Zwiggelaar, and C. Rubin. Tracking mammographic structures over time. In 12th *British Machine Vison Conference*, pages 143–152, 2001.
4. R. Marti, R. Zwiggelaar, and C. Rubin. Automatic point correspondence and registration based on linear structures. *International Journal of Pattern Recognition and Artificial Intelligence*, 16(3), 2002.

Other Application of Digital Mammography

Risk Assessment: the use of Background Texture in Mammographic Imaging

Lilian Blot[1], Erika Denton[2] and Reyer Zwiggelaar[1]

[1] School of Information Systems, University of East Anglia, Norwich, UK
[2] Department of Breast Imaging, Norfolk & Norwich University Hospital, UK

Abstract. We have developed an approach to the separation of background texture and structures in images. This technique is based on the statistical difference between local and median co-occurrence matrices. In this paper we investigate if the classification of mammographic parenchymal patterns can be improved if anatomical structures can be removed from the image and the classification is based only on the background texture information. A comparison of two techniques - one developed by Byng, the other developed by Karssemeijer - applied to the original and reconstructed images is presented. To validate our approach, we use a dataset where each mammogram has been classified by experts using two different approaches: Wolf grades and the six classes described by Boyd.

1 Introduction

Wolfe [6] has shown that mammographic parenchymal patterns provide a strong indicator of the risk of developing breast cancer. This relation between mammographic density and risk has been confirmed by Boyd *et al.* [2]. Since then, automated classification techniques have been investigated and most of these are based on grey-level distributions in the mammographic images [3, 4].

It is our hypothesis that classification can be improved if it is based on the background texture information only and not on a combination of the background texture and other anatomical structures which might be present. In [1] we proposed a method to extract the background texture of the mammographic images and then apply Karssemeijer and Byng *et al*'s model to classify the textured image. In section 3 these results are compared with the results based on the original mammographic images. The dataset used is composed of 263 mammograms from the MIAS database [5] and has been scored by two experts (observation 1 and 2 have been done by the same expert).

2 Background Extraction

We assume that there is a statistical difference between the Grey-Level Co-occurrence Matrices (*GLCMs*) for image regions that include image structures and regions that only contain background texture. The *GLCM* is used as a local descriptor of the image. The method consists of comparing the *GLCM* of

Table 1. Classification results obtained for originals mammograms and reconstructed textures using Wolfe grades with Byng *et al.* algorithm and Karssemeijer approach (in brackets).

	Original Images			Reconstructed Texture			Obs. 3			Obs. 2		
	Ag.	e_{min}	e_{maj}	*Ag.*	e_{min}	e_{maj}	*Ag.*	e_{min}	e_{maj}	*Ag.*	e_{min}	e_{maj}
Obs. 1	0.62 (0.60)	0.29 (0.33)	0.09 (0.07)	0.59 (0.59)	0.33 (0.35)	0.18 (0.06)	0.72	0.14	0.14	0.84	0.13	0.03
Obs. 2	0.64 (0.62)	0.31 (0.33)	0.05 (0.05)	0.61 (0.61)	0.25 (0.33)	0.14 (0.06)	0.67	0.23	0.10			
Obs. 3	0.71 (0.71)	0.20 (0.19)	0.09 (0.10)	0.61 (0.68)	0.22 (0.26)	0.17 (0.06)						

a region of interest (*RoI*) to a set of *GLCM* obtained from a local neighbourhood of this *RoI*. As image structures in mammographic data tend to be of higher intensity than average, only pixels with a grey-level value higher than the mean value of the region of interest are considered by the model. This is the only prior knowledge incorporated in the developed approach. A more detailed discussion of the method can be found in [1].

3 Results

Karssemeijer's and Byng *et al.*'s model have been applied to two sets of images. The first set is composed of original mammograms and the second of their reconstructed background texture. In our experiment we use two classification model: the model described by Wolfe in [6] (see Tab. 1) and the model introduced by Boyd *et al.* [2] further referred to as SCC (see Tab. 2). The mammograms are classified using a k-nearest-neighbours classifiers with a leave-one-out approach.

We have imposed an equal a priori likelihood for each class (i.e. the difference in the sample size of each class has been taken into account by using a correction to the number of neighbours depending on the size of the class sample).

Two error rates are display in the tables. The minor error fraction e_{min} denotes the fraction of mammograms that are classified differently from the ground truth by one density grade. The major error fraction e_{maj} denotes a difference larger than one density grade.

4 Discussion and Conclusion

The main results can be found in Tabs 1 and 2. The results using Karssemeijer's model are similar for original mammograms and reconstructed images. This indicates that the grey-level distribution and first order statistics (the measures used by Karssemeijer) are preserved in the reconstructed texture. However, a degradation is noticed when using Byng *et al.* algorithm. This is due to the fact

Table 2. Classification results obtained for originals mammograms and reconstructed textures using Boyd *et al.* grades with Byng *et al.* algorithm and Karssemeijer approach (in brackets).

	Original Images			Reconstructed Texture			Obs. 3			Obs. 2		
	$Ag.$	e_{min}	e_{maj}	$Ag.$	e_{min}	e_{maj}	$Ag.$	e_{min}	e_{maj}	$Ag.$	e_{min}	e_{maj}
Obs. 1	0.52 (0.44)	0.37 (0.43)	0.11 (0.13)	0.44 (0.44)	0.34 (0.42)	0.24 (0.14)	0.53	0.43	0.04	0.81	0.18	0.01
Obs. 2	0.58 (0.56)	0.37 (0.38)	0.05 (0.06)	0.41 (0.55)	0.37 (0.39)	0.22 (0.06)	0.57	0.40	0.03			
Obs. 3	0.52 (0.45)	0.36 (0.46)	0.12 (0.09)	0.38 (0.46)	0.43 (0.46)	0.19 (0.08)						

that their model is based on a fractal measure which estimate the roughness of the texture. This roughness is more important in fatty mammograms as the linear structures a more visible. As we remove this structural information in the reconstructed texture, the algorithm is less sensitive to the distinction between fatty and dense mammograms using the background texture. The reconstructed background texture is smoother than the original mammogram. We must emphasis that the inter-observer agreement is low and this could also explain the low results of both algorithm when using SCC grades. In addition the agreement using Byng *et al.* model are similar to those obtained from the two radiologist. Finally, Byng *et al.*'s model provides classification results better correlated with the expert assessment than Karssemeijer's model, especially for SCC grades. To conclude, the use of the background texture is not appropriate for the two models discussed in this paper, but its use with the h_{int} representation will be investigated.

References

1. L. Blot and R. Zwiggelaar. Extracting background texture in mammographic images: a co-occurrence matrices based approach. 5th *International Workshop on Digital Mammography*, Toronto, Canada:142–148, 2000.
2. N.F. Boyd et al. Quantitative classification of mammographic densities and breast cancer risk: results from the Canadian national breast screening study. *Journal of the National Cancer Institute*, 87:670–5, 1995.
3. J.W. Byng, N.F. Boyd, E. Fishell, R.A. Jong, and M.J. Yaffe. Automated analysis of mammographic densities. *Phys. Med. Biol.*, 41:909–923, 1996.
4. N. Karssemeijer. Automated classification of parenchymal patterns in mammograms. *Phys. Med. Biol.*, 43:365–378, 1998.
5. J. Suckling et al. The mammographic images analysis society digital mammogram database. In Dance Gale, Astley and Cairns, editors, *Digital Mammography*, pages 375–378. Elsevier, 1994.
6. J.N. Wolfe. Risk for breast cancer development determined by mammographic parenchymal pattern. *Cancer*, 37:2486–92, 1976.

Comparing Two Breast Density Metrics for Risk Assessment

J.J. Heine and J. Kaufhold

Department of Radiology, University of South Florida, College of Medicine 12901 Bruce B. Downs Blvd, Tampa, Florida 33612-4799
heinejj@moffitt.usf.edu

Abstract. Breast cancer risk associated with increased mammographic density has been shown to be at least as important as, if not more important than, breast cancer risk associated with other known risk factors (family history, e.g.). For this reason, a reliable automated density technique may be of great use for risk modeling. In this work two automated methods of assessing density are compared: (1) a method based on a calibrated pixel aggregate tissue composition metric following from tissue phantom measurements, and (2) a method based on random field modeling and probability methods. The comparison is implemented by analyzing full field digital mammography data. This work shows interesting correlations ($r > 0.7$) and relations between the two techniques.

Introduction

Over the past thirty years, many mammographic tissue studies have indicated women with increased proportions of dense breast tissue are at a substantially higher risk of breast cancer compared to women with lesser degrees of density. However, the risk estimates vary widely. Likely, this variation is due in large part to the estimation approach, which includes the physical measurement technique as well as the image formation process. Most often the estimation is made from film mammograms by the radiologist, or more recently with automated methods applied to digitized film mammograms that normally code a pixel as dense or not without gradations. Both of these historical estimates can be considered binary density projections.

In this work, we investigate the quantitative relationships between two methods for estimating breast density from full field digital mammography imagery. One approach, termed the quantitative method (QM), uses a pixel based look-up table (LUT) transformation derived from tissue-equivalent phantom measurements [1]. The QM provides density information relating to the breast tissue volume attributes. The second technique, based on random field probability analysis [2], is referred to as the probability method (PM). The PM provides binary density measurements, where each pixel is labeled either dense or fat.

Image Data

In this work, 74 digital images acquired from a General Electric Senographe 2000D FFDM system are analyzed. The images are 100 micron digital resolution with 14 bit pixel dynamic range. The images correspond to 37 LCC-RCC pairs.

Density Measurements

The QM provides three types of density information (1) percent dense tissue by volume averaged over the projected area, (2) the average dense tissue height measured in cms, and (3) the total dense tissue by volume measured in ccs. These measures will be referred to as x, y and z. This technique is based on phantom measurements that mimic fat and dense breast tissue at various proportions and x-ray transmission lengths. This approach generates a LUT, which provides the appropriate raw image pixel transformation dependent upon the imaging acquisition parameters.

The PM is based on a deconvolution approach and chi-square probability analysis. Each small image region is labeled as dense or not dense; this measure is referred to as p. This technique is a variant of the approach discussed elsewhere [2]; here we have normalized the raw data to the x-ray exposure representation [3] followed by an exponential transform before applying the technique.

Data Comparison

Fig. 1 shows the regression analysis for $p = mx + b$, where p and x are as above. The regression parameters are shown under the plot with the correlation $r = 0.71$. Similarly, considering all of the QM variables, (x,y,z), performing multiple linear regression of the form $p = ax + by + cz + d$ results in a correlation of $r = 0.78$ with partial correlations of 0.71, 0.68, and 0.25, respectively; $(a, b, c, d) = (0.11, 4.1, -0.04, 33.4)$. Similar plots ($r = 0.75$) result when letting $p = f(x,z)$ or $f(y,z)$, which follow from the strong correlation between x and y ($r = 0.93$). The left and right view correlations (contra-lateral comparison of the 37 image pairs) are $r = 0.88$ and $r = 0.81$ for the x and p measures, respectively, which may help to explain part of the correlation differences between the methods.

Conclusion

We would not expect exact agreement between the two techniques since the PM loses most volume information, which is made clear by the multiple regression analysis by considering the (p, z) correlation. However, the resulting correlation is interesting. Since we are concerned with risk modeling, it is interesting to note $dp = 0.18dx$. Assuming a linear relation in risk and density (which may not be the case), this differential relation indicates that an incremental change in risk measured by QM is worth about a 5 fold change in risk measured by PM. Future work includes determining which measure(s) are the best predictors of risk.

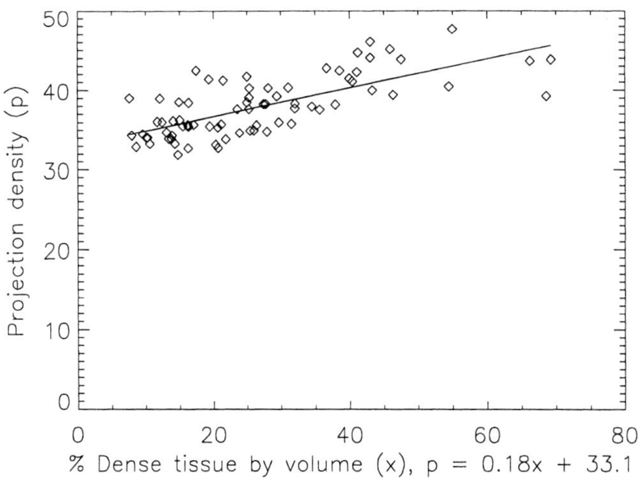

Fig. 1. The scatter plot (diamonds), shows the projection binary density as a linear function (solid) of the density proportion by volume. The linear correlation is r = 0.71.

Acknowledgements

This work was supported in part by U.S. Army Medical Research and Material Command contract DAMD17-99-1-9181 and the Navy Medical Research and Development Command contract 42952.

References

[1] J. Kaufhold, J.A. Thomas, J.W. Eberhard, C.E. Galbo, D.E. Gonzalez Trotter,"A Calibration Approach to Glandular Tissue Composition Estimation in Digital Mammography, submitted *to Med. Phys.*, November, 2001.

[2] J.J. Heine, R.P. Velthuizen, "A statistical methodology for mammographic density detection," *Med. Phys.* 27, 2644-2651 (2000).

[3] S. Vedantham, A. Karellas, S. Suryanarayanan, D. Albagli, S. Han, E.J. Tkaczyk, C.E. Landberg, B. Opsahl-Ong, P.R. Granfors, I. Levis., C.J., D'Orsi, R.E. Hendrick,"Full breast digital mammography with an amorphous silicon-based flat panel detector: Physical characteristics of a clinical prototype," *Med. Phys.* 27, 558-567 (2000).

Assessing the role of quantitative analysis of mammograms in describing breast density changes in women using HRT

Kostas Marias[a], Ralph Highnam[c], Michael Brady[a], Santilal Parbhoo[b], Alexander Seifalian[b]

[a] Robotics Research Group, Engineering Science, Oxford University, Ewert House, Ewert Place, Summertown, Oxford, OX2 7BZ, [b] Department of Surgery, Royal Free and University College Medical School, UCL, London NW3 2QG, [c] MIRADA SOLUTIONS Limited, Oxford Centre for Innovation, Mill Street, OX2 0JX.
kostas@robots.ox.ac.uk

Abstract. We present an update of our investigations into the potential role of quantitative measures of breast density for characterising breast changes, and, in particular, changes due to Hormone Replacement Therapy (HRT). It has been established that long-term use of HRT can increase the risk of breast cancer, a fact that enforces the belief that objective measures of tissue density can be an important development in breast cancer image analysis. A set of 59 mammogram temporal HRT sequences (2 images per patient) were used in our experiments. The clinician's assessment of density changes constituted the ground truth for evaluating the proposed quantitative measures of density change. The measures are based on the h_{int} representation of interesting tissue and their performance (agreement with the expert's description) is also compared to the "interactive thresholding" method that has been used in the past to characterise mammographic density.

1. Introduction

The use of HRT (Hormone Replacement Therapy) in postmenopausal women has created a controversy, especially as its effects are hard to characterise and quantify [1]. Although HRT has several advantages (e.g. reduction of cardiovascular problems, reduction of discomfort during the menopause, prevention of osteoporosis), there is evidence of increased breast cancer risk, especially after long-term therapy. According to [1], the risk increases with the duration of use, while it is reduced after cessation. The increased risk may be due to localized increases in breast density. The breast lobules, ducts and fibrous tissue comprise the breast parenchyma (density).

Oestrogen is a powerful mitogen (for both normal breast epithelium and breast cancer cells) and the induced mitogenic signal is mediated by the hormone receptors [2]. Since there is a variable receptivity to exogenous hormones it can be expected that the density increase should not necessarily have a uniform distribution. An increase in tissue density can have an impact in screening mammography due to the fact that denser breast have a "brighter" mammographic appearance that can mask abnormalities. Kavanagh et al [3] report a significant decrease in mammographic sensitivity and show that HRT users are more likely to have a false-negative report than non-users (odds ratio 1.60).

Clinical studies aim to correlate density changes to an increased risk of cancer or to the type of therapy used, and to assess the possible influence of such localized changes on breast diagnosis. In addition, quantification of temporal changes in women using HRT could be of great clinical value, assisting in a better prognosis for cancer. For these reasons, the development of *objective quantitative measures of density* is of great importance for future research in assessing tissue density. In this paper we suggest mammogram density measures based on a normalized representation of digitised mammograms (section 2) and then we evaluate their agreement with the clinical assessment of changes in a dataset of temporal mammograms of women using HRT (section 3) before concluding with a discussion (section 4).

2. Density Measures

In order to develop objective measures of breast density we need to normalize the mammogram image in order to account for the variability in imaging conditions. This is discussed in the next section (2.1) while in 2.2 we also consider the "area of dense tissue" measure proposed by Boyd et al. [4].

2.1 The h_{int} Representation of Interesting Tissue

Because of the relatively weak control over the image acquisition process, it is difficult to eliminate variability in image characteristics, such as contrast and brightness. Such differences in imaging conditions lead to a complicated functional relationship between the intensities of temporal pairs of mammograms that varies from patient to patient. For this reason, it becomes even more difficult to compare temporal mammograms, consequently to assess changes due to HRT.

The h_{int} representation of interesting tissue, introduced by Highnam and Brady [5], is a method to normalise mammograms, by calculating anatomical information from the mammogram image. In the resulting h_{int} image, each pixel represents the thickness of 'interesting' (non-fat) tissue of the compressed breast above that pixel during acquisition. This effectively provides objective quantitative information about the breast anatomy. Changes of fatty to glandular tissue are precisely changes in non-fatty – i.e. h_{int} – tissue. Hence, h_{int} is the natural representation to use for the quantitative approach needed. By using the h_{int} representation, we propose measures of "interesting" tissue change that reflect the underlying tissue changes due to HRT:

a) The sum of "interesting" tissue:

$$\Delta h_{int}\,(\%) = \frac{S_1(h_{int}) - S_2(h_{int})}{S_1(h_{int})} \cdot 100 \tag{1}$$

b) The index volume of “interesting” tissue:

$$\Delta V_{\text{int}}(\%) = \left(V_1(h_{\text{int}}) - V_2(h_{\text{int}})\right) \cdot 100 \tag{2}$$

Where,

$$S_i(h_{\text{int}}) = \sum_x \sum_y h_{\text{int}}(x_i, y_i) \quad \text{and} \quad V_i(h_{\text{int}}) = \frac{\sum_x \sum_y h_{\text{int}}(x_i, y_i)}{H_i \times A_i} \tag{3}$$

for i=1,2

Where S_1, S_2 are the sum of interesting tissue values in each image, A_1, A_2 the area of the segmented breast region (number of pixels), H_1, H_2 are the heights of the compressed breast in each mammogram and Δh_{int}, ΔV_{int} are the suggested measures of density change.

2. 2 Projected Area

The projected area of glandular tissue has previously been used as a measure of tissue density. This measure is usually acquired by “interactive” thresholding where the clinician increases the image threshold until only the dense part of the mammogram is isolated. Subsequently, the Area % measure is calculated as the ratio of the dense area over the total area of the segmented mammogram (in pixels).

As a measure of breast density, the area of the projected glandular tissue has two basic flaws:

1. It does not calculate the “depth” of the dense tissue, only the 2D area of the projection of the breast parenchyma.

2. The interactive segmentation of the “dense tissue” is a subjective procedure and therefore the measure obtained is not consistent.

In this paper, the Area % is used in conjunction to the suggested h_{int} measures and the experimental results are presented in the next section.

3. Experimental results

Similar to large-scale clinical studies (e.g. in [6]), an experienced clinician described the changes in each HRT temporal mammogram pair. The 59 HRT mammogram sequences were classified into one of three categories by the clinician: involution (density decrease) in 21 sequences, regeneration (density increase) in 21 sequences and no significant change in the remaining 17 sequences.

For each measure, the agreement with the clinician was evaluated according to the sign of the difference of the measure between the 2 mammograms of each sequence, as is described in Table 1. The “no change” category was not considered since it is not clinically useful (only density changes can be related to cancer) and it is not a clear category since there is always a certain degree of change in the breast.

By using this description as the gold standard we evaluated our measures according to the rule presented in Table 1. The results on the agreement between classification based on measures and the clinician are presented in Table 2.

Table 1. The rule to assess mammographic changes due to HRT

Measure change in each mammogram sequence	Physiological change indicated
If $\%\Delta h_{int}$ or ΔV_{int} or $\%\Delta$Area >0	Density Decrease (Involution)
If $\%\Delta h_{int}$ or ΔV_{int} or $\%\Delta$Area <0	Density Increase (Regeneration)

Overall, the measure that performed the best is the Δh_{int} measure, as it gave consistently good results (agreement with clinical "ground truth") in both cases (involution, tissue regeneration pairs). This experiment agrees with the hypothesis that h_{int} is the right representation to use for the quantitative comparison of temporal mammograms.

Table 2. Results on the agreement between the quantitative measures used and the clinician, concerning tissue changes

Density change measure	$\%\Delta h_{int}$	ΔV_{int}	$\%\Delta$Area
Agreement with clinician in "tissue regeneration" pairs	71%	60%	71%
Agreement with clinician in "involution" pairs	81%	86%	57%

In Figure 1, we can see the V_{int} and Area % measures calculated both for the previous and current mammograms of each sequence. It is noticeable that the Area measure tends to be very similar in the "previous" and "recent" curves while the V_{int} captures more efficiently the temporal changes due to HRT. A possible explanation is that the Area measure is only a 2D measure of area, depends on user interaction (user defines global threshold) and does not capture the anatomical changes in dense tissue due to the use of HRT, or equivalently the changes in brightness due to increased or decreased density (that can be confined in the same mammographic area).

4. Discussion

We have developed a method for quantitative description of density changes in mammogram sequences and evaluated the performance of 3 measures by assessing their agreement with a clinician. Although there remains much validation work to do, it is clear from these results that measures based on the h_{int} representation can play the role of objective quantitative descriptors of mammographic density and that measures based on the area of dense tissue alone (e.g. [4]) can fail to capture temporal variations in breast density caused by physiological processes (involution) or due to the use of HRT.

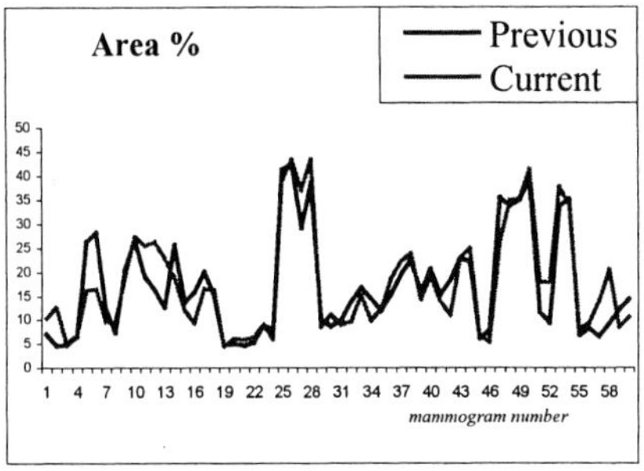

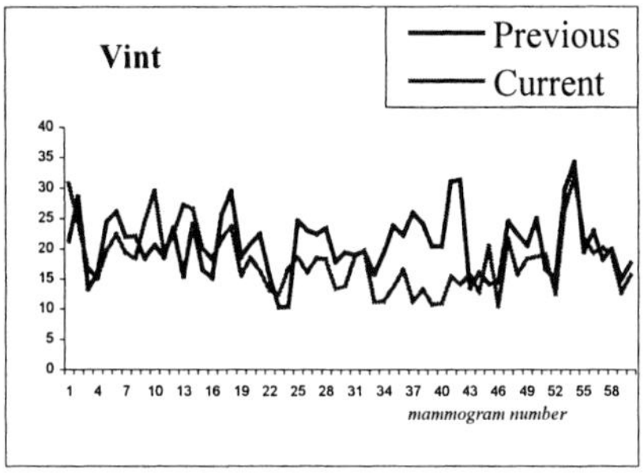

Fig. 1. Quantitative measures of breast density (Area% and V_{int}) over all the mammogram sequences examined. For each sequence there are two mammograms (previous and recent) and the V_{int} measure captures more efficiently the temporal variations in density while the Area % appears to be more "static" probably because it can't capture the changes in tissue density (or the changes of "brightness" in mammogram sequences).

Acknowledgements

The authors would like to acknowledge the Cancer Research UK for supporting this work and Mirada Solutions (http://www.mirada-solutions.com/) for providing the SMF generation software.

References

1. Collaborative Group on Hormonal Factors in Breast Cancer. : Breast cancer and hormone replacement therapy: collaborative analysis of data from 51 epidemiological studies of 52705 women with breast cancer and 108411 women without breast cancer. The Lancet. 350(No. 9084) (1997) 1047-1059
2. Jameson, J.L. (ed.): Principles of Molecular Medicine. Humana Press Inc. New Jersey USA (1998)
3. Kavanagh, A.M., Mitchell, H., Giles, G.G.: Hormone replacement therapy and accuracy of mammographic screening. The Lancet. 22;355 (2000) 270-4
4. Boyd, N.F, Lockwood, G.A., Byng J.W. et al.: Mammographic densities and breast cancer risk. Cancer Epidimiol Biomarkers. 7 (1998) 1133-1144
5. Highnam, R.P., Brady, J.M.: Mammographic image processing. Kluwer Academic Press (1999)
6. Persson, I., Thurfjell, E., Holmberg, L.: Effect of estrogen and estrogen-progestin replacement regimens on mammographic breast parenchymal density. J Clin Oncol. 15 (1997) 3201-7

Subjective and computer-based characterisation of mammographic patterns

Kostas Marias[a], Styliani Petroudi[a], Ruth English[b], Rosie Adams[b], Michael Brady[a]

[a] Robotics Research Group, Engineering Science, Oxford University, Ewert House, Ewert Place, Summertown, Oxford, OX2 7BZ, [b] Breast Care Unit, Churchill Hospital, Oxford OX3 7LJ, UK
kostas@robots.ox.ac.uk

Abstract. We investigate the subjective characterisation of breast patterns and the possibility of automatic classification using computed measurements. Several clinical studies used mammogram pattern classification in order to investigate their relation to breast cancer. However, the establishment of an objective ground truth for pattern classification remains a problem that diminishes the potential of such studies since there is significant variability in the interpretation and coding of the patterns. For this reason, we investigate the observer variability in classifying mammographic patterns as well as the variability between film-screen and computer screen reading with respect to pattern classification. We also investigate the role of quantitative measures in characterising the breast parenchyma, discuss their agreement with the observer and argue that a normalised mammographic representation can improve the correspondence between measures and the perceived mammogram patterns.

1. Introduction

In 1976 Wolfe [1] suggested that the mammographic appearance of the breast could be a risk factor for breast cancer. To evaluate this hypothesis he suggested four categories to characterise the breast parenchyma[1]:

N1: The breast consists mostly of fatty tissue with no ducts visible. This represents an essentially normal breast and is considered low risk of cancer.

P1: This represents a fatty breast with predominant ducts in the anterior portion up to $1/4^{th}$ of the breast. It is also considered low risk.

P2: The breast in involuted with prominent duct pattern of moderate to severe degree, occupying more than $1/4^{th}$ of the breast volume. The visible duct pattern can occupy the entire breast. It is considered high-risk.

DY: The breast parenchyma is dense, which usually denotes connective tissue hyperplasia[2]. It is considered as the highest risk pattern and can appear homogenous due to the overall increased density. The prominent duct pattern cannot be seen.

---

[1] The breast parenchyma comprises the lobules, ducts and the interlobular fibrous tissue

[2] The abnormal increase in the number of normal cells in normal arrangement in a tissue

The P2 and DY patterns are the most likely to develop cancer according to Wolfe [1] and since they are denser they can lower mammographic sensitivity or obscure a lesion on mammography. Figure 1, shows an example of Wolfe's patterns.

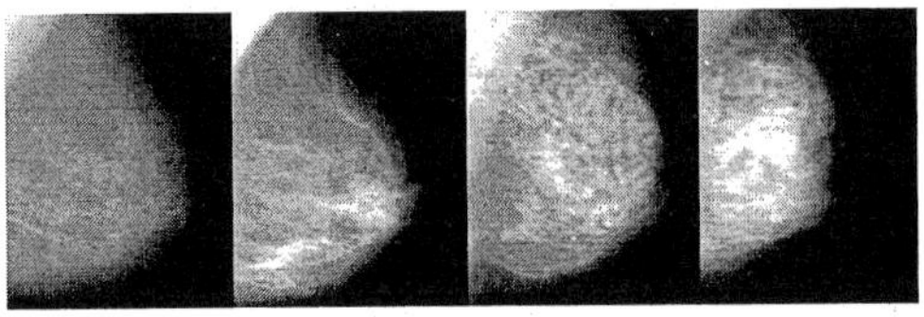

Fig. 1. An example of the Wolfe mammogram patterns (from left to right: N1, P1, P2 and DY)

The American College of Radiologists suggests that breast composition should be reported in all patients using the BI-RADS [2] classification:

I. The breast is almost entirely fat.
II. There are scattered fibroglandular densities.
III. The breast tissue is heterogeneously dense.
IV. The breast tissue is extremely dense.

Mammogram pattern classification can assist clinical studies in defining the role of mammographic appearance as a breast cancer risk. In addition, it can be used to characterise an increase in breast density due to Hormone Replacement Therapy (HRT) that can cause tissue regeneration and even change in breast pattern [3]. However, the classification of mammogram patterns is a subjective task, so it is important to develop an accurate classifier that could automatically report the density class of a given mammogram.

In this paper, we first investigate the observer variability in classifying mammogram patterns (section 2.1). In section 2.2 we discuss the role of quantitative and texture measures for the automatic classification of mammograms, while in section 3 we present some experimental results based on the suggested measures before concluding with a discussion (section 4).

2. Pattern Classification

Before developing method for the automatic classification of the breast parenchyma from the digitised (or digital) mammogram, we consider important to understand the observer variability when using the suggested classification methods (Wolfe, BI-RADS) and the differences when reading directly from the screen vs. film (section 2.1). In section 2.2 we investigate the possibility of computer-based pattern classification.

2.1 Variability in Classification

Two engineers familiar with mammogram patterns and an experienced radiologist classified 132 mammograms using the Wolfe criteria. The radiologist classified the mammograms using both Wolfe and BI-RADS classification. The engineers had previously formed a consensus for classifying the mammograms blinded to the mammograms used in the experiment. The classification results (from the computer screen reading) of all the observers using the Wolfe criteria are shown in Figure 2.a. It is clear that the engineers' classification is similar while there are significant differences between them and the radiologist especially in the P1 and DY classes.

Figure 2.b shows the radiologist's classifications of the 132 mammograms using both the Wolfe and the BI-RADS criteria. For each case the radiologist classified the mammograms reading them from both the films and the computer screen.

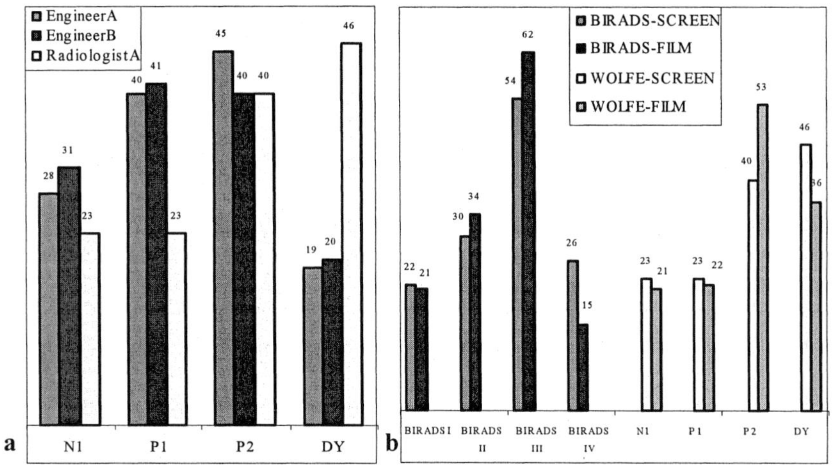

Fig. 2. (a) The classification results of all the observers using the Wolfe criteria, (b) The radiologist classifications using both Wolfe and BI-RADS for both screen and film reading

2.2 Classification Based on Measures

An automatic classifier should depend on robust measures of breast density and texture. Previous efforts to classify mammogram patterns are mostly based on image texture measures (e.g. in [4]). However, differences in imaging conditions lead to complex variations in the mammographic intensity distribution, a fact that diminishes the possible use of texture for mammographic pattern recognition.

For these reasons we use the normalised h_{int} representation of interesting tissue [5] in our experiments. The h_{int} is a quantitative representation of the breast that calculates the height of non-fatty tissue that corresponds to each pixel thus factoring out variations due to differences in image acquisition conditions.

The measures used are:

1. The index volume of "interesting" tissue is defined as:

$$V(h_{\text{int}}) = \frac{\sum_x \sum_y h_{\text{int}}(x, y)}{H \times A} \quad (1)$$

Where A is the segmented mammogram area (excluding the breast edge were the h_{int} is near zero) and H is the height of the compressed breast in each mammogram.

2. Correlation:

$$f_3 = \frac{\sum_i \sum_j ijp(i,j) - \mu_x \mu_y}{\sigma_x \sigma_y} \qquad \mu_{x\,or\,y} = \sum_i ip_{x\,or\,y}(i) \qquad \sigma^2_{x\,or\,y} = \sum_i \left(i - \mu_{x\,or\,y}\right)^2 p_{x\,or\,y}(i) \tag{2}$$

Where $p(i)$ is the probability of grey-level i, and $p(i, j)$ is the 2D probability from the co-occurrence matrix of the image.

3. Results in Automatic Classification

We calculated the measures described in the previous section for the 132 mammograms in our data set. In addition to the V_{int} measure (that is based in the h_{int} representation), we calculate the correlation measure both on the original images and the h_{int} ones. Our principal aim is to understand the significance of various measures for mammogram pattern classification. Since it is difficult (and sometimes unclear to the observer that classifies the patterns) to differentiate P2 from DY (or III and IV in BI-RADS) and P1 from N1 (or I from II), in this experiment we only consider high (P2 and DY or III and IV) vs. low (N1 and P1 or I and II) density classification. Using the V_{int} measure the accuracy in classification was 91% at the V_{int} =21%.

As shown in Figure 3.b, the correlation measure does not show any consistency with the different pattern classes (we use the radiologist's BI-RADS descriptions in this experiment) while in 3.a (h_{int} images) there is a clear separation between the high (III and IV) and low (I and II) density patterns. The accuracy is 88% at f_3=1.7. This clearly indicates the need for normalisation so that texture measures and quantitative measures can become significant and consistent. The result in Figure 3.b is expected since there is no compensation for the variability in imaging conditions and as a result the texture measures are erroneous.

4. Discussion

From the graphs shown in Figure 2, we can conclude that the variability in interpretation and coding is reduced when there is a consensus (as was done by the 2 Engineers). However, as seen in Figure 2.a the perception of the breast patterns can be significantly different and therefore there is a need for a more complete description of these classes as well as the development of standardisation criteria. In addition, as seen in Figure 2.b regardless of the classification method there is a significant difference in film vs. screen classification. Although the classification was performed in a conventional computer screen, the result still addresses an additional issue for the transition to digital mammography and the reading from the screen. Future work in digital mammography may take into consideration the consistency in classifying breast patterns as a mean to evaluate the adequacy of digital systems for mammography.

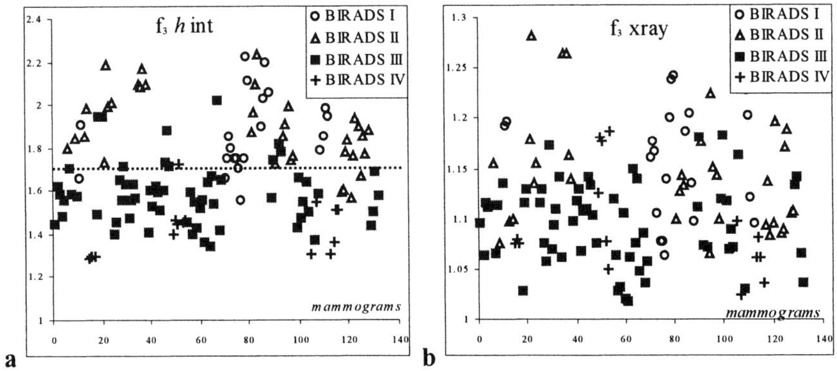

Fig. 3. A simple image texture measure (correlation) calculated in the h_{int} representation of 132 mammograms (a) and in the originals (b). The very good separation between high (III and IV) and low-density (I and II) textures in 3.a makes clear that there is a need for normalisation so that a measure can give significant results.

Finally, the results shown in Figure 3 clearly indicate that the h_{int} normalisation is necessary in order to derive significant measures and develop automatic classifiers of mammogram patterns. So far, our experiments show that a very good discrimination can be achieved between high and low density patterns. However, additional work needs to be done in separating N1 from P1 (or I from II) and P2 from DY (III from IV) and as was discussed in section 2.1 it is necessary to describe patterns more analytically in order to reduce the observer variability and to provide guidelines for the further development of measures that can robustly characterise breast patterns.

Acknowledgements

The authors would like to thank the Cancer Research UK for supporting this work and Mirada Solutions (http://www.mirada-solutions.com/) for the h_{int} generation software.

References

1. Wolfe, J. N.: Breast pattern as an index for developing breast cancer. American Journal of Roentgenology. 126 (1976) 1130-1139
2. ACR.: Illustrated breast imaging reporting and data system (BI-RADS™). American College of Radiology (1998)
3. Sala, E., Warren, R., McCann. J., Duffy, S., Luben, R., Day, N.: High-risk mammographic parenchymal patterns, hormone replacement therapy and other risk factors: a case-control study. Int J Epidemiol. 29(4) (2000) 629-362
4. Miller, P., Astley, S.: Classification of breast tissue by texture analysis. Image and Vision Computing. 10(5) (1992) 277-282
5. Highnam, R.P., Brady, J.M.: Mammographic image processing. Kluwer Academic Press (1999)

The Problem of Image Interpretation in Mammography: How Do Radiologists See What They Think They See?

Claudia Mello-Thoms[1], Calvin F. Nodine[2] and Harold L. Kundel[2]

[1]University of Pittsburgh, Department of Radiology, 300 Halket Street, Suite 4200 Pittsburgh, PA 15213-3180 USA, and [2]University of Pennsylvania, Department of Radiology, 3600 Market Street, Suite 370, Philadelphia, PA 19104
cmellothoms@mail.magee.edu

Abstract: Faulty visual search has been blamed as the primary cause for missed cancers in screening mammography, but eye-tracking studies have shown that 70% of unreported cancers do attract some amount of visual attention. In order to understand how image-based elements are translated into observer-based decision, we use spatial frequency analysis to model the areas in the mammogram that contain reported and unreported lesions. We also derive group profiles for the responses made by experienced mammographers and less-experienced radiology residents when interpreting mammograms. We train a pattern classifier to predict how each radiologist will respond to visually selected areas in new mammogram cases.

1. Introduction

A primary element involved in cancer detection is the radiologist's ability to correctly interpret the information being displayed in the mammogram. The interpretation of medical images involves knowledge about the features of the possible findings and the background, an efficient search strategy, the ability to disambiguate the findings from the breast parenchyma, and plausible decision making criteria to separate true abnormalities from artifacts produced by tissue superposition or image noise [1]. Each one of these factors has different consequences for cancer detection. For example, eye-position monitoring studies have shown that radiologists do not scan the image exhaustively, as it would be expected, considering that they do not know a priori where a cancerous lesion might be hiding [2]. Thus, faulty visual search has been blamed for the radiologists' failure to report a lesion.

Nonetheless, eye position monitoring studies have shown that only 30% of the unreported lesions do not attract any amount of visual attention; all other lesions receive varying amounts of visual dwell [3]. Hence, it is in the processing of this information that radiologists make mistakes. Kundel and Nodine [4] have differentiated these misses into perceptual errors, which occur when the eye lands in the location of the lesion for an insufficient amount of time for accurate recognition of a finding (estimated to be between 800 – 1000 ms [5]), and decision making errors, which occur when the eye stays in the location of the lesion long enough to generate a covert negative decision.

Hence, by studying the radiologists' eye-positions, as they read a mammogram case, we can gain valuable insights into their internal decision making processes, by comparing where they looked with what they reported in the case. We have shown that there exist spatial frequency differences between areas on a mammogram that were correctly reported by the radiologist and the ones that were not (being those either misses or false alarms) [6,7,8]. Moreover, we have shown that energy representations can be derived from visually-selected areas on a mammogram, and they can be used by an Artificial Neural Network to predict if the radiologist will report or not the presence of a finding at the location, based upon how the radiologist responded in the past to similarly structured areas in different mammogram cases.

In this paper we extend our studies to the differences in the decision patterns of experienced mammographers and less-experienced mammography residents, when studying a test set of mammogram cases. We study the consistency of their decisions as a group by comparing the rates of correct predictions made by the ANN. It is our hypothesis that the more experienced readers will be more consistent in their decisions, and this will be translated into better performance by the ANN.

2. Materials and Methods

Seven observers participated in this study. Three observers were experienced mammographers from the Hospital of the University of Pennsylvania (HUP), and four were radiology residents undergoing training at the same institution.

The observers read a test set of 40 two-view (cranial-caudal, CC, and medial-lateral oblique, MLO) mammogram cases. Twenty cases contained at least one malignant lesion which was visible in one- or two-views. All malignancies were biopsy proven. Twenty cases were lesion-free and had been stable for 2 years. The cases were digitized using a Lumiscan Model 100 digitizer (Lumisys Inc, Sunnyvale, CA) with a pixel size of 50μm x 50μm, and a gray level resolution of 12 bits. The two-views were displayed side by side on a single 21'' landscape gray scale monitor (ORWIN, Model DS5000L, Amityville, NY). An expert mammographer marked the x,y coordinates of all cancerous lesions using biopsy results and posterior films. This generated a truth table that was used to score the observers' responses.

The observers were instructed to search for malignancy, and were told to treat benign findings as if they were normal. The experiment was divided in two phases: on the first phase the observers freely examined the case, while their eye-position was being tracked. This phase ended once the observer felt confident to provide an initial impression of the case (namely, 'normal' or 'abnormal'). At that point eye-position monitoring was turned off, and the observer used a mouse-controlled cursor to indicate the nature and location of any malignant findings.

Regions that attracted visual attention on the first phase and that yielded an overt response by the observers (True and False Positive responses), as well as lesion-free regions that attracted prolonged visual dwell (>1sec) but did not elicit an overt response (True Negative responses), and regions that contained a malignant lesion that was not reported by the observer (a False Negative response), were segmented from the mammogram for further processing. Each region extracted corresponded to a 5° visual angle, at a viewing distance of 38cm. This size was chosen because it corresponds to the useful visual field [9].

We chose to process these regions using a system that is based upon the human visual system (HVS), which analyzes images at different scales and orientations. In our system each region is processed using a Wavelet Packets algorithm [10]. The logarithm of the energy of the wavelet decomposition, in each spatial frequency band, is then calculated. This generates a 'local' representation of the area where each decision (overt or covert) was made. Nonetheless, it is important to situate this area in the context of the breast parenchyma against which the decision was made. Hence, in order to create a 'global' representation of the breast tissue, we have averaged, per spatial frequency band, the log-energy values of all the areas that attracted prolonged visual dwell (>1sec), per observer and per case. We reasoned that these areas offered a representation of what each observer deemed as 'interesting features to look at'. In this case the same mammogram could generate very different global representations, depending on where the observer looked.

A feature vector was thus created, which contained 20 features representing the location where the decision was made, and 20 features representing the average breast parenchyma against which the decision was made. To this feature vector we added another feature, namely, a number representing the observer. Our rationale was that it would allow us to follow the decision outcomes made by each observer, and to relate them to the group that the observer belonged to (mammographer or resident).

Analysis of variance (ANOVA) were run on the data set, in order to determine if this representation contained enough information to differentiate amongst the decision outcomes. In addition, we split the data set in two parts: one was used to train an ANN to recognize the decision patterns of each observer, and the other was used to test the ANN's mapping.

3. Results

The first comparison that we made was among the representations of the three types of False Negatives, namely, FNs due to faulty search (FNs), faulty perception (FNp) and faulty decision making criteria (FNd). Table 1 shows the number and type of spatial frequency bands (sfb) where statistically significant differences (as measured by Scheffe's test, $p<0.05$) were found. Throughout this paper local spatial frequency bands contain information related to where the decision was made, whereas global spatial frequency bands contain information related to sampling of the breast parenchyma.

Table 1 shows that no differences could be observed, among the False Negative types, for the residents. Residents made significantly more perceptual errors (on average 42% per resident) than either search or decision making errors (on average, 29% of each per resident). This seems to indicate that residents knew where to look, but they did not know how to correctly process the information displayed in the examined area. On the other hand, mammographers made a similar amount, on average, of perceptual and decision making errors (about 38% of each per mammographer), but they made significantly less search errors (about 25% per mammographer). As the table shows, there were significant interactions in 10 local sfb between decision making and perceptual errors, and in 4 local sfb between perceptual and search errors. This seems to emphasize the conspicuity of local elements as the primary factor for attracting the eye to a given location on a mammogram case, in addition of keeping the eye returning to the location (as measured by cumulative gaze dwell).

Table 1. Number and type of spatial frequency bands containing statistically significant differences among the three types of False Negative decision outcomes.

Pair of FN	Mammographers	Residents
FNs x FNp	4 local sfb	-
FNs x FNd	-	-
FNp x FNd	10 local sfb	-

If we now concentrate on the differences between decision outcomes for both groups, we find the results shown in Table 2.

Table 2. Number and type of sfb where statistically signifiant differences occurred between the pair of decision outcomes shown in the left-column.

Pair of Decision Outcome	Mammographers	Residents
TP x FN	9 local sfb, 4 global sfb	4 local sfb, 4 global sfb
TP x FP	4 local sfb, 1 global sfb	5 local sfb
TP x TN	2 local sfb, 4 global sfb	2 local sfb
FP x FN	6 local sfb, 10 global sfb	4 local sfb, 2 global sfb
FP x TN	-	2 local sfb
FN x TN	4 local sfb	8 global sfb

The conspicuity of local elements seems to be the primary factor in differentiating lesion-containing areas that generated a report by the observer (a TP decision outcome) and the ones that did not (a FN decision outcome). It also seems to be the primary factor involved in the report of a true lesion (a TP decision outcome) versus a lesion-free area that is mistakenly identified as containing a lesion (a FP decision outcome). Moreover, the lack of interactions between FPs and TNs for mammographers could be the result of the small number of FPs made by this group.

If we now split the dataset in two parts, and use one to train an ANN to recognize image characteristics with the decision outcomes that they yield, per group of observers, we obtain the results shown in Table 3.

Table 3 shows that the ANN is consistently better at predicting decision outcome for the mammographers than it is for the residents, suggesting that perhaps the decision structure of the mammographers is more well-defined than that of the residents. In other words, mammographers possess a determined strategy for labeling areas on the image based upon the conspicuity of local elements and the way they sample the breast tissue. For the residents this strategy is still not completely established, which creates some difficulties for the ANN to interpret their data.

Table 3. Percent of correct predictions of the ANN for the testing set, for each of the decision outcomes shown in the left-column.

Decision Outcome	% correct (mammos)	% correct (residents)
TP	74	63
FP	85	70
FN	88	67
TN	94	73

4. Conclusions

Spatial frequency profiling of areas in a mammogram case that attracted visual attention by observers with different experience levels can be used to provide information about the type of decision outcome that a given observer will make in the area. These representations can also be used to derive trends about how different groups of observers respond to the same mammogram cases. Mammographers seem to be better able to balance local information, which represent the area of interest, and global information, which represent tissue sampling. Residents seem more guided by the conspicuity of local elements, and seem to have difficulty in extracting global information to compare with the finding.

Reference

1. Carmody, D.P., Nodine, C.F., Kundel, H.L.: An analysis of perceptual and cognitive factors in radiographic interpretation. Perception 9 (1980) 339-344.
2. Krupinski, E.A.: Visual scanning patterns or radiologists searching mammograms. Academic Radiology 3 (1996) 137-144.
3. Kundel, H.L., Nodine, C.F., Krupinski, E.A.: Computer-displayed eye position as a visual aid to pulmonary nodule interpretation. Investigative Radiology 25 (1990) 890-896.
4. Nodine, C.F., Kundel, H.L.: Using eye-movements to study visual search and to improve tumor detection. RadioGraphics 7 (1987) 1241-1250.
5. Hillstrom, A.P.: Repetition effects in visual search. Perception & Psychophysics 62 (2000) 800-817.
6. Mello-Thoms, C., Dunn, S.M., Nodine, C.F., Kundel, H.L.: An analysis of perceptual errors in reading mammograms using quasi-local spatial frequency spectra. Journal of Digital Imaging 14 (2001) 1170123.
7. Mello-Thoms, C., Dunn, S.M., Nodine, C.F., Kundel, H.L.: The perception of breast cancers: a spatial frequency analysis of what differentiates missed from reported cancers. IEEE Transactions on Medical Imaging 2002 (submitted).
8. Mello-Thoms, C., Dunn, S.M., Nodine, C.F., Kundel, H.L., Weinstein, S.P.: The perception of breast cancer: what differentiates missed from reported cancers in mammography? Academic Radiology 2002 (submitted).
9. Kundel, H.L., LaFollette, P.S.: Visual search patterns and experience with radiological images. Radiology 103 (1972) 523-526.
10. Mallat, S. A wavelet tour of signal processing. Academic Press, San Diego (1998).

Image retrieval system of mammographic masses by using local pattern matching technique

Toshiaki Nakagawa, Takeshi Hara, Hiroshi Fujita, Takuji Iwase[*] and Tokiko Endo[**]

Department of Information Science, Faculty of Engineering, Gifu University
Yanagido 1-1, Gifu 501-1193, Japan
nakagawa@fjt.info.gifu-u.ac.jp
[*]Department of Breast Surgery, Aichi Cancer Center Hospital
Kanokoden 1-1, Tikusa-ku, Nagoya 464-8681, Japan
[**]Department of Radiology, National Hospital of Nagoya
Sannomaru 4-1-1, Naka-ku, Nagoya 460-0001, Japan

Abstract. We proposed a concept of content-based image retrieval and demonstrated the potential usefulness in mammography. The approach incorporated a local-pattern matching method based on Nth-order autocorrelation features with KL expansion (principal components analysis) to retrieve similar mass shadows on digitized screen/film mammograms. We confirmed the tendency that similar mass images were retrieved as the initial studies by using the 75 images of mammographic masses.

1. Introduction

Comparing the previous and similar images with current case is very effective procedure in interpreting by physicians. The purpose of this work is to develop an image retrieval system that searches out the image database for the image resembling to the entered one (query image) and outputs with diagnostic information. Approaches on image retrieval technique well employ the feature-extraction method in many researches. Also in the field of a medical image, some researches are reported on retrieval of the similar image of a lesion based on segmentation technique [1, 2]. Therefore, since the retrieval results depend on the accuracy of the segmentation processing, it is not an effective approach to retrieve images that the object boundaries are difficult to determine strictly. In this research, the technique of extracting the feature from the whole image automatically and performing image retrieval without carrying out the image segmentation is proposed. The simulation experiment using the mammographic mass images was conducted to examine the validity of this technique.

2. Methods

The features were extracted from the query image and the ones within whole database. The images including mass were simply cut from original digitized images in a square form. The autocorrelation features were extracted by counting patterns defined as local patterns consisted of some pixels with various gray level distributions. The example of the local pattern used for the feature extraction is shown in Fig. 1. If the feature extraction is carried out using N pieces of local patterns on each image, the feature vector with N elements is obtained. The feature values of all of the images in database were calculated, and the feature was expressed as a vector in N dimensions. After storing the vector in each image, the KL expansion was used to decrease the number of dimension in feature space to create the retrieval feature space. Next, the Euclid distance among the feature vectors measured on retrieval feature space evaluates the similarity between the query image and the others within the database. The nearest vector from the query image was employed as the retrieval result.

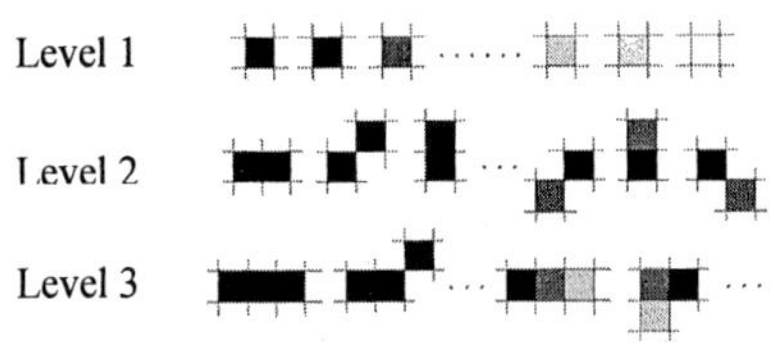

Fig. 1. Local pattern for feature extraction

3. Demonstration of image retrieval on mammographic masses

We evaluated the retrieval methods by using a database of 75 images of mammographic masses. Original images digitized from screen/film mammograms had 4096 gray levels and 100-micrometer sampling pitch. The preprocess to changes gray level into 8 and resolution into 400 micrometers was performed for the mitigation of retrieval condition. Sixty-four kinds (8 at level 1, and 56 at level 2) of local patterns were employed. KL expansion was performed to the extracted amount of the features, and one image in which the Euclid distance had the shortest feature in the retrieval feature space was determined the similar image about each image.

4. Results and Discussion

The retrieval results of the mammographic masses are shown in Fig. 2. The results indicated in the figure were chosen with degree of similar by subjective observation from 75 sets of retrieval results. Although there were many satisfied cases with the difference of density distribution between those images, there were a few results correspond to physician's opinion on the shape and the condition of margin of mass. The rate of coincidence was 29% on the shape, and was 34% on the margin. The reason of this was estimated that the signal-feature of an image is not in agreement with a physician's subjectivity measure. However, it can expect that the system to retrieve an image quantitatively by the degree of similar based on the feature analysis, and can reduce the variation in diagnosis of physicians. Even when it was an inaccurate solution, the retrieved image has a similar impression in many cases. It is estimated that the feature vectors in the retrieval feature space were reflecting the shape of an object image well as this reason, and it may be able to use as diagnostic support.

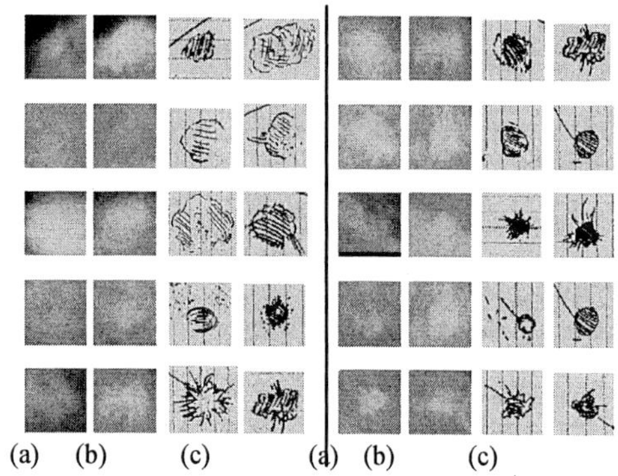

Fig. 2. 10 retrieval results of mammographic mass images. The images of four sheets are (a)a query image, (b)a retrieved one, (c)the sketch of the query image drawn by the physician, and the sketch of the retrieved image in an order from the left.

5. Conclusion

The retrieval technique based on local patterns existing in images was proposed. The experimental results show the effectiveness to retrieve gray-level patterns such as mammographic masses.

Acknowledgements

This work was supported in parts by a grant from the Endo Saijirou commemorative foundation for the promotion of technology (KAI industries, Gifu, Japan), the Grant-In-Aid for Scientific Research from Japan Society for the Promotion of Science, and the Grant-In-Aid for Cancer Research from the Ministry of Health, Labour and Welfare.

References

1. Qi H and Snyder WE, "Content-based image retrieval in picture archiving and communications systems", Journal of Digital Imaging, Vol. 12, No. 2, Suppl 1, pp. 81-83, 1999.
2. Giger ML, Huo Z, Lan L and Vyborny CJ, "Intelligent search workstation for computer-aided diagnosis", Proc. of the 14th International Symposium and Exhibition on Computer Assisted Radiology and Surgery (CARS2000), pp. 822-827, San Francisco, 2000.

Application of dual-energy techniques to digital mammography

Angelo Taibi[1], Sara Fabbri[1], Paola Baldelli[1], Cosimo di Maggio[2], Gisella Gennaro[2], Michele Marziani[1], Alessandra Tuffanelli[1], and Mauro Gambaccini[1]

[1] Dipartimento di Fisica, Università di Ferrara, via Paradiso 12, 44100 Ferrara, Italy
taibi@fe.infn.it
[2] Dipartimento di Scienze Oncologiche, Università di Padova, via Gattamelata 64, 35128 Padova, Italy

Abstract. A dual-energy technique which employs the basis decomposition method is being investigated for application to digital mammography. A three-component phantom was doubly exposed with the digital mammography system manufactured by General Electric. The "low" and "high" energy images were recorded with a Mo/Mo anode-filter combination at 25 kV and a Rh/Rh combination at 40 kV, respectively. The total dose was kept within the acceptable levels of conventional mammography. The first hybrid image obtained with the dual-energy algorithm is presented in comparison with a conventional radiograph of the phantom.

1 Introduction

Early manifestations of breast cancer are often very subtle and are displayed on a complex and variable pattern of normal anatomy that may either obscure or simulate disease. This is particularly important in dense breasts, which belong to approximately 25% of women, because of the complexity of overlying fibroglandular structures. Dual-energy mammography could help to enhance the detectability of lesions by removing this "structure noise". It makes use of two digital images obtained with two different x-ray spectra. By combining these images it is possible to produce hybrid images in which the contrast of relevant structures is preserved while unwanted masking contrast is largely removed [1, 2].

The proposed dual-energy technique for mammography application was previously tested by imaging dedicated phantoms with a compact and tunable quasi-monochromatic source and a digital detector [3]. We are now investigating the potential of such a technique on a GE Senographe 2000D digital unit. By taking advantage of the two anode tracks, namely molybdenum (Mo) and rhodium (Rh), incorporated in the GE unit, two digital mammograms were recorded at "low" and "high" energy. A three-component dedicated breast phantom was doubly exposed with a total dose within the acceptable levels of conventional mammography. In this preliminary study we present the hybrid image obtained with the contrast cancellation algorithm in comparison with the image obtained in standard conditions.

2 Materials and Methods

A three-component breast phantom was specifically designed and built to perform dual-energy analysis. A plexiglas box 5-cm thick is filled with water and plexiglas spheres of 3 different diameters, 8 mm, 12.7 mm, and 22.2 mm, respectively. Five polyethylene spheres are embedded in the phantom as details with a diameter ranging from 3.2 mm to 12.7 mm. Details aside, the phantom is made up of about 65% plexiglas and 35% water. A photograph of the phantom is shown in figure 1. The bigger polyethylene details are clearly visible as white spheres.

The low-energy image was obtained at 25 kV Mo/Mo (HVL=0.294 mm Al) whilst the high-energy image was obtained at 40 kV Rh/Rh (HVL=0.521 mm Al). Figure 2 shows the low- and high-energy spectra attenuated by the phantom. X-ray spectra were obtained via the computer program developed by Boone *et al* [4] which is integrated in the simulation code XOP [5]. The calculation of the mean energy of the x-ray beam which exits the phantom was then performed to determine the linear attenuation coefficients for the dual-energy algorithm. A mean energy of 18.8 keV and 25.5 keV was found for the low- and high-energy output spectrum, respectively. Attenuation coefficients for the basis materials, namely plexiglas and polyethylene, were calculated via the XCOM program [6].

The dual-energy algorithm was implemented as a pluging of ImageJ, a public domain image processing program written in Java [7].

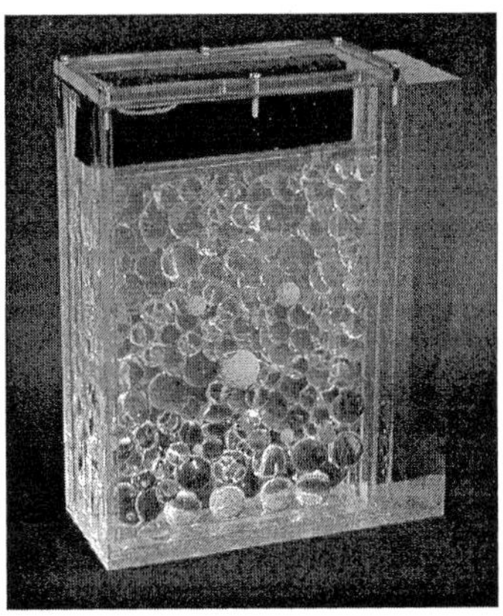

Fig. 1. Photograph of the three-component phantom.

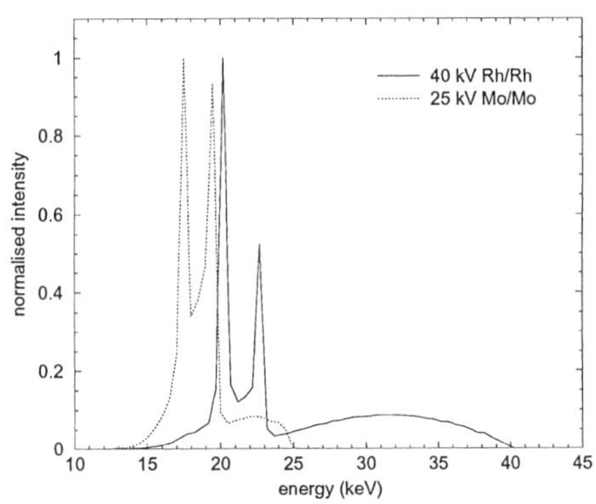

Fig. 2. Calculated x-ray spectra after the attenuation of the phantom.

3 Results and Conclusion

The measured entrance air dose was 9.7 mGy and 4.8 mGy for the "low" and "high" image, respectively. A digital radiograph of the phantom was also recorded in standard conditions, i. e., 28 kV Mo/Mo and the measured entrance air dose was 9.0 mGy. This latter image is shown in figure 3 (left) together with the hybrid image obtained after the application of the dual-energy algorithm (the black circle in the biggest detail is due to an empty cavity inside the polyethylene sphere).

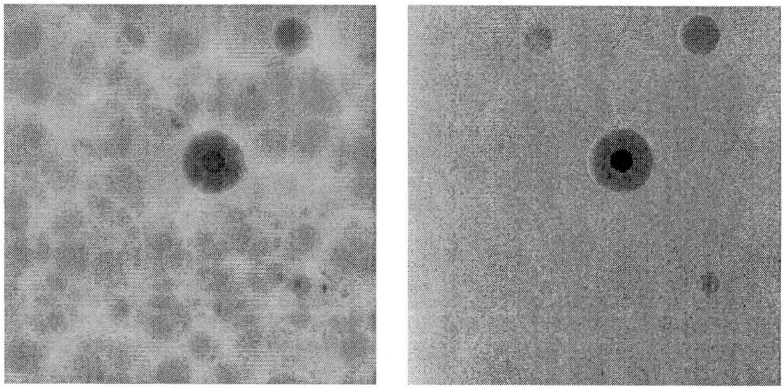

Fig. 3. Left: Radiograph of the phantom obtained at 28 kV. Right: Digital image obtained with the dual-energy technique.

In this preliminary investigation the dual-energy algorithm was directly applied i.e., without correcting for effects of beam hardening and scatter [8, 9]. Although these effects cause miscancellation artifacts it is worth noting that the applied technique satisfactorily succeeded in removing the contrast between water and plexiglas and thereby enhancing the visibility of polyethylene details.

Work is in progress to further investigate and optimize the dual-energy technique for a clinical application.

References

1. R.E. Alvarez and A. Macovski, Phys. Med. Biol. **21**, 733-744, 1976.
2. L. A. Lehmann, R. E. Alvarez, A. Macovski, and W. R. Brody, Med. Phys. **8**, 659-667, 1981.
3. M. Marziani, A. Taibi, A. Tuffanelli and M. Gambaccini Phys. Med. Biol. **47**, 305-313, 2002.
4. J.M. Boone, T.H. Fewell and R. J. Jennings, Med. Phys. **24**, 1863-1874, 1997.
5. M. Sanchez del Rio and R. J. Dejus, SPIE Proc. **3448**, 340 1998.
6. M. J. Berger and J. H. Hubbell, "XCOM: Photon Cross Sections on a Personal Computer," National Institute of Standards and Technology, 1987
7. Program developed at the U.S. National Institutes of Health and available on the Internet at http://rsb.info.nih.gov/ij/
8. H. N. Cardinal and A. Fenster, Med. Phys. **17**, 327-341, 1990.
9. P. C. Johns and R. M. Beauregard, Med. Phys. **21**, 1455-1462, 1994.

An optical method for measuring compressed breast thickness

J. Yang, D. Rico, B. Augustine, G.E. Mawdsley, M.J. Yaffe

Imaging Research, Sunnybrook & Women's College Health Sciences Centre
2075 Bayview Avenue, Toronto ON M4N 3M5 Canada
jyang@swchsc.on.ca

Abstract. Accurate information regarding compressed breast thickness is an important factor for estimating volumetric breast density for breast cancer risk prediction as well as for dose calculation. The thickness display on commercial mammography units does not indicate the effect of tilting and flexing of the plastic compression paddle. We have developed an optical method, which uses a CCD camera, to measure the compressed breast thickness and its spatial variation during mammography. Our results suggest that using this method, the breast thickness can be determined with an average error of about ±2 mm. The accuracy is dependent on CCD pixel size and resolution. The sensitivity is related to the focal distance and projection angle of the CCD camera.

1. Introduction

The transmitted x-ray intensity through the breast is dependent on both the composition of the breast and its local thickness (1). Most current mammography machines have thickness indicators, which give a rough indication of the overall compressed thickness, however do not account for flexing or bending of the plastic compression plate and arm. In addition, the accuracy and precision of such indicators are not reliable, and depend significantly on the applied compression force. Other techniques to measure local thickness have been developed, such as using the magnification of lead markers placed on the top of compression plate (2). This method requires that all markers be shown in the image and does not measure the flexing of the compression plate.

Accurate information regarding compressed breast thickness is an important factor for estimating volumetric breast density as well as for dose calculation (3-5). With commercial mammography units, the actual thickness can differ by as much as one centimeter from the thickness readout. We have developed an optical method, which uses a conventional USB CCD camera to measure the compressed breast thickness and its spatial variation for individual mammograms.

2. Materials and Method

A CCD camera is mounted on the frame of the mammography unit (Fig. 1) and focused on the plastic compression paddle on which a two-dimensional radiolucent pattern with lines in a square grid pattern has been placed.

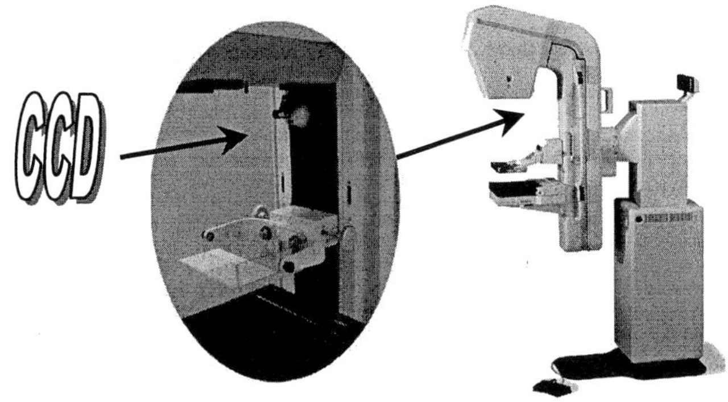

Fig. 1. Mounted CCD camera and mammography machine

The 2D pattern is projected onto the image plane of the CCD camera with a matrix size of 640×480 pixels. For one of squares on the grid pattern, the optical geometry is shown in Figure 2. The camera optical axis has a projection angle α with the central ray axis of the mammography unit. In the figure, S indicates the shift of this grid pattern on the image plane and T is the thickness (elevation) in that corresponding position.

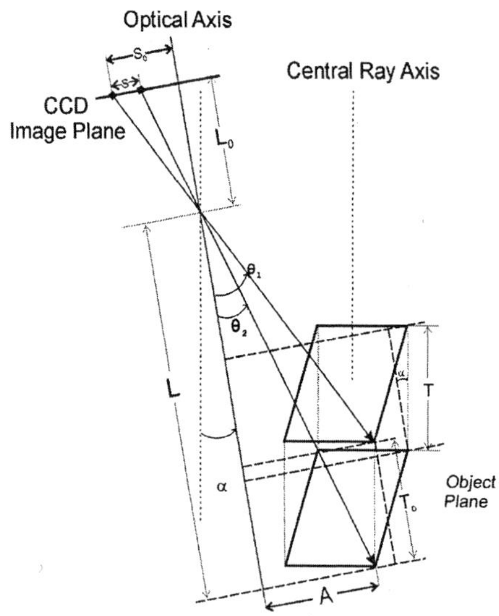

Fig. 2. The optical geometry for one of grid squares (not scaled)

Therefore, $tg(\theta_2) = A/L = (S_0-S)/L_0$ and $tg(\theta_1) = [A+T_0*tg(\alpha)]/(L-T_0) = S_0/L_0$

$$A/L = (S_0\text{-}S)/L_0 \qquad (1)$$

and

$$[A+T_0*tg(\alpha)]/(L-T_0) = S_0/L_0 \qquad (2)$$

Finally,

$$T = T_0/\cos\alpha = S*(L/L_0)[S_0\cos\alpha/L_0 + \sin\alpha] \qquad (3)$$

As seen from Equation 3, the thickness T has a linear relationship to the shift S. For a specified camera position, the measured thickness only depends on the shift of the intersection points of the square grid.

In our study, the pattern was imaged at known compression paddle positions (0~6cm) without any paddle deformation or deflection. The shift of grid marks on the pattern was mapped as a linear function of the paddle height at each x-y coordinate. The thickness at an individual point can be computed from an image of the grid pattern taken by the CCD camera.

3. Results

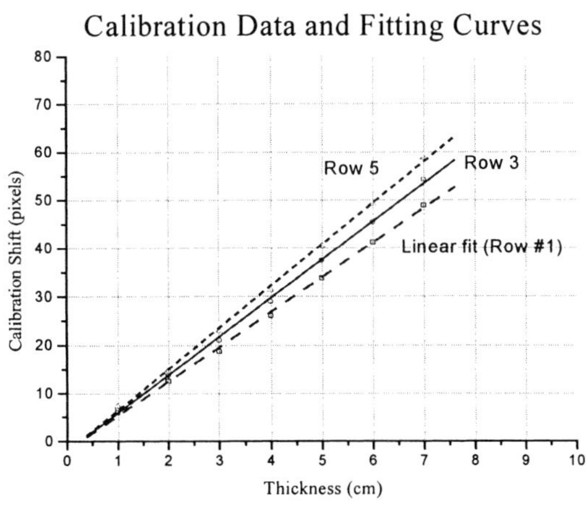

Fig. 3. Calibration data and fitting lines

Using these patterns with the known thickness, shifts (in pixels) are calculated at all intersections of the grid pattern, which are identified as pixel locations (x-y coordinates). The quantitative accuracy of location of grid intersections is about half of the pixel size in the grid plane. Some calibration data are shown in Figure 3 to illustrate the linearity between thickness and pattern shift (S). The method was applied to measure thicknesses of simulated breasts using prosthetic devices as phantoms, under compression (in the range of 5~10daN). With a silicone-filled phantom (Fig. 4), the paddle bulge was identified and measured using the grid shifts and distortion. The relative distortion is shown in an enlarged picture at right.

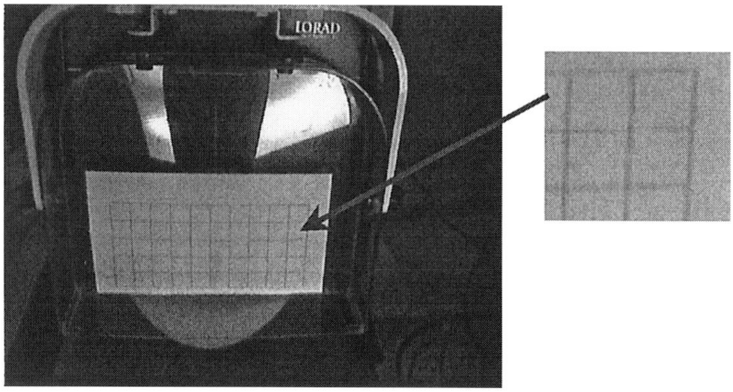

Fig. 4. CCD image of breast phantom under compression

A thickness map was generated using grid shifts based on the linear relationships of Figure 3. The results are shown in Figure 5. As can be seen, the local compression plate position can be determined quantitatively, and shows the two-dimensional thickness distribution of the breast under the compression paddle. There are significant deflection and thickness changes across the breast phantom. From the point where the phantom starts to contact the compression paddle, to the highest point in the image, there is a change in the thickness of about 0.5 cm.

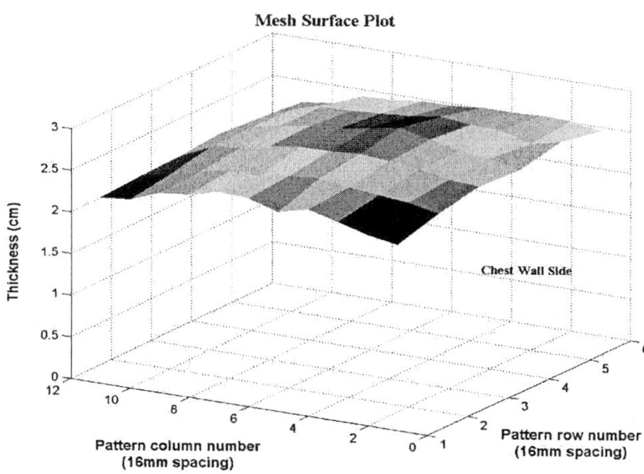

Fig. 5. Thickness map of the compression plate

Our preliminary results suggest that using this method, the breast thickness can be determined with an average error of about ±2mm, based on the linear regression fits of the calibration images (Fig. 3). The accuracy is dependent on CCD pixel size, optical resolution and related to the focal distance and projection angle of the CCD camera. The accuracy may be improved by changing the lens on the camera to reduce the field of view or by using a higher resolution CCD camera.

4. Conclusions

A method for accurately mapping the thickness of the breast has been developed which produces a two-dimensional map of breast thickness and is far less intrusive to the examination or the image than using radiographic markers positioned on the top surface of the paddle. Aside from the presence of the pattern on the compression paddle, there is no other interference with the mammographic procedure. In addition, this method is sensitive to the effects of both paddle tilt and flexing.

Acknowledgments: The authors thank Jill Johns, Imaging Research, Sunnybrook & Women's College Health Sciences Centre, for her assistance in preparing the manuscript.

References

1. Highnam, R.P., Brady, J.M., Shepstone, B.J.: Estimating Compressed breast thickness. Digital Mammography, Kluwer Academic, (1998) 275-278.
2. Burch, A. and Law, J.: A method for estimating compressed breast thickness during mammography. Br J Radiol 68: (1995) 394-399.
3. Pawluczyk, O., Augustine, B., Yaffe, M.J., Rico, D., Yang, J., Boyd, N.F., and Mawdsley, G.E.: A Volumetric Method for Estimation of Breast Density. Submitted to Medical Physics (2002).
4. Law, J., editor: The commissioning and routine testing of mammographic X-ray systems. Institute of Physical Sciences in Medicine, York UK, (1994) 59.
5. Dance, D.R.: Monte Carlo calculation of conversion factors for the estimation of mean glandular breast dose. Phys Med Biol, 35, (1990) 1211-1219.

Volumetric Breast Density Estimation on Digitized Mammograms – A Preliminary Clinical Study

[1]B. J. Augustine, [1]M.J. Yaffe, [1]D. Rico, [1]J. Yang, [1]G. E. Mawdsley, [2]T. Li, [2]J. Wu, and [2]N. F. Boyd

[1]Imaging/Bioengineering Research, SWCHSC, 2075 Bayview Avenue, Toronto, ON M4N 3M5, Canada, [2]Division of Epidemiology and Statistics, Ontario Cancer Institute, 610 University Avenue, Toronto, Ontario M4G 1K9, Canada.
augustin@sten.sunnybrook.utoronto.ca

Abstract. We have developed a method to perform quantitative volumetric analysis of mammographic density (VBD) from digitized screen-film mammograms. The method is being tested on two different ethnic groups of women aged 50 years or older, having greatly different risks of breast cancer. The average VBD in the lower risk group of women was found to be significantly lower than that in the higher risk group. The average entrance exposure (mR) for the lower risk group was also found to be much lower, despite similar average compressed breast thickness obtained for the two groups of women.

1. INTRODUCTION

A relationship between breast parenchymal patterns and breast cancer risk was initially suggested by Wolfe [1] and confirmed by others, e.g. Byrne [2]. Radiologists typically subjectively classify the mammographic appearance using the BIRADS system [3]. Boyd [4] and Byng [5] introduced a quantitative subjective system for assessment of density called Percentage area Density (PD) and showed that women classified into the uppermost category have a six-fold higher risk of getting breast cancer compared to women in the lowest category [4]. We believe that the risk of breast cancer is more likely related to the volume of dense tissue rather than the projected area as measured by PD. Thus, we have developed a technique for breast density quantification based on three-dimensional information about the composition of the breast. The technique is being evaluated in a study of two ethnic groups of women having different risks of breast cancer.

2. MATERIALS AND METHODS

Our approach is to calibrate the imaging system by exposing a specially-designed tissue-equivalent plastic step wedge over a range of exposure parameters employed in mammography [6]. Subsequent variations due to the technique factors, film emulsion and film processing are monitored using an aluminum step wedge, placed adjacent to the breast on the breast support table of the mammography machines. A first-order thickness correction is employed to correct for possible inaccuracies in the thickness readout from the mammography units during each mammogram.

In this study, 111 Caucasian women (higher risk group) and 98 Chinese women recently migrated to Canada (lower risk group) were recruited. All women were aged 50 years or older. Imaging was carried out on three mammography systems at two screening sites. The aluminum step wedge was mounted on the upper corner of the image receptor holders of all three machines. All mammograms obtained on both large and small films from the sites over a period of four months were digitized. For each image, the compressed breast thickness, t_T and the imaging techniques (kV, mAs, anode/filter) were recorded. Shifts in log relative exposure (LRXA) as detected on the aluminum step wedge were used to shift the original (plastic) calibration surface to compensate for variations in exposure conditions or film sensitometry. Finally, the VBD value for each mammogram was calculated. PD measurements also were performed on the two groups of women. PD and VBD were then compared between the two population groups.

Accurate knowledge of the compressed breast thickness is an important factor in the estimation of VBD. To constrain the error in the compressed breast thickness, we identified two parameters on each breast image: 1) the minimum LRXA, which corresponds to the maximum amount of dense tissue and 2) the maximum LRXA which corresponds to the minimum amount of dense tissue. If the maximum LRXA was greater than that for the 100% fat on the calibration surface, the thickness was reduced to match the LRXA for 100% fat on the calibration surface. Similarly, if the minimum LRXA was lower than that for 100% gland on the calibration surface, the thickness was increased to match for 100% gland.

Table 1. VBD estimation on clinical mammograms by machine types (1 & 2), Average kV and mAs used, average breast entrance exposure (mR), and average compressed thickness (t_T) and average percent dense volume (m) for the two groups of women after thickness correction.

	Unit	kV	mAs	mR	t_T_corr (cm)	m_corr (%)
Caucasian	**1**	**26.5**	**184.5**	**1653**	**5.18**	**25.2**
Chinese	**1**	**27.3**	**90.8**	**871**	**4.81**	**18.0**
Chinese	**2**	**26.8**	**73.7**	**948**	**4.63**	**14.1**

3. RESULTS

In total, 209 mammograms (LCC views) were obtained. We found that the VBD was lower in the lower risk group than in the higher risk group both before and after performing the thickness correction, whereas the PD measurements were found to be higher in the lower risk group. Approximately 70% of the images required nothickness compensation. For the 30% of images where thickness corrections occurred, the adjustments were less than 5mm for 25% and under 10mm for the remaining 5%. Table I shows the comparison of the VBD values for the two groups of women sorted by machine type after thickness correction.

4. DISCUSSION AND CONCLUSION

The average kVp used to image the breasts and the average compressed breast thickness were found to be similar in the two groups of women, but the average mAs and breast entrance exposure (in mR) were significantly lower in Chinese women, supporting the lower VBD results obtained for this group. PD measurements obtained for the two groups of women were not consistent with the lower incidence of breast cancer in Chinese women. Thickness inaccuracy in the breast and the change in thickness in the peripheral region is a source of error in the VBD measurements and will be corrected for future studies. However, this preliminary clinical study suggests that VBD may be more relevant than PD for quantifying mammographic density and breast cancer risk. A larger case-control study to evaluate the effectiveness of VBD as a risk indicator is ongoing.

REFERENCES

1. J.N. Wolfe, Risk for breast cancer development determined by mammographic parenchymal pattern, Cancer, 37, 2486-2492 (1976).
2. C. Byrne, Schairer C. et al., Mammographic features of and breast cancer risk, Journal of the National Cancer Institute, 87, 1622-1629 (1995).
3. American College of Radiology (ACR) Breast Imaging Reporting and Data System (BIRADS) Third Edition. Reston, Va: American College of Radiology; (1998)
4. N.F. Boyd, J.W. Byng *et al.*, Quantitative classification of mammographic densities and breast cancer risk: results from the Canadian National Breast Screening Study, J. Natl.Cancer Inst., 87, 670-675 (1995).
5. J.W. Byng, N.F. Boyd *et al.*, The Quantitative Analysis of Mammographic Densities, Phys Med Biol, 39, 1629-1638 (1994).
6. O. Pawluczyk, B.J. Augustine, M.J. Yaffe *et al.*, A Volumetric Method for Estimation of Breast Density on Digitized Screen-Film Mammograms, submitted to Medical Physics (2002).

Enhancement of Microcalcifications in Full-Field Digital Mammography by Energy Subtraction

Diekmann F, Diekmann S, Bick U, Hamm B

Dep. of Radiology, Charité Berlin, Germany
felix.diekmann@charite.de

Abstract. Purpose: To investigate the potential of full-field digital mammography for enhancement of microcalcifications by energy subtraction. Material and methods: Ten breast specimens containing microcalcifications were examined by digital mammography (Senographe 2000D, General Electrics, Milwaukee, USA) at 22kVp and 49kVp without changing the position of the specimens in between. The contrast of 5 microcalcifications relative to a background region of interest was measured in each specimen ((C1-C2)/C1) on the 22 and the 49 kVp images. This contrast was compared to the contrast measured on the image generated by a subtraction algorithm from the 22 and 49 kVp image. Since only specimens were used, there was no need for registration of the images (no movement). Results: The average contrast of the microcalcifications was 0.108 on the 22 kVp images and 0.073 on the 49 kVp images as opposed to 0.168 on the subtraction images. The differences in contrast were statistically significant (Chi2, $p < 0.05$). Conclusions: Full-field digital mammography offers the potential for enhancement of microcalcifications by energy subtraction. Use of simple algorithms is possible especially in examinations of breast specimens.

Introduction:

The advent of direct digital mammography has facilitated the use of such techniques as CAD, contrast-enhanced mammography, energy subtraction, and telemammography. These techniques can also be used with conventional mammography but are clearly more practicable with digital mammography.

Subtraction algorithms are useful not only for the use of CAD systems but also for contrast-enhanced mammography and energy subtraction. While many reports in the literature deal with subtraction and CAD (CAD in follow-up, CAD for comparison with the contralateral side) [1] and, more recently, several study groups have started to investigate contrast-enhanced mammography [2], only little research has so far been done on the use of energy subtraction for differentiating tumors and enhancing microcalcifications. There are two possible explanations for this lack: On the one hand, the subtraction technique can increase radiation exposure in vivo and, on the other hand, the interval between acquisition of two images for assessing microcalcifications is still rather long what leads to movement artefacts. Even minimal patient movement during this interval may impair optimal subtraction. However, since future digital mammography units are expected to provide images of excellent quality at lower doses and will operate with markedly shorter time intervals between two images, investigation of energy subtraction is a worthwhile endeavor in view of future applications in mammography. The aim of the present study is to determine whether the technology already available today has a potential for improving the visualization of microcalcifications by using energy subtraction.

Material and Method:

The study was performed using a digital full-field mammography unit with a detector on the basis of amorphous silicon (Senographe 2000D, General Electrics, Milwaukee, USA). Ten specimens containing microcalcifications were imaged at 22 kVp and 49 kVp. The specimens had been obtained either by vacuum suction biopsy (Ethicon Endo-Surgery and Johnson & Johnson companies, Cincinnati, Ohio) or by open surgery. The fact that specimens were used allowed obtaining the two images without movement in between. The 22 kVp images were obtained at 36 mAs using the molybdenum anode and a filter, the 49 kVp images at 4 mAs using rhodium. All images were acquired with the magnification technique. Subsequently, the two images were subtracted, and the mean contrast of the microcalcifications was calculated on each of the two images as well as on the subtraction image ((C1-C2)/C1). Because of the relatively high dose used in the study, image noise was not taken into account.

Results

The subtraction algorithm used here enhanced the contrast of the microcalcifications. The mean contrast calculated for all calcifications was 0.108 on the 22 kVp images and 0.073 on the 49 kVp images. The contrast was significantly higher at 0.168 on the subtraction images. The contrast enhancement achieved by subtraction is illustrated in Fig. 1, which shows the two images obtained in a specimen and the corresponding subtraction image. Subjective assessment by a radiologist confirmed the higher contrast of the subtraction images. These results suggest that digital full-field mammography allows for enhancing the contrast of microcalcifications by application of energy subtraction. However, a high dose was used in the present study so as not to take into account image noise. The noise already present on the original images is further enhanced on the subtraction image.

Discussion

With digital full-field mammography, it is possible, in principle, to easily and rapidly acquire a series of images with little artifact formation. This is a convenient way of generating subtraction images. Subtraction imaging is already used in contrast-enhanced mammography in some sites and may in the future be applied in other areas such as energy subtraction as well. Ideally, the images used for energy subtraction should be acquired simultaneously and obtained applying X-ray beams with optimized energy spectra. Optimization of energy spectra in digital mammography is an area of research that holds much promise [3]. The use of such optimized procedures in other fields of radiology, though technically very demanding, has allowed for acquiring subtraction images depicting the coronary arteries after peripheral venous injection of contrast medium [4]. In mammography, a digital procedure using storage screens has been described [5] in which a single exposure allows for the read-out and subtraction of images of different exposure. This procedure minimizes the problem of achieving perfect registration of images for reduction of motion artifacts, but dose reduction is still limited by the DQE (detector quantum efficiency) of currently available screens.

Attempts at using energy subtraction for differentiating tissue properties have also been reported in the literature [6]. These investigations show that energy subtraction has a potential for also improving the specificity of mammography in identifying densifications. Initial results of studies investigating energy subtraction for improving the assessment of chest radiographs by subtracting the calcium-containing bone, which is similar to the mammographic technique presented here, suggest that improvements can be expected for diagnostic mammography as well [7].

Conclusion

The results presented here show that energy subtraction has a potential for at least enhancing microcalcifications. Ideally, subtraction should completely eliminate surrounding tissue, leaving only the microcalcifications. Such a procedure would at the same time provide an optimal CAD system for microcalcifications without false-positive or false-negative markers. On the other hand, energy subtraction images for the enhancement of microcalcifications might be obtained as a by?product of subtraction images acquired by contrast-enhanced mammography. In this case, it would certainly be easier to achieve enhancement of microcalcifications rather than a procedure optimized for the depiction of calcifications. Enhancement of microcalcifications by energy subtraction can already be used today for imaging specimens containing very fine microcalcifications. It is thus possible, when vacuum suction biopsy is performed, to inform the pathologist which of the specimens contains such calcifications. However, use of energy subtraction in vivo is impaired by problems arising from movement between two images and the increased noise on subtraction images.

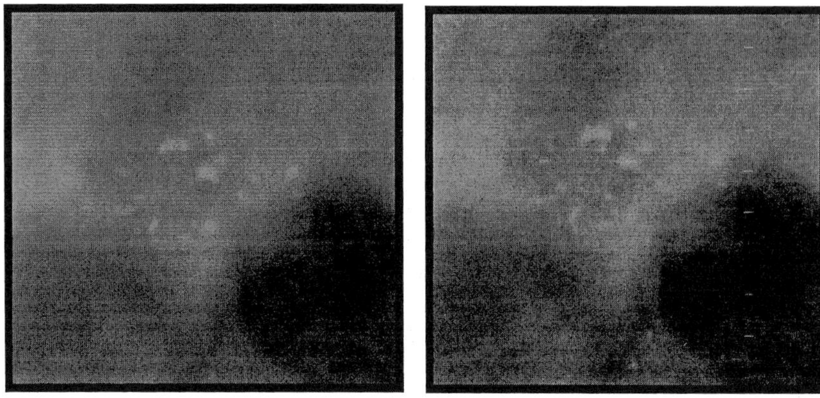

Fig. 1: left: Original image at 22 kVp; right: subtraction image – enhanced Microcalcifications

References

[1] Zheng B, Chang YH, Gur D. „Computerized detection of masses from digitized mammograms: comparison of single-image segmentation and bilateral-image subtraction." Acad Radiol. 1995 Dec;2(12):1056-61

[2] F. Diekmann, S. Grebe, U. Bick, S. Paepke, B. Hamm: „Verbesserte Diagnosefindung durch den Einsatz von Computeralgorithmen in der digitalen Mammographie." Zentralbl Gynakol. 2001 Feb; 123:117-22

[3] Arkadiev, V., et al. (2001) „Aufbau und Charakterisierung eines Röntgen-monochromatormoduls für Mammographiegeräte." Medizinische Physik 2001 (K. Welker & K. Zink, Hrsg.) 123 – 124, Deutsche Gesellschaft für Medizinische Physik, Berlin 2001

[4] Elleaume H, Fiedler S, Esteve F, Bertrand B, Charvet AM, Berkvens P, Benuyer G, Brochard T, Le Dug G, Nemoz C, Renier M, Suortti P, Thomlinson W, Le Bas JF „First human transvenous coronary angiography at the European Synchrotron Radiation Facility." Phys Med Biol. 2000 Sep;45(9):L39-43.

[5] Chakraborty DP, Barnes GT: „An energy sensitive cassette for dual-energy mammography." Med Phys. 1989 Jan-Feb;16(1):7-13.

[6] Asaga T, Mauzawa C, Yoshida A, Matsuura H: „Dual-energy subtraction mammography." J Digit Imaging. 1995 Feb;8(1 Suppl 1):70-3

[7] Kido S, Kuriyama K, Hosomi N, Inoue E, Kuroda C, Horai T: „Low-cost soft-copy display accuracy in the detection of pulmonary nodules by single-exposure dual-energy subtraction: comparison with hard-copy viewing." J Digit Imaging. 2000 Feb;13(1):33-7

Development of a computer-aided sketch system for mammograms

Toshiaki Nakagawa, Takeshi Hara, Hiroshi Fujita, Takuji Iwase* and Tokiko Endo**

Department of Information Science, Faculty of Engineering, Gifu University
Yanagido 1-1, Gifu 501-1193, Japan
nakagawa@fjt.info.gifu-u.ac.jp
*Department of Breast Surgery, Aichi Cancer Center Hospital
Kanokoden 1-1, Tikusa-ku, Nagoya 464-8681, Japan
**Department of Radiology, National Hospital of Nagoya
Sannomaru 4-1-1, Naka-ku, Nagoya 460-0001, Japan

Abstract. We have been developing a computer-aided diagnosis system for mammograms for several years, and some technical approaches to identify lesion areas such as mammographic masses, spicules or clustered microcalcifications have been introduced. The purpose of this study is to develop an automated illustrating system that can be an aid for radiologists when they make a schema for abnormal mammogram. In this system, users (radiologists) can modify the regions displayed on CRT monitor by using a pointing device. Their final schemata were stored after appropriate borders were automatically determined by using defined borders based on automated detection system. As an initial result by employing 430 digitized images, the automated defined region and illustrated images were almost satisfied with what radiologists required.

1. Introduction

With a rapid development of computer technology and its application to medical field, it is significantly required to computerize all medical information. The information includes sketches drawn by radiologists when they make a report of mammogram reading (Fig. 1).

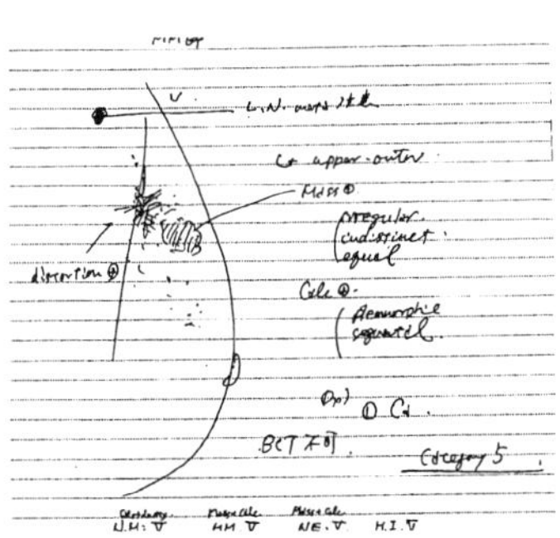

Fig. 1. An example of a sketch of mmammogram drawn by a physician.

However, efficiency of an electronic Medical record (EMR) system decreases because making digital-format sketches drawn on a sheet of paper requires an imagescanner in an ordinary approach in current EMR system. In this work, we propose a new computer-aided sketch drawing (CAS) system, that could be considered as an aid for radiologists to prepare their sketch by partly employing the techniques developed for our computer-aided diagnosis (CAD) schemes in mammography (Fig. 2) [1, 2].

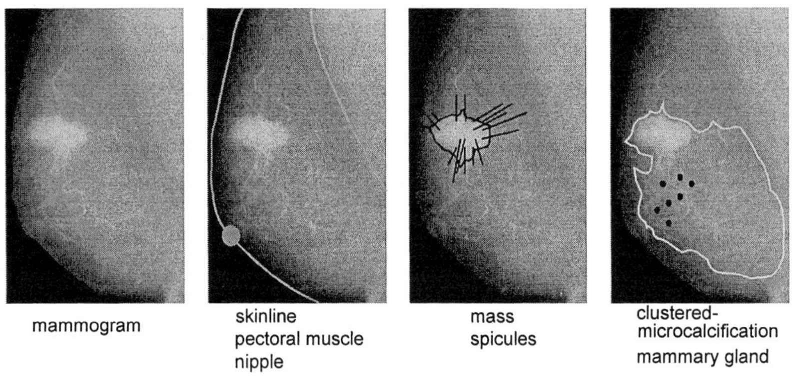

Fig. 2. Identified areas automatically determined by our CAD scheme for mammograms.

2. CAS system

Figure 3 illustrates a concept of CAS system. According to the analyzed (detected) results by our CAD schemes, a primitive sketch is produced automatically with information such as locations and forms of masses, spicules, clustered microcalcifications, mammary gland, pectoral muscles, and nipples. Radiologists sometimes may modify the candidates indicated incorrectly by the CAS system due to false-positive detection of CAD schemes. The modification could be simply done by a simple operation using pointing devices to store.

3. Result

A subjective evaluation was performed by comparing sketches drawn by an experienced physician with those produced by our CAS system. 430 mammograms were used in this study. 50 of 80 sketches by our CAS system including masses were matched to those by the physician. We found that if the borders of masses were extracted clearly by our system, the sketches were tended to match well to the physician's ones. There was a tendency that sketches of masses on high dense area or in low contrast were hardly matched to the physician's ones. However, we achieved feasible results about images with clustered microcalcifications, pectoral muscles, and nipples.

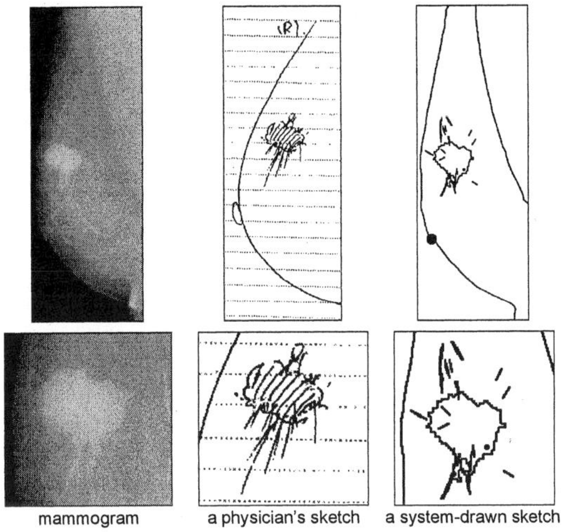

Fig. 3. Mammogram *(left)*, sketch by a physician *(center)*, and that by our CAS system *(right)*.

4. Conclusion

We developed a CAS system that provides radiologists with digital-format sketches automatically drawn by applying region-segmentation techniques developed in our mammogram CAD schemes. An initial result by using 430 images indicated that sketches drawn by the CAS system matched well with physician's ones in most cases of simple images. It is possible to implement an electronic Medical record system more efficiently than the conventional ways in which sketches are drawn on paper sheets by hands.

Acknowledgements

This work was supported in parts by a grant from the Endo Saijirou commemorative foundation for the promotion of technology (KAI industries, Gifu, Japan), the Grant-In-Aid for Scientific Research from Japan Society for the Promotion of Science, and the Grant-In-Aid for Cancer Research from the Ministry of Health, Labour and Welfare.

References

1. Satoshi Kasai, Hiroshi Fujita, Takeshi Hara, et al.: Development of a detection algorithm for masses around thick mammary gland on mammograms, Proc. CAR'98, 213-218, 1998.
2. Miki Goto, Akihisa Morikawa, Hiroshi Fujita, et al.: Automated detection of spicules on digitized mammograms by using multistage pendulum filter, Proc. CAR'98, 880, 1998.

Breast Tissue-Equivalent Contrast Detail, Resolution and Dosimetry Phantom for 3D Imaging

Thomas JA, Schauer DA, Romanyukna A, and Tomon JJ

Uniformed Services University of the Health Sciences
Department of Radiology and Radiological Sciences
4301 Jones Bridge Road
Bethesda, MD 20879-4799
United States of America

Abstract. A tissue-equivalent phantom for measuring contrast detail, high contrast object resolution and glandular dose in 3D has been developed. The phantom consists of homogenous solid slabs with mass attenuation coefficients equivalent to glandular, fat and a 50/50 mixture of glandular and fat. Solid phantom sections have been developed for contrast detail measurements of mass-like objects and different sized calcifications. Removable inserts are provided for TLD measurement at different levels and chest wall to nipple locations. (3D quality measurements and breast dose profiles will be presented for breast tissue compositions ranging from 0% glandular to 100% glandular and thickness from 2 to 8 cm.)

I. INTRODUCTION

Ensuring the highest quality of breast tissue contrast detail and high contrast object resolution represents one of the most serious challenges of tissue imaging. Mammography requires the highest quality of imaging techniques and fine detail over a wide spectrum of object contrasts in order to successful identify cancerous growths in there earliest stages of development. To this end the American College of Radiology (ACR) has established an accreditation program for screen film mammography that uses the clearly detectable components from each group in the breast phantom at a dose of 300 mrad and a net film optical density of 1.0. This paper describes the detail and construction of a tissue-equivalent breast phantom that has been developed for 3D breast imaging. The 3D breast phantom consists of various size slabs of epoxy resins that simulate fat tissue glandular tissue and a 50/50 mix of fatty and glandular tissue. Breast tissue composition varies from woman-to-woman and is characterized by the percentage of adipose and glandular tissue in the breast. Factors such as age and whether or not the woman has been through child berth contribute to the composition of the breast tissue. Breasts are usually defined in terms of the tissue composition into categories such as average, fatty and dense breast. The average breast is assumed to be 50 % adipose tissue and 50 % glandular tissue. While a fatty breast is approximately composed of 30% glandular tissue and 70% adipose tissue and a dense breast is composed of 70% glandular and 30% adipose tissue. The elemental percentage by mass of breast tissue is 10.6% hydrogen, 33.2% carbon, 3.0% nitrogen, 52.7 oxygen, 0.1% sodium, 0.1% Phosphorous, 0.2% sulfur and 0.1% Cl. Based on these percentages of breast tissue elements suitable materials and compounds can be selected to simulate breast tissue as close as practical.

II. DESCRIPTION AND MATERIALS

The 3D phantom consists of slabs of varying thickness and materials for optimal breast-tissue imaging and detail contrast. The slabs are characterized by the type of tissue material that they simulate 100% fatty tissue, 100% glandular tissue, 50%/50% mix and 50%/50% complex. The slabs are fabricated from Plastic water epoxy resin and Table 1 shows the four different types of materials used in the 3D phantom and what percentage of elements in each material. Plastic water resin materials are formulated to maximize breast tissue simulation properties at 20 KeV for mammography. The 50%/50% Complex slab is specially fabricated by first pouring a layer of glandular tissue equivalent then a layer of adipose tissue equivalent followed by another layer of glandular tissue equivalent. Then the layers are mixed by randomly swirling the layers together.

Table 1. 3D Breast Phantom Materials

Slab Type (tissue)	Chemical Composition					
	H	C	N	O	Ca	Cl
100% Adipose	0.0979	0.7144	0.0199	0.1635	0.0013	0.0023
100% Glandular	0.0941	0.6912	0.0184	0.1766	0.0175	0.0014
50%/50% Mix	0.0960	0.7027	0.0193	0.1700	0.0094	0.0019
50%/50% Complex	0.0960	0.7027	0.0193	0.1700	0.0094	0.0019

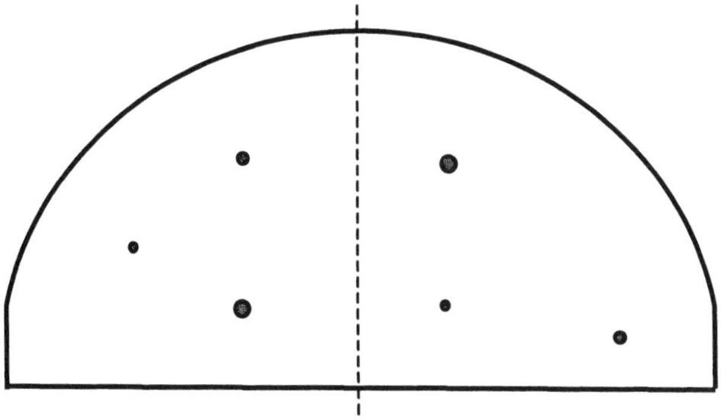

Figure 1. Homogeneous Gland with six masses.

Each of the tissue type slabs for the 3D breast tissue phantom comes in three sizes 1 cm, 0.5 cm, and 0.2 cm. Additionally, each of the slab types contains inserts of either specks or masses of various size distributed in the slab. As an example Figure 1 shows Gland slab with four inserted masses of different sizes.

These tissue phantom slabs can then be placed together to simulate various different breast thickness and breast tissue composition. For example this phantom allows the flexibility to construct a dense breast with the glandular tissue slabs and it also allows for the construction of 50%/50% adipose and glandular tissue breast phantoms. The benefit of this will hopefully be realized in future experiments.

The phantom also contains a breast tissue slab in each of the four tissue materials that has inserts to contain TLD-100H disks or rods. There are three removable machined trays in the breast tissue equivalent slab that can accommodate either 26 TLD-100H disks or rods. The dimensions of the TLD insert is slightly oversized to hold either the 1 mm diameter by 6mm length TLD-100H rods or the 4.2 mm diameter by 0.25 mm thickness TLD–100H disks (Saint-Gobain Ceramics and Plastics). Figure 2 schematically depicts the glandular phantom slab for TLD placement. The construction of this breast tissue equivalent phantom with the TLD insert slab allows for breast dose measurements at various depths within the phantom.

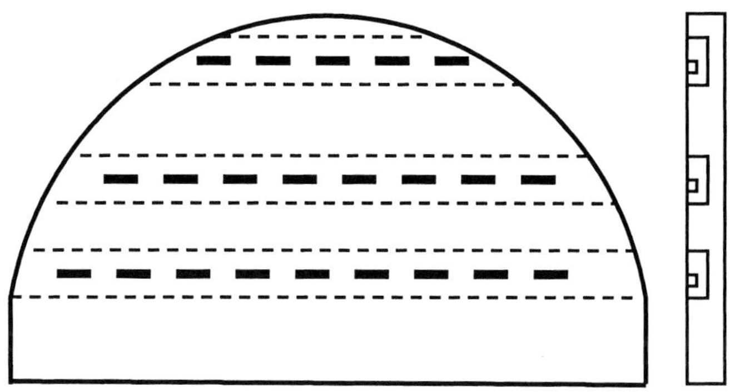

Figure 2. 3D Phantom Slab with TLD-700H Inserts.

III. FUTURE EXPERIMENTS AND PROJECTS

Some of the future experiments and projects that are planned are a determination of whether or not this phantom is acceptable for 3D mammography or is the phantom currently used for screen film mammography better. Measure the typical entrance exposure for an average patient (approximately 4.2 cm compressed breast thickness 50% adipose and 50% glandular composition) and calculate the average glandular dose according to the American College of Radiology Quality Control Manual (ACR). Additional measurements and calculations will be performed for 100% adipose and 100% glandular compositions. Dose profile measurements at varying depths using the TLD-100H disks in the phantom.

Author Index

Subject Index

Druck: Strauss Offsetdruck, Mörlenbach
Verarbeitung: Schäffer, Grünstadt